Dentist's Guide to Medical Conditions, Medications, and Complications

T0337853

Dentist's Guide to Medical Conditions, Medications, and Complications

Second Edition

Kanchan M. Ganda, M.D.

WILEY Blackwell

This edition first published 2013 © 2013 by John Wiley & Sons, Inc.
First edition published 2008.

Wiley-Blackwell is an imprint of John Wiley & Sons, formed by the merger of Wiley's global Scientific, Technical and Medical business with Blackwell Publishing.

Editorial offices: 2121 State Avenue, Ames, Iowa 50014-8300, USA
The Atrium, Southern Gate, Chichester, West Sussex, PO19 8SQ, UK
9600 Garsington Road, Oxford, OX4 2DQ, UK

For details of our global editorial offices, for customer services and for information about how to apply for permission to reuse the copyright material in this book please see our website at www.wiley.com/wiley-blackwell.

Library of Congress Cataloging-in-Publication Data

Ganda, Kanchan M., author.
  [Dentist's guide to medical conditions and complications]
  Dentist's guide to medical conditions, medications, and complications /
Kanchan M. Ganda. – Second edition.
      p. ; cm.
  Revised edition of: Dentist's guide to medical conditions and complications /
Kanchan M. Ganda. 2008.
  Includes bibliographical references and index.
  ISBN 978-1-118-31389-3 (softback : alk. paper) – ISBN 978-1-118-31390-9 (epdf) –
ISBN 978-1-118-31391-6 (epub) – ISBN 978-1-118-31392-3 (emobi)
  I. Title.
  [DNLM: 1. Stomatognathic Diseases–complications.   2. Dental Care for Chronically Ill.
3. Medical History Taking.   4. Pharmaceutical Preparations, Dental–administration & dosage.
5. Pharmaceutical Preparations, Dental–contraindications.   6. Stomatognathic Diseases–drug
therapy. WU 140]
  RK55.S53
  617.6'026–dc23
                                                                                    2013003815

A catalogue record for this book is available from the British Library.

Wiley also publishes its books in a variety of electronic formats. Some content that appears in print may not be available in electronic books.

Cover image: © webphotographeer
Cover design by Maggie Voss

Set in 9.5/12pt Palatino by Aptara® Inc., New Delhi, India
Printed and bound in Malaysia by Vivar Printing Sdn Bhd

1   2013

Dedication

This book is dedicated to all my students, past and present; to my late parents, Amrit Devi and Roop Krishan Dewan; and to my family, for all their encouragement and loving support.

Contents

Acknowledgments

I wish to sincerely thank Bruce J. Baum, D.M.D., Ph.D., Chief of the Gene Therapy and Therapeutics Branch at the National Institute of Dental and Craniofacial Research in Bethesda, Maryland. He was instrumental in mentoring me and motivating me to publish my work, which is now in its second edition. Dr. Baum's vision for dentistry and his confidence that my work would make a difference has been and continues to be very humbling.

Thanks to my former deans at Tufts University School of Dental Medicine—Lonnie Norris, D.M.D, M.P.H., and Dean of Curriculum, Nancy Arbree, D.D.S., M.S.—for making my vision of integrating medicine into the dental curriculum a reality. I was given the flexibility to create a medicine curriculum for our students and integrate this education through all the four years of dental curriculum.

My very sincere thanks to Huw F. Thomas, B.D.S., M.S., Ph.D., our current dean at Tufts University School of Dental Medicine, and to Mark Nehring, M.Ed., D.M.D., M.P.H., the chair of the Department of Public Health and Community Services at Tufts University School of Dental Medicine (my former chair), for their tremendous support in ensuring a rapidly processed sabbatical, so I could complete the second edition of my book. Additionally, I am very grateful to my colleagues Diana Esshaki, D.M.D., M.S., and Patrick McGarry, D.M.D., for their unconditional support in efficiently executing all responsibilities while I was away.

To all the past and present medicine course speakers and rotation directors, specialists in their respective fields of medicine, this unique dental education would have been incomplete without your active participation, dedication, and support. I wish to acknowledge and thank you all for your efforts and endless support.

I also would like to thank my D'14 student Ms. Jaskaren K. Randhawa for her unflagging support and help with the proofing of the material.

I'd like to thank my daughter Kiran, for patiently providing me with around-the-clock technical support. Also, sincere thanks to my daughter Anjali and my husband, Om, both of whom are physicians, for enthusiastically participating in our numerous discussions during which they offered their insights about patient care.

This finest quality second edition would not have been possible without the assistance of my very talented project manager, Ms. Shikha Sharma of Aptara, Inc.,

New Delhi, India. Her professionalism, very friendly personality, expertise, attention to detail made it a very pleasurable experience indeed; she is someone who went above and beyond every step of the way. I am delighted to have been linked with such a talented and knowledgeable individual and I am so extremely satisfied with the final product she created!

Last but not least, I wish to thank all my students, who have been my constant source of inspiration. I never could have experienced the joy of teaching without their active participation and endurance in the learning of medicine!

Kanchan Ganda, M.D.

Introduction: Integration of Medicine in Dentistry

Dental care today holds many challenges for the dental practitioner. Patients are living longer, often retaining their own dentition, have one or more medical conditions, and routinely take several medications.

Along with excellence in dentistry, the practicing dentist has the dual task of staying updated with the current concepts of medicine and pharmacology. They should rightfully be called the "Physician of the Oral Cavity."

The integration of medicine in the dental curriculum has become a necessity, and this integration must begin with the freshman class, so the students can gain maximum benefit and the chance to gain credibility. The integration of medicine is best achieved when done in a case-based or problem-based format and correlated with the basic sciences, pharmacology, general pathology, oral pathology, and dentistry. There needs to be a true commitment and *constant* reinforcement of the integration in *all* the didactic and clinical courses.

The integration of medicine, pharmacology, and medically complex patient care is best achieved when done in a pyramidal process, through the four years of dental education.

The foundation should instill a basic knowledge of:

1. Standard and medically complex patient history-taking and physical examination.
2. Symptoms and signs of highest-priority illnesses, along with the common laboratory tests evaluating those disease states.
3. Anesthetics, analgesics, antibiotics, antivirals, and antifungals used in dentistry.
4. Prescription writing.

"Normal" patient assessment, when stressed in the first year, prepares students to better understand the changes prompted by disease states during the second year of their education, when didactic and clinical knowledge of highest-priority illnesses, associated diagnostic laboratory tests, and the vast pharmacopeia used for the care of those diseases is included. Case-based scenarios should be used to solidify this information.

The progressive learning up to the end of the second year prepares the student to "care" for the patient "on paper." With the start of the clinical years, the student is prepared to apply this knowledge toward "actual" patient care, which occurs typically during the third and fourth years of education.

During the third year, the student should participate in medical and surgical clinical rotations in a hospitalized setting and complete a Hospital Clerkship Program where the student is exposed to head-and-neck cancer care, emergency medicine, critical care, anesthesia, hematology, oncology, transplants, cardiothoracic surgery, and so on. This exposure will widen the student's knowledge, broaden clinical perception, and further enhance the link between medicine and dentistry.

During the clinical years, the students should complete faculty-reviewed medical consults for *all* their medically compromised patients, *prior* to dentistry. This patient-by-patient health status review will help correctly translate their didactic patient-care knowledge in the clinical setting.

The text is a compilation of materials needed for the integration of medicine in dentistry. It is a book all dental students *and* dental practitioners will appreciate both as a read and chair-side.

This text provides information on epidemiology, physiology, pathophysiology, laboratory tests evaluation, associated pharmacology, dental alerts, and suggested deviations in the use of anesthetics, analgesics, antibiotics, antivirals, and antifungals for each disease state discussed.

The student will greatly benefit from the sections detailing history-taking and physical examination; highly expanded clinical and applied pharmacology of dental anesthetics, analgesics, antibiotics, antivirals, and antifungals; stress management; and management of medical emergencies in the dental setting.

Patient Assessment

Routine History-Taking and Physical Examination

GENERAL OVERVIEW

Patient Interview Introduction

The primary job of the dental student starting clinical work is to learn to conduct a patient workup thoroughly and efficiently. The heart of every patient workup is a set pattern done in a sequential order of data collection and analysis.

Patient Workup Sequential Pattern

The sequential pattern of patient workup consists of the following:

1. History and physical examination.
2. Laboratory data collection and analysis.
3. Diagnostic and therapeutic plan formulation.

The first step, the patient interview, or the history, is probably the single most important task in the diagnostic patient workup because of its importance in diagnosis and in the development of a good doctor-patient relationship. The provider should demonstrate a professional manner that will put the patient at ease. During the interview, always listen carefully to the patient. Use interrogation sparingly, or use it later to aid a communicating patient, or to restrict the rare patient who has a tendency to ramble!

Patient Interview Practical Points

Keep your appearance neat and clean. This will help gain your patient's trust. Always introduce yourself when meeting a patient and refer to the patient as "Mr. John Doe" or "Miss Jane Doe." Do not use first names during the initial encounter. Exchange a few brief pleasantries because moving forward, this will help both you and the patient feel comfortable and at ease with one another.

Dentist's Guide to Medical Conditions, Medications, and Complications, Second Edition. Kanchan M. Ganda.
© 2013 John Wiley & Sons, Inc. Published 2013 by John Wiley & Sons, Inc.

Always have a friendly and sincere interest in your patient's problem(s). Always be courteous, respectful, and confidential and show a continued interest while you are with the patient.

Physical Examination Practical Points

Prior to the start of the physical examination let the patient know that you are going to take the pulse and blood pressure and examine the head and neck area. This heads-up will enable the patient to understand that you will be touching him or her. Your attentive and respectful ways will enhance a good doctor-patient relationship.

The physical examination is an art that is learned by constant repetition. There are many styles and methods for conducting the general examination, and every clinician will ultimately choose one examination sequence to go by. Most clinicians, however, prefer the head-to-foot order. When examining any area of the body, it is usually best to follow an orderly sequence of inspection, palpation, percussion, and auscultation. This sequential routine ensures thoroughness.

The physical examination should always be conducted and assessed in the context of the patient's dental and medical history. The range of "normal" varies from patient to patient.

The student needs to become familiar with the use of the stethoscope and the blood pressure cuff. Fumbling with your equipment or the technique during patient examination will cause you embarrassment. The student also needs to practice the head-and-neck exam techniques often on friends or family members to get a good sense of the normal.

History-Taking and Physical Examination: Broad Conclusions

After the history and physical examination is completed, you should, in most cases, be able to answer the following questions:

- The disease states that exist in the patient and whether the patient's problems are acute or chronic.
- The organ systems that may be involved.
- The differential diagnosis of the patient's problems.
- The laboratory tests that will be needed for the evaluation of the disease states.
- Confirmation or exclusion of a diagnosis and/or whether to follow the course of a disease state.

HISTORY-TAKING DETAILS

The purpose of medical history and physical examination is to collect information from the patient, to examine the patient, and to understand the patient's problems. Traditional history-taking has several parts, each with a specific purpose. In order to achieve maximum success, the medical history must be accurate, concise, and systematic.

The following is a standard outline in sequential order of the different components of history-taking. The introductory materials in the health history consist of collecting several types of information from the patient.

Data Collection

The following information is obtained in all patients to gain a basic understanding of the patient:

Date of the visit: Record number:

Name:
(last)   (first)   (middle)
Home address: Home phone:
Business address: Business phone: Cell phone:

Occupation: Date of birth:

Sex: M/F/Transgender/Other
Marital status: S/M/D/W/Partnership
Height:
Weight:
Referred by:

Chief Complaint

The chief complaint states in the patient's own words the reason for the visit, for example, "I have a toothache" or "I need a root canal."

Present History

Present history lists, in clear, chronological order, the details of the problem or problems for which the patient is seeking care. You will determine by interrogation a timeline of the following:

1. When did the patient's problem(s) begin?
2. Where did the problem(s) begin?
3. What kinds of symptoms did the patient experience?
4. Has the patient had any treatment for the problem(s)?
5. Has the treatment had any positive or negative effect on the patient's condition?
6. Has the patient's lifestyle been affected by the problem(s)?

Past History

The past history gives you an insight about the health status of the patient until now. Check with the patient for the presence or absence of diseases by eliciting the **symptoms and signs** associated with the disease states. It is best to access the disease states with the patient in **alphabetical** order to ensure you address each disease state and do not miss anything. Use interrogation to check for the following disease states:

Anemia

Determine the presence or absence of the nutritional, congenital, and acquired or chronic disease-associated anemias.

Bleeding Disorders

Determine the presence or absence of the congenital and acquired types of bleeding disorders.

Cardiorespiratory Disorders

Determine whether the patient has a history of angina, myocardial infarction, transient ischemic attacks (TIAs), cerebrovascular attacks (CVAs/strokes), hypertension, rheumatic heart disease, asthma, tuberculosis, bronchitis, sinusitis, and chronic obstructive pulmonary disease (COPD).

Drugs/Medications

Determine the patient's current medications. Check for prescribed, herbal, and over-the-counter (OTC) medications. Determine whether the patient is currently on corticosteroids or has been on them, by mouth or by injection, for two weeks or longer within the past two years. Check if the patient has known allergies to any drugs, such as NSAIDS, aspirin, codeine, morphine, penicillin, sulpha antimicrobials, bisulfites, metabisulfites, or local anesthetics.

Endocrine Disorders

Check for diabetes, hyperthyroidism, hypothyroidism, parathyroid disorders, and pituitary and adrenal disorders (Addison's disease or Cushing's syndrome).

Fits or Faints

Check for the presence of different kinds of seizures: grand mal epilepsy, petit mal epilepsy, temporal lobe or psychomotor epilepsy, or localized motor seizures.

Gastrointestinal Disorders

Check for oral ulcerations, esophagitis, gastritis, peptic ulcerations, Crohn's disease, celiac disease, ulcerative colitis, diverticulitis, polyps, and hemorrhoids.

Hospital Admissions

Determine the cause or causes for admission and also check if the patient had any history of accidents or injuries. Determine whether the patient was given any anesthesia, either local or general, during the hospital admission. Furthermore, determine whether there were any complications during the hospital admission due to the anesthesia or due to the medical/surgical condition for which the patient was admitted. Determine whether the patient was given a blood transfusion during hospitalization.

Immunological Diseases

Check for lupus, Sjögrens syndrome, rheumatoid arthritis, and polyarthritis nodosa.

Infectious Diseases

Check for infectious diseases of childhood: measles, mumps, chicken pox, streptococcus pharyngitis, rheumatic fever, or scarlet fever. Also check for infectious diseases of adulthood: sexually transmitted diseases (STDs), hepatitis, HIV infection, Methicillin-Resistant Staphylococcus Aureus (MRSA) infection, and infectious mononucleosis.

Jaundice or Liver Disease

If the patient is jaundiced or has had jaundice, determine the cause. Is it due to viral hepatitis, alcoholic hepatitis, or gallstones? Determine whether there is any history of gallbladder dysfunction. Check whether there is any indication of improper liver function.

Kidney Disorders

Determine whether there is any indication of kidney dysfunction, renal stones, urinary tract infections, renal disease, renal failure, or renal transplant.

Likelihood of Pregnancy

Determine the date of the patient's last menstrual period (LMP) and whether the patient is pregnant. Always let the patient know that prior to dental radiographs, you need to know if the patient is pregnant. You need to also know the pregnancy status, as there are certain anesthetics, analgesics, and antibiotics that are contraindicated during pregnancy.

Musculoskeletal Disorders

Check for osteoporosis and other causes of impaired bone metabolism, Paget's disease, osteoarthritis, rheumatoid arthritis, psoriatic arthritis, gout, muscular dystrophy, polymyositis, and myasthenia gravis.

Neurological Disorders

Check for cranial nerve disorders, headaches, facial pains, migraine, multiple sclerosis, motor neuron disease, transient ischemic attacks (TIAs), or cerebrovascular accidents (CVAs) associated neurological deficits, Parkinson's disease, and peripheral neuropathies.

Obstetric and Gynecological Disorders

Check for conditions or diseases that can lead to spontaneous abortions, miscarriages, bleeding, or anemia. Also check for any tumors needing chemotherapy or radiotherapy.

Psychiatric Disease

Check for personality disorders, neuroses, anxiety, phobias, hysteria, psychoses, schizophrenia, dementia, Alzheimer's disease, and posttraumatic stress disorder (PTSD).

Radiation Therapy

Check for any radiation to the head and neck region and the RADS or Gy of radiation received.

Skin Disorders

Lichen planus, phemphigus, herpes simplex, herpes zoster, eczema, unhealed skin lesions, and urticaria (itching of the skin) are conditions that should be checked for.

Tetanus

Determine the patient's immunization status for tetanus, hepatitis, influenza, and pneumonia.

Violence

Check for domestic violence, intimate partner violence (IPV), and elder or child abuse.

Wounds

Determine the patient's wound-healing capacity.

Personal History

In this part of the history, we try to get an insight into the patient's lifestyle, occupation, and habits. In the lifestyle component, an attempt is made to understand what constitutes a typical day for the patient. What does the patient do for recreation, relaxation, and so on? What is the patient's job like? Are there any job-related toxic exposures? Is there any history of alcohol, coffee, or tea intake? How much of these does the patient consume? Is there any history of diarrhea or vomiting?

Is there any history of smoking cigarettes or using "recreational" drugs such as marijuana, cocaine, or amphetamines? Has the patient ever used intravenous (IV) drugs or swapped needles? Has the patient been exposed to any infectious diseases or sexually transmitted diseases (STDs)? Does the patient use any herbal medications or over-the-counter medications?

Does the patient use diet pills, birth control pills, laxatives, analgesics (aspirin, acetaminophen, NSAIDS, and other pain medications), or cough/cold medications?

Family History

Once the patient's medical history has been completed, it is important to assess the health status of the immediate family members. Determine whether certain common diseases run in the family or if a familial disease pattern exists. Determine the age and health of the patient's parents, siblings, and children. If any member is deceased, the cause of death and age at death should always be established.

Presence of diseases with a strong hereditary component or tendency for familial clustering should be determined. These diseases are coronary artery disease (CAD), heart disease, diabetes mellitus (DM), hypertension (Htn), stroke (CVA), asthma, allergies, arthritis, anemia, cancer, kidney disease, or psychiatric illness.

Review of Systems: Overview and Components

Review of systems (ROS) is a final methodical inquiry prior to physical examination. All organ systems not discussed during the interview are systematically reviewed here. It provides a thorough search for further, as yet unestablished, disease processes in the patient. If the patient has failed to mention certain symptoms, the process of ROS helps remind the patient. Also, if you have unknowingly omitted questioning the patient about certain aspects of his or her health, now is the time to include these aspects.

Review of Systems: Assessment Components

Constitutional

Determine whether there is any history of recent weight change, anorexia (loss of appetite), weakness, fatigue, fever, chills, insomnia, irritability, or night sweats.

Skin

Is there any history of allergic skin rashes, itching of the skin, unhealed lesions (probably due to diabetes, poor diet, steroids, HIV/AIDS, an so on)? Is the rash acute or chronic? Is the rash unilateral or bilateral? Does the patient have any history of bruising or bleeding?

Head

Is there any history of headaches or loss of consciousness (LOC)? LOC may be due to cardiovascular, neurologic, or metabolic causes; or it may be due to anxiety.

Is there any history of seizures? Are the seizures generalized (with or without loss of consciousness) or focal? Are there any motor movements? Is there any history of head injury?

Eyes

Check for acuity of vision, history of glaucoma (can cause eye pain), redness, irritation, halos (seeing a white ring around a light source), or blurred vision. Is there any irritation of the eyes or excessive tearing? These symptoms could also be allergy-associated.

Ears

Check for recent changes in hearing, ear pain, discharge, vertigo (dizziness), or ringing in the ears (tinnitus).

Lymph Glands

Check for lymph glandular enlargement in the neck or elsewhere. Are the nodes tender or painless, or are they hot or cold to touch? When did the patient first notice any changes in the nodes? Are the nodes freely mobile, or are they anchored to the underlying tissues?

Respiratory System

Ask if there is any history of frequent sinus infection, postnasal drip, nosebleed, sore throat, or shortness of breath (SOB) on exertion, or at rest. SOB can be due to respiratory, cardiac, or metabolic diseases.

Check for wheezing (may be due to asthma, allergies, and so on) and hemoptysis or blood in the sputum (may be due to dental causes or due to lung causes such as bronchitis or tuberculosis). Check if the cough with expectoration is blood-tinged or is there frank blood in the sputum. Is there any history of bronchitis, asthma, pneumonia, or emphysema?

Cardiovascular System

Is there any history of chest pain or discomfort or palpitations? Have the palpitations been associated with syncope (loss of consciousness)? Is there any history of either hypertension or hypotension? Does the patient experience any paroxysmal nocturnal dyspnea (shortness of breath experienced in the middle of the night)? Is there any shortness of breath (SOB) with exercise or exertion?

Is there any history of orthopnea (SOB when lying flat in bed)? Does the patient use more than one pillow to sleep? Has this always been the case, or has the patient recently started using more pillows?

Is there any history of edema of the legs, face, and so on? Does the patient experience any history of leg pains or cramps? Are the cramps relieved by rest? If so, this is suggestive of intermittent claudication. If the cramping or leg pains are unremitting, it is more likely to be muscular in origin.

Is there any history of murmur(s), rheumatic fever, or varicose veins? Is there any history of hypercholesterolemia, gout, or excessive smoking that can lead to or worsen heart disease?

Gastrointestinal System

Check for a history of bleeding gums, oral ulcers, or sores. Is there any history of dysphagia (difficulty swallowing)? Can the patient point out and describe where the difficulty swallowing exists? Is there any history of heartburn, indigestion, bloating, belching, or flatulence? Is there any history of nausea? Is it related to food? Determine the following:

- **Vomiting:** Is there any associated weight loss? Are there psychosocial factors or medications causing it?
- **Hematemesis (vomiting blood):** Ask for associated ulcer history, food intolerance, abdominal pain, or discomfort.
- **Jaundice:** Is the jaundice due to a viral cause or gallstones?

Is there a history of diarrhea/constipation or any change in color of stools?

Genitourinary System

Is there a history of polyuria (excessive urination) due to diabetes, renal disease, or an unknown cause? Is it a recent change? Is there any history of nocturia (getting up at night to go to the bathroom)? Is this a recent change? Is there any history of dysuria (painful urination)? If dysuria is because of urinary tract infection (UTI), frequency and urgency will also be experienced. STDs will also be associated with similar symptoms. With a positive history of STD, always check to see if treatment for STD was completed. Check for renal stones, pain in the loins, and frequent UTIs.

Menstrual History

Determine the date of the last menstrual period. Never forget to paraphrase this question, as discussed previously. Check for any history of menorrhagia (heavy periods). Check whether the patient uses birth control or oral contraceptive pills and details of the type of contraception. Let the patient know that it is firmly established now that oral antibiotics can only decrease the potency of combined oral contraceptives pills (COCPs) or progesterone-only contraceptive pills when antibiotics cause **severe persistent** diarrhea or vomiting, thus essentially "washing out" the pills. It is only then that the patient will have to use extra barrier protection until the end of the next cycle to prevent pregnancy. It is well documented now that certain medications like Rifampin or antiseizure medications or azole antifungals that **induce** cytochrome P450 enzyme system **do affect** the potency of **just the COCPs** containing estrogen and progesterone, as these medications negatively affect the metabolism of just estrogen and not progesterone. So while on these enzyme-inducer medications in combination with COCPs, the patient will have to use barrier protection to prevent pregnancy. Antibiotics prescribed in the dental setting are not CYP450 enzyme inducers. Always enter a case note in the record stating that the patient has been so informed.

Musculoskeletal System

Check for a history of joint pains and what joints are affected. Is the pain acute or chronic, unilateral or bilateral, and is it in the morning or in the evening? Are there any systemic symptoms? Is there a history of rheumatoid arthritis, osteoarthritis, or gout?

Endocrine System

Check for symptoms associated with diabetes: polyuria (excessive urination), polydypsia (excessive thirst), polyphagia (excessive hunger), or weight change; thyroid: heat/cold intolerance, increased/decreased heart rate or goiter, and adrenals: weight change, easy bruising, hypertension, and so on.

Nervous System

Check for a history of stroke, cerebrovascular accident/stroke (CVA), or transient ischemic attack (TIA). Check for a history of muscle weakness, involuntary movements due to tremors, seizures, or anxiety. Check for history of sensory loss of any kind, anesthesia (no sensation), parasthesias (altered sensation commonly experienced as pins and needles), or hyperesthesias (increased sensations). Check if there is any change in memory, especially a recent change.

History-Taking Conclusion

It is important at this point to collect the relevant data or all positive findings about the patient and then construct a logical framework of the case. You are now able to decide which organ or body area is affected and where to focus on during physical examination.

PHYSICAL EXAMINATION: DETAILED DISCUSSION

Structure and Overview

The history serves to focus on and provides emphasis to the physical examination in the sequence of patient workup. The patient is examined from head to toe, thus ensuring thoroughness and screening for abnormalities. Any specific physical findings suggested because of the history findings are sought.

PHYSICAL EXAMINATION: ASSESSMENT COMPONENTS

The following are components of the physical examination in sequential order.

General Appearance

Note the patient's mental status, ability to interact, speech pattern, neatness, and so on.

Vital Signs: Pulse, Respiration Rate, Blood Pressure, Height, and Weight

Pulse

Note the rate, rhythm, volume, and regularity of the pulse. Count the pulse rate/minute. If the pulse rhythm is irregular, determine whether the irregular rhythm is regular or irregular. An irregularity, more than 5 beats/min, is pathological and should prompt a consult with the patient's MD (normal pulse: 65–85 beats/min).

Respiration Rate

Note the breathing pattern and the respiratory rate (RR)/min **while taking** the pulse, so the patient is unaware and anxiety does not alter the breathing (normal RR: 12–16 breaths/min).

Blood Pressure Overview

Take the blood pressure (BP) in both arms during the patient's first visit. Always obtain two blood pressure readings, taken five minutes apart, during the patient's first visit. If the blood pressure is high, confirm the elevated reading in other arm and then take two more readings at the next visit. An average of three to four readings will determine the mean blood pressure for the patient.

Always ensure that the patient has rested sufficiently in the chair prior to monitoring the BP. Certain physiological states can erroneously raise the blood pressure. Stress, caffeine, heavy meal consumption, improper positioning of the arm, or improper cuff size can alter the BP readings. Normal BP reading: <120/80mmHg in a non-diabetic adult and <140/80mmHg in an adult diabetic

Blood Pressure Recordings and Additional Facts

For a seated patient, place the patient's arm on the armchair and place the arms to the sides for a patient lying down. Fasten the cuff snugly over the arm such that the lower border of the cuff is about $\frac{1}{4} - \frac{1}{2}$ inch above the elbow crease and the rubber tubes are over the brachial artery. The cuff should be at the cardiac level.

Place your fingers on the radial pulse, and as you gradually raise the pressure to 200mmHg, make a mental note of the reading where you lose the pulse. Continue to keep your fingers on the pulse and lower the pressure from 200mmHg to 0mmHg, making a mental note of the pressure where the pulse returns. The pressure where the radial pulse disappears and then reappears is the **same**; this is the patient's **rough systolic pressure**. Next place your stethoscope on the brachial artery and raise the pressure to 30–40mm above the rough systolic pressure. Now gradually lower the pressure and listen for the "tapping" of the Korotkoff sounds. The pressure where the Korotkoff sounds begin is the **true systolic pressure**, and the pressure where the tapping sounds disappear is the **true diastolic pressure**. Always raise the pressure to 200mmHg initially to overcome the **auscultatory gap** that may be present in an occasional hypertensive patient. As shown in Figure 1.1, the "tapping" sounds begin at the true **elevated** systolic pressure, disappear **temporarily**, reappear, and then disappear **finally** at the true diastolic pressure. If you **do not** raise the pressure to 200mmHg, the reappearance of the tapping sounds can erroneously be thought of as the **start** of the tapping sounds.

Current National Institute for Health and Clinical Excellence (NICE) guideline for hypertension states that BP readings showing a difference of 15mmHg or more between both arms is often associated with underlying peripheral vascular or cardiovascular or cerebrovascular disease, as well as increased cardiovascular and all-cause mortality. Therefore, it is advised to routinely check the BP in both arms during patient assessment.

Ambulatory BP monitoring is indicated to evaluate "white coat hypertension." Patient self-check at home is useful for evaluating "white coat hypertension." There should be a 10–20% BP decrease during sleep, and absence of this drop may indicate increased cardiovascular disease (CVD) risk.

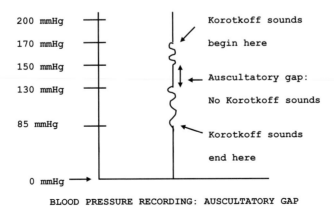

BLOOD PRESSURE RECORDING: AUSCULTATORY GAP

Figure 1.1. Blood pressure recording auscultatory gap.

Hypertension in the elderly: A threshold of <140/90mmHg is considered adequate in patients between 65–79 years of age and a systolic blood pressure (SBP) threshold of 140–145mmHg is reasonable for patients 80 years and older.

Height and Weight

The height and weight of the patient is needed for the calculation of the Body Mass Index (BMI) to determine if a person is underweight, normal weight, overweight, or obese, in addition to the appropriate medication dosage for routine care or during a medical emergency and the radiation dose for dental radiographs.

Examination of the Skin

Note the skin color, temperature, and turgor, and look for skin lesions such as petechiae and bruises.

Examination of the Head

Note the quality of the hair. Is it coarse and dry or thin and sparse? Note the facial symmetry and look for facial edema, butterfly rash, and so on.

Examination of the Ears

Otitis Externa

Otitis externa is external ear infection or inflammation. Do the ear **tug test** by gently pulling on the earlobe. The test is positive if the patient experiences pain during the pinna tug, which indicates infection in that ear.

Otitis Media

Otitis media is middle ear infection or inflammation and is associated with mastoid tenderness. Gently press the mastoid tip with your thumb. The test is positive if the patient experiences pain on slight pressure, indicating otitis media in that ear.

Examination of the Eyes

Xanthelesma

Look for xanthelesma, which is a swelling near the medial end of the eyes. It can be benign or it can be suggestive of hypercholesterolemia. Look for pallor, redness, and yellowing of the sclera by pulling down on the lower eyelid.

Exophthalmus

Exophthalmus or protrusion of the eyeballs can be familial or due to Grave's disease. The lid lag test is **positive** with Grave's disease and **negative** with familial cases of eyeball protrusion.

The Lid Lag Test

Sit in front of the patient and hold the patient's head with your left hand. Then have the patient follow your moving right index finger as it moves from above the face to below the face. The upper eyelid does **not** roll over the eyeball with a positive lid lag test, thus showing the white sclera.

Enophthalmus

Enophthalmus, or sinking in of the eyeballs, can be due to acute starvation, anorexia nervosa, or loss of body mass due to an underlying carcinoma.

Extraocular Movements

Sit in front of the patient and holding the patient's head with your left hand, test for the extraocular movements. Have the patient follow your right index finger and test the patient's ability to look up, down, sideways (both right and left), and diagonally. The superior oblique muscle is innervated by cranial nerve (CN) IV, the lateral rectus muscle is supplied by CN VI, and the remaining muscles are innervated by CN III, as shown in Figure 1.2.

The Light Reflex

To test for the light reflex, maintain the extraocular movements test position and have the patient look straight ahead. Bring a flashlight from the right side and shine it onto the right eye. Bridge the patient's nose with your hand to keep the light from spreading to the other eye. Observe the pupillary constriction in the right eye and also look for a simultaneous constriction in the left eye. The pupillary constriction in the right eye is the **direct** light reflex, and the pupillary constriction in the left eye is the **indirect** or the **consensual** light reflex. Next, follow the same steps using the light from the left side. The afferent nerve for the light reflex is CN II and the efferent nerve is CN III.

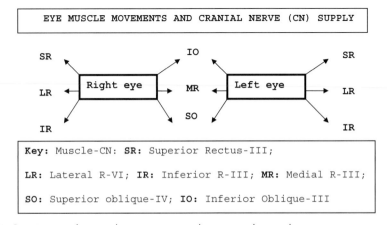

Figure 1.2.   Extraocular muscle movements and associated cranial nerve innervations.

Visual Fields

Maintain the same position as with the light reflex and have the patient look straight ahead. The patient should not move the head, eyes, or gaze during the test. With your arms outstretched, gradually bring your wriggling fingers inward and have the patient inform you at what point in the visual field he or she is able to see your fingers. Test the fields at points above, below, diagonally, and to the sides of the head in a cross and "x" pattern.

Examination of the Nose and Sinuses

Check for sinus tenderness by tapping lightly over the ethmoid, maxillary, and frontal sinuses. Transient flexion of the neck toward the chest can bring out the pain associated with sinusitis.

Examination of the Mouth and Throat

Examine the teeth, gums, mucous membranes, tongue, oropharynx, and roof of the mouth. Gingival hypertrophy, when seen, can be due to puberty, pregnancy, leukemia, and drugs: phenytoin (Dilantin), an antiseizure drug; niphedipine (Procardia), a calcium channel blocker/high blood pressure medication; or cyclosporine (Sandimmune), an antirejection drug for organ transplant.

Examination of the Neck: Lymph Glands, Thyroid, and Trachea

Lymph Glands

Inspect the head and neck region for any lumps or bumps due to lymph node enlargement. Next, proceed with palpation of the lymph nodes. Stand behind or to the side of the patient and feel/palpate the lymph nodes in the neck with the pulp of your fingers. You may do this one side at a time, or both sides at the same time.

Tonsillar nodes are the only nodes that should be palpated **one side at a time**. Simultaneous palpation of both sides can massage the carotid sinus causing bradycardia (slowing of the heart rate). This could cause a problem, particularly in an elderly patient.

Normally, you are unable to feel any nodes. If you do feel some nodes, they should be soft, pea-sized, nontender, and freely mobile. These could be leftover nodes from a past infection. Tender nodes indicate a current infection and this should trigger an assessment of disease-associated symptoms and signs.

Nontender, nonmobile, small, or enlarged nodes with irregular margins are highly suspicious for benign or cancerous tumors.

The preauricular, postauricular, and occipital nodes drain only the superficial tissues. The submental, submandibular, and tonsillar nodes drain superficial and deep tissues.

Bimanual palpation of the floor of the mouth should always be done if the submental and submandibular nodes are enlarged. Using gloved hands, support the floor of the mouth firmly with your left palm under the chin. Place the fingers of your right hand inside the mouth and feel with pressure against the outside hand, the floor and sides of the mouth, noting any enlargements or swellings. Note the shape, size, mobility, and tenderness status of the swelling, when present.

Cervical Nodes

The cervical nodes that collect drainage from the previously mentioned nodes are anterior cervical, posterior cervical, and deep cervical. Firmly gripping the sternocleidomastoid (SCM) muscle, palpate the neck along the anterior border for the anterior cervical nodes, and then palpate along the posterior border for the posterior cervical nodes. The deep cervicals lie **under** the muscle and cannot be palpated.

Nape of the Neck Nodes

The nodes in this area include the trapezius and supraclavicular nodes.

Trapezius Nodes

Stand in front of or behind the patient and palpate on both sides at the nape of the neck, just below the occipital nodes.

Supraclavicular Nodes

Stand in front of the patient and have the patient flex the neck toward the chest. As the patient takes a **deep breath**, use the pulp of your fingers to feel the area behind both the clavicles, adjacent to the suprasternal notch. Deep breathing brings to the surface any enlarged nodes, when present. These nodes are enlarged with liquid tumors or solid tumors affecting the lungs, breast, or upper abdomen. Section XVIII, "Oncology," outlines the head and neck lymphatic drainage disease states.

See Table 51.1 in Chapter 51 to learn more about specific tissues drained by each of the head and neck lymph nodes. The table also outlines direct or indirect drainage into the deep cervical chains.

Thyroid Gland

Use the following techniques:

Inspection: Stand in front of the patient and ask the patient to hyperextend the neck and swallow. Note the free mobility of the thyroid gland in the neck.

Palpation: Palpate the thyroid gland by standing behind the patient. Place your palm on the patient's neck and check whether the gland feels warmer than the surrounding skin. Check whether the surface is smooth. Palpate each lobe separately to note the size and margins of the gland. Move the left gland toward the right, to feel the right margin of the gland. The margin, if felt, should be soft and smooth. Repeat the process on the left side by moving the right gland toward the left.

Auscultation: Occasionally, an arterial bruit may be heard over a highly vascular enlarged gland.

Trachea

The trachea is normally located in the **midline**. Deviation to the right or left may suggest tumor, pneumothorax, or lung collapse.

Examination of the Hands

Check the skin temperature, appearance, and color of the hands, nails, joints, palms, and palmar creases, and look for any deformity. Compare the patient's palm color with the color of your own palms. White palmar creases indicate a hemoglobin level that is less than 50% of normal. Palmar erythema is frequently seen in alcoholics. If the knuckle joints and the proximal interphalangeal joints are swollen and affected bilaterally, it is indicative of **rheumatoid arthritis**. If the distal interphalangeal joints are affected unilaterally, it is suggestive of **osteoarthritis**. Look for and note any changes in the nails.

Examination of the Nails

Clubbing or **convexity** of the nails can be associated with chronic cardiopulmonary diseases. **Spooning** or **koilonychia** can be seen with iron deficiency anemia. **Splinter hemorrhage** in the nails can be associated with subacute bacterial endocarditis (SBE).

Examination of the Back

Inspection

Look for any spinal deformity.

Palpation

The spine should be palpated along the entire length of the spinal column to elicit any areas of tenderness.

Movements

Ask the patient to bend forward, backward, and sideways to check for mobility of the spine. Patients with limitation in movements should be assisted in and out of the dental chair. Rheumatoid arthritis affects the mobility of the cervical spine and the temporomandibular joint (TMJ). Osteoarthritis affects the lumbosacral joint mobility.

Examination of the Lower Extremities

Inspection

Inspect for any skeletal or muscular deformity, varicose veins, joint deformity, and loss of hair on the toes, shin, and feet. Loss of hair occurs due to poor circulation.

Palpation

Palpate the joints for any tenderness or swelling. Also, with the back of your hands, check for the relative warmth of the feet and toes, and indirectly assess perfusion.

Examination of the Lungs or Pulmonary Examination

Inspection

Note the shape and symmetry of the chest. Barrel chest is seen with obstructive lung disease and with emphysema (hyperinflated lungs). Note the rate, rhythm, and regularity of respiration, if not yet assessed. Normal respiration rate for adults is 12–16 breaths/min. Resting shallow tachypnea (rapid shallow breathing) is seen with restrictive lung disease. Hyperpnea (rapid deep breathing) is commonly seen with anxiety, exertion, or metabolic acidosis. The rapid deep breathing as seen in metabolic acidosis is called **Kussmaul's respiration**.

Palpation

Strap or brace the chest with your hands and note the equality of chest excursions on both sides simultaneously, with deep breaths. Test from the apex to the base of the lungs.

Palpation of the Apex of the Lungs

To palpate the apex of the lungs, place your palms on the patient's shoulders and press down firmly as the patient inhales deeply. Check whether the apex of both lungs rises up equally. In the adult patient, a collapsed apex is usually due to tuberculosis (TB).

Percussion

Compare percussion notes at the same intercostal levels over both lung fields. The normal percussion note is resonant. Dullness on percussion is caused by consolidation of the lungs, as in pneumonia, or due to fluid collection, as in pleural effusion. A hyperresonant note occurs with pneumothorax.

Auscultation

Auscultate the right and left lung fields at the same intercostal level for comparison of auscultatory findings. Note the quality of the breath sounds and determine whether any adventitious sounds like rales, ronchi, or wheezes are present. The vesicular breathing pattern as seen in Figure 1.3 is heard over normal lung parenchyma. In this pattern, the inspiration limb is longer than the expiration limb.

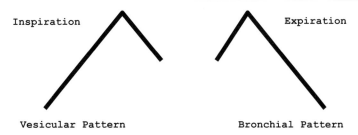

Figure 1.3. Breathing patterns.

Bronchial Breath Sounds

The expiratory sound is higher pitched and louder than that heard with the vesicular breath sounds. Also, the expiratory component is equal to or greater than the inspiratory component (Figure 1.3). Bronchial breath sounds, when heard over the lung parenchyma, are abnormal and indicate underlying disease. Bronchial sounds heard over the bifurcation of the trachea, however, are normal in occurrence.

Adventitious Breath Sounds

Adventitious breath sounds heard on auscultation are:

- **Wheezes**, as with asthma, are whistling sounds caused by constriction of the bronchioles.
- **Rales and ronchi** are crackling sounds indicating presence of fluid in the lungs that can be due to bronchitis or congestive heart failure (CHF). Rales are coarse crackles and ronchi are soft crackles.

Examination of the Cardiovascular System

Inspection

Lay the patient at a 30–40° angle and note the jugular venous pulsation (JVP) in the neck. Normally, the JVP will be seen at or below the clavicle. If the JVP is seen in the neck, it is suggestive of decreased forward flow/cardiac output or increased backward flow. The apex beat, which is usually located in the fifth intercostal space medial to the midclavicular line, is also noted during inspection of the heart. Confirm the apex beat location with your palm during palpation.

Palpation

Locate the carotid pulse with the tips of your fingers along the anterior border of the sternomastoid muscle in the middle of the neck, one carotid at a time. Once located, gently press down and establish the pulse rate per minute. Never use your thumb to feel for pulsations because the thumb has its own pulsation. This can interfere with perceiving the patient's pulsation. Never palpate the carotid at the angle of the mandible because this will compress the carotid sinus and cause the pulse to slow down. This can become problematic in the elderly patient and may result in the patient experiencing dizziness or fainting. Note the pulse rate per minute for each carotid artery. Disparity of pulse rates between the two carotids will require you to auscultate for carotid bruits, as discussed further under "Auscultation."

Palpate the radial pulse at the wrist with the tips of your fingers, but never your thumb. Support the patient's hand in your hand, and with the fingers of your other hand feel the radial pulse, which is located on the side of the thumb. Let the pulse stabilize for a few seconds and then count the rate per minute. Determine the rhythm of the pulse. If there is a rhythm irregularity, assess whether it is regular (regularly irregular rhythm, as in cardiac conduction defects) or irregular (irregularly irregular rhythm as associated with atrial flutter or atrial fibrillation). Palpate over the cardiac area with your palm to feel for the presence of any other pulses or thrills. A thrill is a purring sensation, felt on

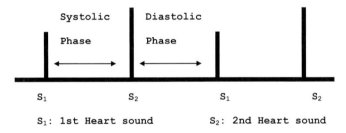

Figure 1.4. Heart sounds: Systolic and diastolic phases.

palpation. Thrills are caused by a loud heart murmur. Murmurs are sounds produced by turbulent blood flow, or they can occur due to vibrating heart valves.

Percussion

Percussion of the heart is done to outline the right and left border of the heart.

Auscultation

There are two associated auscultation techniques:

1. **Carotid Artery Auscultation:** When there is disparity in rates between the two carotids, auscultate over the arteries as the patient **holds** the breath. Turbulence of blood flow in the partially obstructed carotid artery causes a swooshing sound or **bruit** over the carotid artery with the **lesser** pulsation. Holding the breath is important as a bruit, and breath sounds are similar sounding.
2. **Heart Sounds Auscultation:** As shown in Figure 1.4, the first heart sound or S_1 is caused by the **closure** of the **mitral** and the **tricuspid** valves, and the second heart sound or S_2 is caused by the **closure** of the **aortic** and the **pulmonic** valves. The phase between S_1 and S_2 is the **systolic** or **ventricle** contraction phase, and the phase between S_2 and S_1 is the **diastolic** or the **atrial** contraction phase. Auscultation must be done in the four cardiac areas, shown in Figure 1.5. The **aortic** area is located in the **second right** intercostal space, next to the sternum. The **pulmonic** area is located in the **second left** intercostal space, next to the sternum. The **tricuspid** area is located in the third and fourth intercostal spaces; along the left border of the sternum and the **mitral** area is located in the fifth intercostal space, medial to the midclavicular line. The **apex beat** is located in the mitral area.

Systolic murmurs, as shown in Figure 1.6, can be due to aortic stenosis (AS), pulmonary stenosis (PS), tricuspid incompetence (TI), or mitral incompetence/regurgitation (MI). Diastolic murmurs, as shown in Figure 1.7, can be caused by mitral stenosis (MS), tricuspid stenosis (TS), aortic incompetence (AI), or pulmonary incompetence (PI).

Examination of the Musculoskeletal System

Warm, tender elbow joints with subcutaneous nodules are commonly seen with rheumatoid arthritis. Wrists swollen bilaterally are suggestive of rheumatoid arthritis. Palpable

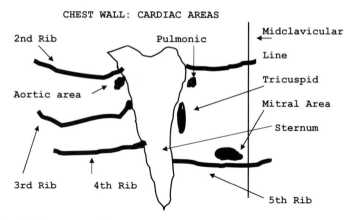

Figure 1.5. Cardiac areas surface anatomy.

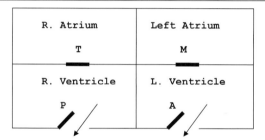

Figure 1.6. Systolic murmurs.

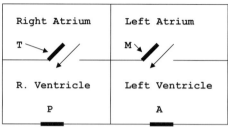

Figure 1.7. Diastolic murmurs.

enlargement of bones in hands, also called **nodules**, is suggestive of osteoarthritis. If the large toe is affected, think of gout. However, an enlarged toe is no longer considered "the classic" gout presentation site, as other areas can and do get affected instead of or before the big toe.

Examination of the Cranial Nerves

Review Table 1.1.

Table 1.1. Cranial Nerve (CN) Examination

CN #:	CN Name:	CN Action:
CN I	**Olfactory**	Causes the sense of smell
CN II	**Optic**	Afferent nerve for vision
CN III	**Oculomotor**	Causes all extraocular muscle movements (except those caused by lateral rectus and superior oblique muscles) and pupillary constriction
CN IV	**Trochlear**	Innervates the superior oblique muscle to move the eye down and in
CN V	**Trigeminal**	Sensory fibers to the face via the ophthalmic, maxillary, and mandibular divisions. Motor fibers to the muscles of mastication, the Temporal and Masseter muscles. **CN V Sensory Exam:** Have the patient **shut** the eyes. Touch the skin in the ophthalmic, maxillary, and mandibular areas with a cotton tip. Sense of touch is intact with optimal sensory function. **CN V Motor Exam:** Put your hands on either side of the patient's face and feel the equality of the Masseter muscle tone as the patient clenches. Next, place your hands on either side of the forehead to test the Temporalis muscles' tone.
CN VI	**Abducens**	Innervates the lateral Rectus muscle and moves the eye laterally.
CN VII	**Facial**	Motor nerve to most facial muscles and anterior tongue taste. Ask the patient to blow, whistle, and frown.
CN VIII	**Acoustic**	Responsible for hearing and balance
CN IX	**Glosso-pharyngeal**	Sensory and motor to pharynx and posterior tongue, plus responsible for taste
CN X	**Vagus**	Motor to the palate, larynx, pharynx; sensory to pharynx and larynx. Test IX and X CNs together. Ask the patient to say a deep "aah." Use flashlight to see if the palate rises equally on both sides.
CN XI	**Spinal Accesory**	Motor nerve to Sternocleidomastoid and Trapezius muscles. To test the Trapezius muscle, stand behind the patient and press down on both shoulders with your hands. Ask patient to shrug against pressure and note equality of tension on both sides. **Sternocleidomastoid test:** Place your palm on patient's **right** cheek and feel the tension in **left** Sternomastoid as the patient tries to turn his face to the right against resistance. Next, test the right sternomastoid muscle.
CN XII	**Hypoglossal**	Motor to tongue. Ask patient to protrude the tongue. It should be in the midline and have no tremors. CN damage causes the tongue to deviate toward the **affected** side.

History and Physical Assessment of the Medically Complex Dental Patient

HISTORY AND PHYSICAL: INTRODUCTION

A medically complex dental patient (MCP) is one who suffers from one or more diseases and who is taking one or more medications for the care of those disease states. The management of the MCP is a multitiered process that requires detailed, organized assessment of several aspects associated with the patient, which can sometimes take more than one dental visit. Every MCP should have a thorough assessment of the medical and dental histories during the first visit. The dentist needs to decide what laboratory tests to obtain from the patient's primary care physician (PCP) and/or the specialist(s). Evaluation of the tests will help determine the control status level of the patient's disease states. The dentist also needs to assess the vital organ status; the patient's American Society of Anesthesiology (ASA) status; the need for stress management; the dental treatment plan; and the final anesthetics, analgesics, and antibiotics (AAAs) that can be safely used during dentistry.

It is important that all pertinent information collected prior to dentistry be incorporated in the patient's record as a separate "medical consultation" summarized case note. This note can then be referenced any time during patient care and should be updated when there is a change in the health history or the list of medications.

MEASURES ESTABLISHED WITH THE COMPLETE HEALTH HISTORY

The complete health history will provide the following:

- The date of the last physical examination.
- The name, address, and telephone number of the primary care physician (PCP) and the specialists.
- The disease state(s) being managed in the patient.

Dentist's Guide to Medical Conditions, Medications, and Complications, Second Edition. Kanchan M. Ganda.
© 2013 John Wiley & Sons, Inc. Published 2013 by John Wiley & Sons, Inc.

The control status of disease state(s) is determined by assessment of appropriate laboratory test results, as with diabetes, or by following standard guidelines, as with blood pressure readings.

Diabetes Assessment Example

To assess diabetes, evaluate the fasting blood sugar (FBS), postprandial blood sugar (PPBS), and the HbA_1C. The well-controlled patient will have FBS: <120mg/dL; PPBS: <160mg/dL; and HbA_1C: <7% (normal: 4–6%).

Hypertension Assessment Example

To evaluate hypertension, assess the blood pressure (BP), and categorize the patient's BP readings as normal, high-normal, mild, moderate, or severe. Determine the following:

- The presence of symptoms of an as yet undiagnosed condition.
- Whether medical emergencies have occurred in past dental visits.
- Whether the patient requires premedication (at a minimum, successive appointments should be scheduled seven days apart when using the same premedication antibiotic).
- The prescribed, over-the-counter (OTC), or herbal medications the patient is taking.

Always confirm whether the patient is compliant with the medications—never presume! Assess the drug-drug interactions (DDIs) between the drugs that the patient is taking and the anesthetics, analgesics, antibiotics, antivirals, or antifungals (AAAAAs) used or prescribed in the dental setting Many of the drugs typically used in dentistry are substrates, inducers, or inhibitors of the CYP450 enzyme system and can be associated with adverse DDIs. By knowing what drugs your patient takes for the underlying disease states, you can help prevent the occurrence of DDIs by prescribing a drug that does not impact the P450 isoform/enzyme involved in the metabolism of that particular drug.

In addition to the CYP enzyme system, metabolism of certain medications can also be affected by transporter proteins that actively transport medications into and out of cells. ATP-dependent efflux drug transporter P-glycoprotein (P-gp) thus affects how drugs are absorbed, distributed, and eliminated by the body. Many P-gp inhibitors are CYP3A4 inhibitors as well. P-gp and CYP3A4 are present in the gut, and this accounts for why some DDIs occur first in the gastrointestinal tract and then in the liver. Drug interactions occurring through CYP isoenzymes mostly involve the P-glycoprotein (P-gp) transporter system too.

Thus, a thorough assessment of all medications is necessary to prevent adverse reactions or drug-related emergencies during dental treatment. Evaluate every drug by assessing its mechanism of action, what condition(s) it treats, and potential DDIs among the drug and the AAAAAs. Digoxin and theophylline are discussed in the next sections as examples to demonstrate the way drugs should be assessed.

Lanoxin (Digoxin) Assessment

Lanoxin (digoxin) is a cardiac glycoside is used to treat congestive heart failure (CHF) and atrial fibrillation (AF). AF is also called **supraventricular arrhythmia**.

Lanoxin (Digoxin) Mechanism of Action

Lanoxin (digoxin) binds to and inhibits the magnesium and adenosine triphosphate (ATP) dependent Na^+ and K^+ ATP-ase, thereby increasing the influx of calcium ions in the cardiac smooth muscle. This increase in calcium ions enhances the myocardial contractility.

Lanoxin (Digoxin) and Local Anesthetics

Ideally, avoid local anesthetics with epinephrine in the presence of digoxin because epinephrine can be counterproductive (Table 2.1). It is safe to use 3% mepivacaine HCL (Carbocaine) or 4% prilocaine HCL (Citanest Plain) instead. However, you may cautiously use the least lipophilic local anesthetic, 4% prilocaine HCL (Citanest Forte) with 1:200,000 epinephrine, maximum two carpules when a local anesthetic with epinephrine is absolutely needed.

Lanoxin (Digoxin) and Analgesics

Avoid aspirin and NSAIDS with digoxin. Aspirin decreases digoxin absorption from the gut and displaces digoxin from the protein binding sites. NSAIDS increase serum digoxin levels by decreasing the renal clearance of digoxin. Use acetaminophen (Tylenol), oxycodone + acetaminophen (Percocet), hydrocodone + acetaminophen (Vicodin), or acetaminophen + 30 mg codeine (Tylenol #3) instead, depending on the needs of the patient and if no contraindications exist to the use of centrally acting pain medications.

Lanoxin (Digoxin) and Antibiotics

Lanoxin (digoxin) is a P-gp substrate and is independent of CYP3A4 action. P-gp inhibits the bioavailability of digoxin and facilitates the renal and biliary secretion of digoxin. Erythromycin or Clarithromycin, when given to patients on chronic digoxin, cause an increase in serum digoxin concentrations, as they are potent P-gp inhibitors.

Table 2.1.   Digoxin and AAAs

AVOID WITH DIGOXIN	USE WITH DIGOXIN
ANESTHETICS: All local anesthetics with epinephrine	**ANESTHETICS:** a. 3% Mepivacaine (Carbocaine) b. 4% Prilocaine HCL without epinephrine (Citanest Plain)
ANALGESICS: a. Aspirin b. NSAIDS	**ANALGESICS:** a. Acetaminophen (Tylenol) b. Tylenol with Codeine (Tylenol #3) c. Tylenol with Hydrocodone (Vicodin) d. Tylenol with Oxycodone (Percocet)
ANTIBIOTICS: a. Clarithromycin (Biaxin) b. Azithromycin (potentiates rhythm issues) c. Tetracyclines	**ANTIBIOTICS:** a. All Penicillins b. All Cephalosporins c. Clindamycin

Azithromycin appears to have little influence on P-gp–mediated digoxin absorption or excretion and would therefore be the safest macrolide to use concurrently with oral digoxin. However, some recent studies have shown that it is best to avoid azithromycin use in patients with underlying cardiac states associated with rhythm issues, myocardial dysfunction, myocardial infarction, angina, cardiac failure, hypertension, hyperlipidemia, diabetes, smoking, obesity, poor diet, and sedentary life style, as azithromycin has been shown to potentially alter cardiac conduction from QTc prolongation and ventricular arrhythmias.

Therefore, avoid macrolides, erythromycin, clarithromycin, and all tetracyclines with digoxin because these drugs increase serum digoxin levels. Use the penicillins, cephalosporins, clindamycin, or azithromycin (when safe to use) instead.

Theophylline (Theo-Dur) Assessment

Theophylline is a xanthine-derivative bronchodilator that is used in the management of moderate to severe asthma. It has a very narrow "therapeutic index," which means that there is a very small dose transition difference between the therapeutic dose and the toxic dose.

Theophylline and Anesthetics

Theophylline can become toxic in the presence of epinephrine. It is advised that you use 3% mepivacaine HCL (Carbocaine) or 4% prilocaine HCL (Citanest Plain) instead.

Theophylline and Antibiotics

Avoid all macrolides because theophylline can become toxic in the presence of macrolides erythromycin, azithromycin, or clarithromycin.

Note that penicillin, aspirin, and NSAIDS can precipitate asthma attacks in some patients. Thus, always check whether the patient is allergic to or has had an adverse reaction with aspirin, codeine, morphine, local anesthetics, sulfa drugs, bisulfites, or penicillin. Avoid the use of those specific drugs.

Over-the-Counter Drugs

Determine the specific over-the counter (OTC) drugs the patient is taking and the frequency of intake. Check if the patient is consuming cough/cold medications, laxatives, diet pills, or herbal medications.

Morphine and Codeine Cross-Reactivity

Check whether the patient was given morphine for pain during past hospitalization. If there was no untoward reaction, the patient could be prescribed codeine during dentistry.

Corticosteroid History

Check whether there is a current or past history of steroid intake for two weeks or longer within the last two years (i.e., the "rule of twos"). If the answer is yes, consult with the patient's physician to determine whether extra steroids are needed for major dental work.

Recreational Drugs

Check whether the patient is using any recreational drugs. Determine whether these drugs will interact with the anesthetics, analgesics, antibiotics, antivirals, or antifungals (AAAAAs) or the patient's medications. Cocaine enhances the action of local anesthetics containing epinephrine. Alcohol enhances the utilization of local anesthetics, resulting in shorter duration of anesthesia. Alcohol also decreases the potency of antiseizure medications. The patient needs to be drug-free **for 24 hours,** and you should **defer** dental treatment in the **intoxicated** patient to avoid accidental needle sticks.

Oral Contraceptives

Oral antibiotics up until now were postulated to interfere with estrogen metabolism by decreasing or destroying the intestinal flora. This concept has been negated by recent evidence-based studies that have demonstrated that only CYP450 enzyme-inducer drugs accelerate estrogen metabolism and impact the efficacy of estrogen containing combined oral contraceptives (COCPs).

Penicillins, cephalosporins, clindamycin, macrolides, tetracyclines, and quinolones do not induce the CYP450 enzyme and consequently do not affect estrogen level. So the patient does not need to be advised about using barrier protection for the short- or long-term use of routine antibiotics prescribed in the dental setting.

How Does the Patient Feel About Dentist Visits?

Presence of anxiety, phobia, or fear calls for stress management during dentistry.

MEASURES ESTABLISHED WITH THE PHYSICAL EXAMINATION

On completion of the medical history, the following are assessed on physical examination:

- Pulse
- Blood pressure
- Respiration
- Height and weight
- Head and neck
- Status of the major systems
- Status of the vital organs

TREATMENT PLAN ASSESSMENT

Complete history and physical examination leads to the treatment plan, which determines the following:

- The final list of AAAs that can be safely used
- Whether the patient needs shorter appointments (ASA-III/IV patients) or appointments that are seven days apart

Table 2.2.   Medical Consultation Case Note Example

Dental Chief Complaint: "My mouth is a mess and I can only eat on one side."
Anticipated Dental Treatment: Full mouth extractions with immediate denture
Age: 59; **Gender:** F; **Ethnicity:** Hispanic; **Allergies:** None
Height: 5'2"; **Weight:** 155lb; **Pulse:** 86/min; **BP:** 125/75mmHg; **Respiration:**
14 breaths/min; **ASA Status:** II
List of Medical Conditions: Depression; social anxiety; Hepatitis C; anemia of chronic illness.
Patient has effectively been in a substance abuse treatment program for 10 months. **Avoid**
narcotics, sedatives, hypnotics, and alcoholic mouthwashes because she is a recovering addict.
Laboratory Tests Requested with Associated Results Against Each Test:
- **LFTs** were "mildly abnormal" per physician
- **CBC w/ WBC differential: WBC:** 6.2: Normal (N);
RBC: 4.26: Low (L); **Hgb:** 13.1: (L); **Hct:** 39.0: (L);
MCH: 30.8: (N); **MCV:** 91.6: (N); **RDW:** 14.1: (N);
Platelet count: 213: (N). **Assessment:** Mild anemia.
List of Medications (Prescribed, OTC, & Herbals) and DDIs:
Zoloft: 250mg/day; Neurontin: 900mg/day; Wellbutrin: 100mg/day; Buspar: 60mg/day;
Trazadone: 150mg HS; Centrum and multivitamin.
Zoloft (Sertraline): SSRI antidepressant. Avoid sedatives, especially Benzodiazepenes. Zoloft
causes bruxism.
- **Anesthetics:** Zoloft increases Lidocaine levels; avoid Lidocaine use.
- **Antibiotics:** No Erythromycin or Clarithromycin.
- **Analgesics:** No NSAIDS (risk of bleeding); no codeine, hydrocodone, or oxycodone (levels
  decreased by Zoloft).
Neurontin (Gabapentin): Used for anxiety disorders. It has an additive effect with sedatives.
Avoid barbiturates and opioid analgesics. It causes xerostomia and dry throat.
- **Anesthetics; Antibiotics:** no contraindication (CI).
- **Analgesics:** No opioid analgesics.
Wellbutrin (Bupropion): Dopamine reuptake inhibitor antidepressant. Causes abnormal taste
and severe xerostomia.
- **Anesthetics:** Use caution with epinephrine as Wellbutrin blocks the reuptake of
  norepinephrine (NE).
- **Antibiotics:** No CI.
- **Analgesics:** No opioid analgesics.
Buspar (Buspirone): Non-benzodiazepine anxiolytic. It causes xerostomia.
- **Anesthetics; Analgesics:** No CI.
- **Antibiotics:** Avoid CYP3A4 inhibitors drugs doxycycline, clarithromycin, and azole
  antifungals.
Trazadone: Serotonin reuptake inhibitor.
- **Anesthetics:** No CI.
- **Antibiotics:** Avoid CYP3A4 inhibitor drugs.
- **Analgesics:** No opioids, oxycodone, or hydrocodone.
- **Centrum multi-vitamin:** No CIs with the AAAs.
- **Need for Premedication:** No.
Final List of Anesthetics Safe for Dentistry:
- 0.5% bupivacaine (Marcaine); 4% prilocaine HCL (Citanest Forte); 3% mepivacaine HCL
  (Carbocaine): Maximum 2 carpules.
Final List of Analgesics Safe for Dentistry:
- Regular or extra-strength Tylenol.
Final List of Antibiotics Safe for Dentistry:
- Penicillins, cephalosporins, or clindamycin.

Table 2.3.   Common Medical Abbreviations

ABBREVIATION	EXPLANATION OF ABBREVIATION
AAA:	Abdominal Aortic Aneurysm
AAF:	African American Female
AAM:	African American Male
ABD:	Abdomen
abx:	Antibiotics
AKA:	Above Knee Amputation
APAP:	Acetaminophen
ARF:	Acute Renal Failure
ASA:	Aspirin
AV:	Atrioventricular
AVM:	Arteriovenous Malformation
AVR:	Aortic Valve Replacement
BKA:	Below Knee Amputation
bx:	Biopsy
c/o:	Complain of
CABG:	Coronary Artery Bypass Graft
CAD:	Coronary Artery Disease
CC:	Chief Complaint
CN:	Cranial Nerves
CP:	Chest Pain
CRF:	Chronic Renal Failure
CRI:	Chronic Renal Insufficiency
CV:	Cardiovascular
CVA:	Cerebrovascular Accident
cx:	Culture
CXR:	Chest X-ray
ddx:	Differential Diagnosis
DJD:	Degenerative Joint Disease
DOE:	Dyspnea on Exertion
EOMI:	Extraocular Muscles Intact
EXT:	Extremities
FH/FHx:	Family History
FOB:	Fecal Occult Blood
GEN:	General
gr:	Grain
GU:	Genitourinary
h/o:	History of
HA:	Headache
Hb:	Hemoglobin
Hct:	Hematocrit
HEENT:	Head, Eyes, Ears, Nose, Throat
HPI:	History of Present Illness
ICD:	Implantable Cardioverter Defibrillator
JVD:	Jugular Venous Distension
LAD:	Lymphadenopathy
LMP:	Last Menstrual Period
LYMPH:	Lymphatic
MDI:	Metered Dose Inhaler
MMSE:	Mini Mental Status Exam
Mmsk:	Musculoskeletal
MVR:	Mitral Valve Replacement

Table 2.3.   Common Medical Abbreviations (*Continued*)

ABBREVIATION	EXPLANATION OF ABBREVIATION
N, V:	Nausea, Vomiting
NAD:	No Acute Distress
NC:	Noncontributory
NDA:	New Drug Application
NEURO:	Neurologic
NKDA:	No Known Drug Allergies
No c/c/e:	No Cyanosis, Clubbing, Edema
No m/r/g:	No Murmurs, Rubs, Gallops
No r/r/w:	No rales, ronchi, wheezes
No T/A/D:	No Tobacco, Alcohol, IV Drug Use
OA:	Osteoarthritis
Palp:	Palpitations
PB:	Phenobarbital
PERRL:	Pupils Equally Round and Reactive to Light
PMH:	Past Medical History
PNA:	Pneumonia
PND:	**If Cardiac:** Paroxysmal Nocturnal Dyspnea
	If Respiratory: Postnasal Drip
PTCA:	Percutaneous Transluminal Coronary Angioplasty
PVD:	Peripheral Vascular Disease
Q.O.D, qod:	Every Other Day
QD:	Every day
qs:	A Sufficient Quantity
qw:	Once per week
R/O:	Rule Out
RCT:	Rotator Cuff Tear
ROS:	Review of System
RRR:	Regular Rate and Rhythm
s/p:	Status Post
SH/SHx:	Social History
SOB:	Shortness of Breath
solv:	Dissolve
SPO2:	Pulse Oximetry
Sptm:	Sputum
TIA:	Transient Ischemic Attack
URI:	Upper Respiratory Infection
VITAL SIGNS:	**T:** Temperature; **HR:** Pulse; **RR:** Respiratory Rate; **BP:** Blood Pressure
wa:	While Awake
WF:	White Female
WM:	White Male
x:	Times

- Whether the patient needs to be given morning or afternoon appointments, depending on when the patient eats. The patient needs to be on a full stomach to prevent hypoglycemia. Never **presume** that the patient has eaten; always **ask** and know **how much** the patient has eaten! Morning appointments are needed for myasthenia gravis patients and for patients needing a steroid boost prior to dentistry.
- If the patient needs to bring his own medications to the dental office, especially when there is a history of asthma, angina, or hypoglycemia.

- Whether stress management is needed using oral or systemic sedation. See Chapter 10 for details.

The Medical Consultation Case Note

The medical consultation case note for the medically compromised dental patient contains an assessment of all pertinent facts (medical status, laboratory tests, medications, and safe AAAs) associated with patient care, and it should be referenced for all appointments. See Table 2.2.

Common Medical Abbreviations

Physicians commonly use a variety of universally recognizable abbreviations in medical records for multiple reasons: to quickly but appropriately log patient-related information, to provide instructions to staff, to transmit orders to the pharmacy, or to provide instructions to their patients.

When a dental provider requests medical information about his or her patient for completion of the medical consult, the physician's office will often send a copy of the patient's entire medical record containing these abbreviations. So you can understand the contents correctly, refer to Table 2.3 for a listing and breakdown of some of the common abbreviations encountered.

Pharmacology

Essentials in Pharmacology: Drug Metabolism, Cytochrome P450 Enzyme System, and Prescription Writing

DRUG METABOLISM OVERVIEW

The liver is the main site for drug metabolism. Drug metabolism often enhances termination of drug action, but on occasion metabolism can lead to bio-activation, as with prodrugs. The drug metabolism process basically introduces hydrophilic functionalities onto the drug molecule to facilitate excretion. When the drug molecule is oxidized, hydrolyzed, or conjugated, the whole molecule becomes more hydrophilic and is excreted more easily.

The liver enzymes induce two drug metabolism pathways known as Phase I and Phase II. These phases are dependent on two factors: hepatic blood flow and metabolic capacity of the liver.

Typical Phase I metabolism includes oxidation and hydrolysis. The microsomal enzymes or cytochromes involved in Phase I reactions are primarily located in the endoplasmic reticulum of the liver cells. Phase I metabolites that are hydrophilic (more water soluble) are readily excreted, and all other metabolites undergo a subsequent Phase II metabolism. The capacity of the liver to metabolize drugs by the Phase I enzyme systems is compromised when the liver is in failure. The metabolic capacity of the liver has to be decreased by more than 90%, before drug metabolism is significantly affected. Phase II metabolism includes glucuronidation and glutathione conjugation of the drug molecule, thus making the drug hydrophilic and ready for excretion. Phase II occurs after Phase I metabolism, and often drugs undergo both Phase I and Phase II metabolism prior to excretion. It is important to note that Phase II can occur independent of Phase I metabolism and Phase II metabolism can still occur even in end-stage liver failure.

Although the liver is the primary site for metabolism, virtually all tissue cells have some metabolic activities. Other organs with significant metabolic activities include the gastrointestinal tract, kidneys, and lungs. When a drug is given orally, it undergoes metabolism in the GI tract and the liver before reaching the systemic circulation. This process is called **first-pass** metabolism. First-pass metabolism limits the oral bioavailability of drugs, sometimes quite significantly. During the first-pass metabolism, after a drug is ingested, it reaches the liver through the hepatic portal system before it reaches

Dentist's Guide to Medical Conditions, Medications, and Complications, Second Edition. Kanchan M. Ganda.
© 2013 John Wiley & Sons, Inc. Published 2013 by John Wiley & Sons, Inc.

the rest of the body. Often, the liver metabolizes these drugs to such an extent that only a small amount of active drug emerges from the liver to enter the systemic circulation. This first pass through the liver thus greatly reduces the bioavailability of the drug. When ingested orally, the first-pass effect of a drug can also be affected by the enzymes of the gastrointestinal lumen, gut wall enzymes, bacterial enzymes, and hepatic enzymes. Thus the drug can be given by alternate routes (IM/IV) if this effect is to be bypassed.

The first-pass effect can be beneficial in some cases, as with prodrugs such as codeine, which gets activated to morphine by first-pass metabolism. Therefore, in this case, Phase I oxidation converts a pharmacologically inactive compound to a pharmacologically active one. Drugs often undergo both Phase I and II reactions before excretion.

CYTOCHROME ENZYME SYSTEM OVERVIEW

Cytochrome P450 refers to a group of heme-containing enzymes that are primarily located in the liver hepatocytes and within the enterocytes in the small intestine. These enzymes are important for drug biotransformation, drug metabolism, and detoxification of endogenous compounds after they have been ingested. This accounts for the high concentrations of these enzymes in the liver and small intestine.

Infants develop a mature hepatic CYP450 enzyme system in the two weeks following birth. CYP450 activity can be temporarily depressed by fulminant infections, or the activity may be affected long term due to celiac disease or cirrhosis of the liver. The elderly may also have a decrease in hepatic CYP450 metabolic activity because of changes in liver blood flow, size, or drug binding and drug distribution with age. The P450 system can be altered by a number of mechanisms, including inhibition and induction, and can vary from person to person. Knowledge of the P450 system is critical in understanding drug metabolism and drug interactions.

Cytochrome P450 Enzyme **Nomenclatures**

Current nomenclature of the cytochrome P450 (CYP) enzymes is three-tiered: CYP followed by a number, representing the enzyme family, followed by a letter representing the subfamily, and then followed by another number representing the individual gene: for example, CYP3A4.

Each enzyme is termed an "isoform" or "isoenzyme." CYP450 enzyme system has eight main P450 isoform groups: CYP1A2, CYP2B6, CYP2C8, CYP2C9, CYP2C19, CYP2D6, CYP2E1, and CYP3A4. CYP2D6 and CYP3A4 are two of the most common enzymes, with the CYP3A4 isoform being the most abundant cytochrome family expressed in the human liver and intestine. Thus CYP3A4 is involved in the metabolism of a greater number of drugs, and consequently a greater proportion of adverse drug-drug interactions (DDIs), than the other CYP isoforms.

As stated previously, CYP enzymes are involved in the oxidative metabolism of a number of drug classes and endogenous substances, including prostaglandins and steroid hormones. Drugs may affect or be affected by one or several isoenzymes, thus accounting for the significant complexity associated with the metabolism of many medications. Cytochrome P450 enzymes metabolize drugs, toxins, and other substances, so they can be safely eliminated from the body. CYP enzymes eliminate drugs by making them water-soluble through a first-phase oxidation process, and if the drug is not completely transformed for elimination, then a second metabolic phase—the conjugation-reaction phase—is triggered to make the drug water-soluble. CYP enzymes account for elimination of commonly prescribed drugs: benzodiazepines, beta-blockers, calcium channel blockers, opioids, statins, selective serotonin reuptake inhibitors (SSRIs), and warfarin (Coumadin), to name a few.

CYP2D6 and CYP2C19 genetic polymorphisms: Of Caucasians, 6–10% are CYP2D6 deficient, whereas others may have high levels of the enzyme. Polymorphism of the gene encoding this enzyme leads to clinical phenotypes showing either extensive or poor drug metabolism. Genetic polymorphism also exists for CYP2C19 expression, affecting 3–5% of Caucasians and 15–20% of Asians. These individuals have no CYP2C19 function, and individuals of Asian and African decent are more likely to be poor metabolizers.

CYP System-Related Terminologies

Substrate: A substrate is a drug or compound on which a particular enzyme acts to metabolize the drug. For example, protease inhibitors idinavir (Crixivan), nelfinivir (Viracept), ritonavir (Norvir), and saquinavir (Fortovase) are substrates for the isoform CYP3A4 and therefore are metabolized by CYP3A4.

Do **not** concurrently prescribe two substrates competing for the same enzyme, as one drug may inhibit or induce metabolism of the other, and an adverse drug interaction may occur. For example, ethanol and acetaminophen (Tylenol) are substrates for CYP2E1; thus when the two are combined, ethanol can adversely affect the metabolism of acetaminophen by causing **increased** NAPQI production. Hence alcoholics can overdose with a therapeutic dose of Tylenol.

Inducer: An inducer of a specific CYP450 isoform increases the amount and subsequent activity of that particular enzyme in the hepatic and small intestinal tissues, thus causing increased clearance of the substrate. This can potentially lead to diminished plasma levels of the active drug that is a substrate for that enzyme. In HIV patients on protease inhibitors, the simultaneous use of the herbal antidepressant St. John's wort significantly decreases blood levels and the antiviral efficacy of the protease inhibitors. This is because St. John's wort is a potent inducer of CYP3A4.

Inhibitor: An enzyme inhibitor reduces the activity of a specific cytochrome P450 isoform to metabolize the substrate, resulting in an accumulation from decreased clearance of the substrate. The toxicity typically seen is identical to what would be seen from an overdose of the substrate drug.

With regard to CYP3A4, it is not just drugs that can inhibit this isoform; it can also be affected by grapefruit juice. Bergamottin, a furan-coumarin, and possibly some other related compounds found in grapefruit juice, both inhibit the action of CYP3A4 and reduce hepatic and intestinal concentrations of CYP3A4, causing the accumulation of a number of CYP3A4 substrates. The ability of grapefruit to lead to excessive plasma concentrations of CYP3A4 substrates was first encountered with calcium channel blockers, where excessive blood levels led to hypotension and peripheral edema.

Drug Transporters

In addition to the CYP enzyme system, metabolism of certain medications can also be affected by transporter proteins that actively transport medications into and out of cells. These transporter proteins are found in various tissues and organs, located on the luminal side of the enterocytes in the small intestines, renal tubular cells, the bile canaliculi, adrenal glands, and on the luminal surface of capillary endothelial cells in the brain. Drug transporters help control access of drugs to the systemic circulation by dictating the amount of drug that can enter the body from the gut lumen. Therefore, they influence how much drug escapes first-pass metabolism in both the gut and the liver.

Transporter proteins are influx or efflux pumps. The influx, or uptake, pumps transport drugs into cells, and the efflux pumps transport drugs out of cells. Efflux pumps control the amount of drug inside a cell. Organic anion transporting polypeptide (OATP) and organic cation transporting polypeptide (OCTP) are examples of uptake transporters. P-glycoprotein (P-gp) is an example of an ATP-dependent efflux transporter that takes drug molecules from the cells and transports the drugs back into the intestinal lumen for excretion. P-gp thus affects how drugs are absorbed, distributed, and eliminated by the body. By transporting many drugs that are substrates of CYP3A4, P-gp helps regulate the amount of drug molecules in the enterocyte, thus preventing CYP3A4 saturation. CYP3A4 concentrations decrease and P-gp concentrations increase from the proximal to distal portions of the gut. P-gp inhibitor drugs will increase the bioavailability of a P-gp substrate by slowing drug excretion, and a P-gp inducer will reduce the bioavailability of a substrate drug by speeding up the elimination of the drug.

Digoxin (Lanoxin) is a P-gp substrate and is independent of CYP3A4 action. P-gp inhibits the bioavailability of digoxin and facilitates the renal and biliary secretion of digoxin. Erythromycin (E-Mycin) or clarithromycin (Biaxin), when given to patients on chronic digoxin, cause an increase in serum digoxin concentrations, as they are potent P-gp inhibitors. Azithromycin (Zithromax) appears to have little influence on P-gp-mediated digoxin absorption or excretion and would be the safest macrolide to use concurrently with oral digoxin.

Hence ATP-dependent efflux drug **transporter P-glycoproteins** affect how drugs are absorbed, distributed, and eliminated by the body. P-gp and CYP3A4 are present in the gut, and this accounts for why some DDIs occur first in the gastrointestinal tract and then in the liver. Drug interactions occurring **through CYP isoenzymes, also most often** involve the P-glycoprotein (**P-gp**) **transporter system**. Many P-gp inhibitors are CYP3A4 inhibitors too.

P-gp substrates: acyclovir (Zovirax) amiodarone (Cordarone), amitriptyline (Elavil), amoxocillin (Amoxil), ampicillin (Omnipen), digoxin (Lanoxin), loperamide (Diamode), methotrexate (Rheumatrex), quinidine (Quinidine Gluconate), valacyclovir (Valtrex), and vinblastine (Velban).

P-gp inhibitors: cyclosporine (Sandimmune), erythromycin (E-Mycin), clarithromycin (Biaxin), iatroconazole (Sporanox), ketoconazole (Nizoral), nelfinavir (Viracept), quinidine (Quinidine Gluconate), reserpine (Serpalan), ritonavir (Norvir), saquinavir (Invirase), tacrolimus (Prograf), and verapamil (Calan).

P-gp inducers: barbiturates, rifampin (Rifadin), and St. John's wort.

Many of the drugs typically encountered in dentistry are substrates, inducers, or inhibitors of the CYP450 enzyme system and can be associated with adverse DDIs. Knowing what drugs your patient takes for underlying disease states can help you prevent the occurrence of DDIs by prescribing a drug that does not impact the P450 isoform involved in the metabolism of drugs the patient consumes routinely.

The substrates, inhibitors, and inducers of the eight most common CYP450 isoenzymes are listed in the following sections. Drugs commonly prescribed in the dental setting, or drugs of importance to the dental setting, have been highlighted in the text following and in Table 3.1.

Table 3.1. Specific CYP Isoenzymes Affecting Drugs Commonly Encountered in Dentistry

DRUGS COMMONLY USED OR ENCOUNTERED IN DENTISTRY:	CYP ENZYME SYSTEM(S) AFFECTING THE DRUG(S):
BENZODIAZEPINES: Alprazolam (Xanax) Diazepam (Valium) Midazolam (Versad) Triazolam (Halcion) Note: **Lorazepam (Ativan)** is the **only** benzodiazepine that is **not** metabolized by any CYP450 enzymes and so is less susceptible to adverse drug interactions.	**All Benzodiazepines are metabolized by CYP3A4** Avoid Benzodiazepines in combination with CYP3A4-associated drugs. Use Lorazepam instead. Benzodiazepines + CYP3A4 inhibitor drugs → Benzodiazepine toxicity Benzodiazepines + CYP3A4 inducer drugs → decreased effectiveness of Benzodiazepine **Diazepam is metabolized by CYP3A4 and CYP2C19** Avoid combining Diazepam with CYP3A4- and CYP2C19- associated drugs.
NSAIDS: Celecoxib (Celebrex) Diclofenac (Voltaren) Ibuprofen (Advil) Naproxen (Aleve) Indomethacin (Indocin) Ketoprofen (Orudis) Piroxicam (Feldene)	**All NSAIDS are metabolized by CYP2C9** **Diclofenac and Ketoprofen** also are inhibitors of **CYP2C9.** **Indomethacin** is additionally metabolized by **CYP2C19** and is also an inhibitor of **CYP2C19**. **Naproxen** is additionally metabolized by **CYP1A2.** Avoid combining the NSAIDS with the corresponding CYP-associated drugs.
ACETAMINOPHEN (TYLENOL):	**CYP 1A2 and CYP2E1 enzymes convert Acepaminophen to NAPQI.** Avoid combining Acetaminophen with CYP1A2- and CYP2E1-associated drugs.
CENTRALLY ACTING ANALGESICS: Codeine/Codeine + Acetaminophen (Tylenol #1–4) Hydrocodone + Acetaminophen (Vicodin) Oxycodone + Acetaminophen (Percocet) Tramadol (Ultram) Meperidine (Demerol) Methadone (Dolophine) Propoxyphene (Darvon): Propoxyphene was recently discontinued because of increased incidence of cardiac arrhythmias and high death rate.	**All listed drugs are metabolized by CYP2D6**. Avoid combination with the appropriate CYP-associated drugs for these analgesics: **Oxycodone** is **not** a prodrug. Oxycodone needs **CYP3A4** enzyme for glucuronidation and **CYP2D6** for elimination. **Codeine, Hydrocodone and Tramadol** are **prodrugs**. **CYP2D6** triggers the following **active forms**: Codeine → Morphine Hydrocodone → O-demethylated Morphine or Hydromorphone Tramadol → O-demethyl Tramadol **Tramadol** is additionally metabolized by **CYP3A4** **Meperidine** is metabolized mainly by **CYP2D6 and CYP2B6** and minimally by **CYP2C19** **Methadone** is primarily metabolized by **CYP3A4, CYP2B6, and CYP2C19**, and minimally by **CYP2D6 and CYP2C9.** **Methadone is also an inhibitor for CYP2D6.** **Propoxyphene (Darvon)** is a substrate **and** inhibitor for **CYP3A4**

(continued)

Table 3.1.   Specific CYP Isoenzymes Affecting Drugs Commonly Encountered in Dentistry (*Continued*)

DRUGS COMMONLY USED OR ENCOUNTERED IN DENTISTRY:	CYP ENZYME SYSTEM(S) AFFECTING THE DRUG(S):
LIDOCAINE (XYLOCAINE):	**Lidocaine** is metabolized by **CYP1A2**, at **low** Lidocaine concentrations and by **CYP1A2 and CYP3A4** at **high** Lidocaine concentrations. Limit the surgical procedure such that smaller total doses of lidocaine are used, particularly when drugs that interfere with Lidocaine cannot be discontinued
CORTICOSTEROIDS: Cortisol (Hydrocortisone) Dexamethasone (Decadron) Methylprednisolone (Medrol): Methylprednisolone is frequently administered in a six-day, 21-dose regimen (a dose-pack), when needed, following major dental surgery to reduce postoperative swelling.	**All listed Corticosteroids are potent substrates and inducers for CYP3A4.** Additionally, **Dexamethasone** is also an inducer for **CYP2D6** and **Prednisone** is an inducer for **CYP2C19**. Steroids cause decreased effectiveness of drugs metabolized by CYP3A4/CYP2D6/CYP2C19, as they are potent inducers. Avoid combining the Steroids with the corresponding CYP-associated drugs.
BARBITURATES: Phenobarbital (Solfoton) Secobarbital (Seconal)	**Barbiturates are potent inducers of CYP2C9, CYP3A4, and CYP1A2** Additionally, **Phenobarbital** is a substrate for **CYP2C19** and an inducer for **CYP2B6 and CYP2C19**. Avoid combining Barbiturates with the corresponding CYP associated drugs.
QUINOLONES: Ciprofloxacin (Cipro) Enoxacin (Penetrex) Norfloxacin (Noroxin) Ofloxacin (Floxin)	**All Quinolones severely inhibit CYP1A2 and moderately inhibit CYP3A4.** Additionally, **Norfloxacin** is an inhibitor for **CYP2D6.** Avoid combining the Quinolones with the corresponding CYP-associated drugs.
METRONIDAZOLE (FLAGYL):	**Metronidazole is an inhibitor for CYP3A4 and CYP2C9.** Avoid combining Metronidazole with the above listed CYP-associated drugs.
MACROLIDES: Erythromycin Clarithromycin (Biaxin) Azythromycin (Zithromax) does **not** affect CYP enzymes	**Erythromycin and Clarithromycin are potent inhibitors of CYP3A4 and CYP1A2.** **Additionally, both are substrates for CYP3A4** Avoid combining Erythromycin and Clarithromycin with CYP-associated drugs.
AZOLE ANTIFUNGALS: Clotrimazol (Mycelex) Ketoconazol (Nizoral) Itraconazole (Sporanox) Fluconazole (Diflucan)	**Clotrimazole** is topical in action but recent studies have shown systemic action causing DDIs from CYP3A4 inhibition, thus raising the hypothesis of **CYP3A4** metabolizing enzyme and/or **P-gp efflux protein** effect at the intestinal level. **Fluconazole** is a **weak** inhibitor of **CYP3A4** and a **potent** inhibitor of **CYP2C9 and CYP2C19.** **Ketoconazole and Itraconazole** are **potent** inhibitors of **CYP3A4, CYP2C9, and CYP2C19.** Additionally, **Ketoconazole** is an inhibitor for **CYP1A2.** Avoid combining Azole antifungals with the above CYP-associated drugs.

Table 3.1. Specific CYP Isoenzymes Affecting Drugs Commonly Encountered in Dentistry (*Continued*)

DRUGS COMMONLY USED OR ENCOUNTERED IN DENTISTRY:	CYP ENZYME SYSTEM(S) AFFECTING THE DRUG(S):
CLOPIDOGREL (PLAVIX):	Clopidogrel is a prodrug. **Clopidogrel is metabolized to its active form by CYP2C19.** Avoid combining Clopidogrel with the CYP2C19-associated drugs.
DOXYCYCLINE (VIBRAMYCIN):	**Doxycycline is extensively metabolized by CYP3A4.** Avoid combining Doxycycline with the CYP3A4-associated drugs.
WARFARIN (COUMADIN): Warfarin is a racemic mixture of **"R"** and **"S"** Warfarin. The S form is 2–5 times more potent that the R form.	The **S form** is primarily metabolized by **CYP2C9.** The **R form** is metabolized by **CYP1A2 and CYP2C19.** Avoid combining Warfarin with the above CYP-associated drugs.

Please reference the CYP drug categories list and Table 3.1 to determine what can and cannot be prescribed in the dental setting, regarding what the patient is already taking for underlying disease states.

For example, naproxen is metabolized by CYP1A2; clarithromycin (Biaxin) and keto-conazole (Nizoral) are CYP1A2 inhibitors. If you plan on prescribing naproxen for pain management and inflammation, you will avoid prescribing clarithromycin or ketoconazole. Dependent on the type of infection, it would be best to opt for a member of the penicillin family or clindamycin (Cleocin) or azithromycin (Zithromax), for a bacterial infection and one of the polyene antifungals, nystatin (Mycostatin) or amphotericin B (Fungizone), if an antifungal is needed.

If the patient is on tramadol (Ultram) for chronic pain, you will not prescribe clotrimazole (Mycelex) or fluconazole (Diflucan) as antifungals, as tramadol is metabolized by CYP3A4, and the azole antifungals are CYP3A4 inhibitors. It would be best to prescribe one of the polyene antifungals, nystatin (Mycostatin) or amphotericin B (Fungizone) instead.

CYP1A2

CYP1A2 substrates: amitriptyline (Elavil), caffeine, chlorpromazine (Thorazine), clomipramine (Anafranil), clozapine (Clozaril), cyclobenzaprine (Flexeril), duloxetine (Cymbalta), estradiol (Estrace), fluphenazine (Prolixin), fluvoxamine (Luvox), haloperidol (Haldol), imipramine (Tofranil), **lidocaine** (Xylocaine), mexiletine (Mexitil), mitrazepine (Remeron), nabumetone (Relafen), **naproxen** (Aleve), olanzapine (Zyprexa), ondansetron (Zofran), perphenazine (Trilafon), **phenacetin** (Saridon) to acetaminophen to NAPQI, propranolol (Inderal), riluzole (Rilutek), **ropivacaine** (Naropin), **(R) warfarin** (Coumadin), tacrine (Cognex), theophylline (Theo-Dur), tizanidine (Zanaflex), triamterene (Dyrenium), sulfamethoxazole (Gantanol), verapamil (Calan), zileuton (Zyflo), ziprasidone (Geodon), and zolmitriptan (Zomig).

1A2 inhibitors: acyclovir (Zovirax), allopurinol (Zyloprim), amiodarone (Cordarone), amitriptyline (Elavil), anastrozole (Arimidex), caffeine, cimetidine (Tagamet), **ciprofloxacin** (Cipro), **clarithromycin** (Biaxin), diltiazem (Cardizem), duloxetine (Cymbalta), **enoxacin** (Penetrex), **erythromycin** (E-myin), **flouroquinolones**, fluvoxamine (Luvox), furafylline, **grapefruit juice**, imipramine (Tofranil), interferon (Intron A), isoniazide (Niazid), **ketoconazole (Nizoral)**, **levofloxacin (Levaquin)**, lomefloxacin (Maxaquin), methoxsalen (Oxsoralen), mexiletine (Mexitil), mibefradil (Posicor), **norfloxacin** (Noroxin), **ofloxacin** (Floxin), oral contraceptives, paroxetine (Paxil), propranolol (Inderal), ritonavir (Norvir), SSRIs, tacrine (Cognex), thiabendazole (Mintezol), ticlopidine (Ticlid), verapamil (Calan), and zileuton (Zyflo).

1A2 inducers: barbiturates, beta-naphthoflavone, **broccoli**, **Brussels sprouts**, **charcoal-broiled foods**, insulin, methylcholanthrene, modafinal (Provigil), nafcillin (Novaplus or Nafcillin), nicotine, omeprazole (Prilosec), phenytoin (Dilantin), primidone (Mysoline), rifampin (Rifadin), and **tobacco smoking**.

CYP2B6

2B6 substrates: bupropion (Wellbutrin), cyclophosphamide (Cytoxan), efavirenz (Sustiva), ifosphamide (Ifex), **meperidine** (Demerol)—a major substrate, **methadone** (Dolophine)—secondary metabolism, and sorafenib (Nexavar).

2B6 inhibitors: clopidogrel (Plavix), orphenadrine (Norflex), prasugrel (Effient), thiotepa (Thioplex), and ticlopidine (Ticlid).

2B6 inducers: phenobarbital, phenytoin (Dilantin), and rifampin (Rifadin).

CYP2C8

2C8 substrates: amodiaquine (Camoquin), cerivastatin (Baycol), paclitaxel (Taxol), repaglinide (Prandin), sorafenib (Nexavar), and torsemide (Demadex).

2C8 inhibitors: anastrozole (Arimidex), fluvoxamine (Luvox), gemfibrozil (Lopid), glitazones (Thiazolidinedione), **ketoconazole** (Nizoral), montelukast (Singulair), omeprazole (Prilosec), quercetin, and trimethoprim (Proloprim).

2C8 inducers: rifampin (Rifadin).

CYP2C9

2C9 substrates: amitriptyline (Elavil), **celecoxib** (Celebrex), **diclofenac** (Voltaren), fluoxetine (Prozac), fluvastatin (Lescol), glibenclamide, glimepiride (Amaryl), glipizide (Glucotrol), glyburide (Diabeta), **ibuprofen** (Advil), irbesartan (Avapro), **lornoxicam** (Xefo), losartan (Cozaar), **meloxicam** (Mobic), **methadone** (Dolophine), nateglinide (Starlix), phenytoin (Dilantin), rosiglitazone (Avandia), tamoxifen (Nolvadex), torsemide (Demadex), **(S) warfarin** (Coumadin), **piroxicam** (Feldene), **(S) naproxen**, suprofen (Profenal), and tolbutamide (Orinase).

2C9 inhibitors: amiodarone (Cordarone), anastrozole (Arimidex), cimetidine (Tagamet), **diclofenac** (Voltaren), disulfiram (Antabuse), fenofibrate (Tricor), **fluconazole** (Diflucan), flurbiprofen (Ansaid), fluvastatin (Lescol), fluvoxamine (Luvox), isoniazide (Niazid), **itraconazole** (Sporanox), **ketoconazole (Nizoral)**, **ketoprofen** (Orudis), lovastatin (Mevacor), **metronidazole** (Flagyl), **miconazole (Micatin)**, oxandrolone (Oxandrin), paroxitine (Paxil), phenylbutazone (Zolandin), probenicid (Benemid), ritonavir

(Norvir), sertraline (Zoloft), **sulfamethoxazole-trimethoprim** (Bactrim), sulfinpyrazone (Anturane), **sulfonamides**, teniposide (Vumon), trogltazon (Rezulin), **voriconazole** (Vfend), and zafirlukast (Accolate).

2C9 inducers: **barbiturates**, carbamazepine (Tegretol), **phenobarbital** (Solfoton), rifampin (Rifadin), and **secobarbital** (Seconal).

CYP2C19

2C19 substrates: amitriptyline (Elavil), carisoprodol (Soma), **chloramphenicol (Chloromycetin)**, citalopram (Celexa), clomipramine (Anafranil), **clopidogrel** (Plavix) – primary metabolism, cyclophosphamide (Cytoxan), **diazepam** (Valium), escitalopram (Lexapro), fluoxetine (Prozac), hexobarbital, imipramine (Tofranil), **indomethacin** (Indocin), **itraconazol** (Sporanox), lansoprazole (Prevacid), **meperidine** (Demerol)— 2C19 is minor substrate, **methadone** (Dolophine), moclobemide (Aurorix), nelfinavir (Viracept), nilutamide (Nilandron), omeprazole (Prilosec), pantoprazole (Protonix), **phenobarbital** (Solfoton), phenytoin (Dilantin), primidone (Mysoline), progesterone (Prometrium), PPIs, proguanil (Chlorguanide), propranolol (Inderal), rabeprazole (Aciphex), R-mephobarbital (Mephytal), **(R) warfarin** (Coumadin), S-mephenytoin (Dilantin), sertraline (Zoloft), Teniposide (Vumon), and venlafaxine (Effexor).

2C19 inhibitors: allicin-garlic derivative, amitriptyline (Elavil), carbamazepine (Tegretol), chloramphenicol (Chloromycetin), cimetidine (Tagamet), felbamate (Felbatol), **fluconazole** (Diflucan), fluoxetine (Prozac), fluvoxamine (Luvox), esomerprazole (Nexium), imipramine (Tofranil), **indomethacin** (Indocin), **itraconazole** (Sporanox), **ketoconazole**, lansoprazole—most potent PPI inhibitor, meclobemide (Aurorix), modafinal (Provigil), omeprazole (Prilosec), oral contraceptives, oxcarbazepine (Trileptal), pantoprazole (Protonix), paroxetine (Paxil), PPIs, probenicid (Benemid), rabeprazole (Aciphex), ritonavir (Norvir), sertraline (Zoloft), ticlopidine (Ticlid), tolbutamide (Orinase), topiramate (Topamax), troglitazone (Rezulin), and **voriconazole (Vfend)**.

2C19 inducers: carbamazepine (Tegretol), norethindrone (Aygestin), **phenobarbital** (Solfoton), phenytoin (Dilantin), **prednisone (Deltasone)**, rifampin (Rifadn), and valproic acid (Depakote).

CYP2D6

Substrates for 2D6: alprenolol (Gubernal), amitriptyline (Elavil), amphetamine, aripiprazole (Abilify), atomoxetine (Strattera), beta-blockers, bufuralol, bupropion (Wellbutrin), carvedilol (Coreg), chlorpheniramine, chlorpromazine (Thorazine), citalopram (Celexa), clomipramine (Anafranil), clonidine (Catapres), clozapine (Clozaril), **codeine**—a prodrug, debrisoquine, desipramine (Norpramin), dexfenfluramine (Redux), dextromethorphan, donepezil (Aricept), doxepin (Sinequan), duloxetine (Cymbalta), encainide (Enkaid), escitalopram (Lexapro), flecainide (Tambocor), fluphenazine (Prolixin), fluoxetine (Prozac), fluvoxamine (Luvox), haloperidol (Haldol), **hydrocodone**—a prodrug, **hydrocodone + acetaminophen** (Vicodin), imipramine (Tofranil), moclobemide (Aurorix), **methadone** (Dolophine), methoxyamphetamine, metoclopramide (Reglan), metoprolol (Lopressor), mexiletine (Mexitil), minaprine (Cantor), mitrazapine (Remeron), nebivolol (Bystolic), nefazodone (Serzone), nortriptyline (Pamelor), olanzapine (Zyprexa), ondansetron (Zofran), **oxycodone** (OxyContin), oxycodone + acetaminophen (Percocet), paroxetine (Paxil), perhexiline (Pexsig), perphenazine (Trilafon), **phenacetin**, phenformin (Fenormin), promethazine (Phenergan), propafenone (Rythmol), propranolol (Inderal), quetiapine (Seroquel), ritonavir (Norvir), risperidone (Risperdol), sparteine, **tamoxifen (Nolvadex)**—a prodrug, thioridazine (Mellaril), timolol (Blocadren), **tramadol** (Ultram)—a prodrug, tranylcypromine (Parnate), trazadone (Desyrel), venlafaxine (Effexor), and zuclopenthixol (Clopixol).

2D6 inhibitors: amiodarone (Cordarone), aripiprazole (Abilify), buproprion (Wellbutrin), **celecoxib** (Celebrex), chlorpheniramine (Chlor-Trimeton), chlorpromazine (Thorazine), clozapine (Clozaril), cimetidine (Tagamet), cinacalset (Sensipar), citalopram (Celexa), clemastine (Tavist), clomipramine (Anafranil), **cocaine**, desipramine (Norpramin), diltiazem (Cardizem), **diphenhydramine (Benadryl),** doxepin (Sinequan), doxorubicin (Adriamycin), duloxetine (Cymbalta), echinacea, **escitalopram (Lexapro)**, fluoxetine (Prozac), fluphenazine (Prolixin), fluvoxamine (Luvox), halofantrine (Halfan), haloperidol (Haldol), hydroxyzine (Vistaril), levomepromazine (Nozinan), lomustine (CeeNU), **methadone** (Dolophine), metoclopramide (Reglan), mibefradil (Posicor), midodrine (Proamatine), moclobemide (Aurorix), nefazodone (Serzone), **norfloxacin** (Noroxin), oral contraceptives, paroxetine (Paxil), perphenazine (Trilafon), propafenone (Rythmol), quinidine, ranitidine (Zantac), risperidone (Risperdal), ritonavir (Norvir), sertindole (Serdolect), sertraline (Zoloft), terbinafine (Lamisil), thioridazine (Mellaril), tricyclic antidepressants (TCAs), valproic acid (Depakote), venlafaxine (Effexor), verapamil (Calan), vinblastine (Velban), vinorelbine (Navelbine), and vistaril (Hydroxyzine).

2D6 inducers: dexamethasone (Decadron) and rifampin (Rifampin).

CYP2E1

2E1 substrates: acetaminophen to NAPQI, aniline, benzene, chlorzoxazone (Parflex), **ethanol**, halothane (Fluothane), isoflurane (Forane), methoxyflurane (Penthrane), sevoflurane (Ulthane), and theophylline (Theo-Dur).

2E1 inhibitors: diethyl-dithiocarbamate and disulfiram (Antabuse).

2E1 inducers: ethanol and isonizide (Niazid).

CYP3A4

3A4 substrates: anti-arrhythmics, **macrolides (except Azythromycin)**, alfentanil (Alfenta), alprazolam (Xanax), amiodarone (Cordarone), amitriptyline (Elavil), amlodipine (Norvasc), aprepitant (Emend), aripiprazole (Abilify), astemizole (Hismanal), atorvastatin (Lipitor), **benzodiazepines**, beta-blockers, boceprevir (Victrelis), buprenorphine (Buprenex), buspirone (Buspar), cafergot, **caffeine**, calcium channel blockers (CCBs), cerivastatin (Baycol), clomipramine (Anafranil), clonazepam (Klonopin), chlorpheniramine (Aller-Chlor), chlorpromazine (Thorazine), clozapine (Clozaril), cilostazol (Pletal), cisapride (Propulsid), citalopram (Celexa), **clarithromycin** (Biaxin), **cocaine, codeine**-N-Demethylation, **cortisol**, cyclosporine (Sandimmune), dapsone (Aczone), **dexamethasone (Decadron)**, dextromethorphan, **diazepam** (Valium), diltiazem (Cardizem), docetaxel (Taxotere), domperidone (Motilium), doxepin (Sinequan), **doxycycline** (Vibramycin), eplerenone (Inspra), **erythromycin (E-Mycin)**, escitalopram (Lexapro), estradiol (Estrogen), ethinylestradiol (hormonal contraceptive), felodipine (Plendil), **fentanyl** (Sublimaze), finasteride (Proscar), flunitrazepam (Rohypnol), gleevec (Imatinib), haloperidol (Haldol), **hydrocortisone (cortisol)**, indinavir (Crixivan), irinotecan (Camptosar), lercanidipine (Zanidip), levacetylmethadole (LAAM), levonorgestrel (Plan B; female sex hormone, oral contraceptive), **lidocaine (Xylocaine)**, lovastatin (Mevacor), **methadone** (Dolophine)—primary metabolism, **meperidine** (Demerol)—major 3A4 substrate, **methylprednisolone** (Medrol), **midazolam** (Versad), mifepristone (Mifeprex)—antiprogesterone, anti-implantation agent, mirtazapine (Remeron), nateglinide (Starlix), nefazodone (Serzone), nelfinavir (Viracept), nifedipine (Procardia), nisoldipine (Sular), nitrendipine (Baypress), ondansetron (Zofran), **oxycodone** (OxyContin), **oxycodone + acetaminophen** (Percocet), paroxetin (Paxil), perphenazine (Trilafon), pimozide (Orap), progesterone, **propoxyphene** (Darvon)—discontinued, propranolol (Inderal), quetiapine (Seroquel), quinidine (Quinidine Gluconate), quinine, risperidone (Risperdol), ritonavir (Norvir), salmeterol (Serevent), saquinavir (Invirase), sertraline (Zoloft), sildenafil (Viagra), simvastatin (Zocor), sirolimus (Rapamune), sorafenib (Nexavar), statins—except pravastatin and rosuvastatin, sunitinib, tacrolimus (FK506/Prograf), tamoxifen (Nolvadex), taxol (paclitaxel), telaprevir (Incivek), telithromycin (Ketek), terfenadine (Seldane), testosterone, torisel (Temsirolimus), **tramadol** (Ultram), trazodone (Desyrel), **triazolam** (Halcion), venlafaxine (Effexor), verapamil (Calan), vincristine (Oncovin), zaleplon (Sonata), ziprasidone (Geodon), zolpidem (Ambien), and zopiclone.

3A4 inhibitors: alprazolam, amiodarone (Cordarone), amlodipine (Norvasc), amprenavir (Agenerase), anastrozole (Arimidex), aprepitant (Emend), atazanavir (Reyataz), atorvastatin (Lipitor), bicalutamide (Casodex), bocepravir (Victrelis), cannabinoids, **chloramphenicol (Chloromycetin)**, cimetidine (Tagamet), **ciprofloxacin** (Cipro), **clarithromycin** (Biaxin), clomipramine (Anafranil), **clotrimazole** (Mycelex), conivaptan (Vaprisol), cyclosporine (Sandimmune), danazol (Danocrine), darunavir (Prezista), delavirdine (Rescriptor), diethyl-dithiocarbamate, diltiazem (Cardizem), **erythromycin (E-mycin)**, **fluconazole** (Diflucan), fluoxetine (Prozac), fluvoxamine (Luvox), fosamprenavir (Lexiva), gestodene, **ginkgo**, **grapefruit juice**, haloperidol (Haldol), imatinib (Gleevec), indinavir (Crixivan), isoniazide (Niazid), **itraconazole** (Sporanox), lopinavir (Kaletra), **ketoconazole** (Nizoral), **metronidazole** (Flagyl), mibefradil (Posicor), **miconazole (Micatin)**, mifepristone (Mifeprex), nefazodone (Serzone), nelfinavir (Viracept), NNRTIs, **norfloxacin** (Noroxin), norfluoxetine (Seproxetine), omeprazole (Prilosec), oral contraceptives, paroxetine (Paxil), pimozide (Orap), **posaconazole (Noxafil)**, **propoxyphene (Darvon)**, protease inhibitors, qestodene, quinidine (Quinidine Gluconate), ranitidine (Zantac), reverse transcriptase inhibitors (RTIs), ritonavir (Norvir), saquinavir (Fortovase), sertindole (Serdolect), sertraline (Zoloft), SSRIs, **star fruit**, telapravir (Incivek), telithromycin (Ketek)—a cidal ketolide antibiotic, troleandomycin (Tao), venlafaxine (Effexor), verapamil (Calan), **voriconazole (Vfend)**, zafirlukast (Accolate), zileuton (Zyflo).

3A4 inducers: barbiturates, carbamazepine (Tegretol), **dexamethasone** (Butazolidine), efavirenz (Sustiva), ethosuximide (Zarontin), **glucocorticoids**, glutethimide (Doriden), griseofulvin (Griseovin), modafinil (Provigil), nevirapine (Viramune), oxcarbazepine (Trileptal), **phenobarbital** (Solfoton), phenytoin (Dilantin), pioglitazone (Actos), primidone (Mysoline), rifabutin (Mycobutin), rifampicin (Rifampin), ritonavir (Norvir), **secobarbital** (Seconal), St. John's wort, sulfinpyrazone (Anturane), topiramate (Topamax), troglitazone (Rezulin).

PRESCRIPTION WRITING

Overview

The goal of accurate prescription writing is to improve patient care and reduce errors. You need to have a good understanding about the specifics of prescription writing because this can help you, your patient, and the pharmacy expedite the dispensing and use of the appropriate medications. You can legally prescribe only those drugs that are appropriate to your practice, and you should prescribe only for patients you see in your practice. Never prescribe for friends or family, as a "favor." Prescribe only those drugs with which you are familiar, and do not allow the patient to dictate what to prescribe!

Do not abbreviate details of the prescription. Write clear and complete instructions in ink and do not use "as directed." Prescribe the correct quantity: for example, five days' supply for most full-course antibiotic therapies or two to three days' supply for analgesics and/or sedatives. Maintain complete records of what you prescribe. Store all controlled substances appropriately and keep necessary records. Communicate telephone orders directly and clearly to a pharmacist when telephoning prescriptions. Establish a rapport with a pharmacist and use him or her as an information source when in doubt.

Establish a good rapport with the patient and explain how to use the prescribed medication. Instruct the patient to: (1) read the label on the prescription container before taking the drug, (2) store the drugs appropriately, (3) use all the medication prescribed, and (4) discard any excess medications after one year. Before you prescribe, you should know the patient's current medical history, current list of medications, and the current status of underlying disease states. You need to check the DDIs among the medications already in use by the patient and what you plan to prescribe, **before** you prescribe. Always confirm and document any history of medication allergies and take that into consideration when writing a prescription. For example, severe allergy to penicillin prevents you from prescribing cephalexin (Keflex), a cephalosporin.

Prescribe doses that are both correct and measurable. Prescriptions should be written using the metric system (gram, g; milligram, mg) and not the apothecary system (grain; dram; ounce, oz). However, you need to be familiar with the metric-to-apothecary or metric-to-household system conversions because a patient may occasionally be on a medication using either the apothecary or household measurements.

Metric, Apothecary, Liquid Weight, and Household Measurement Systems

Metric-to-Apothecary Systems Dry-Weight Measurements

3.89g = 1dram
60mg = 1grain

Liquid Weight Measurements: Metric Versus Household Measurements

15mL = 1Tbsp
5mL = 1tsp
1mL = 15–16drops

Prescription Abbreviations

These are the commonly used abbreviations every provider should know:

qd or od: every day
bid: twice daily
tid: thrice daily
qid: four times daily
ac: before meals
pc: after meals
hs or qhs: at bedtime
disp: dispense
prn: as needed
po: by mouth (orally)
IV: intravenous
IM: intramuscular
stat: immediately
sq or sc: subcutaneous
sig or signa: directions for use
mcg or μg: micrograms

Prescription Writing Regulations

Each state's department of public health decides on the specifics of prescription writing and then publishes the regulations. It is important for you to be familiar with the prescription-writing requirements in your state. Some states require you to have a state prescribing number in addition to a DEA number. The state number does not get listed on the prescription form.

Drug Enforcement Agency Number

You are required by law to register with the Drug Enforcement Agency (DEA) in Washington, to store, dispense, or prescribe drugs, and your prescription forms must contain a space for your DEA number. The DEA license is renewed every three years.

DEA Drug Schedules

The controlled substance act ranks drugs according to their potential for abuse and dependency into categories, called **schedules**. All states in the United States except Massachusetts have five schedules (i.e., Schedules I–V). Massachusetts has six schedules (i.e., Schedules I–VI). The DEA number is required for all controlled substances. Many pharmacies additionally require the DEA number for any telephonically communicated prescription. Scheduled drugs are prescribed for the treatment of cough, diarrhea, mild anxiety, and pain, including postsurgical pain.

DEA Drug Schedule I

Drugs in this category have a significant abuse potential and there are no proven therapeutic indications to prescribe them. **Drugs included in this category**: heroin and marijuana.

DEA Drug Schedule II

Drugs in this category have a high abuse potential and they can be associated with severe psychic or physical dependency. Schedule II controlled substances require a written tamper-proof prescription that must be signed by the practitioner. There is **no federal time limit** within which a Schedule II prescription must be filled after being signed. While some states and many insurance carriers limit the quantity of controlled substance dispensed to a 30-day supply, **there are no specific federal limits** to quantities of drugs dispensed via prescription. Schedule II controlled substances oral order is **only** permitted in an **emergency** situation. The refilling of a prescription for a controlled substance listed in Schedule II is prohibited by law. Prescription records have to be maintained at the pharmacy and at the provider's office.

   Issuing of multiple prescriptions for Schedule II substances: The DEA has revised its regulations regarding the issuance of multiple prescriptions for schedule II controlled substances. Under the new DEA regulations, a provider may issue multiple prescriptions authorizing the patient to receive a total of up to 90-day's supply of a Schedule II controlled substance, provided each separate prescription is issued for a legitimate medical purpose by the appropriate provider; the practitioner provides written instructions on each prescription indicating when a pharmacy can fill each prescription; the practitioner documents that by giving the patient multiple prescriptions, it does not create an undue risk or abuse; that the issuance of multiple prescriptions is in accordance with applicable state laws; and that the individual practitioner follows all other applicable requirements under the Controlled Substances Act and Code of Federal Regulations, as well as any additional requirements under state law.

   It is important to remember that implementation of this change in the regulation when prescribing Schedule II controlled substances should **not** be construed as liberty to issue multiple prescriptions or to see the patient only once every 90 days.

   Faxing prescriptions for Schedule II controlled substances:

- In order to expedite the filling of a prescription, a provider can send a Schedule II prescription to the pharmacy by facsimile, but the Schedule II prescription must be presented to the pharmacist for review prior to the actual dispensing of the controlled substance.
- In an emergency, a practitioner may call-in a prescription for a Schedule II controlled substance by telephone to the pharmacy, and the pharmacist may dispense the prescription provided that the quantity prescribed and dispensed is limited to the amount adequate to treat the patient during the emergency period. Under such circumstances, the prescribing practitioner must send a written and signed prescription to the pharmacist within **seven** days. Also, the pharmacist must notify the DEA if the prescription is **not** received from the provider.

   The following are three exceptions per DEA, for Schedule II facsimile prescriptions:

- A Schedule II prescription fax can serve as the original prescription if a practitioner is prescribing a Schedule II narcotic controlled substance for parenteral, intravenous, intramuscular, subcutaneous, or intraspinal infusion and follows all normal requirements of a legal prescription.
- If a practitioner is prescribing Schedule II controlled substances for residents of long-term care facilities (LTCF).

- If a practitioner is prescribing a Schedule II narcotic controlled substance for a patient enrolled in a hospice care program certified and/or paid for by Medicare under Title XVIII. The prescription should state that it is for a hospice patient and the fax then serves as the original written prescription.

Schedule II drugs used in dentistry: amphetamines, cocaine, codeine in pure form, fentanyl, hydromorphone (Dilaudid), meperidine (Demerol), methadone (Dolophine), morphine, oxycontin, oxycodone, or oxycodone + acetaminophen (Percocet) are Schedule II drugs with medical use and high addiction potential.

DEA Drug Schedule III

Schedule III drugs have a lesser abuse potential than Schedule II drugs. This category includes compounds containing limited quantities of certain opioid and nonopioid drugs. Abuse of these drugs can lead to moderate or low physical dependence or high psychological dependence. A practitioner can call or fax in a Schedule III prescription to the pharmacy. Records need to be maintained, as in Schedule II protocol, but a maximum of **five** refills can be prescribed or dispensed in **six months**.

Schedule III drugs used in dentistry: Codeine compounds, codeine + acetaminophen (Tylenol #1–4), and hydrocodone + acetaminophen (Vicodin), or aspirin, have medical use, moderate addiction potential, and are Schedule III drugs.

DEA Drug Schedule IV

The abuse potential for Schedule IV drugs is less than that with the Schedule III drugs. Abuse is associated with limited physical or psychological dependency. Records need to be maintained, as in Schedule III protocol, and a maximum of **five** refills can be prescribed or dispensed in **six months**.

Schedule IV drugs used in dentistry: Benzodiazepines, diazepam (Valium), flurazepam (Dalmane), midazolam (Versed), pentobarbital (Nembutal), dextropropoxyphene (Darvon), propoxyphene with acetaminophen (Darvocet), and pentazocine (Talwin-NX) have medical use, low abuse potential, and are Schedule IV drugs. In 2010, the US Food and Drug Administration (FDA) withdrew propoxyphene-containing products from the market as new clinical data showed the drug to be associated with potentially serious or even fatal heart rhythm abnormalities.

DEA Drug Schedule V

The abuse potential for Schedule V drugs is less than that with the Schedule IV drugs. Schedule V drugs include preparations containing limited amounts of certain opioids and stimulant drugs, for antitussive (cough), antidiarrheal, and analgesic purposes. Laws and regulations vary by state for drugs in this category. Records need to be maintained, as in Schedule IV protocol, and a maximum of **five** refills can be dispensed in **six months**.

Schedule V drugs: Cough preparations with less than 200mg codeine/mL or per 100 g (Robitussin AC), and promethazine (phenergan) with codeine, have medical use, low abuse potential, and are Schedule V drugs.

DEA Drug Schedule VI

The state of Massachusetts designates an additional category of controlled substances and this sixth category includes all prescription medications that are not already covered in federal Schedules I–V. It is postulated that Schedule VI drugs **may have some addiction potential**, so it is important to consider the medication before prescribing the drug to a patient. Even though tramadol (Ultram) is stated to be a low addiction-potential analgesic, there is evidence that patients with a **history of substance dependence** can experience addictive symptoms with tramadol (ultram) or butalbital with acetaminophen (Fioricet), which in Massachusetts are listed as Schedule VI drugs.

All preparations known as "legend" drugs are included in this category. **Legend** refers to the FDA-required statement: "Caution—federal law prohibits dispensing without a prescription." Records need to be maintained, as in Schedule V protocol, and a maximum of **five** refills can be prescribed in **six months**.

Schedule VI drugs: Butalbital with acetaminophen (Fioricet), cimetidine (Tagamet), penicillin, tolbutamide (Orinase), ibuprofen (Motrin), and idomethacin (Indocin) are drugs included in this category.

Pregnancy Drug Categories A–X

The FDA groups drugs into five categories according to their level of safety for the fetus during pregnancy. Categories **A and B** are considered **safe** during pregnancy. Prior to writing a prescription for a pregnant patient, always know the FDA category for the drug.

Category A

Category A drugs have been used in pregnant women and are proven safe throughout the pregnancy.

Category B

A drug is classified as Category B if animal studies have shown no risk to the fetus but pregnant women have not been tested. Alternatively, animal studies may have shown risk but studies in pregnant women have shown no risk to the fetus in any trimester.

Category C

A drug is classified as a Category C drug if animal studies have shown an adverse effect and pregnant women have not been tested. Alternatively, no studies in pregnant women or animals have been conducted.

Category D

A drug is classified as Category D if studies in pregnant women have shown risk to the fetus. However, the drug may be used in a life-threatening situation if safer drugs are ineffective.

Category X

Drugs in this category have shown positive fetal risk. **Example:** isotretinoin (Accutane)

ELEMENTS OF PRESCRIPTION WRITING

The following sections describe elements of a prescription (Figure 3.1).

Patient Specificity

The prescription should be written for **only** the patient **you** are treating.

Date

The date on which you write the prescription is important because the pharmacy will not honor an undated prescription. The validity of Schedule II prescriptions has been

---

```
              Dental Clinic Prescription Form

Doctor's Name: John Brown, D.M.D

Doctor's Address: One Main Street

                  Boston, MA 02111

Doctor's Telephone #: 617-555-1212

Prescription Date: 01/14/13

Patient's Name: Ms. Jane Doe

Patient's Date of Birth (DOB): 5/5/88

Patient's Address: One Center Street

                  Apt #1

                  Boston, MA 02111

Rx: Amoxicillin (Amoxil), 500mg/capsule,

    for oral infection

Disp: 15 tablets

Sig: Take 1 capsule PO (oral) tid for 5 days

Refill: 0 (zero)

☐: "No substitution"

◉: Label

Practitioner's Signature: Jb

Practitioner's Name Printed: John Brown, D.M.D
```

Figure 3.1. Prescription form for amoxicillin (Amoxil).

discussed. All other scheduled drugs are invalid after six months. Therefore, the date is required for this guideline to be implemented.

Patient's Name, Date of Birth, and Address

Print the patient's name, date of birth, and address very clearly.

Drug Name

Through proper drug reference confirm that the **correct** drug is prescribed for the patient's problem and clearly print the name of the drug. **Example:** Amoxicillin (Amoxil)—generic name (trade name).

Write both the generic and the trade name of the drug, to avoid confusion at the pharmacy. Many drugs have similar-sounding names, such as Lanoxin (digoxin), a cardiac glycoside, versus Levoxyl (levothyroxine), a thyroid hormone! The common antibiotics used in dentistry are all available in generic form and the pharmacist is mandated by law to dispense this form, unless otherwise indicated by you, the provider, in the "no substitution" box.

No Substitution Box

If you do not want to dispense the generic form of the drug, write the trade name of the drug you want to prescribe and check off the **No Substitution** box. This confirms for the pharmacists that you want to prescribe only that particular brand of the drug. **Example:** Amoxil 500mg with the No Substitution box checked off indicates that the pharmacist cannot dispense the generic version of amoxicillin.

Drug Strength

You must clearly list the right drug strength per tablet/capsule/ml. **Example:** Amoxicillin, 500mg/tablet.

Drug Dose

You must clearly indicate the correct dosage schedule and number of times in the day you want the patient to take the drug. **Example:** Amoxicillin, 500mg tid (three times)/day. You avoid confusion by additionally spelling it out as "three times/day." This can be important, especially when prescribing for patients who get easily confused or who do not recall abbreviations well.

Route of Administration

Indicate the correct route of administration. **Example:** Amoxicillin 500mg PO (oral) tid.

Duration of the Prescription

Indicate on the prescription the correct duration for which the drug is prescribed. **Example:** Amoxicillin (Amoxil), 500mg tid × 5 days (for 5 days).

Total Amount of Drug Dispensed

Indicate the total number of tablets you plan to dispense. **Example: Dispense 15 Amoxicillin tablets.**

Total Number of Refills

Points to consider prior to writing refills are drug safety, drug regulations, managed care guidelines, and convenience.

Drug Safety

This should be considered for drugs with high abuse potential. **Example:** Oxycodone + Acetaminophen (Percocet). **No refills.**

Drug Regulations

Some states implement a maximum length of time that certain specific medications can be prescribed (30/60 days). A new prescription is needed in such cases if the drug is to be continued. You need to check with the local state board to know the specifics for your state.

Managed Care Guidelines

Insurance plans often dictate the maximum amount of a drug that can be dispensed at one given time, for the patient to obtain insurance drug coverage.

Convenience

If a patient is getting treated for a stable underlying disease state, a practitioner could write a prescription for 90 days. This option is more commonly used by a medical practitioner and is less commonly used by a dentist because medications for dentistry are usually dispensed short term. If you plan on giving refills, you must write that in the section specified for refills. In the dental setting, antibiotics for premedication prophylaxis often need refills, especially if the patient is to be seen for months at a stretch for several procedures. Determine how much the patient will need and indicate that on the refill line. Do not overprescribe. Write the numerical value and spell it out, to avoid confusion. If you plan on giving no refills, spell that out too. **Example: 0 (zero) refills; 2 (two) refills.**

The patient's name, date, drug, dose, units, quantity, route, frequency, refills, signature, and the "No Substitution" check-off are required by Massachusetts's prescription regulations.

Label Box Check Off and Drug Indication

By law, any specific information about the drug or drug indication that needs to be on the dispensing label is provided by the practitioner in the prescription. The practitioner needs to check off the Label box when this is desired. Drug indication helps the patient and the pharmacy know the reason for which the drug is dispensed. **Example:** Amoxicillin (Amoxil) 500mg/tablet **for oral infection.**

4

Local Anesthetics Commonly Used in Dentistry: Assessment, Analysis, and Associated Dental Management Guidelines

LOCAL ANESTHETIC CLASSIFICATION AND PHARMACOTHERAPEUTICS

There are two distinct types of local anesthetics: amides and esters. Amides are subdivided into amides with epinephrine and amides without epinephrine (Table 4.1).

Classification of Amides with Epinephrine

- 2% lidocaine with 1:100,000 epinephrine (Xylocaine)
- 4% prilocaine HCL with 1:200,000 epinephrine (Citanest Forte)
- 0.5% bupivacaine with 1:200,000 epinephrine (Marcaine)
- 4% septocaine with 1:100,000 and 1:200,000 epinephrine (Articaine)
- 0.5% Ropivacaine with 1:200,000 epinephrine (Naropin)

Amide with Levonordefrin (NeoCobefrin)

- 2% mepivacaine HCL (Carbocaine) with 1:20,000 levonordefrin (NeoCobefrin), a sympathomimetic amine

Classification of Amides Without Epinephrine

- 3% mepivacaine HCL (Carbocaine)
- 4% prilocaine HCL (Citanest Plain)

Classification of Ester Local Anesthetics

- Injectable propoxycaine and procaine (Ravocaine)
- Topical benzocaine

Dentist's Guide to Medical Conditions, Medications, and Complications, Second Edition. Kanchan M. Ganda.
© 2013 John Wiley & Sons, Inc. Published 2013 by John Wiley & Sons, Inc.

Table 4.1. Summary: Local Anesthetics (LAs)

LAs: Generic/Trade Name	LAs: Facts, Advice, or Alerts
AMIDE LA WITH EPINEPHRINE **Amide LA Alerts:**	Use **only 2 carpules** of any LA in compromised patients. **Avoid LAs with epinephrine and epinephrine cords with** Hyperthyroidism; severe coronary artery disease; MAO and Tricyclic antidepressants; Prophylthiouracil (PTU); Lanoxin (Digoxin); Theophylline; bisulfite allergy; G_6PD anemia and with serum creatinine >2mg/dL or CrCl <50/minute. Use 5–10% Aluminum chloride (Hemodent) cords when needed.
2% Lidocaine (Xylocaine) with 1:100,000 epinephrine: Pregnancy Category B	**Concentration/carpule:** 36mg **Lasts:** 60 minutes **Recommended Dose:** 3mg/lb **Healthy adult:** Max. 11.5 carpules
4% Prilocaine HCL (Citanest Forte) with 1:200,000 Epinephrine: Pregnancy Category B	**Concentration/carpule:** 72mg **Lasts:** 2 hours **Recommended Dose:** 2.7mg/lb **Healthy adult:** Max. 5 carpules **Avoid with:** Congenital methemoglobinemia; ASA III/IV status hypoxic states; moderate-to-severe anemia/kidney disease and multiple sclerosis
0.5% Bupivacaine (Marcaine) with 1:200,000 epinephrine: Pregnancy Category C	**Concentration/carpule:** 9mg **Lasts:** 90 minutes or longer **Recommended dose:** 0.6mg/lb. **Healthy adult:** Max. 9 carpules
4% Septocaine (Articaine) with 1:100,000/1:200,000 Epinephrine: Pregnancy Category C	**Concentration/carpule:** 68mg in 1.7mL single use carpule **Lasts:** 45–75 minutes **Recommended dose:** 3.2mg/lb **Healthy adult:** Max. 6 carpules Has 1.5 times Lidocaine potency. Action occurs within 1–3 minutes. **Avoid use in all conditions listed under Citanest Forte.**
NEWER AMIDE LA WITH EPINEPHRINE: **0.5% Ropivacaine (Naropin) with 1:200,000 epinephrine:** Pregnancy Category B	**Concentration:** Available in single dose carpules in 2 (0.2%), 5 (0.5%), 7.5 (0.75%) and 10mg/mL (1%) concentrations. **Lasts:** 120-360 minutes **Healthy Adult Dose:** Surgical anesthesia is 5mg; Minor nerve block dose not to exceed 200mg.
AMIDE WITH LEVONORDEFRIN: **2% Mepivacaine (Carbocaine) with 1:20,000 Levonordefrin (NeoCobefrin):** Pregnancy Category C	**Infiltration/block anesthesia** **Dose:** 36mg/carpule **Healthy adult:** Max. 5 carpules **Avoid with:** Hyperthyroidism, severe coronary disease, MAOIs, bisulfite allergy, G_6PD anemia

(continued)

Table 4.1.   Summary: Local Anesthetics (LAs) (*Continued*)

LAs: Generic/Trade Name	LAs: Facts, Advice, or Alerts
AMIDES WITHOUT EPINEPHRINE:	
3% Mepivacaine HCL (Carbocaine): Pregnancy Category C	**Concentration/carpule:** 54mg **Lasts:** 20 minutes **Recommended dose:** 3mg/lb **Healthy adult:** Max. 7.5 carpules Safe with G_6PD anemia
4% Prilocaine HCL (Citanest Plain): Pregnancy Category B Safe to use in the hypertensive pregnant patient	**Concentration/carpule:** 72mg **Lasts:** 30 minutes **Recommended dose:** 2.7mg/lb Healthy adult: Max. 5 cartridges **Avoid in all conditions listed under Citanest Forte.**
ESTER ANESTHETICS:	
Propoxycaine and Procaine (Ravocaine): Pregnancy Category C	**Concentration/carpule:** 43.2mg **Lasts:** 30-40 minutes **Healthy adult:** Max. 9 cartridges **Not available;** highly allergenic
Topical Benzocaine: Pregnancy Category C	**Avoid in all states listed under Citanest Forte.**

Metabolism of Local Anesthetics

Metabolism of all amide local anesthetics other than septocaine does not begin until those local anesthetics reach the liver where they are metabolized and then, for the most part, excreted through the renal system.

Septocaine (Articaine) is unique among amide-type local anesthetics in the way that it is metabolized. Septocaine is actually a hybrid of both an amide and an ester class anesthetic because of the presence of both an amide and an ester intermediate chain in its chemical composition. Biotransformation of 90–95% of septocaine begins immediately upon the drug entering the blood stream where the plasma carboxyesterase enzymes initiate the metabolic breakdown process via hydrolysis of the ester chain to its primary metabolite, articainic acid, which is inactive. The remainder of septocaine (5–10%) is metabolized in the liver by the hepatic microsomal enzymes. Amides have a high rate of first pass metabolism as the local anesthetic (LA) passes through the liver. Slow absorption from tissue is less likely to result in toxicity. If toxicity occurs, it often results from accidental parenteral injection or due to LA overdose.

Ester local anesthetics are metabolized in the plasma, by plasma cholinesterase, and plasma cholinesterase is **synthesized** in the liver. There is no real advantage to using ester local anesthetics over the amides in a cirrhotic patient. Benzocaine as a topical anesthetic is the only ester used today in dentistry and, as further discussed in this chapter, benzocaine products should not be used in children less than 2 years of age.

Age is one factor that alters the pharmacokinetics of local anesthetics (LAs). The half-life of LAs can be altered in the elderly because of **decreased hepatic blood flow** from disease processes such as liver disease or congestive heart failure (CHF). **These disease**

processes can also impair the ability of the liver to produce enzymes. All these factors contribute to elevated levels of amide local anesthetics in these patients compared to patients with normal liver function.

Hormonal changes during pregnancy are primarily responsible for the enhanced potency of local anesthetics. Thus, pregnancy can also alter the metabolism of LAs, and the dose of LAs should be reduced by 30%, regardless of the trimester of pregnancy.

Factors Affecting Onset and Duration of Local Anesthetics

The onset and duration of action depends on multiple factors:

1. **Tissue pH:** With infection, the pH of the tissue decreases, becoming more acidic. An acidic pH is responsible for the delayed effectiveness or ineffectiveness of the local anesthetic.
2. **Lipid solubility:** The intrinsic potency, onset of action, and duration for a local anesthetic are dependent on the lipophilic-hydrophobic balance and the hydrogen ion concentration. Lipophilic LA molecules have a tendency to bind to membrane lipids. The lipid membrane is a hydrophobic environment. LA duration of action is associated with lipid solubility. Highly lipid soluble LAs have a **longer duration of action** because of decreased clearance and increased protein binding.
3. **Local anesthetic concentration formulation:** The high-concentration local anesthetics prilocaine (Citanest) and septocaine (Articaine) require fewer injections compared to the low-concentration local anesthetics, such as lidocaine. Low-concentration preparations are preferred for use in the pediatric population and 0.5% bupivacaine (Marcaine) should be avoided in children.
4. **Presence of a vasoconstrictor:** By themselves, local anesthetics cause vasodilation, diffuse very rapidly, and last for a shorter duration of time. Presence of a vasoconstrictor improves the duration and depth of anesthesia, thus decreasing the need for more anesthetic use per visit. There are two types of vasoconstrictors used in dentistry: epinephrine and levonordefrin.
   a. **Epinephrine:** Epinephrine is the most common vasoconstrictor added in 1:50,000, 1:100,000, or 1:200,000 concentrations in various local anesthetics. Epinephrine causes vasoconstriction by stimulating the α_1 receptors in the mucus membranes. Epinephrine also affects the β_1 receptors in the heart and the β_2 receptors in the skeletal muscles. Stimulation of the β_1 receptors causes **tachycardia and an increased systolic blood pressure (SBP)**. Stimulation of the β_2 receptors causes vasodilation and a **decreased diastolic blood pressure (DBP)**. The reflex tachycardia triggered by epinephrine becomes an issue in patients with significant cardiovascular disease and should thus be avoided or significantly limited, in such cases.
   b. **Levonordefrin (NeoCobefrin):** Levonordefrin (NeoCobefrin) is a sympathomimetic amine that acts as a vasoconstrictor, producing less cardiac and CNS stimulation than epinephrine. It has a fast onset of action, providing effective anesthesia and has very few side effects. Levonordefrin increases the systolic and diastolic BP but it causes a reflex **bradycardia** (decreased heart rate). Reflex bradycardia is a beneficial side effect in patients with mild-to-moderate cardiovascular heart disease. The potency of 1:20,000 levonordefrin is equivalent to the potency of 1:100,000 epinephrine.

5. **Infiltration versus block anesthesia:** Infiltration anesthesia is more rapid in onset compared to block anesthesia, but it is shorter lasting than block anesthesia.

Local Anesthetics and Cross-Reactivity

True allergy to the amides is very rare. Allergy to one amide does not contraindicate the use of the other amides. A patient may occasionally be allergic to the antioxidant meta-sulfite or bisulfite preservative in the local anesthetic. The preservative maintains the potency of the epinephrine. Switching to an amide without epinephrine is an appropriate option in such situations. There is definite cross-reactivity among the ester local anesthetics. Each ester has a common breakdown allergenic compound, para-aminobenzoic acid, which causes a hypersensitivity reaction.

Local Anesthetic Adjuncts

Epinephrine-containing retraction cords have 8% racemic epinephrine, and they are used to provide adequate bloodless fields during dentistry. Retraction cords mechanically displace gingival tissue causing tissue contraction and hemostasis. The higher the concentration of epinephrine in the cords, the more likely it is that the epinephrine will be systemically absorbed. Epinephrine-containing cords should be **avoided** in the presence of hyperthyroidism, severe coronary artery disease, TCAs or MAOIs, bisulfite allergy, G6PD anemia, and kidney disease associated with serum creatinine >2mg/dL or CrCl <50/min. It is best to use aluminum chloride (a potent astringent) containing cords when epinephrine-containing cords are contraindicated. Five-to-ten percent aluminum chloride (Hemodent) gingival retraction cords are available for use and are considered very safe when used in the medically complex dental patient.

AMIDE AND ESTER LOCAL ANESTHETICS DETAILED DISCUSSION

Amide Local Anesthetics

2% Lidocaine (Xylocaine) with 1:100,000 Epinephrine

- Pregnancy **Category B**
- Concentration per carpule: 36mg lidocaine
- Duration of action: 60min
- Recommended dose for 2% lidocaine (Xylocaine): 3mg/lb
- Maximum number of carpules for a healthy 140lb adult: 11.5

4% Prilocaine HCL (Citanest Forte) with 1:200,000 Epinephrine

- Pregnancy **Category B**
- Concentration per carpule: 72mg prilocaine
- Duration of action: 2h
- Recommended dose for 4% prilocaine (Citanest Forte): 2.7mg/lb
- Maximum number of carpules for a healthy 140lb adult: 5

0.5% Bupivacaine (Marcaine) with 1:200,000 Epinephrine

- Pregnancy **Category C**
- Concentration per carpule: 9mg bupivacaine
- Duration of action: 90min or longer
- Recommended dose for 0.5% bupivacaine (Marcaine): 0.6mg/lb
- Maximum number of cartridges in a healthy 140lb adult: 9

4% Septocaine (Articaine) with 1:100,000/1:200,000 Epinephrine

- Pregnancy **Category C**
- Concentration per carpule: 68mg septocaine in 1.7mL single use carpule
- Duration of action: Depending on the epinephrine concentration, the effects last for 45–75min
- Recommended dose for septocaine (Articaine) 3.2mg/lb
- Maximum number of cartridges in a healthy 140lb adult: 6

Articaine, 4% septocaine, is an amide with a "sulphur-bearing" thiophene ring instead of a benzene ring. Like other amides, 4% septocaine is metabolized in the liver and because it also contains an additional **ester** group, it is metabolized by esterases in blood. It has a half-life of 20 minutes and is rapidly hydrolyzed in the blood, thus decreasing the risk of systemic toxicity when compared with other local anesthetics. Septocaine (Articaine) is 1.5-times **more potent** than lidocaine and has an onset of action within **one to three minutes** of injection. Adverse side effects associated with septocaine in order of frequency include, hypoesthesia, parasthesia, or anesthesia; pain; mandibular nerve injury; and tinnitus. Septocaine is not contraindicated in patients with sulfa allergies and there is no cross-allergenicity between septocaine's sulphur-bearing thiophene ring and sulfonamide antibiotics. Articaine **should not** be given to patients with disease states associated with moderate-to-severe hypoxia or to patients with a history of congenital or idiopathic methemoglobinemia because of the threat of methemoglobinemia. Septocaine contains sodium metabisulfite that may cause allergic-type reactions including anaphylactic symptoms and life-threatening or less severe asthmatic episodes in certain susceptible patients with a history of allergy to metasulfites or bisulfites.

0.5% Ropivacaine (Naropin) with 1:200,000 epinephrine

- Pregnancy **Category B**
- Ropivacaine Hcl (Naropin) injection is **preservative-free** and is available in single dose containers in 2 (0.2%), 5 (0.5%), 7.5 (0.75%), and 10mg/mL (1%) concentrations.
- Ropivacaine has a long duration of action, lasting 120–360 minutes. The maximum dosage of ropivacaine for surgical anesthesia is 5mg; and the dose for minor nerve block should not exceed 200mg.
- Ropivacaine is a long-acting amide local anesthetic that is structurally related to bupivacaine (Marcaine) and mepivacaine (carbocaine).
- Literature shows that ropivacaine has some inherent vasoconstrictive action.
- There is very little published data on the use of ropivacaine in dentistry, but it is suggested that this relatively new addition to the local anesthetic list offers a number of benefits.

- Ropivacaine (Naropin) and bupivacaine (marcaine) have similar clinical profiles, but ropivacaine has fewer cardiac and central nervous system side effects compared to bupivacaine (explained further in the following paragraphs). In efficacy, ropivacaine is between lidocaine (Xylocaine) and bupivacaine (Marcaine).

Toxicity explanation: Medications can contain enantiomers (enantiomers are molecules that contain the same atoms linked in the same way, but they differ in their three-dimensional arrangement (i.e., they are a mirror image of each other), designated with an R for rectus or S for sinister. If these two isomers are in equal concentrations, it is known as a racemic mixture. Epinephrine and bupivacaine (R-bupivacaine and S-bupivacaine) are examples of racemic preparations.

Therefore, racemic preparations result in the patient getting two different medications. It is important to remember that receptors will only allow or be selective to one of the medications, resulting in different pharmacodynamic and pharmacokinetic effects, which include absorption, metabolism, and excretion. One type may result in the desired therapeutic effect whereas the other one may result in undesired effects or be inactive. In general, one enantiomer will show greater potency, a better safety profile, and reduced side effects when compared to the other. S-bupivacaine is almost as potent as the racemic preparation but is less toxic. It takes larger doses of S-bupivacaine to cause cardiac arrest and seizure activity than racemic preparations. **Ropivacaine is a pure preparation containing S-ropivacaine, and ropivacaine has a larger margin of safety.**

- Lipid solubility of ropivacaine is also less than that of bupivacaine and it is cleared via the liver more rapidly than bupivacaine.
- A study conducted by Ernberg and Kopp concluded that ropivacaine **can be** useful for mandibular nerve block but **not** for maxillary infiltration. The study also found that the very long duration of both pulpal and soft tissue anesthesia might be favorable in **reducing** postoperative pain.
- A study by Kennedy et al. indicates that adding epinephrine to ropivacaine results in a 75% success rate of maxillary pulpal anesthesia.
- Ropivacaine at concentrations of 0.5% and 0.75% is an effective local anesthetic for inferior nerve block, providing a rapid onset and prolonged duration of action. It **may be** a suitable local anesthetic without vasoconstrictor for nerve block anesthesia in dental practice.
- The pharmacological action of 0.5% ropivacaine with 1:200,000 epinephrine is equivalent to 0.5% bupivacaine with 1:200,000 epinephrine for maxillary lateral incisor infiltrations.
- Ropivacaine is **not** as effective as lidocaine (Xylocaine) with epinephrine in obtaining pulpal anesthesia after intraligamentary injection, and adverse effects are minor and reversible.
- The motor block is slower in action, less intense, and of shorter duration than an equivalent dose of bupivacaine. This property, along with lower toxicity compared to bupivacaine, enables ropivacaine to be used for surgical anesthesia in 1% concentration strength, thus providing a distinctive advantage over bupivacaine.

2% Mepivacaine (Carbocaine) with 1:20,000 Levonordefrin (NeoCobefrin)

- Pregnancy **Category C**
- Concentration per carpule: 36mg mepivacaine HCL/carpule

- Duration of action: 60min
- Average amount per visit for a healthy adult: 5 carpules
- Average amount per visit for a medically compromised patient: 2

It is available in the United States for **infiltration and block** anesthesia. The anesthetic contains bisulfites to prevent the oxidation of levonordefrin. Avoid use in patients with demonstrated bisulfite allergy and patients with G6PD anemia. Also avoid in patients with a history of hyperthyroidism or severe coronary artery disease and in patients on MAO inhibitors, to prevent a rise in the blood pressure. Systemic injection of the anesthetic can cause bradycardia, decreased cardiac output, anxiety, restlessness, confusion, and seizures. Always aspirate prior to injecting the anesthetic.

3% Mepivacaine HCL (Carbocaine)

- Pregnancy **Category C**
- Concentration per carpule: 54mg mepivacaine
- Duration of action: 20min
- Recommended dose for 3% mepivacaine (Carbocaine): 3.0mg/lb
- Maximum number of cartridges in a healthy 140lb adult: 7.5

4% Prilocaine HCL (Citanest Plain)

- Pregnancy **Category B** local anesthetic
- Concentration per carpule: 72mg prilocaine
- Duration of action: 30min
- Recommended dose for 4% prilocaine (Citanest Plain): 2.7mg/lb
- Maximum number of cartridges in a healthy 140lb adult: 5

The local anesthetic of choice for a **hypertensive** pregnant patient **should be** 4% prilocaine HCL (Citanest Plain) when the dental treatment is cleared by the patient's obstetrician.

Ester Local Anesthetics

Propoxycaine and Procaine (Ravocaine)

These anesthetics are not currently available.

- Ravocaine Pregnancy **Category C**
- Concentration per carpule: 43.2 mg
- Duration of action: 30–40min
- Maximum number of cartridges in a healthy 140lb adult: 9

Topical Benzocaine

Benzocaine, a Pregnancy **Category C** drug, is available as a spray. It is used during medical procedures to numb the mucous membranes of the mouth and throat and in gel or liquid over-the-counter (OTC) products for the relief of teething, canker sores, and irritation of the mouth and gums. Benzocaine sprays in United States are marketed under different brand names such as Hurricaine, Cetacaine, Exactacain, and Topex. OTC Benzocaine gels and liquids are sold under brand names like Anbesol (Wyeth), Hurricaine, Orajel (Del), Baby Orajel (Del), Orabase, and store brands.

Topical Benzocaine Alert

Occurrences of methemoglobinemia were recently reported to the FDA with all strengths of benzocaine gels and liquids, and cases occurred mainly in children aged two years or younger who were treated with benzocaine gel for teething. The signs and symptoms of methemoglobinemia usually appeared within minutes to one or two hours of applying benzocaine. Methemoglobinemia occurred in some cases after the first application of benzocaine, and in other cases it occurred after additional use. The development of methemoglobinemia after treatment with benzocaine sprays was not related to the amount applied. In many cases, methemoglobinemia was reported following the administration of a single benzocaine spray.

Benzocaine products should not be used on children less than years of age. Infants less than 4 months of age, pregnant patients, elderly patients, patients allergic to esters, and patients with glucose-6-phosphodiesterase deficiency, hemoglobin-M disease, NADH-methemoglobin reductase (diaphorase 1) deficiency, and pyruvate-kinase deficiency are at greater risk of developing methemoglobinemia. Adults who use benzocaine gels or liquids to relieve pain in the mouth should be extremely careful and follow package insert instructions closely.

Methemoglobinemia

Methemoglobin is a naturally occurring oxidized metabolite of hemoglobin and physiologic levels (<1%) are normal. Methemoglobinemia occurs when red blood cells (RBCs) contain greater than 1% methemoglobin. Methemoglobinemia is a rare, but serious condition in which the amount of oxygen carried through the blood stream is greatly reduced because methemoglobin does not bind oxygen, and this leads to functional anemia. As levels of methemoglobin rise above 15%, neurologic and cardiac symptoms arise due to hypoxia. Levels above 70% are usually fatal. Therefore, patients who develop methemoglobinemia can appear pale, gray, or with blue-colored skin, lips, and nail beds. They may also experience a headache, lightheadedness, shortness of breath, fatigue, and rapid heart rate.

Most cases of methemoglobinemia occur following exposure to oxidant drugs, chemicals, or toxins. Such drugs fall into two general categories: nitrites or aromatic amines. Benzocaines, lidocaine, prilocaine, and phenazopyridine (Pyridium) are the local anesthetics that can cause methemoglobinemia. Acetaminophen, acetanilid, celecoxib, phenacetin, dapsone, nitrofurans, P-amino-salicylic acid, and sulfonamides are the analgesics and antibiotics that can precipitate methemoglobinemia. Dapsone and benzocaine are drugs that more commonly cause methemoglobinemia. During patient assessment, always check for any known family history of methemoglobinemia, or G6PD deficiency.

Avoid local anesthetics 4% prilocaine or 4% septocaine that promote methemoglobinemia in the presence of any condition causing moderate to severe hypoxia, such as patients with moderate-to-severe anemia, COPD, chronic kidney disease (CKD), or cyanotic congenital cardiac defects.

Methemoglobinemia Treatment

- Supplemental oxygen.
- Methylene blue is the first-line antidote drug.
- Hyperbaric oxygen therapy or packed RBC exchange transfusions are alternative therapies for patients who cannot be treated with methylene blue.
- Additionally, the patient should get dermal decontamination with water rinse, soap scrub, and water rinse again, in addition to gastrointestinal (GI) decontamination with gastric lavage and activated charcoal administration.

LOCAL ANESTHETIC DENTAL ALERTS AND SUGGESTED DENTAL GUIDELINES

The following are dental alerts and guidelines for local anesthetics:

1. Use no more than 2 carpules of local anesthetic per visit in any medically complex patient to avoid excessive use of local anesthetics, epinephrine, and emergencies associated with overuse. Be aware of the lipid solubility of the local anesthetics in use in the medically complex patient. The maximum recommended dose of epinephrine in patients with compromised cardiac status is 40 micrograms (0.04mg) and hyperkalemia exacerbates the cardiotoxicity of local anesthetics. Highly lipid-soluble LAs demonstrate greater cardiac toxicity. Following is the ranking order of LA cardiotoxicity **from lowest to highest:** prilocaine, lidocaine, mepivacaine, ropivacaine, and bupivacaine. Bupivacaine is highly lipophilic and ropivacaine is two to three times less lipid soluble than bupivacaine.

2. Avoid amides with epinephrine in patients presenting with a history of sulfite or bisulfite allergy. Both early and late IgE-mediated reactions can occur with the sulfites. The patient can experience bronchospasm, rhinitis, conjunctivitis, urticaria, or anaphylactic shock.

3. There is no cross-reactivity between the sulpha antimicrobials, sulphur, and the metasulfites or bisulfites. Patients presenting with allergy to the sulpha antimicrobials or sulphur **can be given** epinephrine-containing local anesthetics. It is important to note that patients demonstrating allergies toward the bisulfite preservatives in the local anesthetics **will** give you a history of avoiding consumption of dried fruits, cured meat, and red wine that **also** contain sulfites, so be observant and attentive.

4. A true IgE-mediated reaction to local anesthetics is **rare**. Often, the reaction is due to hyperventilation, vasovagal reaction, numbness of the pharynx from extravasated local anesthetic, or an inadvertent intravascular injection of epinephrine. It is suggested you inject a 0.2mL subcutaneous (SC) local anesthetic challenge and look for a reaction in someone who has never had a local anesthetic or thinks there could be an allergy associated with the local anesthetic. It is safe to proceed with the local anesthetic if there is no reaction within five minutes of the infiltration.

   Treatment of allergic reactions to LAs: As previously stated, allergic reactions to local anesthetics are extremely rare but when they occur, they are treated according to severity of manifestations. Mild cutaneous reactions in adults are treated with diphenhydramine (Benadryl), 25–50mg IV/PO. The pediatric dose for mild reactions is 1mg/kg. The more serious reactions are treated with 0.3 (mL) of 1:1,000 epinephrine, subcutaneous (SC). The patient is closely monitored for any further decompensation. Corticosteroids: 125mg methylprednisolone IV, or 60mg prednisone PO (oral) is given to the patient presenting with a severe allergic reaction associated with respiratory distress and hypotension.

5. Toxicity of the amide local anesthetics can occur with significant liver disease, because of decreased liver enzymes and decreased hepatic blood flow. These factors alter the pharmacokinetics of LAs. So it is not just liver disease that increases the duration of action of the amides, it is also the decreased blood flow that alters the pharmacokinetics of the amides. Dental treatment in a cirrhotic patient must therefore be **simplified** and completed over **multiple** appointments. Treat one area or sextant of the oral cavity at a time, rather than working on different areas of the mouth per appointment. This way, you minimize the total amount of anesthetic used during each visit.

6. **Category B** drugs that are **safe for use** during pregnancy include 2% lidocaine (Xylocaine), 4% prilocaine HCL with 1:200,000 epinephrine (Citanest Forte), or 4% prilocaine HCL (Citanest Plain). Avoid the use of Category B local anesthetic ropivacaine HCL (Naropin) during pregnancy, as there are no adequate or well-controlled studies in pregnant women demonstrating the effects of the drug on the developing fetus.

7. **Category C** drugs that **should not be used** during pregnancy include 0.5% bupivacaine (Marcaine), 4% septocaine with 1:100,000 and 1:200,000 epinephrine (Articaine), 3% mepivacaine HCL (Carbocaine), and 2% mepivacaine (Carbocaine) with 1:20,000 levonordefrin (NeoCobefrin).

8. Old age does not contraindicate the use of local anesthetics. Age is one factor that alters the pharmacokinetics of LAs. The half-life of LAs can be altered in the elderly because of decreased hepatic blood flow from disease processes, such as liver disease or congestive heart failure (CHF). These disease processes can also impair the ability of the liver to produce enzymes. All these factors contribute to elevated levels of amide local anesthetics in these patients, compared to patients with normal liver function. Therefore, use caution with the total number of carpules and the amount of epinephrine or levonordefrin used in elderly patients with compromised liver function or coronary artery disease.

9. Excessive accumulation of prilocaine, septocaine, and benzocaine-associated metabolites can cause methemoglobinemia. These should be avoided in patients presenting with congenital methemoglobinemia. Methemoglobinemia causes cyanosis, which **does not** respond to 100% oxygen.

10. Prilocaine and septocaine have been implicated in causing lingual-nerve associated parasthesias and prolonged anesthesia after dental use, and it can last for eight weeks or longer.

11. Local anesthetics are **not** associated with malignant hyperthermia and are **safe** to use. Inhaled general anesthetics and succinylcholine should be avoided in patients who are genetically predisposed to the condition.

12. Avoid local anesthetics containing epinephrine in patients with a history of hyperthyroidism, patients with severe cardiac and pulmonary disease, and patients on MAOIs (monoamineoxidase inhibitors), tricyclic antidepressants (TCAs), propylthiouracil (PTU), digoxin (Lanoxin), or theophylline.

13. When used in excess, all local anesthetics will cause restlessness, anxiety, confusion, tremors, dizziness, and seizures.

LOCAL ANESTHETIC COMPLICATIONS

Local anesthetics can cause two types of complications: **localized** and **generalized** (local anesthetic and/or epinephrine overdose).

Localized Complications

Localized complications at the site of the injection are:

1. **Pain on injection:** Pain is caused by a dull needle or by rapid injection of the local anesthetic. Use sharp needles, topical anesthesia, and inject slowly to avoid pain on injection. Needle-stick pain can be minimized by pinching the lip or cheek area with your fingers while injecting the local anesthetic, or by stretching the tissue prior to injection.
2. **Burning on injection:** Rapid injections, pH of the local anesthetic, and "warmed" local anesthetic are the main causes. Burning rapidly disappears as the local anesthetic takes effect if the pH is the cause. Rapid injection or an overly "warmed" local anesthetic may cause trismus, edema, or paresthesia. Always store local anesthetics at room temperature in a clean container without alcohol or other sterilizing agents.
3. **Persistent anesthesia or paresthesia:** Anesthesia can persist for days, weeks, or months. Trauma to any nerve or bleeding around a nerve can cause paresthesia. The patient experiences an electric shock sensation throughout the distribution of the nerve. When compared with other local anesthetics, 4% prilocaine (Citanest) and 4% septocaine (Articaine) are often associated with paresthesia, and they should be avoided in patients with multiple sclerosis (MS) and all other disease states associated with neuromuscular dysfunction. Most paresthesias resolve within eight weeks without treatment, though severe damage can be permanent. Reassure the patient and provide frequent follow-up visits to reassess the condition. A highly symptomatic or anxious patient can be given 2mg/5mg/10mg diazepam (Valium) at bedtime.
4. **Trismus:** Prolonged spasm of the jaw muscles is associated with a locked jaw and trismus can become chronic and a problem to manage. The most common etiology is trauma to the muscles or blood vessels in the infratemporal fossa. Low-grade infection following local anesthesia injection can also cause trismus. Symptoms usually develop 1–6 days post treatment. To prevent the occurrence of trismus, decrease multiple needle penetrations in an area and do not inject excessive volumes of the anesthetic solution into a restricted area. The patient can be treated with heat therapy, warm saline rinse, analgesics, and, if necessary, diazepam (Valium). Give 10mg diazepam, bid until the patient is able to tolerate the trismus or has recovered.
5. **Hematoma:** Nicking of an artery or a vein during injection can release blood into the extravascular spaces causing a painful bruise or swelling that persists for 7–14 days. Treatment consists of applying direct pressure at the site of bleeding for about two minutes followed by **icing** the area on the **first** day. Prescribe analgesics and advise the patient to use heat application when needed **after** the first day, to avoid vasodilation and worsening of symptoms.
6. **Infection:** Injecting local anesthetic into an area of infection does not produce optimal anesthetic effect. However, if the local anesthetic is injected under pressure,

bacteria from the local site may be forced into the adjacent tissue. The patient is best treated with antibiotics, heat, analgesics, and benzodiazepines.

7. **Facial nerve paralysis:** Facial palsy can occur when the local anesthetic is introduced into the deep lobe of the parotid gland. Within seconds, the patient will sense a weakening of muscles on the affected side. Treatment: Reassure the patient. The situation will last for a few hours without residual effects. Apply an eye patch to the affected eye after removing the contact lens, when present. Reschedule and follow up.

Generalized Complications

Generalized reactions to local anesthetics can manifest as a local anesthetic overdose or epinephrine overdose reaction. Please refer to Chapter 9 for a detailed discussion of this topic.

Pain Physiology, Analgesics, Opioid Dependency Maintenance Therapies, Multimodal Analgesia, and Pain Management Algorithms

ANATOMY AND PHYSIOLOGY OF PAIN

Introduction

This discussion of the anatomy and physiology of pain will briefly describe the processes that are involved in the generation of acute, chronic, or neuropathic pain sensations. The idea is to provide the practitioner with the basis for the assessment of the type of pain and then to appropriately select interventions for managing the pain effectively.

Nociceptive Pain

Nociception is the normal processing of pain by nociceptors in response to tissue damage and inflammation (noxious stimuli), associated with trauma, surgery, inflammation, infection, and ischemia that could be damaging or potentially damaging to normal tissue. Transduction of pain begins when the free nerve endings (nociceptors) of A-delta and C-fibers of the primary afferent neurons respond to noxious stimuli. The nociceptors are distributed in the somatic structures (skin, superficial tissue, muscles, connective tissue, bones, joints, and blood vessels) and visceral structures (visceral organs such as the liver and the gastrointestinal tract).

A-delta and C Afferent Pain Fibers

The A-delta and C-fibers are associated with different qualities of pain. The myelinated A-delta pain afferent axons are the smallest and slowest of the myelinated axons. A-delta fibers respond to either mechanical or temperature stimuli and produce the acute sensation of sharp, bright pain. The unmyelinated C afferent pain fibers respond to a broad range of painful stimuli, including mechanical, thermal, or metabolic factors. The pain produced is slow, burning, and long lasting.

Dentist's Guide to Medical Conditions, Medications, and Complications, Second Edition. Kanchan M. Ganda.
© 2013 John Wiley & Sons, Inc. Published 2013 by John Wiley & Sons, Inc.

Generation of Pain Impulse to Noxious Stimuli

There are three categories of noxious stimuli: mechanical (pressure, swelling, abscess, incision, tumor growth), thermal (burn, scald), and chemical (excitatory neurotransmitter, toxic substance, ischaemia, infection).

The cause of stimulation may be internal, such as pressure exerted by a tumor, or external, such as a burn. This noxious stimulation causes a release of chemical mediators from the damaged cells including: bradykinin, histamine, potassium, prostaglandin, serotonin, and substance P. These chemical mediators activate and/or sensitize the nociceptors to the noxious stimuli. In order for a pain impulse to be generated, an exchange of sodium and potassium ions (de-polarization and re-polarization) occurs at the cell membranes. This results in an action potential and generation of a pain impulse.

Acute Pain Transmission

Pain transmission process occurs in the following three stages that occur in sequential order:

- **First stage:** The pain impulse is transmitted from the site of transduction along the nociceptor fibers to the dorsal horn in the spinal cord.
- **Second stage:** From the spinal cord, the impulse is transmitted to the brain stem.
- **Third stage:** From the brain stem, the impulse goes through connections between the thalamus, cortex, and higher levels of the brain.

The A-delta fibers and the C-fibers terminate in the dorsal horn of the spinal cord. There is a synaptic cleft between the terminal ends of the A-delta fibers and the C-fibers and the nociceptive dorsal horn neurons (NDHN).

Excitatory neurotransmitters are then released for the pain impulses to be transmitted across the synaptic cleft to the NDHN and these neurotransmitters then bind to specific receptors in the NDHN. The neurotransmitters released are adenosine triphosphate, glutamate, calcitonin gene-related peptide, bradykinin, nitrous oxide, and substance P.

The pain impulse is then transmitted from the spinal cord to the brain stem and thalamus via two main nociceptive ascending pathways. These are the spinothalamic pathway and the spinoparabrachial pathway. When these impulses arrive in the thalamus they are directed to multiple areas in the brain where they are processed.

Acute Pain Perception

Pain perception is the end result of the neuronal activity of pain transmission, and this is where pain becomes a conscious experience. The multidimensional experience of pain has affective-motivational, sensory-discriminative, emotional, and behavioral components. When the painful stimuli are transmitted to the brain stem and thalamus, multiple cortical areas are activated and the following responses are elicited.

The reticular system: This system is responsible for the autonomic and motor response to pain and for warning the person, for example, to automatically remove a hand from a hot surface when it touches the surface. It also has a role in the affective-motivational response to pain such as looking at and assessing the injury to the hand once it has been removed form the hot surface.

Somatosensory cortex: This area of the brain is involved with the perception and interpretation of sensations. It identifies the intensity, type, and location of the pain sensation and relates the sensation to past experiences, memory, and cognitive activities. It identifies the nature of the stimulus before it triggers responses such as: Where is the pain? How strong is the pain? What does the pain feel like?

Limbic system: This system is responsible for the emotional and behavioral responses to pain including attention, mood, and motivation and also with the processing of pain and past experiences with pain.

Acute Pain Modulation

The modulation of pain involves changing or inhibiting transmission of pain impulses in the spinal cord. The multiple, complex pathways involved in the modulation of pain are referred to as the descending modulatory pain pathways (DMPP), and these can lead to either an increase in the transmission of pain impulses (excitatory) or a decrease in transmission (inhibition). Descending inhibition involves the release of inhibitory neurotransmitters that block or partially block the transmission of pain impulses, thereby producing analgesia. Inhibitory neurotransmitters involved with the modulation of pain include: acetylcholine, endogenous opioids (enkephalins and endorphins), gamma-aminobutyric acid (GABA), neurotensin, norepinephirine (noradrenalin), oxytocin, and serotonin (5-HT).

Endogenous pain modulation helps to explain the wide variations in the perception of pain in different people as individuals produce different amounts of inhibitory neurotransmitters. Endogenous opioids are found throughout the central nervous system (CNS) and prevent the release of some excitatory neurotransmitters, such as substance P, thus inhibiting the transmission of pain impulses.

Chronic Pain

Chronic pain can affect the patient's quality of life. It can be caused by alterations in nociception, injury, or disease and may result from current or past damage to the peripheral nervous system (PNS), central nervous system (CNS), or it may have no organic cause.

The exact mechanisms involved in the pathophysiology of chronic pain are complex and unclear. It is postulated that following injury, rapid and long-term changes occur in parts of the CNS that are involved in the transmission and modulation of pain. A central mechanism in the spinal cord, referred to as hypersensitivity or hyperexcitability, may occur. This occurs when repeated and prolonged noxious stimulation causes the dorsal horn neurons to transmit progressively increasing numbers of pain impulses.

The patient can feel intense pain in response to a stimulus that is not usually associated with pain, such as touch. This abnormal processing of pain within the PNS and CNS may become independent of the original painful event. In some cases, as with amputation, the original injury may have occurred in the peripheral nerves, but the mechanisms associated with the phantom pain are generated in both the PNS and the CNS.

Neuropathic Pain

Neuropathic pain can be defined as pain triggered or caused by a primary lesion or dysfunction in the nervous system resulting from trauma, such as complex regional pain syndrome or chronic postsurgical pain; infection, such as postherpetic neuralgia; ischemia, such as diabetic neuropathy; cancer; or chemical influence, following chemotherapy. This type of pain is usually less responsive to standard pain medications.

Some types of neuropathic pain may develop when the PNS has become damaged, causing the pain fibers to transmit pain impulses repeatedly and become increasingly sensitive to stimuli. Neuropathic pain is distinctly different from nociceptive pain and is described as burning, dull, aching, tingling, electric shock-like, or shooting.

Physical and Psychological Assessment of Pain

Anxiety and fear are known to activate the pituitary-adrenal axis, resulting in increased pain perception. Patients experiencing chronic nonfacial pain may also have increased pain perception as the brain neurophysiology may be altered in such patients. A fearful and anxious patient experiences increased pain, which can best be alleviated by appropriate stress management during patient care. As previously discussed, pain can exist even in the absence of a physical cause; consequently, pain assessment should address both the physical and the psychological aspects of pain.

The best treatment course for pain management begins with a good understanding of:

- Characteristic features of the pain, along with the duration, frequency, location, symptoms at onset, pain pattern, and severity/quality of the pain, so that you can better help the patient.
- Past and current pain medication history: all long-acting analgesics or other interventional modalities need to be factored in the decision-making process if the patient is currently on chronic pain therapy.
- The patient's current medical status.
- The patient's vital organs status, which includes the status of the liver and the kidneys.
- Assessment of daily medications for underlying disease states and associated DDIs.
- The biochemical pathways of pain management.
- Assessment of the appropriate analgesic dose and type(s) of analgesic(s) that should be dispensed.

Analgesics are a very important adjunct in dentistry to assure quick recovery from pain. It is best to prescribe analgesics for no more than two to three days, and patients experiencing pain beyond three days should be reassessed before any additional analgesics are prescribed. Having a tight hold on the amount of analgesics you dispense keeps drug addicts away from your practice!

BIOCHEMICAL OPTIONS FOR PAIN MANAGEMENT

Pain control can be achieved using one or more of the following:

- **Nonopioid drugs:** acetaminophen, NSAIDS, aspirin, or celecoxib.
- **Opioids:** morphine, codeine, oxycodone, hydrocodone, oxymorphone, hydromorphone, methadone, fentanyl, meperidine, pentazocine, buprenorphine, and propoxyphene (now withdrawn from the US market).

- **Nonnarcotic opiate agonist:** tramadol (Ultram).
- **Adjuncts:** corticosteroids, benzodiazepines, antihistamine H_1 blockers, muscle relaxants, tricyclic antidepressants (TCAs), and bisphosphonates.

NONOPIOID ANALGESICS

Introduction

Nonopioids were formerly known as "nonnarcotic" analgesics and the opioids were formerly known as "narcotics." Both classes of drugs have varying degrees of central and peripheral action. Nonopioids include acetaminophen and nonsteroidal anti-inflammatory drugs (NSAIDS). Both interfere with prostaglandin synthesis and both have a maximum, or **ceiling**, dose for their **analgesic effect**. NSAIDS do not cause respiratory depression or impair gastrointestinal motility, so NSAIDS are considered an important component with acetaminophen in multimodal pain management, which is discussed further in this chapter.

Acetaminophen (Tylenol)

Acetaminophen Pharmacology

Acetaminophen or paracetamol, a Pregnancy Category B drug, is also known by its chemical name *N*-acetyl-*p*-aminophenol (APAP).

Acetaminophen mechanism of action (MOA): Acetaminophen has both analgesic and antipyretic properties, and although the exact MOA is unclear, it is thought to exert its analgesic activity **centrally** by inhibiting the synthesis of prostaglandins in the CNS and **peripherally** by blocking pain impulse generation. It should be noted that the drug has barely any influence on peripheral prostaglandin synthesis, especially within inflamed tissues. Thus, acetaminophen is devoid of peripheral anti-inflammatory effects that NSAIDS have. Acetaminophen also has a serotonergic (5-HT) mechanism and a cannabinoid agonism mechanism, which may contribute to its analgesic effect. The half-life of Tylenol is two to four hours and the therapeutic dose in a patient who is not medically complex is 3 g/day.

Acetaminophen metabolism: Acetaminophen undergoes metabolism in the liver through three pathways: conjugation with glucuronide; conjugation with sulfate; and oxidation via the CYP450 enzyme pathway, primarily involving CYP2E1. More than 90% of an acetaminophen dose is metabolized by the liver to sulfate and glucuronide conjugates, which are water soluble and eliminated in the urine. Conversion to sulfate is the primary pathway until the age of 10–12years. Glucuronidation is the primary pathway in adolescents and adults. Approximately only 2–4% of an acetaminophen dose is inactivated by glutathione and then excreted by the kidneys.

Tylenol Toxicity

Tylenol is the most commonly overdosed medication. Hepatotoxicity with acetaminophen is most pronounced when dosages exceed the recommended 24-hour dosing and the toxic metabolite NAPQI cannot be adequately conjugated.

Currently, the main cause of acute liver failure in the United States is acetaminophen overdose, which results in thousands of hospitalizations every year, and the only cure in most cases that are detected early is immediate liver transplant. CYP3A4-induced Tylenol hepatotoxicity occurs from the formation of the reactive and toxic metabolite N-acetyl-benzoquinoneimine (NAPQI). Typically, glutathione binds to NAPQI and excretes NAPQI as nontoxic mercapturate conjugates. When glutathione stores are diminished, NAPQI binds to the liver cells causing hepatic necrosis. The conjugate for NAPQI comes from glycogen, and acetaminophen may be toxic for patients with depleted glycogen stores, due to dieting, anorexia, primary liver disease, or medications toxic to the liver. Alcohol, liver disease, starvation, and protein malnutrition **decrease** glutathione levels and **increase** the chances of Tylenol toxicity. Hepatotoxicity due to Tylenol is most pronounced in the **fasting** patient and patients taking drugs primarily metabolized by the liver. Also, alcohol consumption with Tylenol **increases** NAPQI production, so alcoholics **can overdose** even with a therapeutic dose. Acetaminophen use is absolutely contraindicated **with alcohol and** in the presence of **alcohol-associated liver disease.**

Patients consuming three or more servings of alcohol per day should take even less than the FDA's proposed recommended dosage: More than two servings of alcohol per day can increase the risk of liver failure from acetaminophen. Patients who take acetaminophen (Tylenol) in high doses, or simply use it regularly, are also at risk. Therefore, patients suspected of chronic alcoholism should limit their daily acetaminophen intake to **below** 2g in divided doses, rather than the normal daily maximum of 3g. Also, patients with decreased liver function, kidney disease, hepatitis, malnutrition, AIDS, chronic alcohol abuse, or anorexia nervosa may also be at increased risk for liver failure and death when using Tylenol. Acetaminophen may affect the results of blood glucose tests in diabetics as well.

According to an American Pharmacists Association recent news release, the maximum daily dose for single-ingredient Extra Strength Tylenol (acetaminophen) products sold in the United States has been **lowered** from **8** tablets, caplets, gelcaps, or tablespoons per day (4,000mg) to **6** per day (3,000mg), and the dosing interval has **changed from 2 pills every 4–6hours to 2 pills every 6hours.** The FDA has announced that it is taking steps to cut the risk of acetaminophen-associated liver damage and other effects of acetaminophen toxicity. Specifically, the FDA is requesting all makers **of prescription products that contain acetaminophen** to limit the amount of acetaminophen to **325mg** per capsule or tablet. Drug companies have until January 14, 2014, to reduce the amount of acetaminophen in their products to 325mg per capsule or tablet. Tylenol and other acetaminophen-based medications will include warnings that taking more than recommended amounts can cause liver damage, that the products should not be combined with other medications that include acetaminophen, and that acetaminophen is the active ingredient.

Induced acute liver failure resulting from Tylenol toxicity can cause impaired hepatic synthetic function, the extent of which can be judged by monitoring the PT/INR (Table 5.1). The PT/INR is **increased** when the acutely injured liver is unable to produce clotting factors. The Tylenol toxicity prognosis is good when the PT/INR is **normal** in the presence of increased ALT and AST. Renal failure, encephalopathy, and cerebral edema can additionally occur with acute liver failure associated with Tylenol toxicity. An immediate liver transplant is the only treatment in such cases.

Table 5.1. Summary: Acute Acetaminophen (Tylenol) Toxicity-Associated Liver Function Test (LFT) Changes

LFT Marker	Marker Status
Total Protein	Normal
Albumin (A)	Normal
Globulin (G)	Normal
A:G ratio	Normal
ALT/SGPT	>10,000 IU/L; rapidly normal on recovery
AST/SGOT	Increased, but less than ALT
ALT:AST ratio	ALT>AST
GGT	Normal
Alkaline Phosphatase (AP)	Increased
PT/INR	Acutely prolonged with liver failure
Total Bilirubin	Normal
Direct-B	Normal
Indirect-B	Normal

Tylenol Toxicity Symptoms and Signs

Tylenol toxicity can present with an irregular pulse, nausea, vomiting, diarrhea, sweating, abdominal pain, seizures, and coma.

Tylenol Toxicity Laboratory Test Assessment

Tylenol toxicity causes an acute rise in the ALT and AST to >10,000 U/L within 24hours after ingestion or within 8–16hours in very severe cases, and peak levels occur at 48–72 hours. As discussed previously, the PT/INR, serum creatinine, and blood urea nitrogen (BUN) levels must also be assessed.

Tylenol Toxicity Treatment

The first step in management of Tylenol toxicity is gastrointestinal decontamination with activated charcoal. N-acetylcysteine (NAC) given PO (oral) or IV (intravenous) is the antidote, and most patients recover if NAC is given within eight hours of ingestion of the toxic dose. Glutathione levels are replaced by the sulfhydryl compounds from NAC causing reversal of the toxicity.

N-acetylcysteine (NAC) dose: Initial dose: 140mg/kg followed by 70mg/kg every 4h × 17 doses, after the initial dose.

Acetaminophen (Tylenol) Dosing: Avoid Alcohol When Using Acetaminophen

1. **Normal acetaminophen (Tylenol) dose:**
   a. **Regular strength acetaminophen (Tylenol):** 325mg/tablet. Adults and children 12years and older can take 2 tablets every 6hours while symptoms last and the patient should not take more than 8–10 tablets in 24hours.
   b. **Extra-strength acetaminophen (Tylenol):** 500mg/tablet. Adults and children 12years and older can take 2 caplets or gelcaps every 6–8hours while symptoms last and the patient should **not** take **more than 6** caplets or gelcaps **in 24hours.**

2. **Tylenol dose with kidney disease:** Tylenol dose must be adjusted in renal failure because metabolites can otherwise accumulate. The maximum daily dose of acetaminophen should be no more than **2 g/day** in patients with significantly decreased renal function. Use the following guidelines for dosing with kidney disease:

   a. **CrCl >50mL/min or serum creatinine <2.0mg/dL: Dose normally as discussed previously.**

   b. **CrCl 10–50mL/min or serum creatinine >2.0mg/dL to predialysis:** Prescribe 325–650mg **q6–8hours** only; dose interval decided according to the severity of underlying kidney disease.

   c. **CrCl <10mL/min or the renal failure/dialysis patient:** Prescribe 325–650mg **q8hours** only.

3. **Tylenol dose with liver disease:** Use Tylenol with caution in the presence of hepatic impairment. Cases of hepatotoxicity at daily acetaminophen dosages <3g/day have been reported. Limited, low-dose therapy is usually well tolerated with hepatic disease or cirrhosis. Avoid **chronic** use in hepatic impairment. The maximum daily dose of acetaminophen should be no more than **2 g/day** in patients with cirrhosis or chronic active hepatitis. Use the following guideline for dosing with liver disease:

   a. **Chronic inactive hepatitis:** Give Tylenol 325–650mg **q6–8hours**; dose interval decided according to the extent of inactivity of underlying liver disease.

   b. **Chronic active hepatitis or cirrhosis:** Give Tylenol 325–650mg **q8hours**.

IV Acetaminophen

IV Acetaminophen was approved by the FDA in 2010 for postoperative pain management of varying intensities for adults and children, to be used either alone or in combination with opioids either prior to surgery or during the intraoperative period.

IV Acetaminophen Advantages

- IV acetaminophen does **not** have a black box warning and it can be used in the pediatric population.
- It does not cause nausea, vomiting, or respiratory depression, which are typically associated with opioids.
- It does not affect platelets, nor does it cause gastritis and nephropathy that is occasionally seen with NSAIDS
- It has few DDIs and is very rapid in onset **avoiding first-pass in the liver**, thus reducing the potential for hepatotoxicity, and proving to be safe in some patients with underlying liver disease. However, it is **contraindicated** in patients with **severe** liver disease.
- IV acetaminophen can easily be switched to oral acetaminophen once the patient tides over the acute phase.

IV Acetaminophen Vial and Dosing Facts

- No dose adjustment is needed when converting between oral and IV acetaminophen dosing in adults and adolescents.

- IV acetaminophen is dispensed as a 100mL single-use vial containing 1,000mg acetaminophen. The contents do not need to be reconstituted. It is given over 15 minutes and is not combined with any other drug, especially drugs like chlorpromazine and diazepam. Once punctured, the dose of IV acetaminophen must be administered within six hours or otherwise discarded.

IV Acetaminophen Adult and Children Dosing

1. **Adults and children age ≥13years, weighing ≥50kg:** 650mg **q6h** or 1,000mg **q8h**, with 1,000mg being the maximum single dose injected.
2. **Adults and children age ≥13years, weighing <50kg:** 12.5mg/kg **q4–6h** or 15mg/kg **q6h**, with 15mg/kg being the maximum single dose injected.

Nonsteroidal Anti-Inflammatory Drugs (NSAIDS)

NSAIDS Overview and Classification

Commonly discussed members in this category are aspirin, Pregnancy Category C; ibuprofen, Pregnancy Category B; naproxen, Pregnancy Category B; and celecoxib, Pregnancy Category C.

NSAIDS Mechanism of Action

Cyclooxygenase (COX) enzyme is responsible for the formation of prostaglandins, prostacyclins, and thromboxane A_2, with each being involved in the inflammatory response. Thromboxane A_2 is additionally responsible for platelet aggregation. There are two different COX enzymes, COX-1 and COX-2. Both COX-1 and COX-2 convert arachidonic acid to prostaglandin, resulting in pain, fever, and inflammation.

Cyclooxygenase-1 (COX-1) is present in most tissues. COX-1 maintains the normal lining of the stomach and the intestines; it maintains renal perfusion and promotes clotting by maintaining platelet function/cohesiveness. Inhibition of COX-1 is therefore undesirable. Cyclooxygenase-2 (COX-2) is primarily present at sites of inflammation, therefore inhibition of COX-2 is considered desirable.

Nonsteroidal anti-inflammatory drugs (NSAIDS) work by inhibiting prostaglandins. Traditional or "nonselective" NSAIDS, such as ibuprofen and naproxen, inhibit both COX-1 and COX-2. The inhibition of COX-2 accounts for the anti-inflammatory effect of the drugs, whereas the inhibition of COX-1 can lead to NSAIDS-associated toxicity and side effects including ulcers, prolonged bleeding times, and kidney problems.

Aspirin and the traditional NSAIDS very particularly inhibit the vasodilator prostaglandins in the kidneys.

NSAIDS and Vital Organs

NSAIDS are metabolized by the liver via conjugative and oxidation pathways, and patients with liver disease should specifically **avoid** aspirin and ibuprofen. Some NSAIDS are more hepatotoxic than others. Patients with liver cirrhosis are at **increased risk of kidney damage** due to NSAIDS. Therefore, NSAIDS should be avoided in patients with cirrhosis.

NSAIDS and Pregnancy

NSAIDS should generally be avoided during pregnancy, especially during the first and third trimesters. There is risk of miscarriage in the first trimester and a risk of premature ductus arteriosus closure in the third trimester. Prostaglandins keep the ductus arteriosus patent in the fetus, and therefore prostaglandins should **not** be inhibited, especially during the third trimester. If benefits far outweigh the risk and if cleared for use by the obstetrician, ibuprofen or naproxen should **not** be dispensed for more than **48–72hours**. Pregnancy Category B acetaminophen is the safest nonopioid analgesic to rely on as an alternate. Additionally, avoid celecoxib (Celebrex) and Pregnancy Category C/D drugs during pregnancy, and diclofenac potassium (Cataflam) and ketorolac in late pregnancy. Also, NSAIDS can alter the renal cortical function in the mother and decrease the fetal renal output.

NSAIDS Adverse Side Effects

NSAIDS can cause gastric irritability, platelet dysfunction, renal insufficiency, and hepatotoxicity.

   Gastric toxicity: The most common adverse effect of NSAIDS is gastric toxicity, and older adults and patients with a history of peptic ulcer disease are at highest risk for this adverse side effect. Prostaglandins also produce compounds that protect the gastric lining. Once absorbed, NSAIDS inhibit prostaglandin synthesis in the gastric mucosa and subsequent distribution to the gastrointestinal wall. Avoid NSAIDS in patients with bleeding disorders.

   NSAIDS also excessively increase the risk of gastrointestinal bleeding, when combined with warfarin (Coumadin) or clopidogrel (Plavix). This is an important issue, particularly in the elderly and patients on anticoagulant therapy, including patients on low-dose/81mg aspirin. If a patient is at risk for thrombosis, aspirin should not be withdrawn for dentistry.

   Acute renal failure: NSAIDS-associated renal damage is due to selective inhibition of the vasodilator prostaglandins, resulting in unopposed action of vasoconstrictor prostaglandins and consequent reduction in renal blood flow. **Short-term (2–3 days), low-dose NSAIDS use does not cause this side effect.** The risk of renal toxicity with NSAIDS increases with old age and when used in the presence of renal disease, diuretics, cirrhosis, and other nephrotoxic drugs. Prostaglandins are largely responsible for optimal renal perfusion and function; consequently, chronic NSAIDS use can be associated with nephrotoxicity, particularly in patients with compromised renal function. Acute renal failure has been known to occur within 24hours in patients with renal dysfunction and is known to be even more severe in the presence of acute or chronic volume depletion, cardiac failure, liver cirrhosis, ascites, diabetes, or preexisting hypertension. In the presence of renal disease, if the patient's physician approves and when absolutely needed, short-acting low-dose NSAIDS can be prescribed for a maximum of two to three days.

   Platelet dysfunction: NSAIDS **temporarily** affect platelet cohesiveness and the platelets regain their cohesiveness once the NSAIDS have cleared the system. NSAIDS can usually be stopped 24hours prior to major surgery, once cleared by the patient's medical doctor.

Leukotrine overproduction: Aspirin and NSAIDS can cause rhinosinusitis, polyps, and asthma in patients allergic to these medications, by blocking the cyclo-oxygenase-1 enzyme, which triggers an overproduction of leukotrienes. Leukotrienes, in turn, cause bronchoconstriction.

Aspirin

Aspirin is a Pregnancy Category C drug that becomes a Category D drug in the third trimester of pregnancy. Aspirin has an analgesic efficacy equivalent to 5–10mg, IM morphine. When needed, the lowest effective aspirin dose should be used. Aspirin has to be used for several days to maximize effect and achieve optimal plasma levels. Aspirin has analgesic, anti-inflammatory and antipyretic activity. The antipyretic activity is central in action.

Metabolization

Aspirin is mainly metabolized in the liver and excreted through the kidneys. Patients with a creatinine clearance <50mL/min or with serum creatinine >2mg/dL should be given aspirin every six hours (**q6h**) only. **Avoid** aspirin use in patients with **severe liver disease** and in patients on dialysis, with a CrCl <10mL/min.

Alerts

Aspirin and primary hemostasis: When taken daily, aspirin permanently affects platelet cohesiveness for the entire life span of the platelets, which is 10–14 days. Aspirin-associated platelet effect impacts **primary homeostasis,** causing a prolonged Bleeding Time (BT). Aspirin does not affect the platelet count, PT/INR, or the APTT.

The patient's physician must always be contacted prior to any major dental procedure to determine **if and when** the aspirin can be stopped. Consultation with the MD is absolutely necessary as it is the MD who clearly knows the patient's risk for thrombosis. In most cases in the past, adult or baby aspirin was usually stopped seven days prior to the major surgical procedure when the risk for thrombosis was minimal. Most physicians now prefer the continuation of low-dose aspirin, as bleeding can very easily be controlled with pressure, local hemostats, and sutures, plus the majority of patients encountered these days are high risk for thrombosis to begin with. In the presence of high daily doses of aspirin for arthritis care aspirin may have to be stopped for ten days, but with MD approval. When stopped, aspirin should be restarted **1–2 days** after the procedure, so good primary hemostasis is ensured. Tylenol may be substituted in the interim period for pain control.

Aspirin and ibuprofen combination therapy: When given in combination, some studies have shown ibuprofen to competitively inhibit the anti-platelet action of aspirin, whereas other studies have found thromboxane inhibition by aspirin to be reduced by only 1% after ten days of concurrent ibuprofen use.

Routine low-dose aspirin intake is important for patients at increased risk for thrombosis and this effect of ibuprofen on aspirin is important, no matter how small the risk. It is important to note that the anti-platelet action of aspirin occurs **within the hepatic portal system** after absorption. So in situations when you have to prescribe ibuprofen, it is best for the patient to **take daily aspirin on waking up** and **delay** the intake of **ibuprofen by 1–2hours**, so optimal aspirin effect occurs. As per FDA documents, if used occasionally, there is only minimal risk that ibuprofen will interfere with the effect of low-dose aspirin. If you need only a single dose of ibuprofen, the FDA recommends the patient take ibuprofen **8hours before or 30 minutes after** taking a regular (not enteric-coated) low-dose aspirin. **FDA recommendations are only for regular, immediate-release low-dose aspirin (81mg).** The ability of ibuprofen to interfere with the anti-clotting effects of enteric-coated aspirin or larger doses of aspirin, such as an adult aspirin (325mg), is **not** known.

Diclofenac and celecoxib (Celebrex) do **not** have the ibuprofen-associated interaction with aspirin, so when NSAIDS are absolutely needed in the presence of low dose aspirin, diclofenac and celecoxib are more appropriate to dispense.

Aspirin and pregnancy or lactation: Aspirin is a potent prostaglandin inhibitor and theoretical concern for organogenesis in the first trimester, and premature closure of the ductus arteriosus in the third trimester does exist, just as with other NSAIDS. However, no such cases have been found when aspirin has been used for the prevention of preeclampsia. Aspirin should **not** be used during the breast-feeding period.

Dose

Aspirin is available as an 81mg tablet (baby aspirin) and a 325mg tablet (adult aspirin). **Dose:** 325–650mg q4–6h PRN, maximum dose: 4 g/day. Reduce the dose in the elderly and avoid in patients with **hypoalbuminemia and a CrCl <10mL/min** (this is the patient on dialysis).

Ibuprofen and Naproxen

NSAIDS have an analgesic efficacy equivalent to 5–10mg, IM morphine and the lowest effective NSAIDS dose should be used. NSAIDS have to be used for several days to maximize effect and achieve optimal plasma levels. Ibuprofen and naproxen are Pregnancy Category B drugs.

Actions

They have analgesic, anti-inflammatory, and antipyretic activity. The antipyretic activity is central in action.

Metabolism

They are mainly metabolized in the liver and excreted through the kidneys. NSAIDS use must be avoided in patients with any form of kidney or liver disease. The clearance of naproxen is decreased in the presence of chronic hepatitis.

Analgesia Dose

1. **Ibuprofen (Motrin) dose:** 200–400mg PO q4–6h PRN; maximum dose: 1,200 mg/day.
2. **Naproxen (Naprosyn) dose:** 250–500mg PO q8–12h PRN; maximum dose: 1,500 mg/day.

COX-2 Inhibitors

Facts

COX-2 production is induced by inflammation and is associated with pain. COX-2 inhibition has analgesic, anti-inflammatory, and antipyretic activity. The analgesic activity of COX-2 is similar to that of the COX-1 inhibitors. Like the COX-1 inhibitors or traditional NSAIDS, the COX-2 inhibitors also are equally effective in treating inflammation, pain, and fever associated with acute or chronic pain from rheumatoid arthritis and osteoarthritis. Unlike the COX-1 inhibitors, they do not affect the gastric mucosa, but recent studies have shown COX-2 inhibitors **promoting** platelet aggregation. COX-2 inhibitors are Pregnancy Category C drugs that become Category D drugs with prolonged use or with high dosage. Celecoxib has a **sulfa** tail that can cause a reaction and it should be avoided in patients with **sulfonamide** antimicrobial allergy.

Celecoxib (Celebrex) is the only selective COX-2 inhibitor currently available in the United States. Unlike aspirin, which is also an NSAID, COX-2 inhibitors are **not** effective in preventing strokes and heart attacks in patients with high risk for cardiac disease. All other previously available COX-2 inhibitors have now been withdrawn from the US market because of the increased risk for heart attack and stroke. This warning has now also been added to the prescribing label for celecoxib (Celebrex), so patients are aware.

Metabolism

COX-2 drugs are metabolized in the liver and excreted through the kidneys. They have renal effects similar to the COX-1 inhibitors. COX-2 inhibitors should be avoided in the elderly and in patients with renal, hepatic, or cardiac impairment.

Dose

Celecoxib, 100–200mg q12h PRN.

Nonopioid Associated Dental Alerts

- **Postoperative pain management:** NSAIDS can significantly reduce postoperative pain and swelling when used **preoperatively**, prior to prostaglandin synthesis. Prostaglandins already formed are **not** affected, so it is best to provide NSAIDS either **preoperatively** or **before the local anesthesia** numbing effect **dissipates**. A recent clinical trial showed significant pain reduction in patients with irreversible pulpitis when lornoxicam (but not diclofenac potassium) was given prior to an inferior alveolar block anesthesia injection.
- NSAIDS and acetaminophen have a **ceiling effect** as far as **analgesia** is concerned, and any further increase in dose provides **no** additional benefit. Generally, the pain-relieving effect does not increase with higher doses; thus, 400mg of Motrin/ibuprofen has just as much pain relief as 800mg of Motrin/ibuprofen. A person is more likely to suffer a significant stomach problem with the higher dose.
- **Higher dosing** with **any** NSAID is needed to achieve **anti-inflammatory** effect, compared with the dose needed to control pain and fever. Thus 200–400mg ibuprofen every six hours reduces pain and fever, but the patient will need 400–800mg ibuprofen every six to eight hours, if inflammation is to be suppressed. All efforts should

be made not to exceed the maximum antipyretic total daily total dose of 1,200mg and the maximum anti-inflamatory daily total dose of 2,400–3,200mg. My suggestion would be to try to stay at 2,400mg/day in divided doses for management of inflammation as much as possible instead of 3,200mg/day, **for as short a time as possible (maximum two to three days and consume large amounts of water). This way you will avoid any NSAID-related untoward side effects.**

- Postoperative pain can significantly be reduced using ibuprofen 400mg, diclofenac 50mg, codeine 30–60mg with acetaminophen, oxycodone 10mg with acetaminophen, naproxen 500/550mg, or celecoxib (Celebrex) 400mg. It has been found that **NSAIDS are generally better than opioids at routine doses.**
- Patients with poor oral hygiene and cigarette smoking habits experience more pain following dental procedures than those with good oral hygiene or non-smokers.
- **NSAIDS and SSRIs:** Short-term or long-term dispensing of NSAIDS in combination with SSRIs should always be avoided. Chronic NSAIDS use in the presence of SSRIs can lead to GI bleeds, especially in patients with preexisting bleeding conditions. The potential interaction between the SSRIs and NSAIDS should also be appreciated, even for short-term postprocedural use.
- **NSAIDS and tricyclic antidepressants:** NSAIDS combined with tricyclic antidepressants or anxiolytics, along with psychological support, can be useful in treating persistent facial pain of unknown etiology (PFPUE).
- **CYP2D6 inhibitors and inducers:** SSRI antidepressants are potent CYP2D6 inhibitors, thus making codeine less effective when given in combination with SSRIs. Dexamethasone is a CYP2D6 inducer that enhances the conversion of codeine to morphine. So as an alternative, morphine or hydromorphone can be prescribed for pain management to patients on SSRIs or dexamethasone.
- **Xerostomia:** Ibuprofen occasionally causes xerostomia that may increase oral plaque and the incidence of dental caries.
- **DDIs with other drugs:** NSAIDS should also not be combined with methotrexate or lithium, as NSAIDS are known to increase the serum levels of these drugs.
- **NSAIDS and pregnancy or lactation:** There is fair evidence of safety with short-term ibuprofen or naproxen use during the second trimester of pregnancy, but NSAIDS must be avoided in the first trimester to avoid any negative impact on organogenesis and in the third trimester to avoid premature closure of the ductus arteriosus. NSAIDS should not be consumed in large quantities over long periods of time.
- **COX-2 inhibitors associated side effects:** In the presence of risk factors for NSAID use, such as gasterointestinal or cardiovascular disease, use the lowest COX-2 dose possible and for the shortest duration possible. Selective COX-2 inhibitors have been found to **increase** platelet aggregation, so it is best **not** to prescribe to patients with **significant** history of **atherosclerosis.**

OPIOID ANALGESICS

Opioids Pathophysiology

Four classes of opioid receptors have been identified: μ-mu, δ-delta, κ-kappa, and the nociceptin/orphanin FQ (N/OFQ) peptide receptor. Opioids act by binding to opioid receptors on neurons distributed throughout the nervous and immune systems. Most opioids have their primary activity at the morphine, or mu, receptors and are thus designated "mu agonists." Codeine is a prodrug that has very little affinity for the mu receptor.

Opioid receptors are located within the CNS and throughout the peripheral tissues. Opioids have no dose limit or **dose ceiling** for analgesia, so essentially you can keep increasing the dose until relief is obtained, or side effects occur. Most opioids are metabolized in the liver by glucuronidation or by the CYP450 system, and then they are excreted through the kidneys.

Opioids Classification

Opioids can be classified according to their "occurrence" or according to their "action on specific receptors and their dose-ceiling effect. The latter classification is the one that is most commonly used.

Classification by occurrence is as follows:

- **Naturally occurring opioids:** Opium and morphine are the two naturally occurring opioids, with morphine being the primary active component of opium.
- **Semi-synthetic opioids:** Heroin, oxycodone, oxymorphone, hydromorphone (Dilaudid), and hydrocodone are the five semi-synthetic opioids.
- **Synthetic opioids:** Buprenorphine, methadone, fentanyl, meperidine, codeine, pentazocine, and propoxyphene (withdrawn from US market) are the seven synthetic opioids.

Classification according to action on specific receptors and dose-ceiling effect is as follows:

- **Full morphine-like opioid agonists:** Codeine, fentanyl, hydrocodone, hydromorphone, methadone, morphine, oxycodone, oxymorphone, and propoxyphene are members of this group.
- These full agonist members do **not** have a dose-ceiling effect and they do **not** reverse or antagonize the effects of other full agonists when used simultaneously.
- **Partial opioid agonists:** Buprenorphine, a member of this group, **has a ceiling effect** and therefore is less effective as an analgesic at opioid receptors than full agonists.
- **Mixed opioid agonist-antagonists:** Pentazocine (Talwin) is a mixed agonist-antagonist drug. Pentazocine also **has a dose-ceiling** effect and it cannot be combined with opioid agonists, because pentazocine will be antagonistic in action, thus causing the pain intensity to increase.
- **Nonnarcotic opiate agonist:** Tramadol (Ultram). It is important to note that tramadol (Ultram) is **not** classified as a controlled substance.

Opioid Metabolism and the Liver

Adequate liver function, optimal albumin levels, and good blood flow to the liver are essentials for the proper processing of drugs metabolized by the liver. Metabolism is also dependent on whether the drug is a high- or low-extraction drug. High-extraction drugs are efficiently removed from the bloodstream by the liver. Liver disease is thus associated with a decrease in clearance and an increase in plasma concentration and elimination half-life of drugs metabolized by the liver.

The liver is the major site for biotransformation of the opioids, and most of them are metabolized by oxidation. Hepatic metabolism converts drugs into products that are less potent than the original drug, and these products are eventually more easily excreted. However, some products may be more potent than the original drug. The metabolism of opioids is impaired in liver and kidney disease. Liver failure is associated with **decreased oxidation** of opioids and **decreased clearance**, particularly affecting meperidine, propoxyphene, pentazocine, and tramadol. **Lower the dose and prolong the interval** if an opioid has to be used in a patient with liver disease. Use caution with codeine, morphine, and oxycodone because their active metabolites are cleared through the kidneys. Avoid meperidine, propoxyphene, pentazocine, and tramadol with liver or kidney disease. Hydromorphone and fentanyl are recommended for use in liver or kidney failure.

Opioid-Associated Effects and Side Effects

The mu receptor agonists are associated with the following effects and side-effects: pain relief, euphoria and decreased anxiety, respiratory depression, constipation, cough suppression, suppression of corticotropin-releasing factor and adrenocorticotropin hormone, pinpoint pupils, nausea, vomiting, pruritus, lightheadedness, dizziness, dry mouth, mental sluggishness, difficulty urinating, and constipation.

Opioid-associated allergic reaction: It is not uncommon for patients to report previous episodes of nausea as an "allergic reaction." Even though rare, true allergy to opioids is known to occur. Nearly all opioids can trigger degranulation of mast cells leading to direct release of histamine. IgE antibodies have been detected that react with several opioids. In such cases it is best to prescribe pain medications that are not derived from morphine or codeine. Consequently, pentazocine becomes a good choice.

Opioid Antidote

Naloxone (Narcan): Naloxone is a competitive opioid receptor antagonist that acts both centrally and peripherally, affecting the mu, kappa, and delta receptors. When given as an intravenous (IV) injection, naloxone acts immediately to reverse opioid toxicity.

FULL MORPHINE-LIKE OPIOID AGONISTS
Codeine

Codeine in pure form is a Schedule II drug, but combination compounds of codeine are Schedule III drugs.

Codeine Analgesic Efficacy

Tylenol with codeine is **not** stronger than an adequate dose of ibuprofen. The combination is as effective as tramadol and possibly better tolerated. When compared to morphine, codeine is milder but causes more constipation.

Codeine Metabolism and CYP2D6

Codeine is a **prodrug** that is metabolized by **CYP2D6** enzyme to morphine. Thus, codeine is affected by CYP2D6 inhibitor drugs. About 5–10% of Caucasians metabolize codeine **poorly**, and about 1–7% of Caucasians have **increased** CYP2D6 activity, accounting for increased sensitivity to codeine. These "rapid metabolizers" are at increased risk for toxicity because of rapidly escalating morphine levels. Thus, tamoxifen, a CYP2D6 substrate **cannot** be combined with CYP2D6 needing pain medications, oxycodone, codeine, hydrocodone, or tramadol. Morphine would be a good option under such circumstances.

Once metabolized in the liver, codeine is excreted through the kidneys. With liver failure, codeine conversion is impaired, and its analgesic effectiveness is compromised. The active metabolites accumulate in renal failure, and there are reports of serious adverse effects in renal failure patients. **Dose adjustments** are recommended in patients with **hepatic and renal** insufficiency.

Codeine and Pregnancy

Codeine and acetaminophen-codeine have both been assigned Pregnancy Category C. There are no effects of maternal codeine intake during pregnancy on infant survival or congenital malformation rate, but because of the association with acute cesarean delivery and postpartum hemorrhage, there should be a certain level of caution when prescribing codeine toward the end of pregnancy. Acetaminophen is routinely used for short-term pain relief and fever in all stages of pregnancy, and it is safe in pregnancy when used intermittently for short durations. Codeine is the **only** narcotic analgesic that has shown a statistically significant association with teratogenicity, involving respiratory tract malformations. Like other narcotics, codeine rapidly crosses the placenta, and neonatal codeine withdrawal has occurred even in infants whose mothers were taking codeine as cough suppressants for as little as ten days prior to delivery. Acetaminophen-codeine should only be given during pregnancy when benefits far outweigh the risk.

Codeine and Lactation

Codeine is excreted into human milk in small amounts. Nursing infants whose mothers are taking codeine and who happen to be **ultra-rapid metabolizers** of codeine can experience apnea, bradycardia, and cyanosis from high levels of morphine in the mother. However, codeine is considered safe with breast-feeding by the American Academy of Pediatrics.

Codeine Caution

A patient allergic to morphine will always be allergic to codeine due to cross-reactivity.

Codeine Preparations

Codeine is typically used in combination with acetaminophen as:

- Tylenol #1: 7.5mg codeine + 300mg acetaminophen (APAP).
- Tylenol #2: 15mg codeine + 300mg APAP.
- Tylenol #3: 30mg codeine + 300mg APAP: combination prescribed most often.
- Tylenol #4: 60mg codeine + 300mg APAP.

Codeine with Acetaminophen Dosing

1. **Normal dose:** The usual dose is 30–60mg/1–2 tablets q4–6h, maximum 12 tablets/24hours. Do not exceed 3 g/day of acetaminophen.
2. **Dose with kidney disease:**
    a. **CrCl >50mL/min or serum creatinine <2.0mg/dL:** Dose normally, use 30–60 mg codeine. Dispense 1–2 Tylenol #3 q4–6h PRN.
    b. **CrCl 10–50mL/min or serum creatinine >2.0mg/dL to predialysis:** Decrease codeine dose by 50%, use 15–30mg codeine. Dispense 1–2 Tylenol #2 q6h PRN.
    c. **CrCl <10mL/min or in the Renal Failure/Dialysis Patient:** Decrease the codeine dose by 75% and use 7.5–15mg codeine. Dispense 1–2 Tylenol #1 q8h PRN.
3. **Dose with liver disease:**
    a. **Mild or chronic inactive hepatitis:** Dose normally, give 30–60mg codeine. Give 1–2 Tylenol #3 **q4–6h** PRN.
    b. **Moderate-to-severe or active hepatitis:** Dispense 50% dose, give 15–30mg codeine. Give 1–2 Tylenol #2 **q6h** PRN.
    c. **Cirrhosis:** Reduce dose by 75%, give 7.5–15mg codeine. Give 1–2 Tylenol #1 **q8h** PRN.

Morphine

Morphine, hydromorphone, and fentanyl are three very potent, pure opioid agonists. They are named "pure" because they most closely mimic the action of endogenous opioids. All three drugs activate the mu and kappa receptors producing analgesia.

Morphine sulfate (immediate release), a strong, short-acting (3–4hours) opiate agonist, is the drug of choice for severe cancer pain. Morphine is also safe to use over prolonged periods if necessary. The preferred route of administration is oral. Orally administered morphine provides pain relief comparable to that of parenterally administered morphine, which can be achieved if you implement the 3:1 oral-to-parenteral ratio for dosing. The oral dose must be three times the parenteral dose because the oral dose is subject to the first-pass effect in the liver. **Controlled-release morphine** is also now available in tablet form that releases the drug over 8–24hours. This obviates taking the immediate release form every 3–4hours.

Metabolism

Morphine is primarily metabolized to morphine-3-glucuronide (M3G) and morphine-6-glucuronide (M6G) morphine in the liver by urldine-5′-diphosphate (UDP) glucuronosyltransferase, UGT2B7 isozyme. These metabolic products account for approximately 65% of a dose of morphine, with the remaining drug biotransformed to multiple minor species or excreted unchanged. M6G is an opioid agonist and has a potency that is greater than morphine. M3G, on the other hand, is inactive and has been found to have little pharmacologic activity.

Morphine clearance is decreased in liver failure, and renal failure is associated with an accumulation of morphine metabolites. Morphine can thus cause hepatotoxicity and nephrotoxicity.

Uses

Morphine is used in the management of moderate to severe pain. Avoid use in the elderly and in patients with severe pulmonary disease.

Morphine and Pregnancy

Morphine is classified as Pregnancy Category **C** by the FDA. No increased risk of congenital malformations in humans has been associated with use of morphine in pregnancy. Morphine should be given during pregnancy only when benefits far outweigh the risk. Short-term use of the drug is acceptable in the first or second trimester of pregnancy, as the drug is found to have no risk in controlled animal studies. Chronic use of morphine in later pregnancy has been associated with neonatal drug withdrawal, irritability, vomiting, diarrhea, weight loss, and death.

Morphine and Lactation

Morphine is excreted into human milk in trace amounts and adverse effects in the nursing infant are unlikely. Morphine is considered compatible with breast-feeding by the American Academy of Pediatrics.

DDIs Associated with Morphine

Morphine is affected by carbamazepine (Tegretol), diclofenac, naloxone, tamoxifen, tricyclic antidepressants, ranitidine, and rifampin.

Morphine Dose

1. **Normal oral morphine:** 10–20mg q3–4h. The long-acting forms of morphine are given q8–12h.
2. **Normal IV morphine:** 2mg q2–3h.

   Morphine dosing alert: Morphine is a high-extraction drug and its bioavailability increases in patients with advanced liver disease or cirrhosis. The dosing interval of morphine should be increased by 1.5–2 times the regular dosing interval **if you must** use it in a patient with liver disease. Ideally, morphine should **not** be used in the presence of liver and kidney disease.

Hydromorphone (Dilaudid)

Hydromorphone is a Schedule II drug that is more potent than morphine and is used in the management of moderate-to-severe pain. Hydromorphone is preferred over morphine in patients with renal failure to avoid accumulation of toxic morphine metabolites. Patients with hepatic and renal impairment should be started on a lower starting dose of hydromorphone.

Metabolism

Hydromorphone is extensively metabolized in the liver and excreted in the urine.

Hydromorphone and Pregnancy

Hydromorphone is a Pregnancy Category C drug, and according to animal data, the drug may cause fetal harm. It should be used with caution during labor.

Hydromorphone and Lactation

Hydromorphone distributes rapidly from plasma into breast milk and it is best to "pump and dump" the milk while the mother is on hydromorphone.

Hydromorphone Caution

Dilaudid tablets contain metabisulfite, and the drug should not be used in patients with a history of allergy to sulfites or in patients with a history of G6PD anemia. Avoid in elderly patients and in patients with severe pulmonary disease. Hydromorphone **can be used** in kidney or liver failure patients.

Hydromorphone Dose

Hydromorphone can be given orally, or by intravenous, intramuscular, or subcutaneous injections. Dilaudid is available as a 2, 4, or 8mg tablet. The following are the usual doses:

1. **Oral hydromorphone:** 2–4mg q4h.
2. **Parenteral hydromorphone:** The usual starting dose of hydromorphone is 1–2mg subcutaneously (SC) or intramuscularly (IM), every two to threehours as necessary.

Should intravenous (IV) administration be necessary, the injection should be given **slowly**, over at least two to three minutes and the usual starting dose is 0.2–1mg.

Fentanyl

Fentanyl is a Schedule II opioid that is available in transdermal, parenteral, and trans-buccal formulations. Fentanyl is distinctly more potent than morphine, highly lipophilic, and binds strongly to plasma proteins. It is extensively metabolized in the liver by CYP3A4 to inactive, nontoxic metabolites and is affected by CYP3A4 inhibitors.

Uses and Contraindications

Fentanyl is used to treat intolerable adverse effects of other opioids, for pain management in patients unable to take or retain oral analgesia, or for patients with a history of renal failure. Fentanyl should be used with caution in patients with disease-related fever, significant pulmonary disease, other causes of CNS depression, and in elderly and debilitated patients. Adverse effects associated with fentanyl are qualitatively similar to morphine, with less constipation, sedation, and skin reactions. Fentanyl is contraindicated for severe pain requiring rapid analgesic titration and pain unresponsive to morphine or other μ-agonists.

Fentanyl and Pregnancy

Fentanyl has been assigned Pregnancy Category **C**. There are no controlled data for fentanyl use during pregnancy, and the drug should be used during pregnancy only when the benefits far outweigh the risks.

Fentanyl and Lactation

Fentanyl is excreted into human milk and levels achieved in the colostrum are greater than maternal serum levels, especially during the first week of infancy. Even though fentanyl is considered to be compatible with breast-feeding by the American Academy of Pediatrics, it is best to avoid feeding the infant while the mother is on fentanyl.

Fentanyl Patch Preparation Strengths

The drug is dispensed as 25, 50, 75, and 100µg/h fentanyl patches (containing 2.5, 5, 7.5, and 10mg fentanyl).

Fentanyl Patch Alert

The fentanyl transdermal patch needs 6–12hours for onset of action after application, typically reaching steady state in 3–6 days. Once the patch is removed, fentanyl clearance can take up to 24hours.

Fentanyl Dose for Patients on Strong Opioids

Calculate the previous 24-hour dose as mg/day of oral morphine. Divide this value by 3 and choose the nearest patch strength in µg/h. Titrate the dose q72h for optimal relief.

Fentanyl Dose for Opioid Naïve Patients or Patients on Weak or Short-Acting Opioids

Start with 25µg/h patch and titrate the dose q72h for optimal relief.

Oral Transmucosal Fentanyl Citrate

Oral Transmucosal Fentanyl Citrate (OTFC) is used for breakthrough pain in cancer patients who are already on opioids. OTFC has been shown to provide safe and effective treatment for breakthrough pain in 75% of patients. Twenty-five percent of patients either do not achieve analgesia with the highest dose (1,600µg) or they suffer unacceptable adverse effects. OTFC is 100 times more potent than morphine. Some (25–50%) absorption is transmucosal and the rest is via slow gastrointestinal absorption. OTFC becomes effective in 5–10 minutes and the effect lasts for 1–3.5hours, but it can last longer with higher doses. Fentanyl metabolism is **unaffected** by liver disease.

Fentanyl Citrate Side Effects

Fentanyl causes dizziness, nausea, and drowsiness.

OTFC Preparations

OTFC is dispensed as 200, 400, 600, 800, 1,200, and 1,600μg lozenges.

OTFC Dose Titration

There is no relationship between the effective dose of OTFC for breakthrough pain and the dose of opioid being used for background analgesia. Each patient has to be individually titrated to find the appropriate OTFC dose. OTFC is a "lollipop on a stick" containing fentanyl in a hard, sweet matrix, and these OTFC lozenges are expensive. OTFC is used by placing the lollipop against the mucosa of one cheek and constantly moving it up and down, and then doing the same against the other cheek. It is important that the patient follows this practice from one cheek to the other, so the drug is optimally effective. Do not place it on the tongue because this will slow the absorption of OTFC.

The patient uses one 200μg lozenge over 15 minutes, and a second 200μg lozenge is used after 15 minutes if the analgesia is inadequate. The patient should **not** get more than **2** lozenges per episode of pain. The **dose** can be **repeated** for 2–3 pain episodes per day. If this dose is ineffective, then increase to the next-strength lozenge and repeat the same steps previously outlined. The patient is said to have an effective dose when the pain relief occurs with a single lozenge.

Oxycodone and Oxycodone + Acetaminophen (Percocet)

Unlike codeine, hydrocodone, and tramadol, oxycodone is **not** a prodrug. Oxycodone is typically combined with acetaminophen (Percocet) or aspirin (Percodan). Percocet is the only preparation advised for dentistry because Percodan can trigger aspirin-induced platelet dysfunction associated bleeding. Percocet is used for mild, moderate, or severe pain.

Oxycodone is **mainly** metabolized by glucuronidation to noroxycodone and **minimally** by CYP2D6 to oxymorphone for clearance in the urine. The analgesic effect of oxycodone is almost entirely attributed to the parent drug and only a very small amount is demethylated to oxymorphone. Consequently, oxycodone is a **better** choice for patients taking known CYP2D6 inhibitors, as there is only a very small potential for drug-drug interaction between oxycodone and CYP2D6 inhibitor drugs. A percentage (5–10%) of Caucasians lack the CYP2D6 enzyme, which is necessary to convert oxycodone to oxymorphone, and oxycodone should **not** be used in these individuals.

Immediate release (IR) oxycodone is available in tablet form and the action lasts for 4–6hours. **Controlled release oxycodone (Oxycontin)** is also available in tablet form that releases oxycodone over an 8–12hour period. **Sustained release (SR)** tablet form releases oxycodone over 12hours.

Oxycodone Indications and Contraindications

Oxycodone is indicated for mild-to-moderate and severe pain. Prescribe with **caution** and careful **renal impairment** patients, and use with **caution** in the presence of **severe hepatic dysfunction**, in the elderly, and in the presence of **severe** liver, kidney, other causes of CNS depression and significant pulmonary disease. **Limited, low-dose** therapy is usually well tolerated in hepatic disease or cirrhosis. However, cases of hepatotoxicity at daily acetaminophen dosages <3g/day have been reported. Avoid chronic use in the presence of hepatic impairment.

Percocet DEA Schedule

In the pure form or in combination with acetaminophen or aspirin, oxycodone is a Schedule II drug that requires a written prescription. No refills are allowed for oxycodone.

Oxycodone and Pregnancy

Oxycodone is a Category B drug but acetaminophen-oxycodone (Percocet) has been assigned to Pregnancy Category C by the FDA. When compared with other narcotics, oxycodone is considered to be the **safest** narcotic for use during pregnancy. When Percocet is used for a **prolonged** period at term or in high doses, it can become a Category D drug causing breathing difficulty and even death in the newborn. Oxycodone in combination with ibuprofen (Combunox) is **contraindicated** in the third trimester.

Oxycodone and Lactation

Maternal use of maximum dosages of oral narcotics while breastfeeding can cause infant drowsiness, and this holds true for oxycodone too. Oxycodone is excreted into human milk, but the clinical significance in regard to breast-fed infants is unknown. It is best to limit the maximum oxycodone dosage to 30mg daily and closely monitor the infant for any drowsiness or breathing difficulties.

Oxycodone + Acetaminophen (Percocet) Preparations

Percocet is available in the following strengths:

- 2.5mg oxycodone + 325mg acetaminophen (APAP): 2.5/325
- 5mg oxycodone + 325mg APAP (original tablet): 5/325
- 7.5mg oxycodone + 325mg APAP: 7.5/325
- 7.5mg oxycodone + 500mg APAP: 7.5/500
- 10mg oxycodone + 650mg APAP: 10/650

Percocet Dosing

1. **Normal Percocet dose: oxycodone + APAP (Percocet):** 2.5–5mg oxycodone **q4–6h**
   In the healthy adult, depending on the pain intensity: Dispense one 2.5/325 or 5/325 Percocet tablet **q4–6h** PRN. It is better to dispense one 5/325 tablet instead of two 2.5/325 tablets for severe pain, so that the total Tylenol intake can be kept down. Keep the maximum oxycodone dose at 20mg per day and the long-acting forms can be given q8–12h.
2. **Percocet dose with kidney disease:**
   a. **Predialysis: 1**, 2.5/325 tablet **q6h** PRN
   b. **Dialysis: 1**, 2.5/325 tablet **q8h** PRN
3. **Percocet dose schedule with liver disease:**
   a. **Hepatitis: 1**, 2.5/325 tablet **q6h** PRN
   b. **Cirrhosis: 1**, 2.5/325 tablet **q8h** PRN

Hydrocodone and Hydrocodone + Acetaminophen (Vicodin)

Hydrocodone is the most commonly used opioid, and like codeine, hydrocodone is also a **prodrug** and the parent drug has no analgesic effect. Plain hydrocodone is not available. Hydrocodone with acetaminophen (Vicodin) is thought to be **twice** as strong as acetaminophen or any NSAID and has few side effects, but oxycodone with acetaminophen (Percocet), is probably **stronger** than Vicodin and is very similar in its safety and side effects. Hydrocodone gets demethylated in the liver by CYP2D6 to hydromorphone, which then exerts the analgesic effect. One should be cautious using hydrocodone in the presence of CYP2D6 inhibitor and inducer drugs. Administer with **caution** and careful monitoring in patients with **renal failure** and use with **caution** in the presence of **hepatic impairment**. Limited, low-dose therapy is usually well tolerated in hepatic disease or cirrhosis. However, cases of hepatotoxicity at daily acetaminophen dosages less than 3g/day have been reported. Avoid chronic use in the presence of hepatic impairment.

Hydrocodone Uses and Side Effects

Hydrocodone, in combination with acetaminophen or ibuprofen (Vicodin and Lortab, respectively), is used for the management of moderate-to-severe pain, and it is a Schedule III drug. The main side effect of hydrocodone is constipation.

Hydrocodone and Pregnancy

The FDA has assigned hydrocodone and acetaminophen-hydrocodone to Pregnancy Category C. Hydrocodone should be given during pregnancy only when the benefits far outweigh the risks. Hydrocodone bitartrate in combination with ibuprofen (Vicoprofen) is contraindicated in the third trimester of pregnancy.

Hydrocodone and Lactation

No data exist demonstrating the excretion of hydrocodone into human milk, so it is considered safe to dispense during lactation.

Vicodin Preparations

Hydrocodone dose alert: Be cognizant to calculate the total daily dose of APAP, ASA, or NSAID given in combination with hydrocodone so you do **not** exceed the maximum daily dose for APAP, ASA, or NSAID. Some combinations of hydrocodone, for example, contain 750mg of APAP per tablet, and by dispensing eight such tablets daily, you can very quickly reach a daily APAP dose range of 4–6g/24hours. Therefore, my suggestion is for you to opt for oxycodone-acetaminophen instead for the medically complex patient, as the APAP dose in the combination is lower.

1. **Each Vicodin tablet contains:** 5mg hydrocodone + 500mg acetaminophen (APAP).
2. **Vicodin ES contains:** 7.5mg hydrocodone + 500mg APAP.
3. **Vicoprofen contains:** 7.5mg hydrocodone + 200mg ibuprofen. Vicoprofen is particularly useful in the presence of pain and inflammation.

Vicodin Dosing: Do Not Exceed the Maximum Daily Dose for APAP/NSAIDS

1. **Normal dose:** 5–10mg hydrocodone: Give **1–2** tablets **q6h** PRN.
2. **Vicodin dose with kidney disease:**
   a. **Predialysis:** Vicodin, **1** tab **q6h** PRN
   b. **Dialysis:** Vicodin, **1** tab **q8h** PRN
3. **Vicodin dose with liver disease:**
   a. **Hepatitis:** Vicodin, **1** tab **q6h** PRN
   b. **Cirrhosis:** Vicodin, **1** tab **q8h** PRN

Propoxyphene Dextropropoxyphene (Darvon)

Propoxyphene is a weak, short-acting (3–4hours), Schedule IV opioid agonist that was recently taken off the US market because of fatal metabolite-triggered cardiac toxicity and death. I will discuss this drug for the benefit of students taking board exams and providers in countries where the drug is still available.

Propoxyphene levels increase in patients with chronic liver disease or cirrhosis, resulting in hepatotoxicity. Propoxyphene's metabolite norpropoxyphene also accumulates with kidney disease, causing sedation and confusion. **Avoid** dextropropoxyphene (Darvon) or propoxyphene-acetaminophen (Darvocet) in patients with liver and kidney disease.

Propoxyphene and Pregnancy

Propoxyphene is Pregnancy Category **C**. Propoxyphene is best avoided, as several case reports indicate that infants exposed to propoxyphene in utero have been born with a variety of congenital malformations.

Propoxyphene and Lactation

Propoxyphene and its active metabolite, norpropoxyphene, are excreted into human breast milk in small amounts, but the clinical effects in breast-fed infants have not been described. Propoxyphene is considered compatible with breast-feeding by the American Academy of Pediatrics. Propoxyphene preparations: Do not exceed the daily acetaminophen dose/day.

1. **Darvocet N:** 50mg propoxyphene + 325mg acetaminophen. **Dose:** 1–2 tablets q4h PRN, maximum 600mg propoxyphene napsylate/day.
2. **Darvocet N 100:** 100mg propoxyphene + 650mg acetaminophen.

Darvon Dose

One tablet q4h, maximum 600mg propoxyphene napsylate/day.

Meperidine (Demerol)

Meperidine is a Schedule II drug that is **not** considered a first-line opioid analgesic for acute pain. Poor oral absorption and accumulation of normeperidine makes meperidine a very poor choice as an **oral** analgesic and it should **not** be used as such. Meperidine is metabolized in the liver, excreted through the kidneys, and its metabolite, normeperidine, which has a very long elimination half-life, has significant neurotoxic properties. It is a high-extraction drug and its bioavailability increases in patients with advanced liver disease or cirrhosis. Its metabolite normeperidine accumulates with kidney disease causing CNS toxicity. Thus, meperidine should **not** be used in patients with liver disease or kidney disease and in the elderly, as these patients are at increased risk for toxicity from accumulation of the toxic metabolite, normeperidine.

Indications and Contraindications

Meperidine should only be used for the management of moderate-to-severe **acute** pain. It should **not** be used for the management of **chronic** pain in palliative care. Meperidine should not be given to patients on monoamine oxidase inhibitors (MAOIs), as severe respiratory depression, excitation, delirium, and seizures may occur. Be very cautious, as the side effects are **not** reversed by naloxone.

Meperidine and Pregnancy

Meperidine has been assigned to Pregnancy Category **C**. It is frequently used **short term** in pregnancy and during labor. If the drug is administered to the mother shortly before delivery, meperidine and normeperidine cross the placenta very rapidly causing respiratory depression in newborns. Infants of chronic users may experience drug withdrawal. Meperidine should be given during pregnancy only if clearly needed.

Meperidine and Lactation

Meperidine is excreted into human milk and apnea events in breastfed infants **of mothers taking any opiates, including meperidine while nursing, have been known to occur. It is best to** "pump and dump" the milk while the mother is on meperidine.

Meperidine Dosing

1. **Meperidine duration of action:** 2–3hours; oral: 50–100mg q4h PRN.
2. **IV/IM/subcutaneous meperidine:** 25–100mg q4h PRN.
3. **Continuous IV meperidine:** It is administered at a rate of 15–35mg/h.

Methadone

Methadone is a Pregnancy Category **C** drug. Methadone is a highly lipophyllic, strong Schedule II synthetic opioid. It is a μ opioid agonist and a NMDA receptor antagonist. It inhibits the uptake of serotonin and norepinephrine. The plasma **half-life** of methadone varies between **13–36hours**, and although the analgesic activity does not last that long, **the drug accumulates in the blood with repeated dosing**, producing excessive sedation if the dose is not properly adjusted. **Because of its long plasma half-life, adequate pain relief is initially difficult to achieve with methadone alone and rapid dose adjustments are more difficult.**

Methadone is metabolized in the liver, primarily by CYP3A4 and secondarily by CYP2D6, and in the intestines by the CYP3A4 enzyme. It is excreted exclusively in the feces. Grapefruit juice increases methadone levels from CYP3A4 inhibition.

Indications and Contraindications

Methadone is indicated for moderate and severe pain; pain poorly responsive to morphine, especially neuropathic pain; intolerance to morphine or other opioids; in the treatment of heroin addiction; and renal failure.

Side Effects and DDIs

Methadone can trigger fatal cardiac arrhythmias in the presence of hypokalemia and hypomagnesemia. Be cautious when using methadone in patients on SSRIs and TCAs. Carbamazepine, phenytoin, rifampin, barbiturates, and anti-retroviral drugs can induce methadone metabolism, thus decreasing effectiveness of the drug.

Methadone Dosing

Methadone can be given by mouth, per-rectum, or as IV/IM/SC injections. The oral-to-parenteral dose ratio is 2:1. Duration of action initially is 4–6hours and with continued use 8–12hours. Methadone is available as 10mg/mL injection or as 5mg/10mg tablets.

1. **Methadone normal dose:** 2.5–10mg oral/IM/SC q4–12h; the 5mg oral dose given q6–8h, is typical for pain management.
2. **Kidney disease dose:** Give 50–75% of normal dose in the presence of CrCl <10mL/min.
3. **Liver disease dose:** Methadone is **not** recommended for patients with severe liver disease/cirrhosis.
4. **Elderly patient dose:** 2.5mg PO/IM q8–12h.

Oxymorphone (Opana)

Oxymorphone is a Schedule II, Pregnancy Category **C** drug. It is a strong, short-acting (three to four hours) opioid agonist with characteristics similar to those of morphine but it is ten times more potent than morphine. Oxymorphone is not affected by CYP3A4 or CYP2D6 enzymes. Therefore, it is a good alternative in the presence of potent CYP3A4 and CYP2D6 inhibitor and inducer drugs. It is available as immediate- and sustained-release/long-acting formulations. **Oxymorphone dose:** 10mg/day.

PARTIAL OPIOID AGONISTS

Buprenorphine (Subutex)

Buprenorphine is a Pregnancy Category **C** drug that produces agonist/antagonist effects at the opioid mu receptor. Buprenorphine binds less tightly with opioid receptor sites compared with pure agonists, thus producing less effect than pure agonist. Subutex is the sublingual product that containing only the active ingredient buprenorphine hydrochloride. Naloxone has now been added to buprenorphine to guard against intravenous (IV) abuse of buprenorphine by opiate addicts, and this preparation is called Suboxone. Like mixed opioid agonist-antagonists, the patient can develop psychomimetic effects with prolonged or high-dose therapy.

Buprenorphine Dose

The drug reaches agonist ceiling effect at about 12mg and doses greater than 12–16mg do **not** produce any more analgesia. A seven-day buprenorphine supply can be used for cancer-associated pain, and the maximum dose is 20μg/hour.

Mixed Opioid Agonists-Antagonists
Pentazocine (Talwin)

Pentazocine is a Schedule IV Pregnancy Category **C** drug. Pentazocine is the only oral pain medication that produces analgesia by acting as an agonist at the kappa receptors **and** as an antagonist at the mu receptors. Being a kappa agonist, pentazocine has a **ceiling analgesic** effect, and no further analgesia is achieved by increasing the dose beyond 50mg. Because it is a mu receptor antagonist, pentazocine, when combined with other opioids, acts as an opioid antagonist and then impairs pain reduction.

Mixed opioid agonist-antagonists have a high incidence of unpleasant psychomimetic effects, and because of these characteristics, pentazocine is **not** recommended for treatment of **chronic** pain. Pentazocine is most commonly used for postoperative pain in patients who are **opioid-agonist naïve**.

Pentazocine Use

Pentazocine is a good choice for patients with a history of opioid abuse, as it does not provide the euphoric effects that are mediated by traditional mu agonists.

Pentazocine Preparation

Pentazocine is available in combination APAP or in combination with naloxone. Naloxone combination is to prevent injection abuse. Hence if injected, naloxone blocks all effects of pentazocine, rendering it ineffective. When taken by mouth, naloxone is inactive and therefore does not affect the actions of pentazocine.

Pentazocine Dose

50mg q4h PRN or Pentazocine + APAP: 25/650: 1–2 tabs q4h PRN with maximum pentazocine dose of 6g/day and maximum acetaminophen dose of 3g/day.

NONNARCOTIC OPIATE AGONIST
Tramadol (Ultram)

Tramadol is a synthetic analgesic that belongs to the class of drugs known as opioid agonists. Tramadol is an atypical, centrally acting nonnarcotic prodrug analgesic that is **not** considered a controlled substance. Therefore, it can be obtained with a regular prescription. Tramadol causes less respiratory depression and is less addicting when compared with opioids. Tramadol has the same effectiveness as codeine-acetaminophen combinations. Although it is a less-potent analgesic than the "scheduled" narcotics, it is very useful in some chronic pain patients who do not require stronger analgesics, in patients who have a history of substance abuse whose physicians want to avoid scheduled medications, and for opioid withdrawal. It is **not** recommended for patients with a tendency toward **opioid abuse or dependence**.

On ingestion the CYP2D6 enzyme in the liver converts tramadol to its active form O-desmethyl-tramadol, which demonstrates an agonist action on mu receptors. Inactive metabolites of this product are excreted by the kidney. Like tricyclic antidepressants (TCAs), the parent drug inhibits the reuptake of norepinephrine and serotonin, thus proving beneficial in the management of chronic pain.

Tramadol Alert

Avoid tramadol in the presence of **severe** liver or kidney disease and in patients on seizure medications, TCAs, or SSRIs.

Tramadol and Pregnancy

Tramadol has been assigned to Pregnancy Category C by the FDA and animal studies have revealed evidence of embryotoxicity and fetotoxicity.

Tramadol and Lactation

Tramadol is excreted into human milk in small amounts and it is best that tramadol **not** be prescribed to nursing mothers.

Tramadol Preparations

Tramadol (Ultram ER): Tramadol (Ultram ER) is a sustained-release medication and it has the advantage of being used once per day.

Tramadol-acetaminophen (Ultracet): 37.5mg tramadol + 325mg APAP.

Tramadol Dose

50–100mg Ultram PO q4–6h PRN. Maximum tramadol dose per day, in divided doses is 400mg.

OPIOID ALERTS AND SIGNIFICANT FACTS FOR DENTISTRY

The following are alerts and facts that are significant for dentistry:

1. Oral narcotics should be prescribed for only two to three days, and further pain management should be continued with nonnarcotic pain medications.
2. Chronic narcotic use accelerates the liver enzymes causing faster drug metabolism and consequent need for larger and more frequent doses. Physical dependence and tolerance can thus occur with long-term use.
3. Opioids increase alcohol effects, and these substances should not be combined.
4. Avoid opioid analgesic use just prior to birth, because this can cause serious breathing problems in the newborn. However, when used, constant monitoring of the infant is required.

5. Limit use in the lactating patient as opioids pass through the breast milk.
6. Opioid use should be restricted in patients with a history of frequent seizures, severe asthma, COPD, severe emphysema, uncontrolled hypothyroidism, Addison's disease, gallstones, diverticulitis, enlarged prostate, urinary retention problems, drug abuse, and addiction.
7. Do not prescribe opioid analgesics to patients on antipsychotics, CNS depressants, or TCAs because this can cause opioid analgesic toxicity.
8. Morphine, codeine, and meperidine are nonspecific histamine liberators that bind to a specific receptor on the mast cells causing histamine release. Patients with severe symptoms can be given pentazocine or a nonopioid pain medication such as tromethamine (Toradol).
9. Do not combine opioid analgesics with sedating antihistamines, CNS depressants; tricyclic antidepressants (TCAs), muscle relaxants, or warfarin (Coumadin).
10. Do not combine meperidine (Demerol) with monoamine oxidase inhibitors (MAOIs); do not combine Darvocet N or Darvon with antiseizure medications; and do not combine morphine with zidovudin (AZT).
11. Avoid opioid use with H_2 blockers, cimetidine, and ranitidine to prevent DDIs.
12. Patients with renal and hepatic dysfunction show an increased sensitivity to a number of analgesics, particularly narcotics. Therefore, start with lower doses in patients with renal and liver dysfunction until the patient shows adequate dose-response relationship.

ADJUVANTS

Adjuvants are not true analgesics, but they do contribute significantly to pain relief when **used alone or in combination** with other analgesics. They are particularly useful for opioid-insensitive pain and neuropathic pain. **Corticosteroids**, benzodiazepines, antihistamine H_1 **blockers, muscle relaxants, TCAs**, and bisphosphonates **are commonly used adjuvants.**

Corticosteroids

Corticosteroids are powerful, peripheral acting anti-inflammatory agents that have non-selective COX inhibition action and are best used for acute pain or flare-up of a chronic inflammatory problem. Corticosteroids such as Orabase-HCA, Oracort, and Oralone are anti-inflammatory medications that are used to relieve discomfort and redness of the mouth. Corticosteroids can also be prescribed either orally (Medrol pack or prednisone), or in the form of cortisone injections into the soft tissues or joints. The dose equivalencies for the commonly prescribed corticosteroids are 100mg Hydrocortisone = 25mg Prednisolone = 4mg Dexamethasone.

Medrol Dose Pack

Medrol dose pack contains methylprednisolone **tablets** for oral administration. **Each Medrol tablet can contain** 2, 4, 8, 16, or 32mg methylprednisolone. **The initial dosage of Medrol** tablets can range from 4–48mg of methylprednisolone per day, depending upon the specific underlying disease entity that is being treated. Less severe, acute issues, such as acute dental inflammation, require lower tapering doses given over a short period of time (**six** days). The more severe conditions, such as rheumatoid arthritis or lupus, require higher initial doses that are maintained or adjusted until a satisfactory response is seen at the lowest possible dose. Thus, dose requirements vary and need to be adjusted according to the patient's response to the underlying disease states.

Corticosteroid Side Effects

Corticosteroids should be used with caution in the presence of peptic ulceration, diabetes mellitus (can trigger hyperglycemia), cardiac failure (can cause sodium and water retention), and edematous states.

Benzodiazepines

Benzodiazepines, such as diazepam (Valium), lorazepam (Ativan), and oxazepam (Serax), aid in the treatment of pain through their anxiolytic effect. They are also useful for muscle spasm or acute musculoskeletal pain.

Antihistamine H₁ Blockers

Diphenhydramine (Benadryl) acts by blocking the action of histamine. By causing drowsiness, diphenhydramine assists with sleeping. Typically, 25–50mg is used 30 minutes prior to bedtime. Doxylamine (Unisom) 25mg, taken 30 minutes prior to bed, up to a maximum of 100mg, also induces sleep. Doxylamine, in combination with acetaminophen and codeine, is used for pain management.

Muscle Relaxants

Cyclobenzaprine (Flexeril)

Cyclobenzaprine acts by blocking the pain-associated nerve impulses coming to the brain. The recommended dose of cyclobenzaprine is 5mg, three times a day, and based on individual patient response, the dose can be increased to 10mg, three times a day.

Baclofen

Baclofen acts at the spinal level. The drug is started at 5mg/day and cautiously titrated up to a maximum of 100mg/day. The drug must be **withdrawn slowly** to avoid withdrawal symptoms and seizures.

Dantrolene

Dantrolene acts directly on muscles. It is started at 25mg/day and is titrated to a maximum of 400mg/day.

Tricyclic Antidepressants (TCAs)

TCAs act by blocking the presynaptic re-uptake of serotonin and noradrenaline in the CNS, enhancing the action of the descending inhibitory pathways. They have analgesic properties but are more useful as adjuvants or co-analgesics in reducing the total drug dose of opioids and NSAIDS, especially in the management of neuropathic pain, as with diabetic neuropathy. Once-daily dosing at bed time is the optimal way to prescribe TCAs.

Drugs such as amitriptyline, imipramine, or doxepin are started at a dose of 10–25mg at night and increased to 50–100mg. If there is no benefit in one week the given drug is stopped. The adverse effects of TCAs, such as sedation, anticholinergic effects, and postural hypotension, are usually mild when used in the lower doses that are typically recommended for neuropathic pain.

Bisphosphonates

Bisphosphonates reduce pain and skeletal events in patients with bone metastases. They act by inhibiting osteoclast activity and by blocking mineral dissolution, and they are also effective in the treatment of hypercalcaemia associated with cancer. The nitrogen-containing bisphosphonates, pamidronate, ibandronate, olpadronate, and zoledronic acid are more potent than the non-nitrogen-containing compounds etidronate and clodronate. An improvement in pain related to bone disease occurs over time. Bisphosphonates are not recommended for immediate analgesia.

MULTIMODAL ANALGESIA

Pain involves multiple mechanisms, and pain management ideally requires treatment using multimodal analgesic techniques with the aim of improving analgesia by combining analgesics, which demonstrates additive or synergistic effects. A multidisciplinary approach should encompass optimizing the use of preoperative, intraoperative, and postoperative pain control mechanisms. Multimodal analgesia achieves acute and chronic pain relief by targeting pain transmission at multiple levels with the use of analgesics and/or adjuvants in combination.

Pain transmission can be affected by modulating the upward transmission of pain, by altering pain perception at the central level, and by modulating the descending inhibitory pathways. Different drugs act at different sites, and by using multiple drugs one can reduce the total dose of any one drug, thus leading to the reduction of untoward side effects associated with any single drug.

Pain reduction can be achieved by affecting pain transmission pathways in multiple ways including decreasing the nociceptive input with local anesthetics and NSAIDS or by using drugs that act on the spinal cord (e.g., opiates, NSAIDS, and gabapentinoids, which are anticonvulsants that are effective in the treatment of chronic neuropathic pain); with the use of centrally acting drugs such as opiates and acetaminophen; or with drugs that act on the descending pathways such as tramadol or clonidine.

Multimodal analgesia is an approach to **preventing** postoperative pain. It involves administering a combination of opioid and nonopioid analgesics that act at different sites within the central and peripheral nervous systems, to improve pain control while eliminating opioid-related side effects. Use of multimodal analgesia for the prevention of pain in the outpatient setting is one of the keys to improving the recovery process, and it is important in helping patients resume their daily activities as quickly as possible. The "preventive" multimodal analgesic regimen for effective pain management is started in the preoperative or early postoperative period and continued thereafter for three to five days, depending on the extent of the procedure.

Recent clinical studies have shown that when traditional NSAIDS or COX-2 inhibitors were given for three to five days post surgery, significant benefit was achieved with resumption of normal activities, improvements in short-term pain control, and reduced need for opioid-containing oral analgesics. **The combination of acetaminophen and an NSAID has been found to offer superior analgesia compared with either drug alone. Glucocorticoids can also provide beneficial effects when administered in the perioperative setting**, and in appropriate doses, as part of a multimodal analgesic regimen. Other studies have also confirmed that a rational combination of different nonopioid analgesics, when given as part of multimodal analgesia, reduces postoperative pain.

A multimodal analgesic regimen should be adjusted to meet the needs of the individual patient by taking into consideration their preexisting medical conditions, the type of surgery planned, and any previous experiences related to both acute and chronic pain management. The individual differences in pain sensitivity are related to a combination of still poorly understood genetic and environmental factors, which influence central and peripheral modulation of pain signaling.

Opioid analgesics continue to play an important role in the acute treatment of moderate-to-severe pain in the early postoperative period. However, nonopioid analgesics are increasingly being used as adjuvants before, during, and after surgery to facilitate the recovery process after surgery. Because of their anesthetic and analgesic-sparing effects, their ability to reduce postoperative pain with movement, and their ability to not cause any opioid-related side effects, they shorten the duration of the hospital stay and the convalescence period.

Opioid analgesics were once considered the standard approach to preventing acute postoperative pain, but they are now being **replaced** by a **combination of nonopioid analgesic** drugs with diverse modes of action, as part of a multimodal approach to preventing pain after surgery. Efficacy of multimodal analgesic regimens continues to improve, and opioid analgesics are increasingly becoming "rescue analgesics" for acute post-surgery pain. Multimodal analgesia is now becoming the "standard of care" the world over for preventing pain following procedures. Optimal multimodal perioperative analgesic regimens should provide effective pain relief, have minimal side effects, be safe, and be easily managed by the patient and/or a family member once the patient has left the dental setting.

Finally, multimodal analgesia is widely acknowledged to be superior to a single-drug approach. Improved pain relief can be demonstrated along with fewer drug-associated side effects. Multimodal analgesia does **not** decrease complications or length of hospital stay, but it can decrease the occurrence of chronic pain.

Acute Multimodal Pain Management Algorithms in Opioid Naïve and Opioid Dependent Patients

Multimodal Acute Pain Management Facts

A multimodal technique for pain management is now the norm and it includes the administration of two or more drugs that act by different mechanisms for providing analgesia. These drugs may be administered via the same route or by different routes. There is strong evidence to suggest that, when possible, the practitioner should use multimodal pain management therapy. Multimodal pain management allows for better analgesia with lower doses of given medications than if the drugs were used alone. Additionally, a multimodal approach improves postoperative pain relief, increases patient satisfaction, and expedites mobilization.

Preemptive Analgesia

- Postoperative multimodal pain management can start with the administration of drugs preoperatively. Preemptive analgesia prevents the sensitization of the CNS that would normally amplify subsequent nociceptive pain, thus reducing the severity of postoperative pain. It is best to provide the analgesic(s) **prior** to surgery but the next best in order of effectiveness is **intraoperative,** or just **prior to the loss** of anesthesia.
- The American Society of Anesthesiologists (ASA) recommends that unless contraindicated, all major surgery patients should receive an around-the-clock (ATC) regimen of oral or IV acetaminophen and a NSAID for acute postsurgical pain, and the dosages plus duration of therapy should be individualized to be effective while avoiding adverse events. Oral or IV acetaminophen with nonselective NSAIDS/COX-2 selective NSAIDS (COXIBs) should be part of a postoperative multimodal pain management regimen.
- When needed, oral opioids can be combined with acetaminophen, NSAIDS, or COX-IBs, if severe pain is expected or the pain does not improve. Occasionally, the practitioner may opt to use oral opioids only. Be aware that even when used in the treatment of moderate-to-severe pain post surgery, NSAIDS have a significant opioid dose-sparing effect and can therefore reduce opioid-related side effects. If planning on using ketorolac (Toradol), do not use it for more than five days. Acute pain management with opioids should initially be titrated to effect, and then given on a scheduled basis.
- **The short-acting or weak opioid analgesics:** Codeine, immediate-release (IR) oxycodone, hydrocodone, and the nonopioid tramadol are short-acting analgesics. It is best to use short-acting opioids **first** before opting for the more potent immediate release analgesics or sustained-release medications.
- **Immediate-release more potent/stronger analgesics:** Codeine, IR oxycodone, hydromorphone, morphine, methadone, meperidine, oxymorphone, fentanyl, and tramadol are the immediate-release more potent/stronger analgesics. Fentanyl transmucosal (Actiq/Fentora) allows the drug to be absorbed into the blood stream through the oral mucosal lining. Fentanyl transmucosal onset of action is rapid and the drug has FDA approval for cancer breakthrough pain.
- **Sustained release strongest analgesics:** Morphine (MS Contin), hydromorphone, SR oxycodone (OxyContin), fentanyl (Duragesic or Fentanyl Patch), oxymorphone (Opana), and methadone (Methadose) are the strongest sustained-release analgesics.

Multimodal Pain Management Algorithm for Pain

- Combination of an NSAID with acetaminophen provides greater analgesia than does either drug alone, as they both inhibit prostaglandin synthesis but act at different sites. It is because of these differences in methods of action among acetaminophen and NSAIDS that when used in combination, synergistic effects occur. See Figure 5.1.

```
MILD PAIN: ATC¹ nonopioids² Oral/IV Acetaminophen +

NSAIDs + Adjuvants³ OR ATC NSAID only + Adjuvants

MILD-TO-MODERATE PAIN: Oral/IV Acetaminophen + NSAID +

Adjuvants + short-acting/weak analgesic⁴ PRN⁵

MODERATE-TO-SEVERE PAIN: Stop short-acting/weak

analgesic PRN drug and add immediate-release/stronger

analgesics⁶ OR low dose Morphine to the nonopioids +

Adjuvants

SEVERE PAIN: Use sustained-release⁷ drugs ATC +

nonopioids + Adjuvants


KEY: ATC¹: Around-the-clock; Nonopioids²: Oral/IV

Acetaminophen, ibuprofen, naproxen, indomethacin,

ketorolac, or celecoxib. Adjuvants³: Corticosteroids;

Benzodiazepines; Antihistamines; Muscle Relaxants and

TCAs. Short-acting, weak, analgesics⁴: Codeine,

immediate-release (IR) Oxycodone, Hydrocodone and

Tramadol. PRN⁵: As needed. IR stronger analgesics⁶:

Codeine, IR Oxycodone, Morphine, Hydromorphone,

Methadone, Meperidine, Oxymorphone, Fentanyl, & Tramadol

Sustained-release strongest analgesics⁷: Morphine,

Hydromorphone, SR Oxycodone, Fentanyl, Oxymorphone,

Methadone.
```

Figure 5.1. Preemptive multimodal acute pain management algorithms in opioid naïve patients.

- In turn, this combination can decrease the need for opioids, but if pain persists after the optimal dose for each drug has been used, an opioid may be added to alleviate pain. So always begin pain management with nonopioids and add opioids when needed.
- The practitioner must be cognizant not to exceed the daily recommended doses of acetaminophen to avoid liver damage.
- **Non-narcotic analgesic options for mild-to-moderate pain:** Acetaminophen, ibuprofen, naproxen, indomethacin, ketorolac, and celecoxib.
  - **Mild, acute pain protocol:** Oral or IV Acetaminophen and an NSAID are started prior to surgery in a scheduled around-the-clock (ATC) dosing, with or without an adjunct. Sometimes if the pain is tolerable, ATC-NSAID alone may be sufficient.

○ **Mild-to-moderate acute pain protocol:** In addition to the nonopioid analgesics, with or without an adjunct, prescribe a short-acting opioid analgesic on an as-needed basis (PRN).

○ **Moderate-to-severe acute pain protocol:** In the presence of escalating pain, the practitioner should **stop** the short-acting opioid and **add an immediate-acting stronger opioid** or **add a low dose of morphine** to the nonopioids, with or without an **adjuvant**.

○ **Narcotic regimens typically used for moderate-to-severe pain:** codeine, oxycodone, morphine, hydromorphone, methadone, meperidine, fentanyl, and tramadol.

○ **Transdermal patches** provide controlled drug delivery with a lower potential for abuse than oral analgesics. Patches can be applied once every 12–24hours. Conditions like postherpetic neuralgia and chronic cancer pain are routinely treated with transdermal patches. Be aware that when exposed to heat, transdermal patches cause rapid absorption and consequent drug toxicity, so the patient must avoid heat exposure.

○ **Opiate-infused lollipops and buccal lozenges** are other alternative forms of drug delivery used to treat patients with malignant or cancer-associated pain.

○ **Severe acute pain management protocol:** For continuous severe pain, a long-acting or sustained-released opioid is given ATC, with or without nonopioids and with or without an adjunct.

Chronic Pain Management Therapies

● Opioids are prescribed for chronic pain to allow the patient to function normally and not be sedated from the medications.

● When used, a pump delivers medications into the cerebrospinal fluid (CSF) surrounding the spinal cord.

● Most people using chronic opioid therapy do drive. It is up to each individual who is taking narcotics to determine if they are alert enough to drive. If someone taking opioids is involved in a traffic accident, they can be charged with driving under the influence.

● The provider should review the patient's daily opioid intake regimen. The route of delivery may be oral, subcutaneous via syringe pump, transdermal, or spinal via implanted infusion device.

● Patients may be on strong opioids such as morphine sulphate continuous, transdermal fentanyl, transdermal buprenorphine, methadone, or immediate-release preparations such as oral morphine.

Opioid Agonist Treatments (OATs)

Methadone maintenance therapy (MMT) and buprenorphine maintenance therapy (BMT) for opioid dependent patients:

● Most opioids associated with dependence and abuse are the mu-agonists such as heroin, morphine, hydrocodone, oxycodone, and meperidine; the partial mu-agonist such as buprenorphine; or the opioids with no mu-agonism such as pentazocine. Heroin has the greatest potential for abuse because of its rapid onset. Mu receptor agonists with delayed onset of action and longer half-lives (e.g., methadone) have very little impact on mood, and this is the reason why methadone can be used for maintenance therapy instead of the other, more abusive, opioids.

- Mortality rates are significantly reduced from overdose, when patients are treated with methadone or buprenorphine maintenance therapy. MMT and BMT are treatments currently available for opioid-dependent patients to stop drug craving and drug hunger.
- Methadone is a highly regulated Schedule II medication that can be dosed once daily and is only available at specialized methadone maintenance clinics. Buprenorphine (Subutex), the partial mu receptor agonist, binds extremely tightly to the mu receptor. It is a Schedule III drug that has a ceiling effect at which higher doses of the drug cause no additional effects. This **ceiling effect** accounts for why Buprenorphine is **better** than methadone, and also, methadone can be lethal in overdose.
- Naloxone is very effective in treating acute opioid overdose. Orally administered buprenorphine with naloxone (Suboxone) prevents addicts from abusing through injection use. Naloxone is poorly absorbed orally but is well-absorbed intravenously. So when an opioid-dependent patient injects buprenorphine with naloxone, the patient suffers a withdrawal syndrome secondary to naloxone's occupation of the mu receptors.

Multimodal Pain Management Algorithm for Opioid-Dependent Patients

Most patients who are physically dependent on preoperative opioids will need baseline opioid intake in the postoperative period for optimal pain management and to prevent withdrawal reactions. The postoperative baseline opioid requirement is calculated from the preoperative opioid consumption. See Figure 5.2.

- **Opioid-tolerant patients will need larger doses of an opioid to gain adequate pain relief.** Each analgesic regimen should be individualized according to the patient's requirements.
- Postoperative opioids are given parenterally, epidurally, or orally depending on the patient's postoperative physical condition, the extent of the surgical procedure, recovery from the surgical procedure, and if the procedure was done under local or general anesthesia.
- **Preoperative and postoperative NSAIDS and/or adjuvant use will also have significant opioid-sparing effects in this setting.** MMT and BMT therapies **do not** provide sustained analgesia. The analgesic effects last only 4–8hours, and the medications are dosed every 24–48hours. **No evidence indicates that exposure to opioid analgesics during acute pain increases relapse rates.** In fact, the **stress** of unrelieved pain **can trigger relapse.**
- Always alert the MMT/BMT prescribing physician if you end up prescribing any benzodiazepines or opioids because these drugs can be detected in the patient on urine drug screening. Be aware that the combination of opioid agonist treatments (OATs) and other opioids has the potential for respiratory depression, so naloxone should always be available.
- **Always aggressively treat pain with conventional opioid analgesics, and higher opioid analgesic doses at shorter intervals may sometimes be needed. Use**

```
*Continue IR/SR¹ oral opioids preoperatively

*Continue intraspinal opioids via pump intraop.

*Give postop. opioids calculated from preop. opioid

consumption.

•    MMT Patients: MMT + ATC² short-acting opioids³

•    BMT Patients: ATC² BMT q6–8h OR BMT + ATC²

short-acting opioids³ OR stop BMT and add ATC²

short-acting opioids³ OR stop BMT and add MMT +

ATC² short-acting opioids³.

•    Mild Pain: Preop & postop. NSAIDs⁴ + adjuvant⁵

•    Moderate-Severe Pain: Use ATC² short-acting

opioids³

KEY: IR/SR¹: Immediate-release & Sustained Release

opioids. ATC²: Around the clock. Short-acting

opioids³: Codeine, IR Oxycodone, Hydrocodone and

Tramadol. NSAIDs⁴: Ibuprofen, naproxen,

indomethacin, ketorolac, or celecoxib. Adjuvants⁵:

Corticosteroids; Benzodiazepines; Anti-histamines;

Muscle Relaxants and TCAs.
```

Figure 5.2. Preemptive pain management algorithms for patients on methadone maintenance therapy (MMT), buprenorphine maintenance therapy (BMT), or other chronic opioid therapies.

> **continuous scheduled dosing of the opioid rather than as-needed (PRN) dosing. Add short-acting opioid analgesics for MMT patients.**
- Pain management with opioids for BMT patients is complicated because buprenorphine competes with opioid analgesics at the mu receptors. There are several ways in which you can implement pain management in these patients, such as you can request the physician to divide the buprenorphine dose to 6–8hours to take advantage of its short-acting analgesic effects; you can request the physician to continue BMT therapy and titrate a short-acting opioid analgesic; or you can request that the physician discontinue BMT therapy, then temporarily implement opioid analgesia, and finally, restart BMT when opioid analgesia is no longer needed. In the hospital setting, BMT can be replaced with MMT, and then the provider can add short-acting opioids to treat pain. The patient is converted back to BMT, prior to discharge from hospital.
- Patients on oral immediate- and sustained-release opioids should continue taking the medications preoperatively.

- Patients getting intraspinal opioids through an implantable pump should continue with the therapy throughout the perioperative period.
- Patients using transdermal opioid patches should **remove** the patch **prior** to major surgery, to avoid postoperative problems caused by delayed opioid absorption and inflexible dose delivery. Clearly, the patch removal protocol is for anticipated acute pain following major surgery and requires consultation with the patient's physician, to ensure successful and uninterrupted pain management intra and postoperatively. **Immediate-release oral opioid preparations should be provided intraoperatively and postoperatively at equianalgesic doses.** When a dose of one analgesic is equivalent in pain-relieving effects to that of another analgesic, it indicates equianalgesic dosing. This equivalence allows the provider to substitute medications to prevent possible side effects of one of the drugs.
- **Transdermal fentanyl conversion dose calculation to immediate release (IR) oral morphine:** 25μg/h fentanyl patch size, corresponds to <20mg/4h oramorphine; 50μg/h fentanyl patch size, corresponds to 25–30mg/4h oramorphine; 75μg/h fentanyl patch size, corresponds to 40–50mg/4h oramorphine; and 100μg/h fentanyl patch size, corresponds to 55–60mg/4h oramorphine.
- The formula for conversion of oral to IV morphine is 3:1.
- **Conversion dose calculation for morphine to oral immediate release (IR) morphine:** 5mg IM morphine equals 10mg oral morphine; 3.3mg IV morphine equals 10mg oral morphine; 5mg subcutaneous (SC) morphine equals 10mg oral morphine; 1mg epidural morphine equals 10mg oral morphine and 0.1mg intrathecal morphine equals 10mg oral morphine.

FDA SAFETY MEASURES FOR OPIOID MEDICATIONS

- The FDA recently approved a new Risk Evaluation and Mitigation Strategy (REMS) for extended-release (ER) and long-acting (LA) opioid analgesics in the treatment of moderate-to-severe chronic pain to reduce prescription drug abuse, misuse, or over use.
- The drug manufacturing companies are now required to provide FDA-approved and created continuing education (CE) programs to all DEA-registered prescribers ER/LA opioids, with contents on the risks and benefits of opioid therapy plus how to recognize opioid misuse, abuse, and addiction. Provider knowledge assessment and proof of completion of the program is a requirement of this program. The manufacturers also must provide FDA-approved patient education materials regarding safe drug use, storage, disposal, and signs of overdose and subsequent emergency contact instructions.
- The CE programs are mandatory for manufacturers but voluntary or elective for the prescribers. The first such CE program is scheduled for implementation in March 2013. The FDA will audit to ensure that companies achieve FDA-established goals for providers who complete the training, as well as assess the prescribers' understanding of important risk information over time.
- **Drugs requiring REMS:** All morphines (Oramorph), buprenorphine transdermal, fentanyl transdermal (Duragesic), hydromorphone (Exalgo), methadone (Dolophine), morphine and naltrexone combination pill (Embeda), morphine oral (Avinza, Kadian, or MS Contin), SR oxycodone (OxyContin) and oxymorphone (Opana ER).

ANALGESICS SUMMARY

Review Table 5.2.

Table 5.2. Analgesics Summary

Analgesic	Analgesic Doses: All Used PRN

Oral Acetaminophen (Tylenol):
Pregnancy Category B
Strengths available:
325/500mg/tablet
IV Acetaminophen:
	Normal Dose: 325mg/tablet: 2 tabs q6h PRN, maximum 8–10 tablets in 24hours.
	500mg/tablet: 2 caplets/gelcaps q6-8h PRN, maximum 6 caplets/gelcaps/day. Avoid alcohol use.
	Normal Maximum Dose: 3g/day
	Liver Disease Dose: <2g/day
	Chronic Inactive Hepatitis:
	325–650mg **q6-8h**
	Chronic Active Hepatitis or Cirrhosis: 325–650mg **q8h**
	Kidney Disease Dosages:
	  a. S. Creatinine (Cr) <2.0mg/dL: Give normal dose
	  b. S. Cr >2.0mg/dL to Pre-dialysis: 325–650mg **q6-8h**
	  c. Dialysis: 325-650mg **q8h**
	  • Adults and children age ≥13years, weighing ≥50kg: 650mg q6h or 1,000mg q8h, with 1,000mg being the maximum single dose injected.
	  • Adults and children age ≥13years, weighing <50kg: 12.5mg/kg q4-6h or 15mg/kg q6h, with 15mg/kg being the maximum single dose injected.

Aspirin: Pregnancy Category C; Category D in third trimester Strengths available: 81/325mg/tablet	Normal Dose: 325–650mg q4-6h Maximum Dose: 4g/day. Reduce dose in the elderly. Kidney Disease Dose: S. Cr >2mg/dL to Pre-dialysis: Dose Aspirin q6h only. Avoid with cirrhosis and in patients on dialysis. Avoid Aspirin use in Dentistry.
Ibuprofen (Motrin): Pregnancy Category B Strengths available: 200/400/800mg/tablet	Normal Dose: 200–400mg q4-6h Maximum Dose: 1,200mg/day Avoid in Liver and Kidney disease.
Naproxen (Naprosyn): Pregnancy Category B Strengths available: 250/500mg/tablet	Normal Dose: 250–500mg PO q8-12h Maximum Dose: 1,500mg/day Avoid in Liver and Kidney Disease
Celecoxib (Celebrex): Pregnancy Category C; Category D with prolonged use or high dosage. Strengths available: 100/200mg/tablet	Normal Dose: 100-200mg q12h Avoid with Liver or Kidney Disease

Table 5.2. Analgesics Summary (*Continued*)

Analgesic	Analgesic Doses: All Used PRN

Codeine:
Pregnancy Category C
Strengths available:
Tylenol #1:
7.5mg Codeine + 300mg
   Acetaminophen (APAP)
Tylenol #2:
15mg Codeine + 300mg APAP
Tylenol #3: Most prescribed strength.
30mg Codeine + 300mg APAP
Tylenol #4: 60mg Codeine + 300mg
   APAP
	Normal Dose: 30–60mg/1–2 tabs q4-6h. Maximum 12 tabs/24hours and <3g/day of TylenolKidney Disease Dosages:
	a. S. Cr. <2.0mg/dL: Normal dose. Dispense 1–2 Tylenol #3 q4-6h PRN.
	b. S. Cr. >2.0mg/dL to Pre-dialysis: 1–2 Tylenol #2 **q6h**
	c. Dialysis: 1–2 Tylenol #1 q8h
	Liver Disease Dosages:
	a. Mild or chronic inactive Hepatitis: Dose normally: 1–2 Tylenol #3 q4–6h
	b. Moderate-Severe or active Hepatitis: 1–2 Tylenol #2 **q6h**
	c. Cirrhosis: 1–2 Tylenol #1 **q8h**

Morphine: Pregnancy Category C Strength: 10mg/tablet	Normal Dose: Oral: 10–20mg q3-4h. The long-acting forms of Morphine are given q8-12h. IV: 2mg q2-3h Avoid with Liver or Kidney Disease
Hydromorphone (Diluadid): Pregnancy Category C	Normal Dose: Oral dose: 2-4mg q4h Parenteral dose: The usual starting dose of Hydromorphone is 1-2mg subcutaneously (SC) or intramuscularly (IM), every 2 to 3hours as necessary. IV dose: 0.2-1mg injected slowly over 2–3 minutes, q4h Liver/Kidney Disease: Can be used in Liver or Kidney failure
Oral Transmucosal Fentanyl Citrate (OTFC): Pregnancy Category C	Normal Dose: Suck on one 200µg lozenge over 15 minutes. Use another 200µg lozenge after 15 minutes if pain persists. The dose can be repeated for 2–3 pain episodes per day.
Fentanyl Patch:	Dispensed as 25, 50, 75, and 100µg/h Fentanyl patches (containing 2.5, 5, 7.5 and 10mg Fentanyl). **Fentanyl Dose for Patients on Strong Opioids:** Calculate the previous 24h dose asmg/day of oral Morphine. Divide this value by 3 and choose the nearest patch strength inµg/h. Titrate the dose q72h, for optimal relief. **Fentanyl dose for patients on weak/short acting Opioids or Opioid naïve patients:** Start with 25µg/h patch and titrate the dose q72h, for optimal relief.

(continued)

Table 5.2.   Analgesics Summary (*Continued*)

Analgesic	Analgesic Doses: All Used PRN

Oxycodone + APAP (Percocet):
Oxycodone: Pregnancy Category B.
  Acetaminophen + Oxycodone
  (Percocet): Pregnancy Category C
Strengths available:
2.5/325:
2.5mg Oxycodone + 325mg
  Acetaminophen (APAP)
5/325:
5mg Oxycodone + 325mg APAP
  (original tablet)
7.5/325:
7.5mg Oxycodone + 325mg APAP
7.5/500:
7.5mg Oxycodone + 500mg APAP
10/650:
10mg Oxycodone + 650mg APAP
	Normal Dose: One 2.5/325 or 5/325 Percocet
	  tablet **q4-6h**
	Keep the maximum oxycodone dose at 20mg per day
	  and the long-acting forms can be given q8-12h.
	Kidney Disease Dosages:
	  a. Predialysis: One 2.5/325 tab **q6h**
	  b. Dialysis: One 2.5/325 tab **q8h**
	Liver Disease Dose:
	  a. Hepatitis: One 2.5/325 tab **q6h**
	  b. Cirrhosis: One 2.5/325 tab **q8h**

**Hydrocodone + Acetaminophen
  (Vicodin):**
Prganancy Category C
Strengths available:
Each Vicodin tablet contains:
5mg Hydrocodone + 500mg
  Acetaminophen (APAP)
Vicodin ES:
7.5mg Hydrocodone + 500mg APAP
Vicoprofen:
7.5mg Hydrocodone + 200mg
  Ibuprofen.
	Normal Dose: 1–2 tablets **q6h**
	Kidney Disease Dosages:
	  a. Predialysis: 1 tab **q6h**
	  b. Dialysis: 1 tab **q8h**
	Liver Disease Dosages:
	  a. Hepatitis: 1 tab **q6h**
	  b. Cirrhosis: 1 tab **q8h**
	Alert: Do not exceed the maximum daily dose for
	  APAP/NSAID

**Dextropropoxyphene +
  Acetaminophen (Darvocet N or
  Darvocet N 100):**
Pregnancy Category C
Strengths available:
Darvocet N:
50mg Propoxyphene + 325mg
  Acetaminophen.
Darvocet N 100:
100mg Propoxyphene + 650mg
  Acetaminophen.
	Darvocet N Dose:
	1–2 tablets q4h; maximum 600mg Propoxyphene
	  Napsylate/day
	Darvocet N 100 Dose:
	1 tablet q4h; maximum 600mg Propoxyphene
	  Napsylate/day
	Avoid with Kidney/Liver disease
	Alert: Discontinued in the US market.

Meperidine (Demerol):
Pregnancy Category C
Strength: 50mg/tablet
Meperidine should only be used for the
  management of moderate to severe
  acute pain.
	Normal Oral Dose: 50–100mg q4h
	Continuous IV Meperidine: It is administered at a rate
	  of 15–35mg/hr.
	Avoid in Kidney/Liver disease

Tramadol (Ultram):
Pregnancy Category C
Strength available: **Ultracet**
  37.5/325: 37.5mg Tramadol +
  325mg APAP
	Normal Dose: 50–100mg PO q4-6h
	Maximum Tramadol dose per day, in divided doses:
	  400mg
	Avoid in severe Liver and Kidney disease.

Table 5.2. Analgesics Summary (*Continued*)

Analgesic	Analgesic Doses: All Used PRN
Methadone: Pregnancy Category C Methadone is available as 10mg/mL injection or as 5mg/10mg tablets.	Methadone can be given by mouth, per-rectum or as IV/IM/SC injections. The oral to-parenteral dose ratio is 2:1. Duration of action initially is 4–6h, and 8–12h with continued use. **Methadone Normal Dose:** 2.5–10mg oral/IM/SC q4-12hr; the 5mg oral dose given q6-8h, is typical for pain management. **Kidney disease Dose:** Give 50–75% of normal dose in the presence of CrCl <10mL/min. **Liver Disease Dose:** Methadone is not recommended for severe liver disease/cirrhosis. **Elderly Patient Dose:** 2.5mg PO/IM q8-12hr
Oxymorphone (Opana): Pregnancy Category C	**Oxymorphone Dose:** 10mg/day
Buprenorphine (Subutex): Pregnancy Category C	The drug reaches agonist ceiling effect at about 12mg and doses >12–16mg, do not produce any more analgesia. A seven-day buprenorphine supply can be used for cancer-associated pain, and the maximum dose is 20µg/hour.
Pentazocine (Talwin): Pregnancy Category C	**Pentazocine Dose:** 50mg q4h PRN or Pentazocine + APAP: 25/650: 1–2 tabs q4h PRN with maximum Pentazocine dose of 6g/day and maximum acetaminophen dose of 3g/day. **Avoid all** these analgesics in the presence of kidney or liver disease
– Aspirin – NSAIDS – Extra strength Tylenol – Meperidine (Demerol) – Propoxyphene (Darvon) – Pentazocine – Tramadol (Ultram)	
– Regular strength Tylenol – Dose modified Codeine with Tylenol; Oxycodone or Hydrocodone with Tylenol – Hydromorphone (Diluadid) or Fentanyl	These Analgesics **can be used** with Kidney or Liver disease

Odontogenic Infections, Antibiotics, and Infection Management Protocols

ODONTOGENIC INFECTION OVERVIEW AND MANAGEMENT FACTS

Odontogenic infection, when presenting as an abscess, is typically treated, when possible, with incision and drainage (I&D) of the abscess. Antibiotics, pain and fever relief using appropriate analgesics, and removal of the source of infection once the patient has stabilized (e.g., extraction of an infected tooth), are additional steps in the management of odontogenic infections.

FACTORS ASSESSED PRIOR TO ANTIBIOTIC USE

The following factors should be considered, assessed, and evaluated prior to prescribing antibiotics:

- Infection presentation: Determine if the infection is localized or generalized.
- Know the specific organism(s) involved.
- Find out how long the patient has been symptomatic.
- Specific antibiotic facts: Know the half-life, therapeutic window, spectrum of activity, and mechanism of action of the antibiotic. Know if the antibiotic is bactericidal or bacteriostatic. Know where the antibiotic is metabolized and cleared. Know the appropriate dosage and duration of the antibiotic you plan on prescribing. Know the drug-drug interactions (DDIs) between the patient's medications and the antibiotic prescribed, along with the antibiotic side effects, and the immune system status of the patient.
- Know the patient's current liver and kidney status.
- Have in place the mechanisms to maintain the intestinal flora during the antibiotic intake.
- Advice on the water or fluid consumption needed or required with the antibiotic intake. Know if the antibiotic will be affected with food intake.

Dentist's Guide to Medical Conditions, Medications, and Complications, Second Edition. Kanchan M. Ganda.
© 2013 John Wiley & Sons, Inc. Published 2013 by John Wiley & Sons, Inc.

- Consider what negative effect an antibiotic prescription causing severe, persistent vomiting, and/or diarrhea will have in the presence of combined oral contraceptive pill (COCP) intake by the patient.
- Know which antibiotic to use during pregnancy or during breast-feeding.

ODONTOGENIC INFECTIONS: ORGANISMS AND DURATION OF INFECTION

Odontogenic infections usually have a mixed aerobic and anaerobic flora. The most common isolates are gram-positive aerobes, particularly alpha-hemolytic streptococcus. Other isolates include some gram-negative aerobes and a variety of gram-positive and gram-negative anaerobes. Aerobic bacteria are the main isolates in cellulitis-associated infections. The main isolates from abscesses are anaerobic bacteria, particularly bacteroides. In early infections or infections symptomatic for less than three days, the bacteria are predominantly aerobic and gram-positive streptococcus viridans or alpha-hemolytic streptococcus. These organisms respond extremely well to penicillin, clindamycin (the choice for penicillin allergic patients), or cephalosporins. Penicillin VK is the first drug of choice for **early** infections in the non-penicillin allergic patient. Clindamycin or cephalexin (Keflex), are alternate first-choice, early infection drugs, in a severe and mild-moderate penicillin-allergic patient, respectively. As the infection lingers, the patient's defenses take over and the flora changes from being aerobic to becoming anaerobic. Anaerobes are therefore associated with **late** infections or infections symptomatic for more than three days. **Staphylococcus aureus** predominates in **late** infections. However, occasional isolates in early oral infections can also show the presence of staphylococcus aureus. Patients with staphylococcus aureus infection respond extremely well to clindamycin and poorly to penicillin. Clindamycin is the treatment of choice for **late** odontogenic infections. Clindamycin has also **replaced** erythromycin as the drug of choice for patients allergic to penicillin, due to increased bacterial resistance to erythromycin and the increased frequency of CYP3A4 associated DDIs with erythromycin, especially in the medically complex patient that is taking multiple medications.

Periodontal infections are often polymicrobial and anaerobic bacteria predominate. Peri-implant disease is mostly plaque-induced, and bacteria, when isolated, are similar to those associated with periodontal infection. An aerobic flora comprising streptococcus viridans or alpha-hemolytic streptococcus is most commonly associated with dental caries. Dental pulp involvement is associated with a more anaerobic flora. Gram-negative bacilli are more likely to be associated with periapical infections.

Odontogenic Infection and Associated Antibiotic Management Protocol

Infection symptomatic for fewer than three days:

- Immune-competent patients: Start with pen VK/clindamycin (for the penicillin-allergic patient). Use amoxicillin instead of pen VK in the immune-compromised patient.
- Switch to clindamycin (first choice), azithromycin, clarithromycin, penicillin VK, **and** metronidazole (in the immune-competent patient), or amoxicillin **and** metronidazole (in the immune-compromised patient), if there is no response in

24–48 hours. Clarithromycin is also associated with CYP3A4-related DDIs, similar to erythromycin, so my recommendation is to restrict the use of clarithromycin at all times in the medically complex patient who is taking multiple medications.

Infection symptomatic for more than three days:

- Start with clindamycin (first choice).
- Azithromycin, clarithromycin, or pen VK, **and** metronidazole (in the immune-competent patient); amoxicillin and metronidazole (in the immune-compromised patient) are alternate drugs if clindamycin cannot be used.

Periodontal infections:

- Amoxicillin, clindamycin, metronidazole, doxycycline, and tetracycline are antibiotics commonly used for treatment of periodontal infections.

Odontogenic Infection Types

Odontogenic infections can be localized or generalized. Localized infections can present as a dry socket causing pain, swelling, and redness, or as an abscess/localized pus-forming process that can cause fever, malaise, mild prostration, and localized lymphadenopathy.

Generalized/spreading infections can spread into anatomic sites causing cellulitis and septicemia. The patient presents with rapidly progressing fever, chills, malaise, and tachycardia; diffuse swelling at the site of infection; moderate-to-severe prostration; and lymphadenopathy. Always assess the mental status of the patient and patient interactiveness. A spreading infection can be associated with a non-interactive patient status. Also assess the respiratory status in the presence of a generalized infection. Ludwig's angina compromising the sublingual and submandibular spaces should be considered if the patient is experiencing breathing difficulty. Swelling around the eyes or a generalized swelling of the face is localized cellulitis that has the potential for spreading.

Symptoms, Signs, Patient Immunity, and Vital Organ Status

Oral infections cause pain, fever, malaise, minimal-to-significant swelling, and erythema. If the infection is localized and the patient's immunity is adequate, incision and drainage (I&D) and pain medications are all that is needed. Avoid antibiotic use in the **absence** of fever and facial swelling, as the patient's immune system is very capable of eradicating the infection, following I&D. This practice also **reduces** the potential for future antimicrobial resistance. I&D of an abscess improves circulation to the infected tissues and improves the delivery of the minimum inhibitory concentration of the antibiotic to the area, when prescribed. Antibiotics are definitely needed to treat an infection when adequate drainage cannot be achieved, the patient is significantly symptomatic, the infection is spreading (cellulitis) and/or compromising the airways, there is significant lymphadenopathy, and/or the patient is immune compromised. The antibiotic selected should match the organisms that need to be targeted. The practitioner must focus on the patient's immunity and implement the absolute neutrophil count (ANC) guidelines in patients presenting with leucopenia. You can prescribe **either**

Table 6.1. Antibiotics Summary

Antibiotic:	**Antibiotic Doses: Normal/Modified**
Penicillin VK: Pregnancy Category B Strength: 250/500mg/tab	1. **Normal Dose:** 250–500mg PO q6h/qid. **Liver Disease:** No dose alteration. Renal Dose determined using serum creatinine (S.Cr) or creatinine clearance (CrCl). 2. **S.Cr. <2.0mg/dL or CrCl >50mL/min:** Dispense normal dose. 3. **S.Cr 2.0mg/dL to Predialysis or CrCl 10–50mL/min:** 250–500mg q8-12h. 4. **Dialysis:** 250–500 q12-16h.
Liquid Pen VK:	Liquid Pen VK is available as 125mg/5mL or 250mg/5mL strengths. Either strength can be dispensed as 5mL unit dose, available in 100mL or 200mL size bottles. **Adult Rx:** 250–500mg (1–2tsp, 250mg/5mL), q6h/qid x 5 days.
Penicillin G: Pregnancy Category B Strength: 1.2 MU/injection	1. **Normal Dose:** 1.2 million units Penicillin G, IM q12h. 2. **Patient with Both Liver and Kidney Disease:** Use half the normal dose.

Amoxicillin (Amoxyl):
Pregnancy
Category B
Strengths: 250/500/
875mg/capsule
	1. **Normal Dose:**
	  a. 250–500mg PO q8h or 500–875mg PO q12h x 5days.
	  b. **Amoxicillin Oral Suspension:** Powder for oral suspension is available as trihydrate in 125mg/5mL or 250mg/5mL strengths. Either strength can be dispensed as 5mL unit dose and is available in 80mL, 100mL, 150mL or 200mL size bottles.
	  Adult Rx: 250/500mg (1–2tsp, 250mg/5mL), q8h x 5 days.
	  c. **One-day Rx for severe acute infection:** 3g or 6, 500mg capsules twice in 8 hours.
	2. **Premedication:** 2g PO 1h prior to Rx.
	3. **Kidney Disease:**
	  a. **CrCl >30mL/min or a S.Cr <3.3mg/dL:** Dispense the normal dose.
	  b. **CrCl 10–30mL/min or S.Cr >3.3mg/dL to Pre-dialysis:** Prolong the interval and avoid the 875mg tablet: Give 250–500mg PO q12h.
	  c. **CrCl <10mL/min or Dialysis:** Prolong the interval and give 250–500mg PO q24h **after** dialysis.
	4. **Amoxicillin and Liver Disease:** Use normal Amoxicillin dose till compensated cirrhosis. Avoid Amoxicillin use in the presence of decompensated cirrhosis.
	5. **Liver and Kidney Disease:** Can be used. Use renal dose guidelines.

Augmentin: Pregnancy Category B Strength: 250/500mg/capsule	1. **Normal Dose:** 250/500mg q8h. 2. **Kidney Disease:** Decrease total daily dose by 50% with kidney disease.

(continued)

Table 6.1. Antibiotics Summary (*Continued*)

Ampicillin:
Pregnancy
Category B
Strength:
250/500mg/capsule

1. **Normal Dose:** 250–500mg q6h x 5 days.
2. **Ampicillin Oral Suspension:** Powder for Ampicillin oral suspension is available as trihydrate: 125mg/5mL or 250mg/5mL. Either strength is dispensed as 5mL unit dose in 80mL, 100mL, 150mL, or 200mL size bottles. Ampicillin oral suspension is also dispensed as 500mg/5mL; 5mL unit dose, in 100mL size.
3. **Premedication Dose:** 2g IV/IM 30 minutes prior to procedure.

Dicloxacillin:
Pregnancy
Category B
Strength:
250/500mg/capsule

1. **Normal Dose:** 250–500mg qid x 5 days.
2. **Kidney Disease:** Use 50% of the normal daily dose.

Cephalosporins:
Cephalexin (Keflex):
Strength:
250/500mg/capsule
All Cephalosporins are
   Pregnancy
Category B

1. **Cephalexin (Keflex):**
   a. **Normal Dose:** 250–1,000mg q6h/qid x 5 days, maximum 4g/day.
   b. **Cephalexin Oral Suspension:** Powder for Cephalexin oral suspension is available as monohydrate: 125mg/5mL or 250mg/5mL, 5mL unit dose, available in 100mL and 200mL size bottles.
      Adult Rx: 250–1,000mg liquid, q6h/qid x 5 days, maximum 4g/day.
   c. **Kidney Disease Dose:** q12h or q24h.

Cefadroxil (Duricef):
Strength
250/500mg/capsule

2. **Cefadroxil (Duricef):**
   a. **Normal Dose:** 1–2g/day in 2 divided doses x 5days.
   b. **Cephadroxil Oral Suspension:** Cephadroxil oral suspension is dispensed as monohydrate: 125mg/5mL, 250mg/5mL, or 500mg/5mL, available in 50mL and 100mL size bottles.
      Adult Rx: Typically, 1–2g/day liquid, in two divided doses x 5 days.
3. **Premedication Prophylaxis with Cephalexin or Cefadroxil:** 2g PO 1h prior to procedure.
4. **Cefazolin (Ancef):** 1g IV/IM 30 minutes prior procedure.

Ceftriaxone (Rocephin):
Injection

5. **Ceftriaxone (Rocephin):** 1g IV/IM 30 minutes prior to the procedure.
6. **Kidney and Liver Disease:** All Cephalosporins can be used with **50%** total daily dose reduction.

Clindamycin (Cleocin):
Pregnancy
Category B
Strengths:
 150/300mg/tablet
Note: 150/300mg PO is a
   static dose;
   150/300mg IV/IM is a
   cidal dose;
   600mg PO or IV/IM is a
   cidal dose

1. **Normal Dose:** 150–450mg q6-8h/qid PO x 5 days. Best to prescribe the lower dose, 150mg tid or q8h to minimize adverse side effects.
2. **Clindamycin Oral Suspension:** Clindamycin as granules for oral suspension is dispensed as palmitate: 75mg/5mL in 100mL size bottle.
   1. **Adult Rx:** 2–4tsp/dose, tid x 5 days; best to dispense 2tsp/dose, to minimize adverse side effects.
3. **Refractory Cases of Periodontal Infection**: 600mg/day x 7 days.

Table 6.1. Antibiotics Summary (*Continued*)

	4. **Premedication Prophylaxis:**
	  a. 600mg PO 1h prior to treatment.
	  b. 600mg, IV 30 min before procedure.
	5. **Hepatitis:** No dose change.
	6. **Cirrhosis:** Decrease total daily dose by 50%.
	7. **Kidney Disease:** No dose change with kidney disease or renal failure.
	8. **Kidney and Liver Disease:** Can be used with a 50% total daily dose reduction.

Azithromycin (Zithromax/Z-pak): Pregnancy Category B Strength: 250/500/ 600mg/immediate release tablet	**Azithromycin:** 1. **Azithromycin Normal 5-day Dose:** 250mg bid or 500mg HS on day one, then 250mg/day for the next 4 days. 2. **Azithromycin Normal 3-day Dose:** 500mg/day x 3 days. 3. **Azithromycin and Kidney Disease:** No dose change. 4. **Azithromycin and Liver Disease:** No dose adjustments with mild or moderate liver disease and either reduce daily dose or better yet, avoid with severe liver disease. 5. **Azithromycin extended-release suspension (Zmax):** Dispensed as 2g/60mL. The entire 60mL is a onetime dose. 6. **Oral suspension:** Liquid Azithromycin is dispensed as 100 or 200mg/5mL liquid. 7. **Intravenous preparation:** Dispensed as ypholized Azithromycin 500mg/10mL vial.
Clarithromycin (Biaxin): Pregnancy Category C Strength: 250/500mg/immediate release tablet; 500mg extended-release tablets, and 125/250mg/5mL granules for oral suspension.	**Clarithromycin:** 1. **Clarithromycin Normal Dose:** 250 or 500mg bid for 5 days. 2. **Clarithromycin and Kidney Disease:** Decrease the total daily dose by 50%. Best to avoid 3. **Clarithromycin and Liver Disease:** Can be used with normal dose in mild liver disease and dose reduction with moderate–severe liver disease, **only if** kidney status is normal. **Premedication Prophylaxis with Both:** 1. Azithromycin or Clarithromycin, 500mg PO 1h prior to procedure.
Metronidazole (Flagyl): Pregnancy Category B: Metronidazole is safe after 14 weeks gestation: Safety prior to 14 weeks has not been established. Strength: 250/500mg/capsule	1. **Normal Dose:** 250mg q6h or 500mg q8h x 5 days. Best to give lower dose. (250mg) instead of the 500mg dose, to minimize dry mouth and metallic taste. 2. **Alternate Rx for bacterial Infection:** 7.5mg/kg BW (Max. 1g), q6h x 7 days. 3. **"Poor Man's Augmentin":** 250/500mg Pen VK/Amoxicillin + Metronidazole 250mg q6h or 500mg q8h x 5 days. 4. **Pseudomembranous Colitis Treatment:** 250/500mg q8h x 14 days. Repeat one more cycle if infection persists. 5. **Kidney Failure/Dialysis:** 500mg PO q12h, given after dialysis. 6. **Mild Liver Disease**: Normal dose. Moderate/severe Disease: Use 50% total daily dose. 7. **Liver and Kidney Disease:** 250mg q12h.

(continued)

Table 6.1. Antibiotics Summary (*Continued*)

Tetracycline HCL: Pregnancy Category D Strength: 250/500mg per capsule	**Tetracycline HCL:** 1. **Tetracycline HCL Normal Dose:** 250mg qid PO on empty stomach x 5 days. 2. **Tetracycline and Liver/Kidney Disease:** Avoid with liver or kidney disease or both liver and kidney disease.
Doxycycline (Vibramycin): Pregnancy Category D Strength: 50/100mg per capsule	**Doxycycline:** 1. **Doxycycline, 100mg/capsule Normal Dose:** 200mg PO 2 hours prior to bed on day one; 100mg, also 2 hours prior to bed/day for days 2–10. 2. **Doxycycline, 50mg/capsule Normal Dose:** 100mg PO 2 hours prior to bed, on day one; 50mg, also 2 hours prior to bed/day for days 2–10. 3. **Doxycycline with Liver/Kidney Disease:** Normal dose. 4. **Kidney and Liver Disease:** Normal dose. 5. **Doxycycline Oral Suspension:** Powder for oral suspension is dispensed as monohydrate: 25mg/5mL in 60mL size bottle in syrup form or 50mg/5mL, in 30mL or 473mL size bottles. **Adult Rx:** 100mg/200mg loading dose, followed by 50mg/100mg/dose liquid Doxycycline x 10 days.
Vancomycin (Vancocin) HCL Pulvules: Pregnancy Category C **Oral Vancomycin:** 125/250mg per pulvule **IV Vancomycin:** Pregnancy Category C	1. **Vancomycin HCl pulvules for Pseudomembranous Colitis:** 125mg 4 times/day x 10–14 days. Second recurrence is treated with oral vancomycin tapered over 4 weeks, with or without pulse dosing. Pulse dosing prescription: 125mg oral Vancomycin is given q2-3 days, for 2–8 weeks. 2. **Vancomycin for Systemic Infections:** 7.5mg/kg BW or 500mg–1 g IV q6-12h. Kidney Disease: Avoid. Liver Disease: No dose change.
Tigecycline: Pregnancy Category D	**Tigecycline dose:** Recommended dose is 50mg every 12 hours after a 100mg loading dose. If a patient has severe hepatic impairment, a dose of 25mg every 12 hours should be given after a loading dose of 100mg. Doses are given intravenously over 30–60 minutes.
Daptomycin: Pregnancy Category B	**Daptomycin Dose:** Daptomycin is given at a dose of 4mg/kg IV, once daily and dose adjustment is necessary in the presence of renal dysfunction.
Linezolid: Pregnancy Category C	**Linezolid Dose:** **Adults:** 600mg oral/IV, q12h; **Pediatric:** 10mg/kg oral/IV, q8h.

bactericidal or bacteriostatic antibiotics to patients with **mild or moderate** leucopenia-associated **ANC values**. However, **only bactericidal** antibiotics can be used if the patient is presenting with **ANC <500 cells/mm**. The patient's vital organ status or functioning capacity of the liver and the kidneys must also be assessed when prescribing an antibiotic. The liver could affect antibiotic metabolism and the kidney could affect drug elimination.

The liver is the major site of drug metabolism, and knowing how drugs are processed by the liver helps the practitioner make better prescription choices when treating a patient presenting with hepatitis or cirrhosis. Hepatic drug metabolism can be broadly classified into Phase I and Phase II metabolisms. These phases are dependent on two factors: hepatic blood flow and metabolic capacity of the liver. Most of the Phase I metabolism occurs in the cytochromes and involves a number of transformations, including oxidation and methylation, so the parent drug becomes more water soluble to facilitate renal excretion. Fluoroquinolones and flucloxacillin are antibiotics metabolized via this route, as are acetaminophen and corticosteroids. The capacity of the liver to metabolize drugs by the Phase I enzyme systems is compromised when the liver is in failure. The metabolic capacity of the liver has to be decreased by more than 90% before drug metabolism is significantly affected. Phase II metabolism includes glucuronidation and glutathione conjugation. Phase II occurs after Phase I metabolism, **or** it can occur on its own. Phase II metabolism can still occur even in end-stage liver failure. Drugs with first-pass metabolism in patients with decompensated liver cirrhosis require reduction in oral dosages. It is important to note that drug-induced hepatotoxicity is often poorly tolerated by patients with cirrhosis. Consequently, drugs that are metabolized by the liver and/or have potential hepatotoxicity should be avoided and are usually contraindicated in patients with chronic liver disease.

It is important to note that sometimes potentially hepatotoxic drugs may have to be used in patients with liver cirrhosis based on the clinical needs and when no other alternatives are available. The drug dosing is then individualized depending on factors like the patient's nutritional status, renal function, and DDIs. Therefore, it is very important to frequently monitor the liver function as well.

Hydrophilic and lipophilic solubility characteristics of antibiotics (more details follow) can alter drug pharmacokinetics caused by pathophysiological changes common to critical illness. Many hydrophilic antibiotics are excreted unchanged by the kidney, and therefore elimination is limited in renal failure and dosing has to be altered. Many lipophilic antibiotics produce metabolites that require renal elimination, and these metabolites can accumulate in the presence of kidney disease. As such, it is best to be safe and use an antibiotic that clears through the kidney without involving the liver if the patient has hepatitis or cirrhosis, and vice versa, if the patient has underlying kidney disease.

The response to infection(s) largely depends on the patient's medical status and his/her ability to ward off or fight the infection. Diabetes, chemotherapy, radiotherapy, neutropenia, status post splenectomy, chronic steroid use, systemic lupus erythematosus (SLE), HIV/AIDS, compromised hepatic/renal status, leukemia, or severe anemias, are some of the disease states where the patient may respond poorly to an infection. These systemic conditions must be **simultaneously** addressed and controlled with the help of the patient's physician as you manage the odontogenic infection.

ANTIBIOTIC PHARMACOTHERAPEUTIC CONSIDERATIONS AND FACTS FOR ODONTOGENIC INFECTIONS

Antibiotics and Dose-Selection Criteria

The patient's weight or physical characteristics should always be considered when making a decision about what antibiotic dose to prescribe. There is strong evidence that the metabolism and clearance of antibiotics can be affected by the patient's body mass. According to current adult antibiotic dosing practices, an obese patient gets the same antibiotic dose as a very lean patient, even though the body sizes are significantly different. Just as pediatric dosing has always been guided by the patient's body weight, adult dosing should also, for optimal efficacy, take body mass into consideration. Obesity can affect the distribution, protein binding, metabolism, and clearance of antibiotics. This issue is now gaining even more attention because of the increasing prevalence of obesity and antibiotic resistance the world over, making broad standards for antibiotic dosing no longer optimal for all body types. Significantly obese patients may actually need larger doses for an antibiotic to be effective, and underweight patients may actually need lower doses, to decrease the incidence of opportunistic infections, particularly yeast overgrowth in female patients and intestinal flora washout, which can occur with larger-than-required antibiotic doses or when antibiotics are prescribed for longer duration than necessary. When selecting the antibiotic dose, it is my suggestion that you use 140lb as a cutoff. As an example, prescribe 250mg pen VK qid/four times per day, for a patient under 140lb and 500mg qid for a patient over 140lb. Be vigilant when treating a significantly obese patient, as one such patient may not respond adequately to the >140lb dosing and may need to have a further increase in dose, as previously discussed.

Occasionally, a patient can be prescribed a **loading dose** of the antibiotic to achieve an effective dose in the bloodstream quickly before dropping down to a maintenance dose. This becomes particularly important when treating the patient who has a significant septic infection and/or inflammation. Loading dose is a function of volume of distribution of a drug and the desired drug plasma concentration achieved. Inflammatory mediators associated with sepsis cause damage to vascular endothelium, and fluid leaks out into the extravascular space. Loading doses of hydrophilic antibiotics such as β-lactams (penicillins and cephalosporins), glycopeptides (vancomycin), and aminoglycosides (Gentamycin) are **required** in presence of **increased** sepsis-associated extravascular space, smaller volume of distribution, and increased clearance occurring in severe sepsis. Lipophilic antibiotics have greater affinity for fatty tissue, greater volume of distribution, greater protein binding, deeper tissue penetration, and are more likely to be metabolized in the liver. With lipophilic antibiotics such as macrolides, linelozid, fluoroquinolones, and rifampicin, the inflammatory process is less important compared to underlying obesity. Thus, the obese patient will require higher than predicted macrolide dosing for targeted plasma concentration in the initial stages of sepsis. Hydrophilic antibiotics have a much lower protein binding and are more likely to be excreted unchanged by the kidneys.

Minimum Inhibitory Concentration

The minimum inhibitory concentration (MIC) is the smallest concentration of an antimicrobial needed to stop bacterial growth. The MIC needs to be maintained for a period of time to completely eradicate the bacterial infection, and, in turn, this correlates with the duration for which an antibiotic is prescribed. Most infections respond in about two days when treated with an appropriately selected antibiotic. Once the patient responds, the antibiotic should be continued for an additional two to three days to prevent rebounding of the infection. It is more common now to prescribe antibiotics for five days instead of the typical seven days, as this decrease in the duration of antibiotic intake helps preserve the normal balance and ecosystem of the intestinal flora.

Antibiotic Half-Life

The half-life of a drug determines the dosage length or time period for which the drug is prescribed. Penicillin has a shorter half-life when compared with amoxicillin or azithromycin (Zithromax). Penicillin is prescribed qid (four times/day) or q6h (every six hours), as opposed to amoxicillin, which is prescribed tid (three times per day) or q8h (every eight hours). Azithromycin (Zithromax) is taken once a day for three to five days, depending on pill strength. The effect of azithromycin (Zithromax) lasts for about seven days.

Therapeutic Window

For any drug to be effective there is a desired therapeutic concentration range at which the drug needs to be maintained. Above this range the drug becomes toxic, and below this range the drug is not effective.

Antibiotic Spectrum of Activity

Antibiotics may be classified as "narrow spectrum," "broad spectrum," or "extended spectrum," based upon their range of effectiveness.

Narrow-spectrum antibiotics: Narrow-spectrum antibiotics are active against a limited group of microbes and exhibit lower toxicity to the host. The spectrum of activity includes mostly gram-positive bacteria and few, if any, gram-negative bacteria. **Penicillin** is a narrow-spectrum antibiotic with just these properties.

Narrow-spectrum antibiotics are used for the treatment of a specific infection when the causative organism is known. In doing so, the narrow-spectrum antibiotic does **not** kill as many of the normal microorganisms in the body as the broad-spectrum antibiotic would. Thus, a narrow spectrum antibiotic has the advantage of causing **less** superinfection and **less** bacterial resistance, as it deals with only the specific bacteria it targets. The disadvantages of narrow spectrum antibiotics are that they can be used only if the causative organism is identified. So if the drug is not chosen very carefully, the antibiotic may not actually kill the microorganism causing the infection. Narrow spectrum antibiotics should always be the **first** choice when treating oral infections that may be early/simple/infections of less than three days' duration **or** late/complex/infections of more than three days' duration, as the bacterial spectrum is frequently easy to establish by knowing the location, duration, and severity of infection. **Narrow spectrum members** include penicillin VK, azithromycin, clarithromycin, clindamycin, erythromycin, and vancomycin.

Broad-spectrum antibiotics: Broad-spectrum antibiotics successfully treat a wider range of both gram-positive and gram-negative systemic, enteric, and urinary tract pathogens. They tend to have higher toxicity to the host, and may be used to treat a variety of bacterial infections. They are of importance in the treatment of potentially serious illnesses where the patient can become significantly ill and/or succumb if the broad-spectrum antibiotic is not initiated quickly. Broad-spectrum antibiotics are also useful for drug-resistant bacteria that do not respond to other, narrower-spectrum antibiotics. In superinfections where there are multiple types of bacteria causing illness, this warrants either a broad-spectrum antibiotic or combination antibiotic therapy.

A clear advantage to the use of broad-spectrum antibiotics, when compared with narrow spectrum antibiotics, is that there is less of a need to identify the infecting pathogen with real certainty before starting treatment. On the other hand, a broad-spectrum antibiotic will have a more profound effect on the normal intestinal flora; there is potential for drug resistance and an increased risk of developing childhood asthma if a child has received broad-spectrum antibiotics during the first year of life.

An ideal antimicrobial medication should be highly toxic to the microbe, nontoxic to the host, not interfere with the ability of the host to fight other diseases, and not lead to the development of drug resistance. **Broad-spectrum members** include amino-glycosides, amoxicillin + clavulanate potassium (Augmentin), amoxicillin, ampicillin, carbenicillin, cephalosporins, chloramphenicol, ciprofloxacin, dicloxacillin, levofloxacin, streptomycin, sulfonamides, and tetracyclines. Broad-spectrum members amoxicillin and ampicillin are also sometimes labeled **"extended spectrum"** penicillins because they are effective against almost all gram-positive organisms and some gram-negative bacteria, thus falling short compared to the other broad spectrum members, but with a wider spectrum compared to the narrow spectrum antibiotics. See Table 6.2.

It is best to target early infections (infection symptomatic less than three days), with penicillin VK in the immune-competent patient, amoxicillin in the immune-compromised patient, and clindamycin in the penicillin-allergic patient. It is best to treat late infections (infection symptomatic more than three days) with clindamycin, azithromycin, clarithromycin, or pen VK plus metronidazole or amoxicillin plus metronidazole, as previously discussed.

Bactericidal and Bacteriostatic Activity

Bactericidal drugs kill bacteria by inhibiting the bacterial cell wall synthesis, so bactericidal drugs kill cells that are actively growing. Bacteriostatic antibiotics are protein-synthesis inhibitors that prevent bacterial growth, and thus allow the patient's immune system (host phagocytic activity) ultimately to eradicate the bacteria. Cidal and static antibiotics should never be prescribed together because with the cidal drugs needing active bacterial growth and the static drugs stopping bacterial growth, a cidal drug is made **less** effective in the presence of a static drug.

On occasion you may encounter an oral infection in a patient on a long-term, daily, single-dose antibiotic: for example, tetracycline or minocycline (bacteriostatic drugs) for acne management. You will need to prescribe a bacteriostatic antibiotic from **another** antibiotic family to treat the oral infection, such as clindamycin or azithromycin, which are also bacteriostatic. The newly prescribed static antibiotic can be taken **along** with the tetracycline/minocycline. However, a **six-hour interval** must be maintained between the static tetracycline/minocycline and a cidal antibiotic, such as single-dose amoxicillin that you might plan on using for premedication prophylaxis.

Another scenario for antibiotic selection could be that you encounter a patient taking the bactericidal drug trimethoprim-sulfamethoxazole (Bactrim), once every morning for Pneumocystis Jirovecii pneumonia (formally called PCP pneumonia). An early oral infection in a patient who is not allergic to penicillin can be treated with bactericidal antibiotic amoxicillin, as the patient is immune compromised. Late infections require clindamycin, but this will be incorrect as it is a bacteriostatic antibiotic that will need to be taken three or four times per day, and one of the doses will interfere with Bactrim. Alternatively, you could go ahead with amoxicillin + metronidazole or azithromycin,

Table 6.2.   Antibiotics: Mechanism of Action, Solubility Characteristics, and Spectrum of Activity

Antibiotic	MOA: Bactericidal or Bacteriostatic	Solubility Characteristics: Hydrophilic Or Lipophilic	Spectrum of Activity: Narrow, Broad or Extended Spectrum
Aminoglycosides	Cidal	Hydrophilic	Broad
Amox + Clavulanic acid	Cidal	Hydrophilic	Broad
Amoxicillin	Cidal	Hydrophilic	Extended
Ampicillin	Cidal	Hydrophilic	Extended
Azithromycin	Static	Lipophilic	Narrow
Cephalosporins	Cidal	Hydrophilic	Extended
Chloramphenicol	Static	Lipophilic	Broad
Clarithromycin	Static	Lipophilic	Narrow
Clindamycin	**Oral 150mg or 300mg dose:** Static **Any IV/IM dose or 600mg oral:** Cidal	Lipophilic	Narrow
Daptomycin	Cidal	Hydrophilic	Narrow
Dicloxacillin	Cidal	Hydrophilic	Broad
Erythromycin	Static	Lipophilic	Narrow
Linezolid	Static	Lipophilic	Narrow
Metronidazole	Cidal	Lipophilic	Narrow
Penicillin VK	Cidal	Hydrophilic	Narrow
Quinolones	Cidal	Lipophilic	Broad
Sulfonamides	Static	Hydrophilic	Broad
Tetracyclines	Static	Lipophilic	Broad
Tigecycline	**Mostly Static; Cidal and Static for Strep. Pneumoniea**	Lipophilic	Broad
Vancomycin	Cidal	Hydrophilic	Narrow

once per day, but given at least six hours apart from Bactrim. My suggestion is for the patient to take Bactrim in the morning and azithromycin in the evening, so both antibiotics work optimally for the patient.

Protein Synthesis Inhibitors

Bacteria have ribosomal subunits 30S and 50S. Specific bacteriostatic antibiotics selectively target these subunits. Tetracycline, streptomycin, and kanamycin target the 30S subunit; erythromycin, chloramphenicol, and clindamycin target the 50S subunit.

Antibiotic Resistance Mechanism

Bacterial resistance to the penicillins occurs through the production of beta-lactamase, which has the ability to break the beta-lactam ring structure of penicillin. This prevents penicillin from reaching its binding sites. Penicillin is ineffective against gram-negative infections because it cannot penetrate the multilayer gram-negative bacterial cell wall. Beta-lactamase stable antibiotics, augmentin (amoxicillin + clavulanic acid), and clindamycin are antibiotics that work against the beta-lactamase–producing bacteria. Clavulanic acid has the beta-lactam ring that acts as a decoy for the enzyme. The enzyme destroys this ring, thus letting amoxicillin target the bacteria.

Antibiotic Drug-Drug Interactions

The DDI could be with dietary items, as with tetracycline and metal cations. When tetracycline is taken with milk of magnesia, Tums, or Mylanta, it gets precipitated out in the gastrointestinal tract. The antibiotic does not get absorbed and never reaches the bacteria.

Antibiotics and Allergy

Always ask the patient about allergies to antibiotics. Determine whether the reaction was mild, moderate, or severe. Clindamycin is the antibiotic of choice for a patient allergic to penicillin VK or any other member of the penicillin family. The penicillins and the cephalosporins share a common chemical structure; consequently, patients presenting with severe or anaphylactoid-type allergy to the penicillins can have 5–15% cross-reactivity with the cephalosporins. Clindamycin, azithromycin (Zithromax), or clarithromycin (Biaxin) are alternate drugs that can be prescribed instead.

Antibiotics and Intestinal Bacterial Flora

Any antibiotic, when used in large doses or for prolonged periods, has the potential to eradicate the intestinal bacterial flora, cause diarrhea, clostridium difficile overgrowth, and pseudomembranous colitis. It is suggested that you always appropriately dose antibiotics, match antibiotic spectrum of activity to the type of organisms involved so the infection is rapidly eradicated, and recommend the use of probiotics or acidophilus-containing yogurt with the antibiotic, because this will maintain the bacterial flora and minimize or prevent this very untoward side effect.

Antibiotics and Water/Fluid Consumption

Always have the patient drink 6–8 glasses of water when taking an antibiotic. This will help flush the kidneys and prevent adverse effects caused by poor antibiotic clearance and accumulation of toxic metabolites. Always remember that dehydration impairs the renal clearance of drugs.

Oral Antibiotics and Oral Contraceptives

Routinely, oral contraceptives are absorbed into the bloodstream and delivered to the liver. They are inactivated in the liver and delivered back to the gut where the intestinal bacteria reactivate the birth-control pill thus rendering it effective. Oral antibiotics can only decrease the potency of combined oral contraceptive pills (COCPs) or progesterone-only contraceptive pills when antibiotics cause severe persistent diarrhea or vomiting, essentially "washing out" the pills. It is only then that the patient will have to use extra barrier protection until the end of the next cycle to prevent pregnancy. It is now well documented that certain medications such as rifampin, antiseizure medications, or azole antifungals that induce cytochrome P450 enzyme system, do affect the potency of just the COCPs containing estrogen and progesterone, as these medications negatively affect the metabolism of estrogen and not progesterone. So while on these enzyme-inducer medications in combination with COCPs, the patient will have to use barrier protection to prevent pregnancy. Antibiotics prescribed in the dental setting are **not** CYP450 enzyme inducers and do **not** affect COCP potency, and **routine** antibiotic use **not** associated with severe persistent diarrhea or vomiting does **not** call for warning the patient about extra barrier protection post antibiotic use. Always enter a case note in the record stating that the patient has been so informed.

Antibiotics and Breast-Feeding

Minimize the use of antibiotics with breast-feeding because of the risk of altering the baby's intestinal flora. Excessive or inappropriate use of antibiotics may promote growth of resistant pathogens. As previously discussed, there is an increased risk of developing childhood asthma in children who receive broad-spectrum antibiotics during their first year of life, so be careful as you prescribe. When antibiotic use is absolutely needed, have the patient take the antibiotic **after** the feed or have the mother "pump and dump" the breast milk for the duration of antibiotic intake.

ANTIBIOTICS USED IN DENTISTRY

Antibiotic Classification

Antibiotics can be classified in accordance with:

- **Spectrum of activity** (e.g., narrow-spectrum or broad-spectrum antibiotics)
- **Solubility characteristics**
- **Chemical structure**

Classification by Solubility Characteristics

Antibiotics can be classified according to solubility characteristics into hydrophyllic and lipophyllic antibiotics. Hydrophilic antibiotics are mostly affected with the pathophysiological changes seen in critically ill patients with increased volumes of distribution and altered drug clearance related to changes in creatinine clearance. Lipophilic antibiotics have lesser volume of distribution alterations but may develop altered drug clearances.
  Examples of hydrophilic antibiotics:

- **Aminoglycosides:** amikacin, arbekacin, gentamicin, kanamycin, neomycin, netilmicin, paromomycin, rhodostreptomycin, streptomycin, tobramycin, and apramycin.
- **β-lactams:** penicillin derivatives and cephalosporins.
- **Glycopeptides:** vancomycin, teicoplanin, telavancin, bleomycin, ramoplanin, and decaplanin.
- **Polymyxins:** colistin.

Examples of lipophilic antibiotics:

- **Fluoroquinolones:** ciprofloxacin, clinafloxacin, gatifloxacin, levofloxacin, lomefloxacin, norfloxacin, ofloxacin, sparfloxacin, and trovafloxacin.
- **Macrolides:** erythromycin, azithromycin, and clindamycin.
- **Lincosamides:** lincomycin and clindamycin.
- **Tigecycline:** an injectible antibiotic that is structurally similar to tetracycline.

Antibiotic Classification by Chemical Structure

- *β*-**lactams: Penicillin derivatives:** penicillin VK, penicillin G, amoxicillin, amoxicillin + clavulanic acid (Augmentin), ampicillin, dicloxacillin, benzathine penicillin, nafcilin, oxacillin, and methicillin. **Cephalosporins:** cephalexin (Keflex), cephadroxyl (Duricef), cephazolin (Ancef), ceftriaxone (Rocephin), cephalothin, cephapirin, cephradine, cefaclor, cefamandole, cefonicid, ceforanide, cefotetan (Cefotan/Apatef), cefoxitin (Mefoxin), cefuroxime, cefcapene, cefdaloxime, cefditoren, cefetamet, cefixime, cefmenoxime, cefodizime, cefoperazone, cefotaxime, cefpimizole, cefpodoxime, ceftibuten, cefclidine, cefepime, cefluprenam, cefozopran, cefpirome, and cefquinome.
- **Lincosamides:** clindamycin.
- **Macrolides:** erythromycin, azithromycin, clarithromycin, dirithromycin, and telithromycin.
- **Nitroimidazoles:** metronidazole (Flagyl).
- **Tetracyclines:** tetracycline HCL, doxycycline (Vibramycin), minocycline, and oxytetracycline.
- **Glycopeptides:** vancomycin.
- **Glycylcycline:** tigecycline.
- **Fluoroquinolones:** ciprofloxacin, levofloxacin, clinafloxacin, gatifloxacin, lomefloxacin, norfloxacin, ofloxacin, sparfloxacin, and trovafloxacin.
- **Aminoglycosides:** gentamicin, amikacin, kanamycin, streptomycin, tobramycin, and neomycin.
- **Dichloroacetic Acid Derivative:** chloramphenicol.
- **Lipopeptides:** daptomycin.
- **Oxazolidinones:** linezolid.
- **Sulfonamides:** sulfadiazine, sulfadoxine, sulfamethizole, sulfamethoxazole, sulfanilamide, sulfasalazine, sulfisoxazole, and dapsone.

Generally, penicillins, cephalosporins, clindamycin, macrolides, metronidazole, tetracyclines, and vancomycin are the antibiotics used in the dental setting and only specific members from each class that are used in dentistry will be discussed here in great detail. Penicillins, cephalosporins, clindamycin, fluoroquinolones, macrolides, tetracyclines, and aminoglycosides are most often used in the medical setting. Additional drug classes have been included to complete the list; to provide the dental student taking board exams with updated information on antibiotics that were of importance once; and to provide the dental practitioner with information on antibiotics gaining greater importance in the management of specific and sometimes serious systemic infections.

PENICILLINS

Overview

The penicillins are the oldest class of antibiotics and they have a common chemical structure that they share with the cephalopsorins. The two groups are classed as the beta-lactam antibiotics and are bacteriocidal in action. The penicillins can be further subdivided. The natural pencillins are based on the original penicillin G structure; penicillinase-resistant penicillins, especially methicillin and oxacillin, are active even in the presence of the bacterial enzyme that inactivates most natural penicillins. Aminopenicillins, such as ampicillin and amoxicillin, have an extended spectrum of action compared with the natural penicillins; extended spectrum penicillins are effective against a wider range of bacteria. These generally include coverage for Pseudomonas aeruginosa.

Penicillins are hydrophilic, beta-lactam **bactericidal** antibiotics that cause death of the bacteria by inhibiting the cell wall synthesis and are therefore known as cell-wall synthesis inhibitors. Gram-negative bacteria are generally less susceptible to cell-wall synthesis inhibitors, compared with the gram-positive bacteria, because cell wall synthesis inhibitor antibiotics fail to reach the cell wall as they are blocked by the gram-negative outer membrane. Penicillins cross the placenta and are distributed in the breast milk. This is an important point to remember especially when prescribing any one of the penicillins to a lactating mother. All penicillins primarily have a **renal** elimination. Penicillins can cause an allergic reaction in some patients. Allergy toward one member of the penicillin family indicates allergy toward all other members of the family. Allergies are more common with parenterally administered penicillins, and less common with the orally administered penicillins. When planning on using any of the penicillins in the renal-compromised patient, you need to reduce the total daily **dose or increase** the dosing **interval**. My suggestions always are to keep the pill or dose strength unchanged, but prolong the interval of intake as it is less confusing and easier to implement. Alternatively, you could use a drug like clindamycin instead. Clindamycin can be safely used in a renal-compromised patient, even in the presence of dialysis or end-stage renal disease (ESRD). You can also use the full dose of azithromycin to treat an infection in a renal-compromised patient, because azythromycin has minimal urinary excretion. All oral penicillins should be taken **one hour prior** to eating **or one hour after eating**, to prevent binding of the penicillins to food and avoid acid inactivation.

Penicillin Types

- **The Natural Penicillins:** The natural penicillins are based on the original penicillin-G structure. Penicillin-G types are effective against gram-positive strains of streptococci, staphylococci, and some gram-negative bacteria such as meningococcus. Members include, penicillin VK, penicillin G, procaine penicillin G, and benzathine penicillin.
- **AminoPenicillins:** AminoPenicillins such as amoxicillin and ampicillin have an extended spectrum of action compared with the natural penicillins. Extended-spectrum penicillins are effective against a wider range of bacteria.
- **Penicillinase-resistant Penicillins:** Penicillinase-resistant penicillins, particularly dicloxacillin, nafcilin, oxacillin, and methicillin, are active even in the presence of the bacterial enzyme that inactivates most natural penicillins.

The natural form of the drug is penicillin G, and it is a narrow spectrum drug with limited action against gram-negative bacteria. The semisynthetic forms, amoxicillin and ampicillin, are derived from penicillin G and are broad-spectrum drugs that target both gram-positive and gram-negative bacteria. Penicillin and penicillin-derived drugs have a characteristic beta-lactam ring structure that is used to disrupt bacterial cell wall synthesis.

Many bacteria produce enzymes called beta-lactamases or penicillinases, which can destroy the beta-lactam ring structure. To prevent the breakdown of the drug by bacterial enzymes, clavulanic acid is often added to semisynthetic penicillins, such as the combination of amoxicillin and clavulanic acid, which is marketed as Augmentin. Other cell-wall inhibitors include cephalosporin, vancomycin, and bacitracin.

Penicillin VK

Penicillin VK Spectrum of Activity

Penicillin VK is a **narrow-spectrum bactericidal** antibiotic that is effective against most gram-positive bacteria and only targets a few gram-negative cocci. Pen VK has a large therapeutic window and minimal drug interactions, if any. Being a narrow-spectrum antibiotic, pen VK causes minimal disturbance to the intestinal flora. Pen VK is an ideal antibiotic for treating infections that have been symptomatic for less than three days.

Penicillin VK: Drug Uptake and Clearance

After oral ingestion, peak serum levels occur within one hour and almost the entire drug is excreted unchanged through the kidneys. The dose must be adjusted in renal failure. **Penicillin VK is in Pregnancy Category B.**

Penicillin VK Dosing

1. **Penicillin VK prescription for adults and children older than 12 years of age:**
   a. **Rx: Pen VK:** 250mg or 500mg/tab
      Disp: 20 tablets
      Sig: 250mg or 500mg q6h/qid × 5days
   b. **Liquid pen VK dosing:** Liquid Pen VK is available as 125mg/5mL or 250mg/5mL strengths. Either strength can be dispensed as 5mL unit dose, available in 100mL or 200mL size bottles.
      Adult Rx: 250–500mg (1–2tsp, 250mg/5mL), q6h/qid × 5 days.
2. **Pen VK with kidney disease:**
   a. **In the presence of serum creatinine <2.0mg/dL or the CrCl is >50mL/min:** Pen VK is dosed normally at 250–500mg PO **q6h**. As previously stated, by prolonging the interval but keeping the pill strength the same as in a healthy patient, you end up decreasing the **total** dose intake **for** the **day.**
   b. **In the presence of CrCl 10–50mL/min or serum creatinine between 2.0mg/dL to predialysis:** Pen VK is dosed at 250–500mg **q8-12h.**
   c. **In the dialysis patient:** Pen VK is dosed at 250–500 **q12-16h.**
3. **Pen VK with liver disease:** No dose alteration is needed.

Penicillin G

Penicillin G Facts

Penicillin G, a **narrow-spectrum** antibiotic, is mainly excreted through the kidneys when the renal status is normal. If the renal status is compromised, the liver becomes the major route of excretion via bile. Penicillin G **can be prescribed** for treatment of infection with a 50% total daily dose reduction in a patient with a compromised liver **and** kidney status. **Penicillin G is in Pregnancy Category B.**

Penicillin G Dose

1.2 MU (million units) penicillin G, IM q12h.

Amoxicillin

Amoxicillin Spectrum of Activity

Amoxicillin is broad-spectrum penicillin, but on occasion, amoxicillin may also be listed as extended-spectrum penicillin. It is **less** effective against gram-positive cocci compared to pen VK and has a **similar** coverage to penicillin against anaerobic bacteria. It does provide coverage against **gram-negative enteric** bacteria, which is of importance in the immune-compromised patient, but oral infections in the immune-competent patient do not require this coverage.

Amoxicillin Drug Uptake

Amoxicillin is **better absorbed** from the gut and has **more stable** blood concentrations over time, compared to penicillin. Amoxicillin is metabolized in the liver and excreted through the kidneys, and the dose must be adjusted in the renal-compromised patient.

Amoxicillin Use

Amoxicillin is **the** antibiotic recommended by the American Heart Association (AHA) for the prevention of subacute bacterial endocarditis (SBE) in patients not allergic to the penicillins. Amoxicillin can be prescribed for infections symptomatic for less than three days, but because it is an extended-spectrum antibiotic, it is suggested that you prescribe pen VK instead in the immune-competent patient. This conscious effort to prescribe a narrow spectrum antibiotic will prevent the occurrence of antibiotic resistance. However, amoxicillin should be considered the first drug of choice when treating oral infections in an immune-compromised, non-penicillin allergic patient, because gram-negative enteric bacteria may be present at the infection site. **Amoxicillin is in Pregnancy Category B.**

Amoxicillin Prescriptions

Amoxicillin is prescribed tid (three times per day) or q8h (every 8hr) because it has a longer half-life compared with pen VK. Amoxicillin can be prescribed in the following ways:

1. **Oral infection Rx:**
   a. **Rx: Amoxicillin** 250, 500, or 875mg/capsule

Disp: Variable.

Sig: 250/500mg q8h or 500–875mg PO q12h × 5days.

Note: The 875mg tablet should not be used in patients with CrCl <30mL/min or the patient with a serum creatinine >3.3mg/dL.

b. **Amoxicillin oral suspension:** Powder for oral suspension amoxicillin is available as trihydrate in 125mg/5mL or 250mg/5mL strengths. Either strength can be dispensed as a 5mL unit dose and is available in 80mL, 100mL, 150mL, or 200mL size bottles.

Adult Rx: 250/500mg (1–2tsp, 250mg/5mL), q8h × 5 days.

2. A high-dose, one-day, short-course of amoxicillin can be used for treatment of a **very symptomatic acute** dento-alveolar abscess. The one-day course has been found to be as effective as the conventional five-day, 250mg qid course of penicillin VK.

Rx: Amoxicillin 500mg/capsule.

Disp: 12 capsules.

Sig: Take 3g (6, 500mg capsules) amoxicillin twice for one day only, keeping an 8h interval between the two doses.

3. **Amoxicillin for premedication prophylaxis:**

Rx: Amoxicillin 2g PO 1h prior to procedure

4. **Amoxicillin dose guidelines with kidney disease:**

a. **CrCl >30mL/min or a serum creatinine <3.3mg/dL:** Dispense the normal dose of amoxicillin, 250–500mg PO **q8h.**

b. **CrCl 10–30mL/min or a serum creatinine >3.3mg/dL to predialysis:** Prolong the interval and avoid using the 875mg tablet. Rx: 250–500mg PO **q12h.**

c. **CrCl <10mL/min or dialysis:** Prolong the interval: **Rx:** 250–500mg PO **q24h.** The dose during hemodialysis is the same as that given for CrCl <10mL/min and the dose must be given **after** completion of dialysis on the days of dialysis.

    Note: When treating an infection in a renal-compromised patient who is not yet on dialysis, you need to prescribe reduced-dose amoxicillin for **five days.** But once the patient is on dialysis, you can prescribe a **single** 2g amoxicillin dose if the patient needs amoxicillin for premedication prior to dentistry. Remember that this dose is given for treatment that is scheduled on the "off-day" of dialysis, and the drug can do no harm as the patient has end-stage kidney disease. The drug will be completely cleared when dialysis occurs the next day. However, you **cannot** use amoxicillin premedication prophylaxis dose **in the predialysis renal-compromised patient**, because the drug will not be cleared appropriately, resulting in accumulation.

5. **Amoxicillin dose with Liver disease:** The dose of Amoxicillin does not need to be adjusted even in the presence of compensated cirrhosis but you must avoid Amoxicillin use with decompensated cirrhosis.

Amoxicillin can be used in a patient with **both** kidney and liver disease, with dose adjustments according to the renal guidelines.

Amoxicillin-Clavulanic Acid (Augmentin)

Augmentin Spectrum of Activity

The beta-lactamase (penicillinase) inhibitor potassium clavulanate extends amoxicillin's spectrum of activity to include beta-lactamase–producing strains of staphylococcus aureus, haemophilus influenzae, and many strains of enteric gram-negative bacilli.

Amoxicillin plus clavulanic acid (Augmentin) is therefore classified as a broad spectrum antibiotic. This combination is useful for the oral treatment of bite wounds, otitis media, sinusitis, some lower respiratory infections, and urinary tract infections.

Augmentin Adverse Effects

Augmentin can very easily wash out the intestinal bacterial flora, causing a higher incidence of diarrhea and other gastrointestinal symptoms compared with amoxicillin alone. Therefore, Augmentin can increase the effectiveness of warfarin (Coumadin). It is suggested that you minimize the use of Augmentin because of its side effects and cost. **Augmentin is in** Pregnancy Category **B**.

Augmentin Dosing

Each Augmentin capsule contains 125mg clavulanic acid and 250/500/875mg amoxicillin.

1. **Rx: Augmentin** 250mg or 500mg/tablet
   Disp: 15
   Sig: 250/500mg q8h × 5days
2. **Augmentin dose with kidney disease:** Decrease the total daily dose by at least 50% in renal-compromised patients.

Ampicillin

Ampicillin Spectrum of Activity and Overview

Ampicillin is a semisynthetic penicillin, and, like amoxicillin, it is classified as a broad-spectrum or extended-spectrum antibiotic. It is as effective as penicillin G in pneumococcal, streptococcal, and meningococcal infections.

Ampicillin is also active against many strains of salmonella, shigella, proteus mirabilis, and escherichia coli along with most strains of haemophilus influenzae. Some strains of H. influenzae, however, are now resistant to ampicillin, and the drug is not effective for the treatment of infections caused by penicillinase-producing staphylococci. Aminoglycosides or quinolones plus a beta-lactum with significant gram-negative coverage are now more effective against pseudomonas infection, when compared with ampicillin alone.

Adverse Effects

Rashes are more frequent with ampicillin than with the other penicillins.

Drug Uptake

Take ampicillin one hour prior to or one hour after a meal to ensure proper absorption. Ampicillin does concentrate in the bile, but the major excretion occurs through the kidneys. Use caution in the presence of liver disease. **Ampicillin is in** Pregnancy Category **B**.

Ampicillin Dosing

1. **Rx: Ampicillin** 250mg or 500mg/capsule
    Disp: 20 capsules
    Sig: 250–500mg q6h × 5days
    b. Ampicillin oral suspension: Powder for ampicillin oral suspension is available as trihydrate: 125mg/5mL or 250mg/5mL. Either strength is dispensed as 5mL unit dose in 80, 100, 150, or 200mL size bottles. Ampicillin oral suspension is also dispensed as 500mg/5mL; 5mL unit dose, in 100mL size.
    Adult Rx: 250–500mg liquid, q6h × 5days.
2. For premedication prophylaxis in patients unable to take oral preparations
    Rx: Ampicillin 2.0g, IV/IM 30min prior to procedure
3. **Ampicillin dose with kidney disease:** The total daily dosage of ampicillin should be **decreased** by at least 50% in the renal-compromised patient.

Dicloxacillin

Dicloxacillin is a beta-lactamase–resistant, broad-spectrum, semisynthetic penicillin that is effective against penicillinase-producing staphylococcus infection.

Dicloxacillin Drug Alert

Dicloxacillin increases the effectiveness of anticoagulants.

Dicloxacillin Dosing

1. **Normal dose:** 250–500mg qid × 5days
2. **Dicloxacillin dose with kidney disease:** As with all penicillins, use dicloxacillin with caution in the renal-compromised patient and decrease the total daily dose by at least 50%.

CEPHALOSPORINS
Cephalosporins Spectrum of Activity and Overview

Cephalosporins, like the penicillins, contain a beta-lactam chemical structure and are cell-wall synthesis inhibitors. Consequently, there are patterns of cross-resistance and cross-allergenicity among the drugs in these classes. They are classified as hydrophilic, **broad-spectrum** antibiotics that are completely cleared through the renal system. Cephalosporins generally have a wide therapeutic index, and the dose-lowering guidelines for cephalosporine in the presence of renal dysfunction are consequently less stringent when compared with those in place for aminoglycosides in the presence of kidney disease. Patients with combined liver and kidney disease need **greater** reduction in dose than do patients with isolated renal dysfunction.

Cephalosporins are grouped into "**generations**" by their antimicrobial activities. Each generation has a broader spectrum of activity than the one before. In addition, cefoxitin is highly active against anaerobic bacteria, which offers utility in treatment of abdominal infections. Cephalopsorins are usually the preferred agents for surgical prophylaxis.

The first generation of cephalosporins has excellent coverage against most gram-positive organisms and poor coverage against most gram-negative organisms and anaerobes. The first-generation members include cefadroxil, cefazolin, cephalexin, cephalothin, cephapirin, and cephradine.

The second generation of cephalosporins has an expanded gram-negative spectrum, in addition to the gram-positive spectrum of the first-generation cephalosporins. Significant variation exists among the second-generation cephalosporins in regard to their spectrums of activity against gram-negative bacteria; hence susceptibility testing is generally required to determine sensitivity. The second-generation members include cefaclor, cefamandole, cefonicid, ceforanide, cefotetan (Cefotan/Apatef), cefoxitin (Mefoxin), and cefuroxime.

The third generation of cephalosporins has much more expanded gram-negative activity, but some members of this group have decreased activity against gram-positive organisms. They have convenient dosing schedules, but they are expensive. The third-generation drugs cross the blood-brain barrier and may be used to treat meningitis and encephalitis. Third-generation members include cefcapene, cefdaloxime, cefditoren, cefetamet, cefixime, cefmenoxime, cefodizime, cefoperazone, cefotaxime, cefpimizole, cefpodoxime, ceftibuten, and ceftriaxone.

The fourth generation of cephalosporins includes extended-spectrum drugs with similar activity against gram-positive organisms, as with first-generation cephalosporins. They have a greater resistance to beta-lactamases than the third-generation cephalosporins. Many fourth-generation cephalosporins can cross the blood-brain barrier and are effective in the management of meningitis. The fourth-generation members include cefclidine, cefepime, cefluprenam, cefozopran, cefpirome, and cefquinome.

The first-generation cephalosporins have very good bone penetration and increased activity against staphylococcus aureus. They are an excellent choice for joint prosthesis prophylaxis. Cephalosporins should **not** be prescribed to patients with an anaphylactoid reaction toward penicillins because there is 5–15% cross-reactivity with the cephalosporins.

The first-generation cephalosporins dispensed in oral dose form are cephalexin (Keflex) and cephadroxyl (Duricef). Cephazolin (Ancef) is also a first-generation **injectable** drug, recommended by the AHA for premedication prophylaxis in penicillin-allergic patients unable to take oral medications. As of April 2007, AHA has added a third-generation cephalosporin, ceftriaxone (Rocephin), to its list of injectable premedication antibiotics for penicillin-allergic patients unable to take oral medications.

Cephalosporins Adverse Effects

Cephalosporins and the other broad-spectrum antibiotics can wash out the intestinal bacterial flora, decrease vitamin K absorption, and cause increased bleeding, particularly in patients on warfarin (Coumadin).

Cephalosporins Drug Use

The first-generation drugs are excellent at treating **early** oral infections because they have excellent coverage against most gram-positive organisms and poor coverage against most gram-negative organisms and anaerobes. This accounts for the first-generation cephalosporins **not** being effective for **late** infections. The first-generation cephalosporins are considered a good second alternative to clindamycin for treatment of early oral infections in **nonanaphylactoid**, penicillin-allergic patients. **Cephalosporins are in** Pregnancy Category B.

Cephalosporins Prescriptions

1. a. **Rx: cephalexin (Keflex), 250 or 500mg/capsule**
        Disp: Variable
        Dose: 250–1,000mg PO q6h/qid × 5days, maximum 4g/day
          The renal dosing of Keflex should be q12h or q24h, in the presence of kidney disease.
    b. **Cephalexin oral suspension:** Powder for cephalexin oral suspension, is available as monohydrate: 125mg/5mL or 250mg/5mL, 5mL unit dose, available in 100mL and 200mL size bottles.
        Adult Rx: 250–1000mg liquid, q6h/qid × 5 days, maximum 4g/day.
2. a. **Rx: Cephadroxyl (Duricef), 250 or 500mg/capsule**
        Disp: Variable
        Dose: 1–2g/day PO in two divided doses × 5days
    b. **Cephadroxyl oral suspension:** Cephadroxyl oral suspension is dispensed as monohydrate: 125mg/5mL or 250mg/5mL or 500mg/5mL, available in 50mL and 100mL size bottles.
        Adult Rx: Typically, 1–2g/day liquid, in two divided doses × 5days.
3. **For premedication prophylaxis:**
    a. **Cephalexin or cephadroxyl:** 2g PO, 1h prior to procedure
    b. **Cephazolin (Ancef):** 1g, IV/IM 30min prior procedure
    c. **Ceftriaxone (Rocephin):** 1 g IV/IM, 30min prior to the procedure
4. **Cephalosporins and Kidney Disease:** Almost all of the cephalosporins used for management of odontogenic infections are excreted unchanged by the kidneys. Reduce the total daily dose of cephalosporins by 50% in a renal-compromised patient. Cephalosporins can be used in a patient with **both** kidney and liver disease but with a 50% total daily dose reduction.

LINCOSAMIDE GROUP ANTIBIOTIC, CLINDAMYCIN

Clindamycin Spectrum of Activity and Overview

Clindamycin is a lipophilic, narrow-spectrum antibiotic that is very effective against gram-positive and anaerobic gram-negative bacteria. It is used primarily to treat infections caused by susceptible anaerobic bacteria, including infections of the respiratory tract, skin, and soft tissue. In patients with hypersensitivity to penicillins, clindamycin may be used to treat infections caused by susceptible aerobic bacteria as well. Clindamycin has excellent tissue penetration and it is used to treat bone and joint infections, particularly those caused by Staphylococcus aureus. Clindamycin (Cleocin HCL) is often used in the treatment of serious infections caused by susceptible anaerobic bacteria and is very effective for endodontic infections or dental abscesses involving bone and/or soft tissue not responding adequately to penicillin. Clindamycin is a protein-synthesis inhibitor that targets the 50S ribosomal subunit. Clindamycin also has a stimulatory effect on the host immune system. At **low** doses (150 or 300mg oral), for treatment of infections, clindamycin is bacteriostatic in action. At **high** doses (600mg oral), as with the AHA-recommended antibiotic prophylaxis or when dosed at 150 or 300mg, intravenous (IV)/intramuscular (IM), clindamycin is bactericidal in action.

Clindamycin Drug Uptake

Peak clindamycin levels are attained in about one hour after oral ingestion. Clindamycin attains high levels in the saliva, gingival tissue, and bone, as previously stated. The half-life of clindamycin is two to three hours. Clindamycin is **partially** metabolized in the liver and intestinal mucosa. The metabolites are excreted through the kidneys, feces, and bile.

Clindamycin Adverse Effects

Pseudomembranous colitis due to clostridium difficile overgrowth after the first few pills of clindamycin, or even months after taking a full course, has been cause for concern for a very long time. However, recent literature **downplays** this side effect and states that clindamycin **does not** cause the pseudomembranous colitis when used appropriately in an outpatient setting. The literature further states that not just clindamycin but **any** antibiotic that washes out the intestinal bacterial flora can cause pseudomembranous colitis.

In the presence of antibiotic-induced colitis, the offending antibiotic should be stopped, and metronidazole (Flagyl) or vancomycin pulvules (oral vancomycin) should be prescribed to treat the infection associated with clostridium difficile.

Clindamycin Drug Uses

In the early stages of oral infections the bacterial population is more aerobic, and in the late stages it switches from aerobic to anaerobic. This is the reason why clindamycin is *the* drug of choice for treatment of oral infections symptomatic for more than three days. Clindamycin 600mg PO (oral) is the drug of choice for joint prosthesis prophylaxis, in penicillin-allergic patients. **Clindamycin is in** Pregnancy Category **B**.

Clindamycin Prescriptions

1. a. **Rx: Clindamycin**, 150 or 300mg/tablet
      Disp: Variable
      Dose: 150–450mg q6-8h/qid PO × 5days
      Note: At this dose, clindamycin is static in action. It is best to prescribe the lower dose of clindamycin, **150mg, tid or q8h** because this **minimizes** the adverse side effects. Clindamycin serum levels are known to exceed the MIC for bacterial growth for at least 6h after consumption of the recommended dose.
   b. **Clindamycin oral suspension:** Clindamycin as granules for oral suspension is dispensed as palmitate: 75mg/5mL in 100mL size bottle.

> **Adult Rx:** 2–4tsp/dose, tid × 5days; best to dispense 2tsp/dose, to minimize adverse side effects.

2. **Refractory cases of periodontal infection**: These patients are best treated with 600mg/day of **clindamycin** × 7days.
3. **Premedication prophylaxis:**
   a. **Clindamycin:** 600mg PO, 1h prior to treatment. This is a cidal dose.
   b. **Clindamycin** 600mg, IV 30min prior to procedure. This is a cidal dose.
4. **Clindamycin and liver disease:**
   a. **Hepatitis:** The full dose of clindamycin can be used in the presence of nonacute, nonfulminant hepatitis.
   b. **Cirrhosis:** Decrease clindamycin total daily dose **by 50%** in patients with liver cirrhosis.
5. **Clindamycin and kidney disease:** No dose change is needed in the presence of kidney disease or renal failure.

Clindamycin can be used with a 50% total daily dose reduction in a patient with **both** kidney and liver disease.

MACROLIDES

Macrolides Overview and Spectrum of Activity

Macrolides are considered lipophilic, **narrow-spectrum** antibiotics, and the members include: erythromycin, azithromycin, clarithromycin, dirithromycin, and telithromycin. The new macrolides azithromycin, clarithromycin, dirithromycin, and telithromycin are semisynthetic derivatives of erythromycin, with structural modifications to improve tissue penetration and broaden the spectrum of activity. Although azithromycin and erythromycin are in Pregnancy Category B, the other members are in Pregnancy Category C. Azithromycin and clarithromycin are the two new macrolides currently encountered in the dental setting.

Macrolides are mainly active against gram-positive cocci (staphylococci and streptococci) and bacilli and, to a lesser-extent, gram-negative cocci. Azithromycin has increased gram-negative coverage, compared with erythromycin and clarithromycin. Erythromycin, also a narrow-spectrum antibiotic, was used to treat chlamydia, diphtheria, syphilis, acne, and penicillin-resistant streptococcal infections. In general, azithromycin and clarithromycin are effective against the most frequently isolated bacteria causing pharyngitis, otitis media, sinusitis, tonsillitis, throat infections, laryngitis, bronchitis, pneumonia, typhoid, and urinary tract infections. Azithromycin rapidly penetrates tissues, concentrating more in infected tissues, compared with uninfected tissues. Macrolides are used to treat respiratory-tract related infections such as pharyngitis, sinusitis, and bronchitis, as macrolides have a high level of lung penetration. Additionally, they are used for treatment of genital, gastrointestinal tract, and skin infections.

Erythromycin is metabolized in the liver and excreted mainly through the feces and bile. Some minimal excretion also occurs through the kidneys. Azithromycin elimination occurs primarily in the feces as the unchanged drug, and urinary excretion of the drug is minimal. Azithromycin undergoes some hepatic metabolism, with the majority of the drug being excreted in bile and, to a lesser extent, urine. Azithromycin has no liver cytochrome enzyme involvement. Although the drug is generally well tolerated and associated with few adverse effects, therapy with azithromycin should be administered cautiously in patients with severe liver and/or severe biliary disease. The clinical significance of possible drug accumulation is unknown. When compared with normal hepatic function, the serum pharmacokinetics of azithromycin for patients with mild-to-moderate liver function impairment is unchanged. **No** azithromycin dose adjustment is necessary for patients with **mild-to-moderate** liver function impairment. However, in these patients urinary recovery of azithromycin does appear to increase, possibly to compensate for reduced hepatic clearance. In conclusion, no dosing modifications are necessary in patients with mild or moderate hepatic impairment, and even though the potential for hepatotoxicity is rare, azithromycin should be used with caution in end-stage liver disease/cirrhosis. Either reduce the daily dose or avoid using azithromycin altogether.

Clarithromycin is metabolized in the liver by the cytochrome P450 3A4 (CYP3A4) enzymes to the active 14-hydroxy form and six additional products. Thirty to forty percent of an oral dose of clarithromycin is excreted in the urine either unchanged or as the active 14-hydroxy metabolite. The remainder is excreted into the bile. In patients with moderate-to-severe renal impairment, creatinine clearance <30mL/min, the dose of clarithromycin should be reduced. In patients with moderate-to-severe hepatic impairment and normal renal function, there is less metabolism of clarithromycin to the 14-hydroxy form and increased renal excretion of unchanged clarithromycin. Therefore, dosing modifications are necessary for these patients. Clarithromycin is used in the treatment of bacterial pharyngitis, tonsillitis, acute maxillary sinusitis, and acute bacterial exacerbation of chronic bronchitis, pneumonia, and skin infections.

Clarithromycin can be given with food and does not cause the gastrointestinal upset associated with erythromycin. Azithromycin immediate-release suspension and tablet can be taken with or without food. Azithromycin extended-release suspension (Zmax) should be taken either one hour prior to or two hours after a meal. Taking extended-release azithromycin too close to meals will impair absorption.

Erythromycin and clarithromycin suppress the cytochrome P4503A4 enzyme in the liver and gut. The 3A4 enzyme metabolizes many useful therapeutic drugs and is also involved in the conversion of some prodrugs into active functional metabolites. With suppression of the 3A4 enzyme, the non-metabolized drugs accumulate in the liver and become toxic, whereas the prodrugs are rendered ineffective.

Azithromycin **does not** affect the P4503A4 enzyme. In rare cases, azithromycin has been associated with allergic reactions including angioedema, anaphylaxis, dermatologic reactions such as Stevens-Johnson syndrome, and toxic epidermal necrolysis. Azithromycin can cause severe diarrhea, and oral and vaginal yeast infections in some patients. Avoid azithromycin use in myesthenia gravis patients.

Azithromycin and sudden cardiac arrhythmia: It is well documented that clarithromycin and erythromycin can increase the risk of serious ventricular arrhythmias and both antibiotics have been associated with an increased risk of sudden cardiac death. A recent study has shown azithromycin to be potentiating altered cardiac conduction from QTc prolongation and ventricular arrhythmias. According to the study, the five-day azithromycin therapy showed a small absolute increase in cardiovascular deaths, particularly among patients with a high baseline risk of cardiovascular disease. **Factors accounting for increased risk included underlying cardiovascular disease, smoking, obesity, poor diet, and sedentary life style.** It is important for providers to know that the study did not find increased cardiovascular death risk to persist after the five-day supply of antibiotic ended. Patients who have taken azithromycin in the past should be aware of this important new complication being associated with azithromycin.

It is best to avoid azithromycin use in patients with underlying cardiac states associated with rhythm issues, myocardial dysfunction, myocardial infarction, angina, cardiac failure, hypertension, hyperlipidemia, diabetes, and the aforementioned associated risk factors.

Erythromycin is no longer used in the dental setting. Bacterial resistance, severe gastrointestinal upsets, and DDIs associated with the cytochrome P4503A4 enzyme were all cause for the loss in popularity of erythromycin. Additionally, erythromycin can aggravate the weakness experienced by patients with myasthenia gravis.

Azithromycin and clarithromycin are recommended as alternates for SBE prophylaxis by the AHA, in the penicillin-allergic patient. Both of these drugs are also used in the management of odontogenic infections symptomatic for more than three days in the penicillin-allergic patient. Because clarithromycin is associated with several DDIs, it is suggested that you use azithromycin instead, always confirming that there are no underlying cardiac issues as previously discussed.

Drugs Interacting with Azithromycin, Erythromycin, and Clarithromycin

DDIs can occur between azithromycin (Zithromax) and the following drugs: aluminum/magnesium-containing antacids (Maalox/Mylanta/Gelusil), carbamazepine (Tegretol), cyclosporine (Sandimmune), digoxin (Digitek/Lanoxin), ergot alkaloids, nelfinavir (Viracept), phenytoin (Dilantin), quinine (Qualaquin), tacrolimus (Prograf), theophylline (Theo-Dur), triazolam (Halcion), and warfarin (Coumadin).

Drugs interacting with erythromycin and clarithromycin are theophylline, oral anticoagulants, lanoxin (Digoxin), methylprednisolone, phenytoin sodium (Dilantin), carbamazepine (Tegretol), cyclosporine (Sandimmune), and ergot alkaloids.

Erythromycin and azithromycin are Pregnancy Category B drugs. Clarithromycin is in Pregnancy Category C.

Macrolides Prescriptions

Macrolides for premedication prophylaxis: Give azithromycin or clarithromycin, 500mg PO one hour prior to the procedure.

Azithromycin Preparations and Dosing

- **Oral tablets:** As 250, 500, or 600mg immediate-release tablets.
- **Azithromycin extended-release suspension (Zmax):** Dispensed as 2gm/60mL. The entire 60mL is a one-time dose.
- **Oral suspension:** Liquid azithromycin is dispensed as 100 or 200mg/5mL liquid.
- **Intravenous preparation:** Dispensed as lypholized azithromycin 500mg/10mL vial.

1. **Rx:** five-day supply: **azithromycin** 250mg/capsule.
   Disp: 6 capsules.
   Sig: 250mg bid or 500mg hs on the first day, and then 250mg/day for the next four days.

I prefer dispensing the five-day, low daily dose azithromycin to lean patients weighing <140 lbs.

2. **Rx: three-day supply: azithromycin** 500mg/capsule
   Disp: 3 capsules
   Sig: 500mg/day × 3 days
3. **Azithromycin and kidney disease:** Use full-dose azithromycin in the renal-compromised patient.
4. **Azithromycin and liver disease:** No dose modifications are necessary in patients with mild or moderate hepatic impairment, and even though the potential for hepatotoxicity is rare, azithromycin should be used with caution in end-stage liver disease/cirrhosis. Either reduce the total daily dose or avoid using azithromycin altogether.

Clarithromycin Preparations and Dosing

Clarithromycin is available as immediate-release tablets (250 or 500mg), extended-release tablets (500mg), and granules for oral suspension (125 or 250mg/5mL).

1. **Rx: Clarithromycin** 250 or 500mg/cap
   Disp: Variable
   Sig: 250 or 500mg bid × 5 days
2. **Clarithromycin and kidney disease:** It is best to **avoid** clarithromycin use in the renal-compromised patient, but, if needed, use the following guidelines:
   a. CrCl 30–60mL/min or a serum creatinine <3.3mg/dL; decrease the total daily dose by 50% and **give 250mg q12h.**
   b. CrCl <30mL/min or a serum creatinine >3.3mg/dL to predialysis; decrease the total daily dose by 75% and **give 125mg q12h.**
   c. In presence of CrCl <10mL/min or dialysis dose clarithromycin at **125mg q24h.**
3. **Clarithromycin and liver disease:** In patients with **mild** liver disease in the presence of **normal** renal function, **no dose change** is needed. With **moderate-to-severe** hepatic impairment and **normal** renal function, there is less metabolism of clarithromycin to the 14-hydroxy form, and increased renal excretion of unchanged clarithromycin. **Therefore, dosing modifications are necessary for these patients.**

NITROIMIDAZOLES: METRONIDAZOLE (FLAGYL)

Metronidazole (Flagyl) Spectrum of Activity and Overview

Metronidazole, a narrow-spectrum bactericidal member of the nitroimidazole family, is rather lipophilic and is effective against obligate anaerobic bacteria. Metronidazole kills bacteria by interfering with their ability to make new DNA. Metronidazole is used for treatment of trichomoniasis, amebiasis, giardiasis, Gardnerella vaginitis, and anaerobic bacterial infections only. The anaerobic organisms have the ability to metabolize metronidazole to its active form within the anaerobic cells. Metronidazole is metabolized in the liver and excreted through the kidneys and feces. Bacterial resistance to metronidazole is very rare.

Metronidazole (Flagyl) in combination with pen VK/amoxicillin is often dispensed when the patient's infection does not respond to penicillin or amoxicillin alone when you are treating a mixed aerobic and anaerobic bacterial infection. This combination is called the "poor man's augmentin." Metronidazole is also available for intravenous administration in the treatment of anaerobic bacterial infections.

Metronidazole is the first drug of choice for the treatment of an initial bout or first recurrence of mild or moderate clostridium difficile infection (CDI)–associated pseudomembranous colitis.

Metronidazole Adverse Effects

Frequent: Nausea, headache, dry mouth, and metallic taste.
Occasional: Vomiting, diarrhea, insomnia, weakness, stomatitis, vertigo, paresthesia, rash, urethral burning, and phlebitis at the injection site.
Rare: Seizures, encephalopathy, ataxia, leukopenia, and pancreatitis.

Metronidazole and DDIs

Metronidazole interferes with the metabolism of alcohol with a consequent buildup of acetaldehydes, resulting in vomiting and extreme nausea. This disulfiram or Antabuse-type reaction occurs when metronidazole is combined with alcohol. The alcohol metabolite of metronidazole has 30% activity of the parent compound. Accumulation of the alcohol metabolite of metronidazole in patients with renal dysfunction contributes to nephrotoxicity. Provide dose adjustment or avoid using metronidazole in patients with renal impairment. The patient should not consume alcohol when taking metronidazole and must continue to avoid alcohol for an additional 48 hours after the last dose.

Metronidazole increases the effect of anticoagulants. There is decreased effect of metronidazole with Antabuse pentobarbital. There is possible increased toxicity with cimetidine. Metronidazole inhibits the excretion of lithium, which leads to lithium toxicity and consequent renal damage.

Metronidazole (Flagyl) is in Pregnancy Category B. Metronidazole is safe for use after 14 weeks gestation: Safety prior to 14 weeks has not been established.

Metronidazole Prescriptions

For treatment of anaerobic infection or in combination with 250mg pen VK or 250mg amoxicillin:

1. **Rx: Metronidazole (Flagyl),** 250 or 500mg/tab
   Disp: Variable
   Sig: 250mg q6h or 500mg q8h × 5 days
      It is best to dispense the **lower dose** (250mg) of metronidazole instead of the 500mg dose to minimize the dry mouth and metallic taste
2. Alternate metronidazole prescription for bacterial infections:
   Rx: Metronidazole 7.5mg/kg BW, maximum 1g
   Sig: Take q6h × 7 days
3. Treatment of an initial or first recurrence of mild or moderate c. difficile–associated pseudomembranous colitis, per CDC guidelines:
   Rx: Metronidazole (Flagyl), 500mg/tab

Disp: Variable

Sig: 500mg q8h × 10–14 days. Repeat treatment once more if infection persists after the initial 14-day treatment.

4. **Metronidazole (Flagyl) and kidney disease:**
   a. Predialysis: No dose adjustment is needed.
   b. Renal failure/dialysis: Dose adjustment is required only in the presence of renal failure/dialysis. Metronidazole should be dosed at 500mg PO **q12h** instead of q8h and given **after** the dialysis.
5. **Metronidazole (Flagyl) and liver disease:**
   a. Mild liver disease: Prescribe the normal metronidazole dose.
   b. Moderate-to-severe liver disease: Metronidazole total daily dose should be decreased by at least **50%**.

Metronidazole can be used in the presence of **both** liver and kidney disease but with a **reduced dose** (250mg q12h).

TETRACYCLINES

Tetracyclines Spectrum of Activity and Overview

Tetracyclines got their name because they share a chemical structure that has four rings. Tetracyclines are broad-spectrum, lipophilic antibiotics that inhibit the bacterial 30S ribosomal subunit. Tetracycline members include doxycycline, minocycline, oxytetracycline, and tetracycline HCL. Tetracyclines are used to treat gram-positive and gram-negative rods and cocci, aerobes and anaerobes, bacterial infections such as mycoplasma that lack a cell wall, Rocky Mountain spotted fever, Lyme disease, cholera, acne, and some protozoan infections. Because they have such a wide spectrum of activity, they destroy the normal intestinal micro-flora, often producing severe gastrointestinal dysfunction. Consequently, superinfections of tetracycline-resistant proteous, pseudomonas, and staphylococcus, as well as yeast infections, can also result. Tetracyclines may cause increased photosensitivity and tetratogenic changes in the newborn when given during pregnancy, and pregnant women should never be prescribed tetracyclines. Children younger than 8 years old should not use tetracyclines, especially during periods of tooth development, because tetracyclines cause bone deformity and permanent staining of the teeth. All tetracyclines are concentrated in the liver and excreted via bile into the intestine, where they are reabsorbed and then ultimately eliminated through the kidneys.

Doxycycline is bacteriostatic in action against a wide range of both gram-positive and gram-negative organisms. Doxycycline is rapidly and almost completely absorbed from the gastrointestinal (GI) tract after oral administration, and it is partially inactivated in the gastrointestinal tract by chelation. The drug is cleared unchanged by renal and fecal excretion. Thus, the liver is not involved in the metabolism of Doxycycline. Doxycycline also does not require any renal clearance.

Tetracycline HCL, on the other hand, has a large renal clearance. Tetracycline HCL is contraindicated in a patient with liver disease, kidney disease, or both liver and kidney disease. Tetracycline HCL should be taken on an empty stomach, but doxycycline can be taken with nondairy foods a few hours before bedtime.

Tetracyclines Adverse Effects and DDIs

The following are adverse effects and DDIs for tetracyclines:

1. The beneficial bacteria in the gut are destroyed and secondary infection with candidiasis can occur. Tetracycline HCL can also cause **Fanconi syndrome**, which presents as aminoaciduria, phosphaturia, acidosis, and glycosuria.
2. All oral antacids—milk of magnesia, Tums, Mylanta, bismuth subsalicylate, zinc sulfate, and iron—impair the absorption of the tetracyclines, causing the tetracyclines to precipitate on ingestion. Maintain a gap of at least **two hours** between the ingestion of a tetracycline with any of these metal cations.
3. The tetracyclines potentiate the effects of warfarin (Coumadin) and prolong the PT/INR.
4. A decreased doxycycline effect occurs with barbiturates, carbamazepine (Tegretol), and phenytoin sodium (Dilantin).
5. Tetracyclines decrease the effects of oral contraceptives and increase the effects of digoxin, lithium, and methotrexate.

Tetracycline and doxycycline are in Pregnancy Category D.

Tetracyclines Dosing

Subantimicrobial dose (SD) doxycycline (Periostat 20mg): Subantimicrobial dose (SD) doxycycline (Periostat 20mg) effectively treats periodontitis by reducing inflammation via its anticollagenolytic, antimatrix-degrading metalloproteinase, and cytokine down-regulating properties. Doxycycline is used to help treat periodontal disease.

   Acne therapy: Doxycycline, in combination therapy with a topical retinoid, is used effectively for the treatment of acne vulgaris. Treatment with subantimicrobial dose of doxycycline at 20mg twice daily can significantly reduce the number of inflammatory and noninflammatory lesions in patients with moderate facial acne. It is well tolerated, has no detectable antimicrobial effect on the skin flora, and does not result in an increase in antibiotic resistance. Studies also show that doxycycline 20mg is an effective maintenance dosage in patients with inflammatory acne.

1. a. **Rx: doxycycline**, 100mg/capsule
        Disp: 11 capsules
        Sig: 200mg PO 2h prior to bed, on day 1, and then 100mg 2h prior to bed/day: days 2–10.
    b. **Rx: doxycycline**, 50mg/capsule
        Disp: 11 capsules
        Sig: 100mg PO 2h prior to bed, on day 1, and then 50mg 2h prior to bed/day: days 2–10. I prefer dispensing the 50mg/capsule prescription to patients weighing <140 lbs.
2. **Doxycycline oral suspension:** Doxycycline powder for oral suspension is dispensed as monohydrate: 25mg/5mL in 60mL size bottle in syrup form or 50mg/5mL, in 30mL or 473mL size bottles.
    Adult Rx: 100mg/200mg loading dose, followed by 50mg/100mg/dose liquid Doxycycline × 10 days.
3. **Doxycycline and kidney/liver disease:**
    a. No doxycycline dose change is needed with kidney or liver disease.

b. Doxycycline can be used **without** dose alteration in a patient who has both kidney and liver disease.

4. **Rx: Tetracycline HCL** 250mg/capsule, on an **empty** stomach
   Disp: 20 capsules
   Dose: 250mg qid × 5days

5. **Tetracycline HCL and kidney disease:** Avoid tetracycline HCL use with kidney disease, but if absolutely needed, use the following creatinine clearances/creatinine guidelines:
   a. **CrCl 50–80mL/min or serum creatinine between 1.25–2.0mg/dL:** Dose tetracycline HCL **q8–12h**
   b. **CrCl 10–50mL/min or serum creatinine between 2.0mg/dL to predialysis:** Dose tetracycline HCL **q12–24h**
   c. **CrCl <10mL/min or dialysis:** Dose tetracycline HCL q24h

GLYCOPEPTIDES: VANCOMYCIN (VANCOCIN)

Vancomycin Spectrum of Activity

Vancomycin is a hydrophilic, narrow-spectrum, glycopeptide antibiotic that is used for the treatment of infection caused by gram-positive bacteria particularly. Vancomycin acts by inhibiting the bacterial cell-wall synthesis. Vancomycin is an effective alternative to the penicillins for prophylaxis against endocarditis caused by streptococcus viridans or enterococci, for serious staphylococcal infections, infections caused by diphtheroids, in the treatment of pseudomembranous enterocolitis caused by c. difficile, and for penicillin-resistant pneumococcal infections. Vancomycin is also the drug of choice for the treatment of infections caused by methicillin-resistant staphylococcus aureus (MRSA) and epidermidis.

The intravenous (IV) form of vancomycin is used for the management of all systemic all infections. Intravenous (IV) vancomycin dose should be significantly reduced and, better yet, **avoided** in the presence of renal disease, because there is rapid accumulation of metabolites. Vancomycin is minimally metabolized by the liver and no change in drug dose is needed for liver disease.

Oral vancomycin can be life saving in patients with antibiotic-associated colitis due to clostridium difficile. Oral vancomycin is used when metronidazole (Flagyl) use is contraindicated in the presence of liver disease or alcoholism or when two, 14-day courses of metronidazole have been ineffective. Oral vancomycin is the **first** drug of choice for a **second** recurrence or **severe** c. difficile infection (CDI)–associated pseudomembranous colitis.

Vancomycin Adverse Drug Reactions

The following are adverse drug reactions associated with vancomycin:

1. **Frequent:** Thrombophlebitis, fever, chills.
2. **Occasional:** Eighth-nerve damage can occur, especially with large or continuous doses of more than ten days, in the presence of renal damage, in elderly patients, or in the presence of neutropenia.

3. **Rare:** Peripheral neuropathy, urticaria. If vancomycin is injected into a vein too quickly, it can cause the flushing associated with "red-neck" syndrome; a rash over the neck, face, and chest; wheezing or difficulty breathing; and a dangerous decrease in blood pressure.

Vancomycin DDIs

Increased nephrotoxicity occurs when vancomycin is used with aminoglycosides and cephalosporins. Vancomycin is in Pregnancy Category C.

Vancomycin Dosing

1. **Vancomycin HCl pulvules/oral vancomycin:** The **first-line** therapy for an **initial** or recurrence of **severe** CDI disease.
   Rx: Vancomycin 125mg/pulvule
   Dose: 125mg qid ×10–14 days. This regimen is topical in action and is ineffective for any systemic infection.
   Second recurrence is treated with oral vancomycin tapered over 4 weeks, with or without pulse dosing. Pulse dosing prescription: 125mg oral vancomycin is given q2–3 days, for 2–8 weeks.
2. **Systemic infection:**
   Rx: Vancomycin 7.5mg/kg BW or 500mg–1g injected IV, every 6–12hr.

GLYCYLCYCLINE

Tigecycline Facts

Tigecyclines, a glycylcycline class of antibiotics in Pregnancy Category **D**, are structurally related to minocycline. Similar to minocycline, tigecycline is lipophilic and binds to the bacterial 30S ribosome, blocking the entry of transfer RNA. Tetracyclines have developed widespread resistance, and the glycylcyclines were developed to help overcome these resistance mechanisms. Alterations to the tetracycline structure allow tigecycline to maintain activity against tetracycline-resistant organisms, including resistant gram-positive organisms such as penicillin-resistant Streptococcus pneumoniae, methicillin-resistant Staphylococcus aureus (MRSA) and Staphylococcus epidermidis (MRSE), and vancomycin-resistant Enterococcus (VRE) species. Tigecycline is more active against the methicillin-resistant strains of these organisms. Tigecycline has demonstrated improved activity against Streptococcus species, including penicillin-susceptible, penicillin-intermediate, and penicillin-resistant strains of Streptococcus pneumoniae. Tigecycline also has improved activity against Enterococcus species when compared with the other tetracycline agents. Tigecycline is approved for the treatment of complicated skin and skin structure infections (cSSSI) and complicated intra-abdominal infections caused by susceptible organisms. Therefore, tigecycline is used when coverage is needed for resistant gram-positive organisms as well as gram-negative and anaerobic organisms. It is not be used for patients who are not at risk of resistant infections or in patients who have infections sensitive to vancomycin. It is far superior to minocycline or tetracycline HCL. Tigecycline is **bacteriostatic** against Escherichia coli,

Klebsiella pneumoniae, Enterococcus faecalis, and Staphylococcus aureus. It has **bacteriostatic and bacteriocidal** activity against Streptococcus pneumoniae.

Tigecycline Side Effects

Adverse effects are mild and include nausea, vomiting, and diarrhea. Hyperbilirubinemia has been known to occur more often with tigecycline, along with the development of acute pancreatitis.

Tigecycline Pharmacology

Tigecycline is highly protein bound; it is not extensively metabolized, but a slight amount of metabolism may occur via glucuronidation. Tigecycline has an elimination half-life of approximately 36 hours. It is mainly eliminated as unchanged drug; larger amount of metabolites are excreted in the bile and feces and smaller amounts are excreted as unchanged drug in the urine. Based on pharmacokinetic studies, no dosage adjustment is required based on age, sex, or race. Dosage adjustments are **not** recommended in patients with mild or moderate hepatic impairment. Patients with severe hepatic impairment should receive a 100mg loading dose of tigecycline followed by a maintenance dose of 25mg every 12 hours. Similarly, **no** dose adjustments are recommended in patients with impaired renal function or patients with ESRD on hemodialysis.

Tigecycline Dose

The recommended dose of tigecycline is 50mg every 12 hours after a 100mg loading dose. If a patient has severe hepatic impairment, a dose of 25mg every 12 hours should be given after a loading dose of 100mg. Doses are given intravenously over 30–60 minutes.

Tigecycline Associated DDIs

Tigecycline does not inhibit or induce the hepatic cytochrome P450 enzyme system, so it does not alter the metabolism of drugs that are metabolized by this system nor do drugs that inhibit or induce the P450 enzymes affect it. Tigecycline does minimally affect the clearance of the R- and S-isomers of warfarin. No dosage adjustment is recommended for patients getting warfarin and tigecycline but the INR should be monitored more frequently while on tigecycline.

FLUOROQUINOLONES

Fluoroquinolones Facts

The fluroquinolones are synthetic antibacterial agents, and can be readily interchanged with traditional antibiotics. An earlier related class of antibacterial agents, the quinolones, was not well absorbed and could be used to treat only urinary tract infections. The fluroquinolones, which are based on the older group, are broad-spectrum bacteriocidal drugs that are chemically unrelated to the penicillins or the cephaloprosins.

They are well distributed into bone tissue and are so well absorbed that, in general, they are as effective by the oral route as by intravenous infusion.

Fluoroquinolones are Pregnancy Category **C**, lipophilic, broad-spectrum, bacteriocidal, nucleic acid inhibitor antibiotics that treat gram-positive, gram-nagative, acid fast, fungi, and viral infections. They block the replication of DNA or prevent its transcription into RNA. The synthetic fluoroquinolones (Ciprofloxacin) inhibit DNA gyrase, an enzyme needed for bacterial DNA replication. Because of their excellent absorption, fluoroquinolones can be administered by intravenous or oral routes. Fluoroquinolones are used to treat most common urinary tract infections, skin infections, and respiratory infections, such as sinusitis, pneumonia, and bronchitis. The older quinolones are not well absorbed and are used to treat mostly urinary tract infections. Ciprofloxacin is commonly prescribed for cases of anthrax, sexually transmitted diseases, respiratory infections, and urinary tract infections.

Fluoroquinolone members include ciprofloxacin, levofloxacin, clinafloxacin, gatifloxacin, lomefloxacin, norfloxacin, ofloxacin, sparfloxacin, and trovafloxacin. Ciprofloxacin is the most commonly used antibiotic in this class, but it is ineffective for oral infections with a predominant anaerobic flora, particularly those found in complex infections or infections that last longer than three days.

Fluoroquinolones Side Effects

Fluoroquinolones are relatively safe, and the most common side effects include nausea, vomiting, diarrhea, and abdominal pain. Less common but serious side effects include headache, confusion, dizziness, phototoxicity, and convulsions.

AMINOGLYCOSIDES

Aminoglycosides Facts

Aminoglycoside members, streptomycin, gentamicin, and neomycin, are hydrophilic, broad-spectrum, Pregnancy Category **C/D** drugs that block the initiation of translation and cause the misreading of mRNA. The aminoglycosides stop bacteria from making proteins and are bacteriocidal in action. These drugs are effective against gram-positive and aerobic gram-negative bacteria. They are typically used to treat gram-negative infections and they may be used with the penicillins or cephalosporins to enhance bacterial coverage. Aminoglycosides must be injected and are generally given for short time periods. They have the narrowest therapeutic range of any of the antimicrobial family. Accordingly, they require precise administration and monitoring of serum levels. All aminoglycosides are excreted very slowly in the urine over weeks, following discontinuation of therapy. This accounts for the accumulation of any of these compounds in the presence of renal disease. Accumulating compounds cause irreversible nephrotoxicity and ototoxicity, and it is important to note that these untoward side effects can be delayed in onset.

Aminoglycoside Side Effects

The major side effects associated with the aminoglycosides are irreversible ototoxicity (from causes not clearly understood or defined) and nephrotoxicity due to direct damage to the renal cortex.

Aminoglycoside Members

Members include amikacin, gentamicin, kanamycin, neomycin, streptomycin, and tobramycin. Aminoglycoside uses: Streptomycin is used to treat bubonic plague, tularemia and tuberculosis. Gentamicin is less toxic and is used to treat infections caused by gram-negative rods, such as E. coli, pseudomonas, salmonella, and shigella.

DICHLOROACETIC ACID DERIVATIVES

Chloramphenicol

Chloramphenicol is a toxic, lipophilic, bacteriostatic, Pregnancy Category **C**, broad-spectrum, synthetically produced antibiotic that inhibits bacterial protein synthesis by binding to 50S subunit of the bacterial ribosome, thus preventing peptide bond formation by peptidyl transferase. It has both bacteriostatic and bactericidal action against H. influenzae, N. meningitidis, and S. pneumoniae. Due to its high toxicity, chloramphenicol use is limited to treating typhoid fever and brain abscesses.

Chloramphenicol Side Effects

Side effects include bone marrow damage and aplastic anemia, which is irreversible. The drug is also known to cause **"Gray baby syndrome"** in newborns when the baby presents with vomiting, flaccidity, decrease in RBCs, gray skin color, and shock.

LIPOPEPTIDES

Daptomycin

Lipopeptides are natural compounds, and the antibiotic member currently in clinical use is daptomycin (Cubicin). Daptomycin is a Pregnancy Category **B**, hydrophilic, narrow-spectrum bactericidal antibiotic that attacks the integrity of cell membranes. Daptomycin is unable to permeate the outer membrane of gram-negative bacteria, thus its spectrum is limited to gram-positive organisms only. It is very effective against gram-positive organisms, including a number of highly resistant species of S. aureus (including MRSA) and enterococci (including VRE), when compared with vancomycin. The drug has a significant post-antibiotic effect, with growth inhibition occurring up to six hours after drug exposure. Bacteria associated with endocarditis or foreign body infections may be better inhibited by daptomycin compared to vancomycin or nafcillin. It appears to be more rapidly bactericidal than vancomycin. Daptomycin is approved for the treatment of complicated skin and soft tissue infections.

Daptomycin Dose

Daptomycin is given at a dose of 4mg/kg IV, once daily, and dose adjustment is necessary in the presence of renal dysfunction.

Daptomycin Side Effects

Primary toxicity associated with the drug includes reversible dose-related myalgias and weakness. Renal failure, hepatitis, and peripheral neuropathy are other adverse drug reactions with the antibiotic.

OXZOLIDINONES

Linezolid

Linezolid, a Pregnancy Category **C**, lypophylic, narrow-spectrum, bacteriostatic member of the oxazolidinones family is effective against gram-positive bacteria. Linezolid (Zyvox) was the first antibiotic member approved by the FDA. Linezolid attacks the proper assembly of the two ribosomal subunits, 30S and 50S. Linezolid has a unique structure and mechanism of action, which targets protein synthesis at an exceedingly early stage; hence cross-resistance with other commercially available antimicrobial agents is unlikely. It is primarily effective against gram-positive bacteria that have developed resistance to the older antibiotics; for the treatment of MRSA and vancomycin resistant enterococci (VRE) infections; and as an alternative for resistant gram-positive infections, especially pneumonia. The pharmacokinetic parameters of linezolid in adults are not altered by hepatic or renal function, age, or sex to an extent requiring dose adjustment. Linezolid is metabolized independent of the cytochrome P450 (CYP450) enzyme system; consequently, linezolid does **not** interact with medications that stimulate or inhibit CYP450 enzymes.

Linezolid Side Effects

Nausea, vomiting, diarrhea, and rash are frequently encountered side effects with linezolid. Blood dyscrasias (thrombocytopenia), headache, constipation, dizziness, peripheral neuropathy, optic neuropathy, and lactic acidosis are late onset side effects associated with the drug.

Linezolid Dose

Adults: 600mg oral/IV, q12h. **Pediatric:** 10mg/kg oral/IV, q8h.

SULPHONAMIDES

Sulphonamides are hydrophilic, bacteriostatic, broad-spectrum antibiotics that disrupt bacterial metabolism by acting as competitive inhibitors to PABA, a precursor molecule used to synthesize folic acid that bacteria need for nucleic acid synthesis. Most sulfonamides are readily absorbed orally and topically, when applied to burns. Sulfonamides are distributed throughout the body. They are metabolized mainly by the liver and excreted by the kidneys. Sulfonamides compete for bilirubin-binding sites on albumin. Most sulfonamides are Pregnancy Category **B**, broad-spectrum antibiotics that are synthetically produced and effective against gram-positive and many gram-negative organisms. However, use near term and in breast-feeding mothers is contraindicated. If used during pregnancy or in neonates, these drugs increase blood levels of unconjugated bilirubin and increase risk of kernicterus in the fetus or neonate. Sulfamethoxazole and trimethoprim combination (Bactrim and Spectra) is in Pregnancy Category **C**. Sulfonamides enter breast milk. Resistance is widespread, and resistance to one sulfonamide indicates resistance to all, and sulfonamides are contraindicated in patients who have porphyria.

Sulphonamide Members

Systemic use members include sulfadiazine, sulfadoxine, sulfamethizole, sulfamethoxazole, sulfanilamide, sulfasalazine, sulfisoxazole, and dapsone. Sulfonamides available for topical use include silver sulfadiazine (Silvadene) and ophthalmic sulfacetamide (Bleph-10).

Sulfasalazine is used orally for inflammatory bowel disease. Sulfasalazine can **reduce** intestinal absorption of **folate (folic acid)**, so this drug may trigger folate deficiency in patients with inflammatory bowel disease, which also reduces absorption, especially if dietary intake is also inadequate.

Sulfonamides are most commonly used in combination with other drugs, such as sulfamethoxazole and trimethoprim combination (Bactrim and Spectra), for UTI therapy. Bactrim is known to cause hyperkalemia.

Topical sulfonamides can be used to treat the burns (silver sulfadiazine) and superficial ocular infections (ophthalmic sulfacetamide). Always confirm sulfa allergy history in the burn victim prior to using silver sulfadiazine in the dental setting for burns sustained in the work environment.

Dapsone is an antibacterial bacteriostatic antibiotic member that targets a broad spectrum of gram-positive and gram-negative organisms. It is used to treat acne vulgaris, dermatitis herpetiformis, idiopathic thrombocytopenic purpura leprosy, lichen planus, mucous membrane pemphigoid, and for falciparum malaria, pneumocystis pneumonia (PCP), and toxoplasmosis prophylaxis. Agranulocytosis, aplastic anemia, hemolysis, methemoglobinemia, and hepatitis are the dose-related side effects associated with dapsone, and these side effects are more severe in patients with G6PD deficiency anemia.

Sulfonamides Side Effects

Adverse effects can result from oral and sometimes topical sulfonamides. Effects include hypersensitivity reactions (such as rashes, Stevens-Johnson syndrome, vasculitis, serum sickness, drug fever, anaphylaxis, angioedema), oliguria, anuria, photosensitivity, agranulocytosis, thrombocytopenia, and, in patients with G6PD deficiency, hemolytic anemia.

INFECTION MANAGEMENT PROTOCOLS

I've outlined step-wise management protocols of common infections that patients can present with:

Universal Infection Coverage

When in doubt, second- or third-generation cephalosporins are a good choice for many bacterial infections. Antimicrobial coverage includes gram-positive, gram-negative, and strict anaerobic species. Examples of this class include cefmetazole, cefuroxime, cefoxitin, cefotetan, cefamandole, and ceftriaxone.

Anaerobic Infection Coverage

Metronidazole is the antibiotic with good anaerobic coverage and remains the antibiotic of choice for such infections.

Pseudomonal Infection Coverage

Antibiotics with activity against P. aeruginosa include aminoglycosides, ceftazidime, ciprofloxacin, imipenem, levofloxacin, meropenem, and ticarcillin. If serious pseudomonal infection is suspected, double coverage is recommended. The two agents chosen should be from different classes. For example, the combination of ticarcillin/tobramycin is good.

MRSA Infection Coverage

True community-acquired MRSA is a different strain of Staph. aureus and although it is resistant to methicillin, it is susceptible to many common treatment regimens. Vancomycin should be used initially for any suspected severe infection, including endocarditis. In cases of severe infection, other newer agents may be used instead of vancomycin. Such patients may receive linezolid or daptomycin instead of vancomycin. Treatment with vancomycin or the newer drugs should be continued until cultures exclude MRSA or, in the presence of MRSA, prove its sensitivity to other agents. Minor infections with non-nosocomial-type community-acquired MRSA may be treated with a penicillinase-resistant penicillins (Oxacillin, Dicloxacillin), first-generation cephalosporins, trimethoprim-sulfamethoxazole (TMP-SMZ), or tetracyclines.

Non-MRSA Gram-Positive Cocci Infection Coverage

If the patient has no risk factors for the nosocomial-type MRSA, antibiotics effective against S. aureus, such as nafcillin, trimethoprim-sulfamethoxazole (TMP-SMZ), and clindamycin may be used to treat gram-positive cocci infections.

Gram-Negative Sepsis Coverage

Coverage for gram-negative bacteremia is provided by using **two** antibiotics demonstrating good gram-negative activity. Usually a third-generation cephalosporin plus a fluoroquinolone or an aminoglycoside are used. Examples of such coverage include ceftriaxone and gentamicin, or cefmetazole and ciprofloxacin. Combination antibiotics should not be from the same class.

Sinusitis Infection Coverage

- Acute sinusitis typically presents with nasal congestion, purulent nasal discharge, and facial pain. In the immunocompetent host, antibiotics are initially unnecessary.
- Initial treatment should consist of topical decongestants used every four hours, steam inhalations, saline flushes, and having the patient sleep in a semi-upright position to facilitate drainage when the maxillary sinuses are involved.

- Antibiotics should be used in toxic-appearing patients, those in whom initial therapy fails, and in patients with comorbid conditions. Trimethoprim-Sulfamethoxazole (TMP-SMZ) for three days is as effective as a traditional ten-day course of the antibiotic.

Pharyngitis Infection Coverage

- Acute pharyngitis is most commonly caused by viruses. However, to prevent rheumatic fever and its complications, group A beta-hemolytic streptococcal (GABHS) pharyngitis should be recognized and treated.
- Even in the presence of the rapid streptococcal antigen detection test, which is highly specific but lacking sensitivity, a throat culture should always be sent, and follow up with the patient 48 hours later. Be advised that immediate antibiotic therapy is warranted when GABHS acute pharyngitis is highly suspected and the patient has no cough.
- Single-dose benzathine penicillin is recommended for GABHS pharyngitis or tonsillitis, in the acute care/emergency room setting, clearly for compliance reasons. The recommended dosage is 600,000 units intramuscularly (IM) for patients weighing 27kg or less, and 1,200,000 units for patients weighing more than 27kg.
- The twice-daily dosing is as effective as the four-time daily dosing when oral penicillin is used, and it is given for a full ten-day course, which is necessary for eradication of the infection. Oral azithromycin 500mg for the first dose, followed by 250mg PO daily for four days, is the treatment of choice for patients with penicillin allergy.
- Steroids like dexamethasone, betamethasone, or prednisone have been shown in studies to shorten the clinical course of pharyngitis when co-administered with antibiotics as adjuvant therapy to prevent overwhelming bacteremia. Steroids are not recommended in patients who are pregnant or have a history of HIV, oral candidiasis, or ulcerative pharyngitis.

Human Bite Coverage

- Human bites are treated with amoxicillin/clavulanate 500mg bid × 5 days.
- Less costly alternatives include doxycycline 100mg bid, penicillin V 500mg bid/qid, or trimethoprim-sulfamethoxazole (TMP-SMZ) bid.
- The patient should have a follow-up in 24 hours.
- Passive immunization for hepatitis B with immune globulin (HBIG) 0.06mL/kg IM is also advised.

Antifungals Commonly Used in Dentistry: Assessment, Analysis, and Associated Dental Management Guidelines

POLYENE AND AZOLE ANTIFUNGALS: OVERVIEW, FACTS, AND PRESCRIPTIONS

Two distinct classes of antifungal medications used in dentistry are the polyenes and the azole antifungals.

Polyene Antifungals: Mechanism of Action

Polyenes bind with ergosterol in the fungal cells and form holes, causing cell death due to the leaking out of the cell contents.

Polyene Drug Classifications

Polyene drugs include:

1. Nystatin (Mycostatin): topical and oral nystatin
2. Amphotericin B (Fungizone): oral and IV amphotericin B

Azole Drugs Classification

Azole drugs are classified as:

1. **Imidazole antifungals:** clotrimazole (Mycelex) and ketoconazole (Nizoral)
2. **Triazole antifungals:** fluconazole (Diflucan) and itraconazole (Sporanox)

Imidazole and Triazole Antifungals: Mechanism of Action and Facts

Imidazole and triazole antifungals inhibit the CYP450 enzyme, thus preventing the formation of ergosterol and fungal cell membrane synthesis.

Dentist's Guide to Medical Conditions, Medications, and Complications, Second Edition. Kanchan M. Ganda.
© 2013 John Wiley & Sons, Inc. Published 2013 by John Wiley & Sons, Inc.

Fluconazole and itraconazole, the **newer** azole antifungals, generally have **fewer** side effects. They are used a lot more for treatment of fungal infections in the immune-compromised patient compared to ketoconazole. They both affect the fungal cell membrane a lot more than ketoconazole. Hence lower doses are needed for optimal effectiveness.

Topical and Oral Nystatin

Nystatin Facts

The topical and oral forms of nystatin are **not** absorbed on ingestion and consequently are not associated with any DDIs. The oral form is used to treat oral or esophageal fungal infections. Both forms of nystatin are commonly used in HIV/AIDS patients with a low CD_4 count, in patients undergoing chemotherapy, and in patients in whom azole anti-fungals are contraindicated. Nystatin is in Pregnancy Category B. Nystatin suspension is the drug of choice for patients experiencing xerostomia.

Nystatin (Mycostatin) Prescriptions

1. **Nystatin oral suspension for oral candidiasis:**
   Rx: Nystatin oral suspension 100,000 units/mL.
   Disp: 473mL (1 pint) bottle (14-day supply).
   Sig: Use 1tsp or 5mL, qid. Rinse and hold in the mouth as long as possible before swallowing. There should be **no** eating or drinking for 30min after use.
   Note: Nystatin suspension is also dispensed as a 60mL bottle.
2. **Nystatin oral suspension for soaking of dentures/partials:**
   Rx: Nystatin oral suspension 100,000 units/mL.
   Disp: 473mL (1 pint) bottle.
   Sig: Add 5–10mL of 1:100,000 units nystatin to half cup of water and soak the dentures overnight daily for 14days. Rinse the dentures before use.
3. **Nystatin pastille prescription for oral candidiasis:**
   Rx: Nystatin 200,000 units/pastille.
   Disp: 70 pastilles.
   Sig: Dissolve 1 pastille in the mouth 4–5 times/day for 14days. Do not eat for 30min after use.
4. **Nystatin (Mycostatin) cream:** The cream can be applied to the dentures before insertion or can be used for angular chielitis.
   Rx: Nystatin 100,000 units/g.
   Disp: 15g or 30g tube.
   Sig: Apply to affected area 4–5 times/day, for 2 weeks and do not eat or drink for 30min after use.

Amphotericin B (Fungizone)

Amphotericin B Facts

Amphotericin B is available for oral and intravenous (IV) use and it is a Pregnancy Category B drug.

The oral form is used for the management of oral candidiasis. As an oral preparation it is nontoxic. IV amphotericin B is used for systemic fungal infections.

Amphotericin B Mechanism of Action

The mechanism of action is almost similar to, but more complex than, nystatin. IV use can cause a histamine-like reaction causing nausea, vomiting, headaches, hypotension, and chills.

Amphotericin B Metabolism

The half-life of amphotericin B is 24hours and it is metabolized in the kidneys. Amphotericin B can be associated with severe or irreversible nephrotoxicity. Avoid all nephrotoxic drugs and corticosteroids with amphotericin B. Hepatotoxicity, leukopenia, thrombocytopenia, arrhythmias, and cardiac failure can occur with amphotericin.

Amphotericin B Dosing

1. **Topical amphotericin B:**
    Rx: 3% topical amphotericin B
    Disp: 20g tube.
    Sig: Apply to the affected area 3–4 times/day, for 2–4 weeks.
2. **Oral amphotericin B**
    The oral forms are poorly absorbed. Oral amphotericin B is dispensed in capsule or suspension form.
    Rx: Amphotericin B 500mg/capsule or amphotericin B suspension: 500mg/mL.
    Disp: 56 capsules or 56mL suspension.
    Sig: Take 500mg capsule PO qid for 2 weeks or use 1mL of the suspension, swish and swallow qid for 2 weeks.
3. **Intravenous (IV) amphotericin B:**
    a. **IV amphotericin B normal dose:** 0.25–1.5mg/kg, q24h for 2 weeks.
    b. **IV amphotericin B dose for GFR <10mL/min or dialysis:** Prolong the interval and dose at q24–36h.
    c. **IV amphotericin B and liver disease:** No dose adjustment needed.

Clotrimazole (Mycelex)

Clotrimazole Facts

Clotrimazole is available as a cream and a troche. Clotrimazole has been assigned to Pregnancy Category **C** by the FDA when given as oral troches, and Pregnancy Category **B** when used intravaginally or topically. It can cause teratogenic changes in the first trimester and it is best to avoid using the oral form during pregnancy. The oral absorption of the drug is erratic. It is metabolized in the liver and alcohol use is discouraged with the drug. It is contraindicated in the presence of liver disease. Benzodiazepine use with clotrimazole should be avoided because clotrimazole can cause significant elevation of benzodiazepine level due to its inhibitory action of CYP450 enzyme.

Clotrimazole (Mycelex) Prescriptions

1. **Rx: Clotrimazole (Mycelex) cream:**
   Disp: 15g tube.
   Sig: Rub into the affected area 2–3 times daily for 2 weeks.
2. **Rx: Clotrimazole (Mycelex) troches,** 10mg/troche.
   Disp: 70 troches (14-day supply).
   Sig: Dissolve 1 troche in the mouth 5 times daily and *swallow the saliva*. There should be no eating or drinking for 30min after use.

Ketoconazole (Nizoral)

Ketoconazole is an imidazole antifungal that has a strong affinity for fatty tissue. It is a Pregnancy Category C drug.

Ketoconazole Mechanism of Action

Ketoconazole interferes with the synthesis of fungal ergosterol through inhibition of CYP3A4 enzyme.

Ketoconazole and H_2 Blockers, Antacids, or Vitamin Supplements

Ketoconazole needs an acidic pH for absorption, and H_2 blockers or proton pump inhibitors impair the absorption of ketoconazole. Keep a **two-hour** interval between ketoconazole and the H_2 blocker/proton pump inhibitor for optimal effectiveness. Antacids and vitamin supplements chelate ketoconazole and impair absorption. Keep a **two-hour** interval between these agents and ketoconazole.

Ketoconazole Dosing

1. **Normal dose:** 200–400mg q24h.
2. **Dose with kidney disease:** No dose alteration is needed with kidney disease.
3. **Dose with liver disease:** 50% dose reduction is needed with liver disease.

Fluconazole (Diflucan)

Fluconazole Facts

Fluconazole (Diflucan) is a triazole antifungal that is metabolized in the liver and significantly excreted through the kidneys. It is used for the treatment of local and systemic fungal infections. It is available as a topical agent, a capsule for oral use, and an intravenous (IV) preparation for systemic use. It inhibits the CYP450 enzyme, and benzodiazepines should not be used in combination with fluconazole. It can be taken with meals.

Fluconazole and Pregnancy/Breast-Feeding

Fluconazole is a Pregnancy Category C drug, and very high concentrations of the drug appear in breast milk. It is contraindicated if the patient is pregnant or breast-feeding.

Fluconazole and Kidney or Liver Disease

Decrease the dose by 50% in patients with GFR <50mL/min or s. creatinine >2mg/dL-predialysis. Decrease the dose by 50% in mild liver disease. Avoid fluconazole in patients with moderate or severe liver disease.

Fluconazole and Cardiac Conduction

Fluconazole is contraindicated in patients with impaired cardiac conduction.

1. **Fluconazole (Diflucan) prescription for refractory oral or systemic candidiasis:**
    Rx: Fluconazole (Diflucan) 100mg/capsule.
    Disp: 15 capsules.
    Sig: Day 1: Take 2 capsules. Days 2–14: Take 1 capsule daily.
2. **Fluconazole (Diflucan) treatment for esophageal candidiasis:**
    Rx: Fluconazole (Diflucan) 100mg/capsule.
    Disp: Variable.
    Sig: 100mg qd (maximum 400mg qd) for 14–21days.

Itraconazole (Sporanox)

Itraconazole Facts

Itraconazole (Sporanox) has a wider range of activity compared to fluconazole. The oral solution is better absorbed compared to the capsules. The oral or the IV form can be used for the treatment of blastomycosis, aspergillus infection, histoplasmosis, and onychomycosis. Only the IV form is used for the treatment of life-threatening fungal infections. **Sporanox dose**: 200mg/day.

Antifungals and Pregnancy

During pregnancy, use only topical antifungals and avoid systemic antifungal preparations, particularly in the first trimester. **Category B drugs showing no risk during pregnancy include** nystatin (Mycostatin) and amphotericin B. **Category C antifungals that must be avoided during pregnancy include** clotrimazole (Mycelex, Lotrimin), fluconazole (Diflucan), itraconazole (Sporanox), and ketoconazole (Nizoral).

Antivirals Commonly Used in Dentistry: Assessment, Analysis, and Associated Dental Management Guidelines

ACYCLOVIR, VALACYCLOVIR, AND FAMCICLOVIR OVERVIEW AND FACTS

Common Features

Acyclovir and valacyclovir are purine nucleoside analogues and both drugs act against herpes simplex 1 and 2 (cold sores and genital herpes, respectively), varicella zoster (shingles and chicken pox), and the Epstein-Barr virus (infectious mononucleosis).

Neither acyclovir nor valacyclovir cures the viral infection, but they do decrease the symptoms and signs associated with the viral infection. Both drugs can be taken with or without food, and it is best to take the drug around the **same time** every day. The elderly patient should be given a lower dose of either drug, compared to the normal, healthy patient.

Acyclovir (Zovirax) and Valacyclovir (Valtrex) Mechanism of Action

Both drugs impair viral growth by inhibiting replication of the viral DNA. The virus-infected cells absorb more of the drugs compared to the normal cells. Thus, the active form of the drug is available longer where needed, enhancing the efficacy of the drugs.

Acyclovir (Zovirax) and Valacyclovir (Valtrex) Clearance

Kidney

Both drugs are excreted mainly by the kidneys, and the dose should be decreased in the presence of renal dysfunction. The dose of acyclovir or valacyclovir should be repeated after hemodialysis.

Liver

No dose modification is needed with any form of liver disease.

Dentist's Guide to Medical Conditions, Medications, and Complications, Second Edition. Kanchan M. Ganda.
© 2013 John Wiley & Sons, Inc. Published 2013 by John Wiley & Sons, Inc.

Acyclovir (Zovirax) and Valacyclovir (Valtrex) Drug Resistance and Side Effects

Resistance can occur with overuse of acyclovir or valacyclovir and it is best to use these drugs short-term and only when needed. Nausea, vomiting, and diarrhea can occur with both drugs.

Acyclovir

Acyclovir (Zovirax) Facts

Avoid acyclovir with amphotericin B, bactrim, aspirin NSAIDS, zidovudine (AZT/Retrovir), or prograf.

Acyclovir Preparations

- Acyclovir tablet: 400mg/800mg per tablet
- Acyclovir capsule: 200mg/capsule
- Acyclovir suspension: 200mg/5mL: 473mL/bottle
- Acyclovir ointment: 5% cream: 15g tube

Acyclovir Prescriptions

1. **Two weeks of acyclovir therapy for primary herpes simplex infection or for cold sores lasting 1–2 weeks, as seen in the immune-compromised patient:**
   Rx: 200mg 5 times per day × 14days
2. **a. Acyclovir for herpes zoster infection:**
   Rx: 800mg 5 times per day × 7days
   b. Acyclovir for herpes zoster infection with kidney disease:
   Rx: GFR 10–25mL/min or s. creatinine >3 mg/dL to predialysis: Dose 800mg **q8h**
   Rx: GFR <10mL/min or dialysis: Dose 800mg **q12h**
3. **a. Five-day acyclovir intermittent therapy for cold sores lasting less than one week as seen in the immune-competent patient:**
   Rx: 200mg **q4h** or 5 times per day × 5days
   b. Five-day acyclovir intermittent therapy with kidney disease for cold sores lasting less than one week, as seen in the immune-competent patient:
   Rx: GFR <10mL/min or dialysis: Dose 200mg **q12h**
4. **a. One-year acyclovir chronic suppressive therapy with normal kidney status:**
   Rx: 400mg bid/tid or 200mg tid × 1 year; reevaluate after 1 year
   b. One-year acyclovir chronic suppressive therapy with kidney disease: GFR <10mL/min or dialysis:
   Rx: Dose 400mg **q12h** or 200mg **q12h**

Valacyclovir

Valacyclovir (Valtrex) Facts

Valacyclovir is a prodrug that gets converted to acyclovir, its active form. Valacyclovir should not be prescribed with SSRIs, because SSRIs inhibit the 2D6 enzyme needed to activate the drug. It has a longer duration of action compared to acyclovir; thus, the drug is taken more infrequently. Avoid using valacyclovir with cimetidine (Tagamet) or probenecid (Benemid).

Valacyclovir Preparations

- 500mg/caplet
- 1g/capsule

Valacyclovir Prescriptions

1. **Valacyclovir prescription for recurrent herpes simplex (cold sores lasting less than one week/shorter duration cold sores):**
    Rx: 2g bid × 1 day
2. **Valacyclovir prescription for first/initial/primary herpes simplex infection (patient is highly symptomatic):**
    Rx: 1g bid × 10days
3. **Five-day valacyclovir prescription for recurrent herpes simplex infection (for cold sores lasting for 1–2 weeks/longer duration cold sores):**
    Rx: 500mg bid × 5days
4. **a. Herpes zoster infection treatment with valacyclovir (Valtrex):**
    Rx: 1g tid × 7days. Begin Valtrex when symptoms begin or within 48h of the rash.
    b. Herpes zoster treatment with valacyclovir (Valtrex) in the presence of kidney disease:
    Rx: GFR <30mL/min or s. creatinine >3mg/dL to predialysis: 1g q24h
5. **Valacyclovir (Valtrex) Chronic Suppressive Therapy: For chronic cold sores/ Zoster suppression:**
    This prescription should be dispensed for any type of herpes recurrences.
    Rx: Valtrex caplet, 500mg/caplet
    Disp: Dispensed for 6 months to 1 year according to the patient's immunity
    Sig: 500mg OD (once a day) or bid

Famciclovir (Famvir)

Famciclovir Facts

Famciclovir is a Pregnancy Category **B** antiviral drug that is active against the herpes viruses, including herpes simplex 1 and 2 (cold sores and genital herpes) and varicella-zoster (shingles and chickenpox). Famciclovir is a prodrug that is converted to penciclovir, which is then active against the viruses. Famciclovir has a longer duration of action and it can be taken fewer times each day. A 50–75% dose reduction is recommended in patients with end-stage renal disease (ESRD). Patients on hemodialysis should get famciclovir after the dialysis. No dose adjustments are needed in patients with cirrhosis. Famciclovir should **not** be prescribed with SSRIs, because SSRIs inhibit the 2D6 enzyme needed to activate the drug.

Famciclovir Dosing

Famciclovir can be taken with or without food. It is available in tablet form in strengths such as 125, 250, and 500mg. The recommended doses are:

1. Recurrent cold sores in immune-competent patient: 1,500mg as a single dose.
2. Recurrent genital herpes in immune-competent patient: 1,000mg every 12 hours for one day.

3. Suppression of recurrent genital herpes in both populations: 250mg twice daily.
4. Herpes zoster/shingles in both populations: 500mg every 8 hours for 7 days.
5. HIV-infected patients (cold sores or genital herpes): 500mg three times daily for 7 days.
6. a. Famciclovir dosing in kidney disease with GFR (40–59mL/min/1.73m^2):

    Herpes zoster: 500mg q12h.

    For other regimens: No changes needed.

    b. Famciclovir dosing in kidney disease with GFR (20–39mL/min/1.73m^2):

    Herpes zoster: 500mg q24h.

    Recurrent genital herpes (GH): 125mg q24h.

    GH suppression: 125mg q12h.

    c. Famciclovir dosing in kidney disease with GFR (<20mL/min/1.73m^2):

    Herpes zoster: 250mg q24h.

    Recurrent GH: 125mg q24h.

    GH suppression: 125mg q24h.

    d. Famciclovir dosing in patients on dialysis:

    Recurrent genital herpes or suppression: 125mg after each dialysis.

    Herpes zoster or genital herpes in HIV patient: 250mg after each dialysis.

Acute Care and Stress Management

Management of Medical Emergencies: Assessment, Analysis, and Associated Dental Management Guidelines

MEDICAL EMERGENCIES OVERVIEW, FACTS, AND TOOLS

Every practitioner is aware that at one time or another, medical emergencies can happen. With proper assessment and care, however, the emergency can be successfully triaged and optimally managed. Prevention of medical emergencies is the key, and every effort should be made to assess each patient thoroughly prior to dental treatment. Steps should be incorporated to prevent emergencies from happening, and this section discusses and details how to deal with these emergencies.

Prevention of Medical Emergencies

Preventive measures implemented to avoid medical emergencies in the dental setting include thorough assessment of the medical history, thorough physical examination, and appropriate treatment planning.

Thorough Medical History Assessment

Thorough medical history assessment should establish the following:
- The patient's current medical status
- The current list of medications used daily or PRN (as and when needed): including all prescribed and over-the-counter (OTC) medications
- The patient's compliance with medications
- Any history of medical or surgical complications requiring hospitalization within the past two years
- Any history of allergies, particularly to anesthetics, analgesics, antibiotics, antivirals, antifungals, and latex, which are all used or encountered in the dental setting
- Any history of corticosteroid intake, currently or within the previous two years
- Any history of experiencing adverse reactions or negative feelings about visiting a dentist, such as anxiety, fear, or avoidance
- Personal habits, alcohol intake, and "recreational" drug use

Dentist's Guide to Medical Conditions, Medications, and Complications, Second Edition. Kanchan M. Ganda.
© 2013 John Wiley & Sons, Inc. Published 2013 by John Wiley & Sons, Inc.

Thorough Physical Examination Assessment

A thorough physical examination should include an assessment of the following:

- General physical appearance
- Vital signs: pulse, blood pressure, respiration rate, temperature, height, and weight
- Examination of the head and neck
- Assessment of the cardiovascular system
- Assessment of the respiratory system

Assessment of the Treatment Plan

Assessment of the treatment plan should include the following:

- Assessment of the type of anesthetics, analgesics, antibiotics, antivirals, and antifungals that can be safely used during dentistry
- Assessment of whether the patient needs to be premedicated prior to dentistry
- Assessment of whether shorter appointments or appointments at least seven days apart are needed, if the patient is to be premedicated prior to dentistry using the same premedication antibiotic for all visits
- Assessment of whether the patient has presented for treatment on a full stomach; the appointment should occur only after the patient has eaten
- Assessment of whether the patient needs to bring emergency medications for all dental visits: nitroglycerin, inhalers, or sugar pills
- Assessment of whether stress management is needed prior to dentistry

Preparation or Training for Medical Emergencies

Preparation or training for medical emergencies should include the following:

- Acquire CPR certification or ACLS training
- Participate in continuing education courses in emergency medicine, annually
- Know how to access/contact the emergency medical system (EMS) for the dental office in the event of an emergency
- Conduct practice drills in the dental office, making it a team effort
- Have an automated external defibrillator (AED), oxygen tank, and an emergency kit in the dental office with updated medications; know the location and contents of the emergency kit plus how to use the medications, the AED, and how to open the oxygen tank

Emergency practice drill highlights:

- During emergency practice drills always go to where the emergency equipment is located and have participants bring the equipment to the mock-emergency site.
- Review all steps necessary in managing an actual emergency.
- Clearly remind all participants that the new American Heart Association (AHA) Health-Care Provider (HCP) basic life support (BLS) guidelines have moved away from the previous "A-B-C" (Airway-Breathing-Circulation) protocol to the new "C-A-B" (Circulation-Airway-Breathing) protocol. Remind all participants that one no longer has to "look, listen, and feel," as these steps waste precious time and are not

helpful in reviving a collapsed patient. Have participants demonstrate their CPR skills, so the information stays current.

- Run a mock emergency drill with a patient and provider, and have participants respond to the provider's call for help. Observe if the correct provider and bystander tasks are appropriately completed as outlined. Once the drill is completed, provide feedback and correctional steps, if needed, to the provider and bystanders.
- During the drill, the first person or the provider encountering the emergency should call for help and stay to assess and assist the patient.
- The person or provider calling for help follows a structured form of communication so the information gets transmitted correctly to those providing assistance. Remember that the communication needs to be concise and organized, as this standardizes discussion among all participants.
- The person or provider encountering the emergency provides information about the emergency situation, any or all background information, and patient assessment information using the following formula:
  - **Situation:** Why help is needed or what the concern is.
  - **Background:** Information about the patient's current code status, the course of the emergency, and the patient's present medical history and/or present social history.
  - **Assessment:** The patient's vital signs and what problems he/she is experiencing with the vital signs.
- Bystanders responding to the call for help must immediately disperse and bring in the emergency equipments including oxygen; they should assist the provider, call EMS, and direct EMS to the emergency site when they arrive.
- Recommendations will be provided by the EMS or triage team(s), who will indicate what best treatment(s) will help with the care, what additional consults or tests are needed once the patient is stable, and if the patient needs to be transferred for hospitalization.

Common Medications Used During Medical Emergencies

The following medications are used in a medical emergency (list given in alphabetical order):

- Aminophylline (250mg/10mL): In addition to aminophylline, metaproterenol (Alupent) or albuterol (Proventil) are the most common inhalers found in emergency drug kits. The patient places either inhaler into the mouth and compresses the spray vial to express the bronchodilator while inhaling. Then the patient slowly exhales to disperse the medication in the bronchi. Bronchospasm usually resolves within 30 seconds to one minute of inhaler use.
- Aromatic ammonia: The white wrap turns pink when ammonia vapors form after the vaporole is crushed or cracked open.
- Aspirin: Uncoated 81mg and 325mg tablets. Aspirin is part of the prehospital treatment for suspected heart attack victims. Two 81mg tablets or one 325mg aspirin tablet chewed and swallowed is recommended in any patient who is suffering chest pain for the first time. Ensure that the patient has no allergy to aspirin, no underlying bleeding disorders, and no history of peptic ulceration.
- Cimetidine (Tagamet): H_2 blocker: 300mg IV/IM/PO.

- Dextrose ($D_{50}W$): 50mL, 50% dextrose.
- Diazepam (Valium): 5mg/mL vial. Newer kits also contain Midazolam (Versed) in 1mg/mL or 5mg/mL vials.
- Diphenhydramine (Benadryl): H_1 blocker: 50mg/mL. Diphenhydramine (Benadryl) is the histamine blocker most commonly found in emergency drug kits and it is used in the management of allergic reactions that are not life threatening and in the management of acute anaphylactic reactions, after epinephrine has been used.
- Epinephrine: 1:10,000: Administer 0.3mg IV slowly in a hypotensive patient. **Only an emergency room physician or emergency personnel responding to the emergency should administer this.**
- Epinephrine: 1:1,000 dilution: Administer 0.3–0.5mL SC/IM. Epinephrine is dosed in a 1:1000 (0.3 mg) concentration and must be available in a preloaded syringe. The faster the patient gets epinephrine during an acute anaphylactic reaction, the greater is the chance of survival. It is not uncommon to need more than one dose. Therefore, in addition to the preloaded syringe, the emergency kit should contain 1 mL cartridges of epinephrine 1:1000.
- Famotidine (Pepcid): H_2 blocker: 20mg IV/PO.
- Glucagon: 1mg injected IM in the deltoid muscle.
- Glucose: Oral glucose.
- Hydrocortisone sodium succinate (Solu-Cortef): 100–200mg IV/IM.
- Lidocaine.
- Morphine sulfate.
- Naloxone (Narcan): 0.4mg IV.
- Nitroglycerine (NTG) tablet: 0.3mg sublingual (SL). This is given every five minutes up to a maximum of three tablets **after confirming, each time**, that the systolic BP is maintaining above 115 mmHg. Some emergency kits may have nitroglycerine lingual spray instead of nitroglycerine tablets. It is actually better to have nitroglycerine lingual spray in the emergency kit instead of nitroglycerine tablets, as it has a longer shelf life compared to NTG tablets. The nitroglycerine is sprayed onto the patient's tongue and it is as effective as the NTG tablets. The potency of one spray is equal to the potency of one sublingual tablet (0.3mg/tablet).

Emergency Equipment and Adjuncts

Emergency equipment and adjuncts should consist of the following:

- Artificial airways: oropharyngeal and nasopharyngeal airways.
- Airway adjuncts: endotracheal tubes and laryngoscope.
- Ambu-bag: self-inflating, bag-valve mask that provides 100% oxygen.
- Syringes.
- Tourniquets.

Oropharyngeal Airways

Measure from lips to the angle of jaw to determine the size of oropharyngeal airway needed. Insert the airway inverted and turn it upright as you reach the back of the tongue. This holds the tongue off the throat. Oropharyngeal airways are tolerated only by the unconscious patient without a gag reflex.

Cricothyrotomy Needle

A thirteen-gauge cricothyrotomy needle is occasionally inserted to access the airway at a point **below** an upper airway obstruction. This is done by inserting the wide-bore needle through the cricothyroid membrane. This form of care should be provided **only** by emergency personnel.

Endotracheal Intubation

A cuffed tube is passed through the vocal cords utilizing direct laryngoscopy, and the tube is placed in the trachea.

Oxygen

With a nasal cannula you can give 1–6L/min of oxygen. This provides the patient with 24–44% oxygen. Through a simple mask you can deliver 40–60% oxygen, and a non-rebreather mask can deliver 90–100% oxygen.

The Basics of Support: Airway, Breathing, and Circulation (The ABCs)

The new American Heart Association (AHA) Health-Care Provider (HCP) basic life support (BLS) guidelines have moved away from the previous "A-B-C" (Airway-Breathing-Circulation) protocol to the new, "C-A-B" (Circulation-Airway-Breathing) protocol. One no longer has to "look, listen, and feel" as these steps waste precious time and are not helpful in reviving a collapsed patient. This should be followed by reassessment of the patient's status, use of medications, and transfer to the hospital if needed, for definitive therapy.

CLASSIFICATION OF MEDICAL EMERGENCIES

It is always best to classify medical emergencies according to the patient's presenting symptoms. Once you focus on the specific presenting symptoms you are able to triage and implement the proper care for the patient immediately.

Syncope Attack

Multiple factors can cause syncope, but some factors can cause syncope more commonly than others:

- **Common Causes:** The more common causes of syncope attacks are vasovagal syncope, orthostatic hypotension, hyperventilation syndrome, and hypoglycemic reaction or coma.
- **Less Common Causes:** The less common causes of syncope are transient ischemic attack (TIAs), cerebrovascular accident (CVA/stroke), cardiac arrest, hyperglycemia, and acute adrenal insufficiency.

Chest Pains

Chest pains can occur with angina, myocardial infarction, or hyperventilation. Angina can be stable angina/angina of effort, unstable angina, acute coronary insufficiency (pre-infarction angina), and atypical/coronary artery spasm/Prinzmetal's angina.

Respiratory Distress

Respiratory distress can occur from foreign body obstruction, asthma, or hyperventilation.

Adverse Drug Reactions

Adverse drug reactions can be associated with anaphylaxis/allergy, local anesthetic, **and/or** epinephrine overdose.

Seizures

Seizures can be due to grand mal epilepsy, hypoglycemia, or hyperventilation.

VASOVAGAL SYNCOPE

Vasovagal Syncope Predisposing Factors

Predisposing factors for vasovagal syncope include anxiety, fear, and sight of blood; hot and humid surroundings; upright position without movement; prolonged motionless standing for a period of time; and age (patients in their teens to early forties). Males are more often affected than females.

Vasovagal Prodrome Stage

There is a definite prodrome stage when the patient feels that a collapse is imminent: This is the fright and flight response. It lasts for ten seconds to a few minutes. Anxiety, tachycardia, perspiration, light-headedness, and blurred vision are commonly experienced.

Vasovagal Syncope Stage Vital Signs

Bradycardia with hypotension is *the* classic finding on physical examination. This is the only syncope where a *drop* in the blood pressure (BP) is associated with bradycardia and *not* tachycardia. Tonic-clonic activity may occur.

Vasovagal Postsyncope Stage

Recovery occurs within a few seconds. There may be some headache, dizziness, nausea, vomiting, pallor, and perspiration that may persist for a few minutes to a few hours. The patient may try to sit up on recovery. Discourage this from happening.

There is no postsyncope confusion. Confusion could occur if the patient falls during the emergency and knocks his/her head. This should prompt you to activate the emergency medical system (EMS) and transfer the patient to the nearest emergency room (ER) for evaluation of a head injury.

Vasovagal Syncope Treatment

Immediately put the patient in a supine position. Crack open a vial of ammonia (smelling salts), and hold it away from your face to prevent you from inhaling the vapors! The white covering of the vial turns pink once the ammonia vapors are released. Next, lean forward and have the patient inhale the vapors. The patient will immediately start showing movement. Reassure the patient on recovery. Assess the clarity of the mental status by having the patient respond to some common-knowledge questions. Observe for 30–60 minutes with the patient lying down.

Vasovagal Syncope and Suggested Additional Steps of Care

During an emergency always monitor the pulse using one of the most accessible arteries: radial, brachial (in children), or carotid. Use the following guidelines to get an instant perception of the blood pressure level:

1. Inability to feel the radial pulse during an emergency indicates that the systolic blood pressure (SBP) is **less** than 80 mmHg.
2. Inability to feel the brachial pulse during an emergency indicates the SBP is **less** than 70 mmHg.
3. Inability to feel the carotid pulse during an emergency indicates the SBP has dropped **below** 60 mmHg.

Steps to Interrupt a Vasovagal Syncope Attack

Occasionally you will find yourself facing a patient who has denied anxiety and the need for stress management during an initial medical history assessment visit. Now, when you are ready to inject the local anesthetic, you may find this patient clenching the sides of the dental chair and looking quite pale.

Immediately stop the treatment, reassure the patient, and put the chair in a horizontal or slight head-down position. Have the patient open and close the fists and perform bicycling movements with the legs. This will move the blood from the extremities and toward the heart. Stress management should always be provided for future visits in patients who have experienced vasovagal syncope in the dental setting.

ORTHOSTATIC HYPOTENSION

Orthostatic Hypotension Predisposing Factors

Normally when a person stands up from a sitting or lying-down position, the vasoconstriction response maintains the cerebral blood flow. An elderly patient is more likely to experience orthostatic hypotension (OH), because in the elderly patient, the erect vasoconstrictor action upon standing is slow in onset. Patients on antihypertension, antidepression, and anti–Parkinson's disease drugs often experience orthostatic hypotension as a side effect of the medications. OH can also occur due to increased vasodilation right after IV sedation or nitroglycerine use and it is more common in diabetics with autonomic neuropathy.

Orthostatic Hypotension Prodrome Stage

There is no prodrome stage with OH and the patient feels **normal** prior to the syncope.

Orthostatic Hypotension Syncope Stage Vital Signs

The syncope occurs with rapid change from a lying-down position to an upright position. There is a precipitous drop in the blood pressure. The pulse is normal or slightly elevated from baseline values. The patient regains consciousness when becoming horizontal as circulation to the brain is maintained.

Orthostatic Hypotension Pretreatment Diagnosis

In a suspect case for orthostatic hypotension, monitor the BP and pulse in a lying-down and **immediate** upright position. You can diagnose OH if the systolic blood pressure (SBP) drops by 20–30 mmHg or the diastolic blood pressure (DBP) drops by 10–15 mmHg upon standing and the pulse rate increases by 10–15 beats/min.

Orthostatic Hypotension Prevention Strategy

At the end of the appointment have the patient sit upright in the dental chair for a few minutes and then assist the patient out of the chair. Steady the patient until the patient feels stable standing upright.

HYPERVENTILATION SYNDROME

Hyperventilation Syndrome Predisposing Factors

Anxiety and fear are the most common predisposing factors.

Hyperventilation Syndrome Pathophysiology and Clinical Features

Rapid and deep breathing occurs because of severe anxiety and fear. This rapid breathing causes a washout of CO_2 and the PCO_2 goes below normal (35–45 mmHg). The PO_2 stays in the normal range. Generalized vascular involvement, affecting the cerebral, coronary, and gastrointestinal circulation occurs.

Hyperventilation Syndrome Effect on the Cerebral Circulation

Involvement of the cerebral circulation causes the patient to experience headache, confusion, and visual disturbances. The patient feels as if a collapse is imminent, but it doesn't occur.

Hyperventilation Syndrome Effect on the Coronary Circulation

Involvement of the coronary circulation causes the patient to experience severe tightness of the chest and angina-type pains.

Hyperventilation Syndrome Effect on the Gastrointestinal Circulation

Involvement of the gastrointestinal circulation causes the patient to experience nausea, vomiting, and a lump-in-the-throat feeling (globus hystericus).

Hyperventilation Syndrome Additional Clinical Features

The patient never loses consciousness, although the feeling of light-headedness persists. Tingling, numbness, and paresthesia in the perioral area and the extremities are experienced. Carpopedal spasm, tremors, and muscle twitching occur because of a fall in the ionized serum calcium in the arterial blood.

Hyperventilation Syndrome Vital Signs

The pulse, blood pressure, and respiration rate are markedly elevated from baseline, and the respiratory rate is more than 25–30 breaths/min.

Hyperventilation Syndrome Treatment

Activate the EMS (emergency medical system) if the vital signs are markedly elevated and you have an uncooperative patient. Give the patient an upright or a semi-sitting position in the chair, fan the patient, and loosen the clothing. Encourage rebreathing with the patient's cupped hands over his/her mouth and nose or breathing into a paper bag. Never use a plastic bag because it can suffocate the patient. Breathing into cupped hands or a paper bag will help the patient rebreathe the exhaled CO_2. Approximately 10–15mg diazepam is administered IV if rebreathing is not helpful or the patient is uncooperative. Do not give more than 0.1mg/kg body weight of Valium during the emergency. Alternately, midazolam (Versed) can be injected intramuscular (IM), dosed at 70–80 mcg/kg, or intravenous (IV), which is usually dosed at 0.5–1mg but not to exceed 2.5 mg. Midazolam should always be titrated slowly; administer over at least two minutes and allow an additional two or more minutes to fully evaluate the sedative effect of the drug.

Never use any oxygen during a hyperventilation emergency.

HYPOGLYCEMIA

Hypoglycemia can occur in both the diabetic and the nondiabetic patient. The brain is totally dependent on an adequate glucose supply for its energy requirements.

Hypoglycemia Predisposing Factors

Hypoglycemia can be caused by acute starvation, alcohol bingeing, increased insulin, or oral hypoglycemic drugs intake.

Hypoglycemia Clinical Features

Hypoglycemia reaction is very rapid in onset and can progress from mild to moderate to severe in seconds.

Hypoglycemia Mild Stage

During this stage the patient experiences restlessness, irritability, and excitement and shows lack of cooperation. Nausea is quite pronounced and the patient experiences extreme hunger.

Hypoglycemia Moderate Stage

Perspiration is very apparent and the palms and soles are wet, cold, and clammy. Shivering with hair on end occurs.

Hypoglycemia Vital Signs

Tachycardia associated with a bounding pulse occurs in the initial stages of excitement and irritability. The respiration rate is normal, or it could be slightly increased in the mild stage. The blood pressure is elevated initially, but then it starts to drop when no treatment is initiated. The gag reflex is very prominent in the late, moderate stage. If left untreated the patient goes into the severe stage of hypoglycemia, becoming glassy-eyed and quite unresponsive. Tonic-clonic seizures may occur and the patient can become unconscious. During the unconscious stage the BP drops and hypotension occurs along with bradycardia and hypothermia.

Hypoglycemia Treatment

Assess the ABCs and position the patient accordingly. Give the conscious patient a semi-sitting position if the BP is **maintained** and the patient stays **connected** with you in conversational response. Give a horizontal position when, in spite of being conscious, the patient **fails to communicate well** with you.

Administer oral glucose gel, liquid sugar, Glucola, or apple or orange juice in the mild stage. It is best to use baby apple juice because it does not need to be refrigerated. The juice has a long shelf life as long as it is unopened. A baby juice product is also less likely to suddenly disappear because someone was thirsty! The use of orange juice is not advised in an uncontrolled diabetic with preexisting kidney disease because of the high potassium content in orange juice. The potassium from the orange juice can worsen the persisting hyperkalemia associated with kidney disease. Orange juice, however, can be used in the renal-compromised patient with normal potassium levels or in the nondiabetic patient experiencing hypoglycemia.

Once the patient has recovered from a mild reaction, have the patient eat some complex carbohydrate foods such as whole-wheat/rye crackers with cheese or whole-wheat/rye crackers with peanut butter. The fiber in the complex carbohydrates helps keep the sugars in the stomach longer and prevents a relapse.

Administer 50mL of $D_{50}W$ IV **slowly**, at the rate of 10mL/min, in the moderate-to-severe stage. If you are unable to establish an IV line, give 1mg glucagon IM in the deltoid muscle.

Administer oxygen by mask at a flow rate of 4–6L/min. Activate EMS if you have not yet done so, particularly when seizures occur or if the recovery is sluggish.

Hypoglycemia: Additional Suggested Recovery Facts and Alerts

Once an insulin-dependent diabetic has completely recovered from a hypoglycemic reaction and has been well compensated, dental treatment can continue if the patient feels comfortable going ahead with the dentistry planned for the day. Dental treatment must be **discontinued** if a diabetic on oral hypoglycemic drugs develops a hypoglycemic reaction. Oral hypoglycemic drugs can cause the patient to have **rebound hypoglycemia** four to six hours after an initial hypoglycemic reaction. Once the initial reaction is treated in the dental office, the patient should be sent to the ER for monitoring and steady maintenance of the blood sugar levels.

Another fact to remember is, if the patient is taking β-blockers for hypertension or benign tremors and so on, all the symptoms of hypoglycemia are usually absent **except** for perspiration, because β-blockers **blunt** hypoglycemic symptoms. The blunting effect is more **severe** with the **nonselective** β-blockers compared to selective β-blockers.

TRANSIENT ISCHEMIC ATTACKS (TIAS)

The hallmark feature of TIA is that the patient never really loses consciousness. TIAs are associated with temporary cerebral ischemia and no permanent brain damage. Symptoms last for a few seconds to a few minutes—occasionally for a few hours—and resolution of all symptoms occurs within 24 hours.

Transient Ischemic Attacks Predisposing Factors

Predisposing factors for TIAs are hypertension, diabetes, hyperlipidemia, or atrial fibrillation.

Transient Ischemic Attacks Clinical Features

The patient experiences tingling, numbness, or weakness of the limbs or hands and feet. Slurred speech, loss of speech, drooling, blurring of vision, and disorientation can also occur.

Transient Ischemic Attacks Vital Signs

The pulse is rapid and bounding and the BP is elevated.

Transient Ischemic Attacks Treatment

Activate the EMS if this is the first TIA attack for the patient or if it is a worsening attack for a patient with a past history of TIAs. Give the patient an upright position and monitor the vital signs. Try to calm an agitated patient. Do not use oxygen if the patient has no breathing difficulty because the oxygen will promote vasoconstriction and worsen the TIA symptoms. If this is not the first attack, observe the patient for some time and determine by communicating with the patient if this attack is any different from the past attacks. Once the symptoms have subsided, send the patient home as long as the TIA is no different when compared with the ones experienced by the patient in the past. However, if there is a change in the severity, or the symptoms experienced are new, the patient must be sent to the ER for further evaluation and monitoring for potential stroke/CVA.

CEREBROVASCULAR ACCIDENT

Cerebrovascular accident (CVA)/stroke is associated with permanent neurological damage. CVA may be due to cerebral ischemia, infarction, or intracranial hemorrhage. True syncope is rare. However, intracranial hemorrhage invariably results in sudden loss of consciousness and is associated with an increased morbidity and mortality rate.

Cerebrovascular Accident Predisposing Factors

Predisposing factors to CVA are similar to those for TIAs.

Cerebrovascular Accident Clinical Features

Fear and anxiety in the dental setting may lead to the elevation of the BP in susceptible patients. All stroke patients experience headaches that may be mild, moderate, or severe. CVA due to ischemia or infarction is associated with mild-to-moderate headaches. True syncope rarely occurs at the onset with ischemia or infarction. Intracranial hemorrhage or CVA associated with a ruptured aneurysm causes excruciating headaches and sudden loss of consciousness. This type of CVA is associated with increased morbidity and mortality. Dizziness, vertigo, nausea, vomiting, and progressive sensory and/or motor dysfunction are experienced with all forms of strokes.

Cerebrovascular Accident Vital Signs

The pulse is usually bounding with a thrombus or an embolism and may be normal or slow in association with an intracranial hemorrhage. The BP is elevated with stroke from any cause. Respiration is slow and shallow.

Cerebrovascular Accident Treatment

Activate the EMS. Maintain an upright position for the conscious patient and a supine position with the head **slightly elevated** with a neck role (to prevent a further increase in the intracranial pressure) for the unconscious patient.

Monitor vital signs and maintain the ABCs. Do not use oxygen if the patient is breathing adequately. Increased levels of oxygen can cause further vasoconstriction and worsening of symptoms. Oxygen should be given **only** to an unconscious patient experiencing true breathing difficulty. Always rule out airway obstruction due to improper positioning prior to administering oxygen. Once stable, immediately transfer the patient to the hospital.

CARDIAC ARREST OF UNKNOWN ORIGIN

The patient is unresponsive with no palpable pulse.

Cardiac Arrest Predisposing Factors

The predisposing factors are ventricular fibrillation or arrhythmia, severe myocardial infarction, drug overdose, or foreign body airway obstruction.

Cardiac Arrest Clinical Features

Loss of consciousness occurs within three to five seconds, and brain damage can occur within four to six minutes without treatment.

Cardiac Arrest Unresponsive Patient Management

Health-Care Provider Basic Life Support

In 2010, the American Heart Association (AHA) came out with significant new recommendations for layperson and health-care provider (HCP) basic life support (BLS) and advanced cardiac life support (ACLS). The new guidelines have moved away from the previous "A-B-C" (Airway-Breathing-Circulation) protocol to the new, "C-A-B" (Circulation-Airway-Breathing) protocol. One no longer has to "look, listen, and feel," as these steps waste precious time and are not helpful.

The major HCP BLS steps are:

1. **Responsiveness:** Check for responsiveness by shaking and asking the patient, "Are you okay?"
2. **Emergency medical system (EMS) and automated electrical defibrillator (AED):** Activate the EMS and have the AED brought to the site of emergency.
3. **Circulation:** Use **less than 10 seconds** to check the carotid pulse in a collapsed patient. If the pulse is present, then do the head-tilt–chin-lift and provide support with **rescue breathing, once every 5–6 seconds**. If the pulse is absent, first do compressions and then follow-up with ventilation. There is no change in the AHA recommendation for compression-to-ventilation ratio of **30:2** for single rescuers of adults, children, and infants in the health-care setting. However, **chest compressions**, not airway management, are now the **first-priority**, so the oxygen-rich blood that is present in the lungs can get into the circulation and reach the heart and the brain immediately. Prioritizing the airways causes a valuable delay in starting chest compressions. Per AHA recommendations, airway management in the form of **2 ventilations** should begin after the first cycle of **30 chest compressions** has been completed **over 18 seconds**.

    Per new AHA guidelines, pulse checks should be minimized for health-care providers because they cause interruptions and delays in chest compressions. Therefore, use **less than 10 seconds** to check for the pulse, and if no pulse is found then chest compressions should be restarted immediately. After the first cycle of **30:2**, proceed to check the pulse using no more than 10 seconds, and then continue chest compressions at the rate of **100 compressions per minute**. Compress the chest to a depth of **2 inches** in adults, and **1.5 inches** in children and infants. Chest compressions must begin before clearing the airway. Avoid leaning on the chest so the chest can return to its starting position every time as there needs to be complete chest recoil between compressions.

The chest compressions should be continued for as long as possible without the use of excessive ventilation. Minimizing interruptions in chest compressions leads to better outcomes, including spontaneous return of circulation and subsequent survival. Switch compression and ventilation tasks every 2 minutes to minimize any ventilation interruption.

4. **Defibrillation:** When needed, connect the AED and shock the patient. Defibrillation is the most appropriate way to treat cardiac arrest from ventricular fibrillation (VF). However, when waiting for personnel and equipment to arrive, chest compressions should begin immediately in the unresponsive patient with no pulse. Extensive research has shown that chest compressions and early defibrillation, but not airway management, is the best first-step in managing ventricular fibrillation (VF) or pulseless ventricular tachycardia (VT).

5. Establish an IV line with normal saline. Give $D_{50}W$ IV and naloxone (Narcan), 0.4 mg IV. Whenever you are unaware of the exact etiology of the collapse and unresponsiveness, you need to treat it as if it were a hypoglycemia reaction and narcotic overdose. These are two emergency states that can cause brain damage if not treated promptly. In the event the cause is something different, the $D_{50}W$ IV and naloxone will not adversely affect the patient. Repeat the Narcan injection and the dextrose drip if you see a clinical response. If you are unable to establish an IV line, give Narcan IM, 0.4 mg. If hypoglycemia is strongly suspected, give glucagon 1mg IM in the deltoid muscle.

HYPERGLYCEMIA

Hyperglycemia affects only diabetic patients. Poor control and/or poor compliance lead to hyperglycemia. Infection, inflammation, trauma, and bleeding can exacerbate the hyperglycemia and can progress to hyperglycemic coma.

Hyperglycemia Clinical Features

Hyperglycemia takes a few hours to a few days to develop. The patient is red in the face, the skin is warm and dry due to dehydration, and the patient has a ketone smell. The mouth is dry and the patient experiences intense thirst. Abdominal pain often occurs.

Hyperglycemia Vital Signs

The pulse is rapid but weak. The BP is decreased. The respiration is deep and rapid. This is the classic Kussmaul's breathing, which is an abnormal breathing pattern characterized by rapid and deep breathing. It is often seen in patients with metabolic acidosis. The patient has a ketotic, fruity smell.

Hyperglycemia Treatment

Activate the EMS. Management of the syncope is supportive while the patient is in the dental office. Give the patient a horizontal position in the chair. Monitor the vital signs. Start an IV line with normal saline and give 4–6L/min oxygen. The EMS and ER will manage the hyperglycemia with insulin and treat the underlying cause precipitating the hyperglycemia.

ACUTE ADRENAL INSUFFICIENCY

Acute Adrenal Insufficiency Etiology

Acute adrenal insufficiency occurs with acute infection, inflammation, trauma, massive bleeding, or **failure to give** steroids in susceptible patients when there is a **need** to follow "the rule of twos."

The rule of twos: Ask whether the patient is currently on steroids or has been on corticosteroids for two weeks or longer within the past two years. You must go back two years in the history because it can take **two weeks to two years** for the adrenal glands to return to **normal** function.

Acute Adrenal Insufficiency Clinical Features

The patient experiences extreme fatigue, muscle cramps, muscle weakness, mental confusion (due to hypoglycemia), nausea, vomiting, and severe abdominal pain. The deteriorating condition progresses rapidly without treatment, leading to coma.

Acute Adrenal Insufficiency Vital Signs

The respiration is slow and shallow. The BP falls very rapidly and the pulse is rapid and very weak.

Acute Adrenal Insufficiency Treatment

Activate the EMS and immediately give the patient a supine position. Assess the airway, breathing, and circulation (ABCs) and monitor the vital signs. Establish an IV line and start 5% glucose in normal saline. Give 100mg hydrocortisone IV STAT (immediately) followed by hydrocortisone q6h: Total dose given is 100–200mg/24 hr. The hydrocortisone is given until the patient is stable. Give oxygen at a flow rate of 4–6L/min.

ANGINA PECTORIS

Angina Pectoris Clinical Features

Activity precipitates an attack. With the start of the attack the patient is unable to continue with activity, immediately stands still, and is hunched over with the fist across the chest. Tightness or discomfort experienced in the chest occurs for less than 10–15 minutes, and usually lasts about 2–5 minutes in most cases. The discomfort experienced may or may not radiate. If it does radiate, it can go toward the jaw, the left arm, the back, or the upper abdomen. This pain radiation can happen with unstable angina, too. The patient can be quite apprehensive if this is a first angina attack, but apprehension level is less if the patient has experienced angina before. Sweating can be significant depending upon the intensity of the attack.

Angina Pectoris Vital Signs

The pulse is markedly increased and bounding, and the BP is elevated. Some dyspnea or respiratory difficulty may occur.

Angina Pectoris Treatment

Activate the EMS if this is a first attack for the patient or it happens to be a worsening attack for a patient with a past history of angina attacks. Place the patient in an upright position.

Treat with nitroglycerine (NTG) tablets. Start with one 0.3mg nitroglycerine tablet sublingual (SL). Always confirm that the tablet produces a burning sensation under the tongue and a flushed feeling going to the head. This indicates that the pill is potent. Repeat with a second or third nitroglycerine tablet at five-minute intervals, as long as the patient experiences pain and the systolic BP is **above** 115 mmHg prior to each tablet use.

You can give a total of three 0.3mg nitroglycerine tablets at five-minute intervals. Do not go beyond three nitroglycerine tablets even if the pain continues and the BP is elevated. This patient needs to be sent to the ER immediately for further evaluation and care. Give oxygen 4–6L/min with the start of the treatment because this facilitates recovery.

Note that some emergency kits may contain nitroglycerine lingual spray instead of nitroglycerine tablets. Actually, it is better to have the spray in the emergency kit instead of nitroglycerine tablets because the spray has a longer shelf life (one year) than nitroglycerine tablets, which have a maximum shelf life of six weeks once used. The nitroglycerine is sprayed **without shaking the bottle**. The patient should not inhale the spray. The spray is as effective as the tablets and the potency of one spray is equal to the potency of one sublingual tablet (0.3mg/tablet). Questioning of the patient for burning sensation and flushed feeling, along with BP assessment prior to the next dose, are the same as those previously outlined for nitroglycerine tablets.

Protocol for Nitroglycerine lingual spray use is as follows:

- To use nitroglycerin spray, hold the container upright and bring the container as close to the patient's mouth as possible. Press down firmly to release the spray **onto or under your tongue** and then have the patient close the mouth.
- Do not let the patient swallow right after spraying a dose, nor should you allow the patient to spit or rinse the mouth for 5–10 minutes after using the nitroglycerin spray.
- A spray may be repeated every 3–5 minutes if the pain continues, but do not use more than 3 sprays in 15 minutes. Always ensure that the SBP is above 115 mmHg, prior to re-spraying. If chest pain continues after a total of 3 sprays, activate EMS for immediate medical attention and patient transport to the emergency room.

Angina Treatment Alerts

The shelf life of nitroglycerine tablets is six months, unopened, and six weeks, once the bottle has been opened. The shelf life is further shortened when the pills are exposed to light and agitated constantly in the bottle. Always confirm that the patient experiences a burning and tingling sensation when using nitroglycerine, either in pill form or spray.

Check the BP and confirm that the systolic blood pressure is elevated. If the systolic blood pressure goes **below** 115 mmHg with nitroglycerine pill or spray, activate the EMS and stop using any further NTG. This BP drop typically occurs with unstable angina and one should always consider progression to myocardial infarction (MI) as one of the potential causes. With conversion to MI, the blood pressure drops and the pulse becomes rapid and thready (low volume). The pulse may become irregular. In this situation, place the patient in a horizontal position, maintain the ABCs, supply oxygen, and wait for the EMS to arrive. Management of this state is the same as that outlined for an MI attack.

Note that if there has been no response to nitroglycerine in the past, the patient could be given 10–20mg niphedipine (Procardia) sublingual (SL), as this could be Prinzmetal's angina.

Nitroglycerine and Erectile Dysfunction: Drug Combination Alert

Drugs use to treat erectile dysfunction (ED)—sildenafil citrate (Viagra), tadalafil (Cialis), and vardenafil HCL (Levitra)—cause significant vasodilatation. Profound vasodilatation can occur when even a single nitroglycerine tablet or spray is given to a patient who has used an ED drug in the past 24–48 hours, and this significant vasodilatation can cause a precipitous drop in the BP. Therefore, this patient must be sent to the ER for proper assessment, management, and triage for successful outcome of care. The vasodilatation caused by Viagra lasts for 24 hours and that caused by Cialis and Levitra lasts for 48 hours.

MYOCARDIAL INFARCTION

Myocardial Infarction Risk Factors

Risk factors include past history of angina or coronary artery disease, uncontrolled hypertension, any past history of thrombotic episodes (stroke or a previous MI), heavy smoking and excessive alcohol consumption, obesity, or hypercholesterolemia.

Myocardial Infarction Clinical Features

MI pain lasts for more than 10–15 minutes and it is a "crushing" type of chest pain. The pain can be precipitated with or without activity. The patient looks pale and acutely distressed. There is tightness of the chest and excruciating pain that may or may not radiate. If it does radiate, it can go toward the lower jaw or left arm, and sometimes the right arm, back, or upper abdomen. Along with the chest pain, the patient often experiences palpitations, profuse sweating, restlessness, anxiety, lightheadedness, cold and clammy skin, a feeling of impending doom, nausea, vomiting, and abdominal bloating. The patient may attribute the nausea, vomiting, and abdominal bloating to a gastrointestinal problem and may not seek help in a timely manner.

Myocardial Infarction Vital Signs

The patient is short of breath and the respiration is shallow. The pulse is rapid, thready (low volume), and highly irregular. Occasionally, bradycardia can occur. The BP is decreased, compared to normal baseline readings.

Myocardial Infarction Medical Management

Activate the emergency medical system (EMS). Lay the patient down to assess the airway, breathing, circulation (ABCs), and monitor the vital signs. The first line of management for a suspected case of MI is administering **m**orphine, **o**xygen, **n**itroglycerine, and **a**spirin (MONA).

Start 4–6L/min of oxygen by mask. Immediately, give one 0.3mg tablet nitroglycerin sublingual or use one nitroglycerine spray on or under the tongue, as long as the SBP is **above** 115 mmHg. Also give 162mg or 325mg aspirin crushed under the tongue or have the patient chew or swallow the aspirin. The aspirin will immediately thin the blood by decreasing the platelet cohesiveness. Do not use enteric-coated aspirin because that will delay absorption.

The EMS will establish an IV line, start 5% dextrose in water, and give 2–5mg morphine intravenous, every 5–15 minutes until the pain subsides. Respiration rate during morphine administration must always be maintained at more than 12 breaths/minute. Once the pain is stabilized with morphine, the patient is moved to the hospital.

At any time during transportation or otherwise, cardiac arrest can occur with acute MI. Cardiopulmonary resuscitation (CPR) will maintain the patient until an automated electrical defibrillator (AED) can be used to evaluate ventricular tachycardia or ventricular arrhythmia. The AED will revive the cardiac rhythm in such circumstances.

FOREIGN BODY OBSTRUCTION (FBO)

Foreign Body Obstruction Facts

No noise or respiratory sound is heard in total laryngotracheal obstruction. Stridor, cough, cyanosis, and wheezing occur in partial laryngotracheal obstruction or bronchial obstruction. The victim grabs at the throat and experiences intense fear.

Foreign Body Obstruction Treatment

Activate the EMS immediately. Perform the Heimlich maneuver and continue doing it until the FBO is expelled or the patient becomes unconscious. Straddle over the supine patient and do 6–10 abdominal thrusts, after doing a head-tilt–chin-lift, if the patient becomes unconscious.

Next, proceed to do a finger sweep followed by ventilation of the patient. Repeat the thrusts, sweep, and ventilation until you are successful or EMS has arrived.

Additional care can be provided with epinephrine, steroids, albuterol or metaproterenol in order to open the airways and decrease inflammation. Cricythyrotomy with the cricothyrotomy device or a thirteen-gauge needle may be done, if the Heimlich maneuver is unsuccessful.

ASTHMA

Asthma Types

Extrinsic asthma is typically the allergy-associated asthma. Intrinsic asthma is the nonallergy-associated asthma and it is frequently precipitated by infection in the lung(s).

Acute Asthma Clinical Features

Acute asthma is typically associated with shortness of breath (SOB), wheezing on inspiration and/or expiration, cough with or without expectoration, and labored breathing. Cyanosis, intense fatigue, and mental confusion can occur in severe cases.

Asthma Vital Signs

Initially and very transiently the respiratory rate (RR) is normal, but as the asthma progresses the RR becomes rapid. The pulse and the BP are both elevated.

Asthma Treatment

Activate the EMS in severe cases, or if this is an initial attack. Immediately give the patient an upright position in the chair. The patient will prefer to sit hunched over as this helps the patient breath better.

As a first choice, use the patient's own bronchodilator. If this is not possible, have the patient use the metaproterenol (Alupent) or albuterol (Proventil) spray from the emergency kit. Alternately, give 0.3–0.5 ml, 1:1,000 epinephrine, SC/IM if nothing else is available. If the patient's pulse is less than 120–130 beats/min and the BP is less than 140/90 mmHg, epinephrine may be repeated twice at twenty-minute intervals, following the pulse and BP guidelines. Give oxygen at a flow rate of 4–6L/min. In refractory cases, slow infusion of 6mg/kg IV aminophylline, diluted in 50–100mL saline and 100–200mg IV hydrocortisone sodium succinate, are also given.

ANAPHYLAXIS/ALLERGY

Anaphylaxis/Allergy Clinical Features

The patient experiences a sinking feeling, intense itching, hives, and flushing over the face and chest. Rhinitis, conjunctivitis, nausea, vomiting, abdominal cramps, and perspiration also occur. Additionally, the patient experiences palpitation, tachycardia, substernal tightness, coughing, wheezing, and dyspnea. The patient initially looks pale and then, in extreme cases, cyanosis and laryngeal edema can occur. The blood pressure (BP) drops rapidly and loss of consciousness or cardiac arrest can occur in severe cases.

Anaphylaxis/Allergy Treatment

Give the patient a supine position. Establish an IV line with normal saline and give 0.3–0.5mL 1:1,000 epinephrine, SC/IM. Epinephrine may be repeated every 3–5 minutes until improvement occurs. In the severely hypotensive patient, **only emergency personnel** can **slowly** give 1:10,000 epinephrine, 0.3mL IV. Once epinephrine has stabilized the pulse and the BP, inject 50mg diphenhydramine (Benadryl) IV **plus** 300mg cimetidine (Tagamet) **or** 20mg famotidine (Pepcid) IV. Cimetidine and famotadine are H_2 blockers. Additionally, give 100–200mg hydrocortisone sodium succinate (Solu-cortef) IV. Metaproterenol spray can also be used for refractory cases to open the airways. Oxygen is given at a flow rate of 4–6L/min.

When the acute phase is over, the patient is given 50mg diphenhydramine and/or 300mg cimetidine/20mg famotidine (Pepcid) **PO q6h for next 48–72 hours**. Premature withdrawal of the H_1 with or without the H_2 blocker can cause a hypotensive reaction because excess histamine is still in the circulation. Nonsedating fexofenadine HCL (Allegra), cetirizine HCL (Zyrtec), or loratadine (Claritin) can be used instead of the sedating Benadryl, for 48–72 hours in the post-recovery period.

Fexofenadine (Allegra) dose: 60mg bid or 180mg once daily in healthy patients, or 60mg once daily in patients with decreased renal function. **Cetirizine HCL (Zyrtec)**

dose: 10mg daily in healthy patients or 5mg daily in renal or hepatic compromised patients. **Loratidine (Claritin) dose:** 10mg tablet or 2 teaspoonfuls (10 mg) of syrup once daily in healthy patients or 10mg every other day in patients with liver or renal insufficiency.

LOCAL ANESTHETIC OVERDOSE

Duration of the local anesthetic overdose reaction is very short because of quick redistribution and biotransformation of the anesthetic.

Local Anesthetic Overdose Clinical Features

The patient experiences agitation, confusion, excitement, talkativeness, apprehension, slurred speech, muscle twitching, and tremors. Headache, light-headedness, visual disturbance, and a flushed feeling can also occur. Numbness of the tongue and numbness around the perioral area may also occur. Disorientation, drowsiness, and tonic-clonic seizures may occur in progressive cases.

Local Anesthetic Overdose Vital Signs

The pulse, BP, and respiratory rate are all increased.

Local Anesthetic Overdose Treatment

Activate EMS in severe cases. Give the patient a semi-sitting position. Reassure the patient and ask him/her to hyperventilate. Inject 10mg diazepam (Valium) IV slowly or midazolam (Versed) dosed at 0.5–1mg but do not exceed 2.5mg IV slowly if seizure occurs. Give oxygen in severe cases. Perform CPR with cardiac arrest.

EPINEPHRINE OVERDOSE REACTION

Epinephrine Overdose Clinical Features

The patient experiences anxiety, fear, restlessness, throbbing headache, tremors, perspiration, weakness, dizziness, and pallor.

Epinephrine Overdose Reaction Vital Signs

The pulse is rapid and bounding. The respiratory rate is increased and respiratory difficulty is experienced. The BP is elevated.

Epinephrine Overdose Reaction Treatment

Position the patient in a semi-sitting or upright position. Reassure the patient and monitor the vital signs. Administer oxygen at a flow rate of 4–6L/min.

SEIZURES

A typical grand mal seizure attack is always associated with the ictal/seizure phase. A prodromal phase may or may not precede the ictal/seizure phase.

Prodromal Phase

The prodromal phase occurs hours to days before the seizure and it can last for several minutes to several hours. The patient can experience increased anxiety, depression, a low feeling, or tunnel vision. This phase does not occur in every patient. However, if the patient does experience specific symptoms that herald a seizure, those specific symptoms **will always precede** the ictal/seizure phase in the patient.

Seizure or Ictal Phase

The seizure/ictal phase can have four components: the aura, tonic, clonic, and flaccid phase. A typical tonic-clonic seizure lasts for no more than two minutes.

Aura Phase

The aura is not present in every patient, but if it does exist, the aura symptoms experienced **repeat** with every seizure that occurs. The aura lasts for a few seconds only. The patient can see, hear, taste, or smell something specific, like a rotten egg taste or sulfur smell, and verbalizes this during this phase. These are abnormal sensations experienced, but the patient is **unaware** of their presence when questioned later, upon recovery. The patient may, however, recount their presence during history-taking if someone present during a past attack had informed the patient about having experienced those symptoms. Do not remove the patient from the chair during this phase. The patient is conscious but unaware of the surroundings. Immediately give the patient a horizontal position, push the tray away, and call for help. You and an assistant should stand on either side of the chair and provide passive restraint to prevent the patient from falling.

Tonic Phase

In this phase the patient gives out a loud cry and becomes very rigid and hyper-extended after taking in a deep breath. There is loss of consciousness and the patient turns blue from holding the breath. If the patient was initially standing, the patient falls to the ground. You may want to, but **do not** hold the patient down during the tonic phase, because you can injure the patient's spine. This phase lasts for less than a minute.

Clonic Phase

The clonic phase follows the tonic phase. The patient starts breathing and the limbs start to flay. The flailing is initially rhythmic and then becomes arrhythmic toward the end of the phase. Again, do not hold the patient down because fractures may occur. This phase **also** lasts for about one minute or less and it is then followed by the postictal or the flaccid phase.

Flaccid Phase

The entire body becomes limp during this phase. Frothing occurs at the mouth, the tongue falls back and the patient starts to "grunt." There is always incontinence of the bowel and/or the bladder during this phase. Incontinence does **not** occur with seizures due to other causes: drug reaction, hypoglycemia, and so on.

Seizure Treatment

Activate the EMS. Keep the patient in a supine position. Prevent injury during the tonic, clonic, and flaccid phases. Once in the flaccid phase, monitor the vital signs. Perform a head-tilt–chin-lift and turn the head to the side. Use suction and actively remove all secretions to clear the airway. Give oxygen at a flow rate of 4–6L/min by mask. Once the airways have been cleared during the flaccid phase, confirm that the patient has regained consciousness. It is very important to shake the patient and have the patient respond to your questions. It is not uncommon for the patient to go into a deep sleep once the seizure ends. Pinch an unresponsive patient to see whether a painful stimulus can awaken the patient. If there is no response, the patient is in the **status epilepticus**, which is a phase of ongoing seizures and one where the patient continues to remain unconscious. The EMS has to transfer such a patient to the nearest emergency room after injecting diazepam (Valium) or midazolam (versed) IV slowly during one of the flaccid phases to stop the constant seizure activity; 5–10mg diazepam (Valium) or midazolam (Versed) dosed at 0.5–1mg but not to exceed 2.5 mg, is injected IV, over 1–2 minutes, and 50mL of $D_{50}W$ IV is also given if hypoglycemia is suspected. There is a 15% mortality rate with status epilepticus.

Oral and Parenteral Conscious Sedation for Dentistry: Assessment, Analysis, and Associated Dental Management Guidelines

CONSCIOUS SEDATION OVERVIEW

Conscious sedation is what makes dentistry "painless" for the phobic patient or the patient fearful of the dental environment. Elimination of pain and anxiety management are usually the first considerations for patients experiencing fear or phobia toward dentistry. Conscious sedation is an extension of care beyond these measures. Sedation dentistry helps make dental procedures virtually painless. Conscious sedation is not just reserved for the fearful patient. It is also an important option for patients with developmental disabilities and movement disorders so that dentistry can be completed effortlessly. Anesthesiologist-administered general anesthesia for dentistry is not a part of conscious sedation and should be confined to a hospital setting only.

SEDATION CLASSIFICATIONS

Types of sedation include:

1. Anesthesiologist-administered deep sedation
2. Intravenous (IV) sedation or deep conscious sedation
3. Inhalation conscious sedation
4. Oral conscious sedation

Anesthesiologist-Administered Deep Sedation

This type of sedation is to be administered only by an anesthesiologist. The patient has partial or complete loss of protective reflexes, and there is inability to maintain a patent airway independently and at all times. The patient is not easily aroused and the patient is unable to respond to verbal commands or physical stimulation.

Dentist's Guide to Medical Conditions, Medications, and Complications, Second Edition. Kanchan M. Ganda.
© 2013 John Wiley & Sons, Inc. Published 2013 by John Wiley & Sons, Inc.

Intravenous (IV) Sedation or Deep Conscious Sedation

Most oral surgeons and some trained dentists use this technique. It requires certification by the state board of dentistry. IV sedation is provided using a single drug, usually one of the benzodiazepines. The dose is titrated to match the patient's needs and underlying vital organ status. More can be injected for immediate effect when the dose wears off. Fixed dose or bolus dose drug use is highly discouraged. Drugs used for this type of sedation are more effective when given intravenously than when the same drugs are taken orally. There is a more profound amnesia associated with this sedation technique.

Inhalation Conscious Sedation

Inhalation sedation is provided by using titrated doses of $O_2 + N_2O$. The patient usually falls asleep during the procedure. There is some amount of amnesia and analgesia.

Oxygen/nitrous oxide sedation is the most frequently used sedation in dentistry. This type of sedation requires special delivery and scavenging systems for the gases. The patient should not have had any recent upper respiratory tract infections (URTIs) prior to this type of sedation.

All bodily functions remain normal with this type of sedation and the patient is able to breathe on his own. The patient will often fall asleep and experience some degree of amnesia. Dental inhalation sedation works well for mild-to-moderate anxiety. It has a rapid onset, there is flexibility of duration, and it can be used for any appointment length. The dentist has absolute control because it is easy to titrate the level of sedation, which may be altered moment to moment. The recovery is quick and there are very few side effects. There is an analgesic effect experienced and the patient can resume normal activities immediately.

The disadvantages of dental inhalation sedation include severe anxiety, which may require a deeper level of sedation, plus it is not indicated for patients with respiratory problems such as severe asthma, significant emphysema, or COPD.

Oral Conscious Sedation

This type of sedation is patient-administered, safe, and easy to monitor. The patient takes oral benzodiazepines prescribed by the dentist. The patient invariably falls asleep, and deep relaxation is experienced with this method of sedation. All bodily functions remain normal and the patient is able to breathe on his/her own, often falling asleep. Some degree of amnesia is common. The disadvantage of oral sedation, however, is that the level of sedation for each patient is not predictable. Someone must drive the patient to and from the dental appointment and there is no analgesic effect.

Inhalation and Oral Conscious Sedation: Additional Facts

Oral conscious sedation and inhalation sedation are the two most common types of sedation techniques used by most dental practitioners doing sedation dentistry, outside of the oral surgery setting. Conscious sedation is not light general anesthesia. In fact, there is a huge difference between conscious sedation and the unconscious state associated with general anesthesia. In conscious sedation the patient maintains all bodily functions independently, including airway, circulation, and responsiveness to verbal commands and/or stimulation. The sedation level is reached when slurring of speech occurs.

The types of phobias experienced by the patient may dictate the type of conscious sedation used. A patient experiencing injection-needle associated phobia may need to be induced with $O_2 + N_2O$, prior to IV sedation.

PATIENT SELECTION AND INSTRUCTIONS FOR CONSCIOUS SEDATION

Proper patient selection is very important when deciding on dentistry with sedation. Sedation may not work for all patients. You must do a thorough history and physical examination and assess the patient's weight, baseline vital signs, mental status, allergy status, airway status, past history of any significant anesthesia outcome, current medical conditions, current medications (many drugs may interfere with the metabolism of sedatives, resulting in prolonged CNS effects), laboratory tests, the patient's vital organ status, DDIs among the patient's medications and the sedation medications, and the patient's ASA status.

The American Society of Anesthesiology Status

The American Society of Anesthesiology (ASA) status establishes the patient's overall **cardiopulmonary status** (Table 10.1). The ASA status is determined in all patients undergoing surgery using either local or general anesthesia. The cardiopulmonary status is determined by assessing the patient's capacity to walk up a flight of stairs or walk two blocks.

Note that patients with arthritis may not be able to climb stairs. The ASA status in these patients is established by determining the patient's capacity to walk a block or two. Additionally, an ASA III or IV patient will experience significant breathing difficulty when made to lie down horizontally in the dental chair. These patients will also state that they need to be propped up on multiple pillows when in bed, so they can breathe comfortably and without difficulty.

Sedation and the Medically Compromised Patient

When deciding on sedation for a medically compromised patient, the dentist must know the total number of medical conditions that are being treated, the level of control of each disease state, and the patient's cardiopulmonary ASA status. These facts need to be accounted for, prior to assessing the type of conscious sedation that will be safe for the patient (Table 10.2).

Conscious Sedation Contraindications

Conscious sedation is contraindicated in patients with moderate-to-severe liver or kidney disease; patients with moderate-to-severe respiratory disease and COPD; patients

Table 10.1. The ASA Classification

ASA Status	Task Performance Climbing a Flight of Stairs
ASA I	The normal or well-controlled patient reaches the top of the stairs effortlessly.
ASA II	The patient is winded upon reaching the top and has to rest to feel comfortable.
ASA III	The patient gets winded and stops frequently while climbing, but does reach the top.
ASA IV	The patient is very winded and unable to climb.

Table 10.2. Medically Compromised Patient: Disease Associated ASA Status and Conscious Sedation Guidelines

ASA Status	Disease Status	Comments
ASA I	Patient has no known systemic disease.	Conscious sedation is OK. No primary care physician (PCP) consult is required.
ASA II	Single, mild, or well-controlled systemic disease.	Same as ASA I, but get laboratory tests to confirm disease control.
ASA III	Multiple or moderately controlled systemic diseases.	Get PCP consult. Review patient's lab tests, medications, and DDIs with the conscious sedation medication(s).
ASA IV	Poorly controlled systemic diseases.	CS done by anesthesiologist in a hospitalized setting.

with acute narrow-angle glaucoma; patients with unstable arrhythmias; frail, debilitated, and elderly patients; pregnant patients or nursing mothers; and significantly compromised developmentally disabled patients.

Conscious Sedation Patient Instructions

Each patient must be completely evaluated prior to conscious sedation, and conscious sedation is not for **all** patients. ASA I and ASA II patients are the lowest-risk populations; ASA III patients need for you to have a PCP consult, to determine if conscious sedation is right for the patient. The informed consent must be obtained prior to the procedure and start of conscious sedation. Prior to conscious sedation, inform the patient and the person transporting the patient about post-sedation discharge and give follow-up instructions.

There should be no intake of solid food or full liquids for at least 6–8hours prior to sedation. No clear liquids should be consumed for at least 3–4hours prior to the sedation. However, it is best to have the patient fasting or nil-by-mouth (NPO) for conscious sedation. Patients must be monitored before, during, and after a procedure.

VITAL PARAMETERS AND CONSCIOUS SEDATION

The vital parameters that need to be monitored during conscious sedation are baseline vital signs, oxygen saturation level, heart rate and rhythm, and level of consciousness.

Vital Parameters Timeline Protocol

The timeline protocol for monitoring vital parameters is as follows:

1. **Monitor and document the vital parameters every 5 minutes:** during administration of the medication(s), during the sedation period, and during the recovery period.
2. **Monitor the vital parameters every 15 minutes** once the parameters return to baseline in the post-sedation period or if it has been 30 minutes since the last medication was given. The endpoint for monitoring is when the patient regains consciousness and achieves pre-sedation vital parameters status.

Conscious Sedation Recovery Alerts

Take immediate action when there is

1. A ±20% change in the pulse or blood pressure (BP).
2. Change in the cardiac rhythm.
3. Drop in the oxygen saturation by ≥5% below baseline.
4. Dyspnea/apnea/hypoventilation experienced by the patient.
5. Patient experiences sweating.
6. Inability to arouse the patient.
7. A need to maintain the patient's airway mechanically.

Conscious Sedation and the Aldrete Scoring System

The Aldrete scoring system should be used during conscious sedation to determine the patient's ability to follow commands, to maintain respiratory and circulation status, to determine consciousness level, and to determine the patient's ability to maintain color (Table 10.3).

Patient Assessment Alerts

The following are patient assessment alerts:

1. Document the patient's ability to maintain an open airway; this is established by checking the level of consciousness and arousal status.
2. Breathing should be assessed through the use of continuous pulse oximetry and by observation of the respiratory rate, depth of respiration, and breathing effort.
3. Maintain an IV line throughout the recovery stage of sedation.
4. You must be ACLS certified and have functional resuscitation equipment available at all times (Table 10.4).

Table 10.3. The Aldrete Scoring System

Function:	Aldrete Scoring System Points
Activity:	Voluntary movement of all limbs to command: 2 points
	Voluntary movement of two extremities to command: 1 point
	Inability to move: 0 points
Respiration:	Patient breaths deeply and coughs: 2 points
	Dyspnea or Hypoventilation: 1 point
	Apnea: 0 points
Circulation:	BP +/−20 mmHg from preanesthesia BP: 2 points
	BP >20–50 mmHg from preanesthesia BP: 1 point
	BP >50 mmHg of pre-anesthesia BP: 0 points
Con-sciousness:	Fully awake: 2 points
	Arousable patient: 1 point
	Unresponsive patient: 0 points
Color:	Pink: 2 points
	Pale or Blotchy: 1 point
	Cyanotic: 0 points
On Discharge:	Total score must be 9–10 at end of monitoring.
	Patient must retain oral fluids on discharge.
	Patient should be able to void on discharge.

Table 10.4. Emergency Resuscitation Equipment

Emergency Equipment	Emergency Equipment Specifics
Oxygen	System capable of delivering 100% at 10L/minute for 30 minutes
Suction	Powerful suction
Airway Management	All sizes face masks, endotracheal tubes, laryngoscopes, oral, and nasal airways
Monitors	Pulse oximeter, cardiac monitor, blood pressure (BP) device
Resuscitative Equipment/ Medications	Emergency Equipment: Emergency drug card, ACLS protocols, ambu-bag, defib-rillator with EKG recording capability
	Emergency Drugs: Naloxone (Narcan), Flumazenil (Mazicon), and Epinephrine

COMPLICATIONS OF CONSCIOUS SEDATION

Complications associated with conscious sedation are:

- Respiratory depression and hypoventilation
- Cardiac complications and hypotension
- Inadequate analgesia or amnesia

Respiratory Depression and Hypoventilation

This complication presents as shallow respirations and decreased oxygen saturation. It is treated with oxygen and airway management. Perform the head-tilt–chin-lift. This will often improve ventilation and oxygen saturation. Provide oxygen by nasal cannula throughout the procedure and increase the flow when the oxygen saturation is low. Encourage the patient to take deep breaths.

If the oxygen saturation remains low, use the 100% non-rebreathing face mask. Bag the patient with an ambu-bag if the respiratory status is compromised. Continue to bag the patient until the oxygen saturation improves. Use an artificial airway (nasal or oral), if the patient is unable to maintain an airway. This ensures that the patient is breathing and that there is adequate oxygen saturation. The nasal airway may be more tolerable than an oral airway. To determine the airway size, use the following guidelines:

1. **Nasal airway size:** Measure distance from the tip of patient's nose to the earlobe.
2. **Oral airway size:** Measure distance from the corner of patient's mouth to the earlobe.

Respiratory depression can progress to respiratory arrest. If the patient stops breathing, begin artificial respirations immediately and intubate the patient.

Cardiac Complications and Hypotension

Hypotension is corrected by putting the patient in the "Trendelenburg" (head-down) position. Hypotension is also corrected by giving IV fluids. Aggressive drug treatment will be needed if there is no improvement with change of position. Call for **help** if there is no improvement. Cardiac arrhythmias can potentially occur as a complication of conscious sedation. Cardiac arrhythmias must be recognized and treated immediately.

Call the emergency medical system (EMS) if you have not already done so. Begin CPR immediately if the patient arrests. Use the Aldrete scoring scale to determine the patient's status.

Inadequate Analgesia or Amnesia

The dose of amnesic or analgesic drugs is based on the patient's weight. As a general rule, the elderly need less of these drugs and muscular young men need more of these drugs. Allow sufficient time for the drugs to work.

CONSCIOUS SEDATION DRUGS CLASSIFICATION AND FACTS

The most common drugs used for conscious sedation are the benzodiazepines, opioid narcotics, and barbiturates (Table 10.5).

Benzodiazepines Used for Conscious Sedation

- Midazolam (Versed): IV or Oral. The liquid form is most used in children.
- Triazolam (Halcion): The oral form is most used in adults.
- Diazepam (Valium): IV or oral.
- Lorazepam (Ativan): IV or oral.

Triazolam (Halcion), diazepam (Valium), and lorazepam (Ativan) are the most-used bendodiazepines for oral conscious sedation. Benzodiazepines are contraindicated in the morbidly obese patient, the pregnant patient, the fragile elderly patient, patients receiving treatment for gastroesophageal reflux disease (GERD)/peptic ulcer with H_2 blockers, and patients who are on psychiatric medications for depression or schizophrenia.

Opioid Narcotics Used for Conscious Sedation

The most common opioids used are:

- Meperidine (Demerol)
- Morphine, hydromorphone (Dilaudid)
- Fentanyl (Sublimaze)

Opioids produce the most reliable pain control. Always determine the patient's history of drug use prior to giving opioids. Chemically dependent patients need higher doses of opioids. Doses are adjusted to meet the patient's individual needs.

Avoid opioids in moderate-to-severe asthma or airway obstruction states. Start low, go slow, and avoid large bolus doses. Dose levels are maintained after desirable levels of analgesia and sedation are achieved. Narcotic opioids provide analgesia, sedation, and elevation of pain threshold.

Barbiturates Used for Conscious Sedation

The drugs most often used are:

- Pentobarbital (Nembutal)
- Secobarbital (Seconal)

Table 10.5.   Dosages: Stress Management Medications and Reversal Drugs

Medication:	Dosages: Oral (PO); Intramuscular (IM); Intravenous (IV)
BENZODIAZEPINES:	
Midazolam (Versad):	Most common route: IV **Initial IV dose:** 0.5–1mg; initial adult dose should not exceed 2.5mg **Maintenance dose:** 0.25–1mg **Total IV dose:** 5mg **IM Dose:** 0.075mg/kg IM, maximum 30mg **Single Oral Dose:** 0.25–0.5mg/kg 30–40 minutes prior to treatment. Max: 20mg
Triazolam (Halcion):	**Adult Oral Dose:** 0.25mg hs (bed time) the night prior and 0.25mg 1h before the dental treatment (Rx) **Healthy older patient oral dose:** 0.125mg hs and 1h prior to Rx. Max: 0.25mg/day
Diazepam (Valium):	**IV Dose:** Initial dose: 2.5–5mg. Titrate in 1.5mg increments until desired effect **Healthy Elderly IV Dose:** 1.25–2.5mg Titrate in increments of 1.0mg **Oral Dose Under Age 50:** 5–10mg hs; 5–10mg PO 1h prior to Rx. Max: 10mg PO **Lean and petite patient OR healthy person above age 50:** 2–5mg hs; 2–5mg PO 1h prior to Rx. Max: 5mg or less
Lorazepam (Ativan):	**Adult Dose:** 1–2mg PO hs the night prior; 1–2mg PO 30min to 1h prior to Rx
OPIOID NARCOTICS:	
IV Morphine:	**Dose:** 2–5mg IV. Give 1–2mg increments over 30 seconds every (q) 5–10 minutes
Hydromorphone (Diluadid):	**IV Dose:** 0.1–0.5mg increments over 30 seconds q5-10 minutes; Max: 1.5mg PO Dose: 2mg 1h prior to procedure
Fentanyl (Sublimaze):	**Adult Dose:** IV/IM 75–150 μg, start dose at 1–2 μg/kg if used alone
Meperidine (Demerol):	**IV Dose:** 25–100mg: Give in 10mg increments over 30 seconds q5-10 minutes **IM Dose with IM Hydroxyzine (Vistaril):** 50–75mg Meperidine + 25mg Vistaril
BARBITURATES:	
Pentobarbital	**Oral Dose:** 100–200mg hs **IM Dose:** 150–200mg **IV Dose:** 100mg q 1–3 minutes **Maximum IV dose:** 200–500mg
Secobarbital (Seconal):	**Oral Dose:** 100mg hs **IM Dose:** 100–200mg **IV dose:** 50–250mg
BENZODIAZEPINES ANTIDOTE:	
Flumazenil (Romazicon):	**IV Dose:** 0.1–0.2mg IV over 15 seconds **Follow-up dose:** 0.2mg. Repeat at one-minute intervals until 1mg is given.
NARCOTIC ANTIDOTES:	
Naloxan (Narcan):	**IV Dose:** 0.1–0.2mg. Repeat in 3 minutes with no improvement. Use no more than 0.5mL over 2 minutes. Max: 0.8mg.

MIDAZOLAM (VERSED)

Midazolam is the more commonly used short-acting drug compared with diazepam (Valium), due to its higher level of water solubility. It is three to four times more potent per milligram dose than diazepam. It can be used alone or with a narcotic. Reduce the dose of midazolam by a third when combining it with an opioid. It can be given IV, IM, PO, or nasally. The most common route used is IV.

Midazolam is given slowly over two or more minutes. Never give it as a single large bolus dose. Rapid or excess IV doses can cause respiratory depression or arrest, and the use of this drug requires special training. Active metabolites of midazolam can accumulate in patients with kidney disease, causing prolonged sedation.

Midazolam (Versed) Dose

Initial IV Versed Dose

0.5–1.0mg. The initial dose should not exceed 2.5mg in a healthy adult and it should be titrated to the desired effect. Slurring of speech is an excellent indicator of an adequate dose.

Versed Maintenance Dose

0.25–1.0mg. Once sedation is achieved, additional doses should be 25% of the dose required to produce the sedation end point.

Total IV Versed Dose

Total dose should not exceed 2.5mg.

Intravenous Versed Pharmacology Facts

Sedation will occur within 3–5 minutes, and the duration of action is 1–6 hours. The half-life ranges from 1.2–12.3 hours. Patients should not drive on recovery.

Intramuscular Midazolam (Versed)

Give 0.075mg/kg Versed IM. The maximum dose should not exceed 30mg. Onset of action occurs in 15 minutes and the duration of action is 2–3 hours.

Oral Midazolam (Versed)

Adult Oral Midazolam (Versed) Dose

Give 0.25–0.5mg/kg Versed as a single dose pre-procedure, up to a maximum of 20mg and administer it 30–45 minutes prior to the procedure.

Pediatric Oral Midazolam (Versed) Dose

Children under 6 years of age, or patients that are less cooperative, may require as much as 1mg/kg as a single dose. 0.25mg/kg Versed may be sufficient for children 6–16 years of age.

IV Midazolam (Versed) Adverse Reactions

Adverse reactions from IV midazolam (Versed) are hiccups, nausea, vomiting, oversedation, headache, coughing, and pain at the injection site.

Midazolam (Versed) Lower Dose Alert

Give the lower dose of midazolam (Versed) to healthy patients over 60 years of age and patients receiving narcotics. Avoid in patients with acute narrow-angle glaucoma.

Midazolam (Versed) and Diazepam (Valium) Shared Properties

Both these drugs have antianxiety, anticonvulsant, sedative, muscle relaxant, and amnesic properties.

TRIAZOLAM (HALCION)

Triazolam is available as 0.125mg and 0.25mg tablets. Onset of action is rapid and occurs within 15–30 minutes. Halcion has the shortest half-life when compared to diazepam (Valium) or lorazepam (Ativan). It is ideal for sedative hypnotic use. Active metabolites of triazolam can accumulate in patients with kidney disease, causing prolonged sedation.

Halcion and DDIs

Halcion should not be combined with the following drugs:

- Tegretol and Dilantin: These drugs are CYP3A4 inducers and they decrease Halcion levels.
- Azole antifungals, ciprofloxacin, erythromycin, clarithromycin (Biaxin), and doxycycline: These drugs are CYP3A4 inhibitors and they increase Halcion levels.

Triazolam (Halcion) Adult Oral Dosage

Give the patient 0.25mg triazolam hs (bedtime) the previous night and give 0.25mg one hour before the dental procedure. The half-life of Halcion is 1.5–5.5hours and the maximum adult dose is 0.5mg/day.

Triazolam (Halcion) Healthy Older Patient Oral Dose

Give 0.125mg hs the previous night and the same dose one hour prior to the procedure. The maximum dose for a healthy older adult is 0.25mg/day.

DIAZEPAM (VALIUM)

Diazepam (Valium) Facts and Pharmacology

Diazepam can also be used alone or in combination with a narcotic. Reduce the dose of diazepam by a third when combining with an opioid. Diazepam can be given IV or PO. Diazepam intramuscular (IM) is very painful and for this reason it is contraindicated. The IV dose can range from 2–20mg in a healthy adult, but 10mg or less is usually sufficient.

Initial IV Diazepam Dose

The initial IV dose of diazepam is 2.5–5mg. Titrate in increments of 1.5mg for desired effect. Slurring of speech is an excellent indicator of an adequate dose.

Healthy Older Patient IV Diazepam Dose

The dose is 1.25–2.5mg. Titrate in increments of 1mg. Sedation after IV injection occurs within 3–5 minutes. Peak action is seen in 15–30 minutes. Duration of action is 15–60 minutes and the half-life is 32–90 hours. Patients should avoid fine motor or cognition skills post treatment. Diazepam is irritating to the tissues, so inject through a large vein. Do not dilute Valium or mix it with other medications because it will precipitate. Active metabolites of diazepam can accumulate in patients with kidney disease, causing prolonged sedation.

IV Diazepam (Valium) Adverse Reactions

Adverse reactions that can occur are venous thrombosis, phlebitis, apnea, and hypotension. Avoid diazepam (Valium) in patients with narrow-angle glaucoma.

Oral Diazepam (Valium)

Diazepam is a very effective oral anxiolytic for use in stress management.

Oral Premedication Diazepam (Valium) Dosage

Diazepam Average Adult Sedation Dose

5–10mg hs, the night before the appointment, and 5–10mg, 30–60 minutes prior to the appointment. Use the 2–5mg dose hs and one hour prior to treatment, for the lean, petite, or healthy patients over 50 years of age. Use only if the patient can be **escorted** to and from the dental office. The conscious sedation policy does not apply when the premedication doses are used. Avoid oral sedation with diazepam in the debilitated elderly patient.

Oral Diazepam Use for Anxiety, Sedation, and Skeletal Muscle Relaxation in Adults

Oral diazepam is available in the following strengths: 2mg, 5mg, or 10mg tablets.

Oral Diazepam Antianxiety Dose

2–10mg, 2–4 times per day.

Healthy Older Patient Antianxiety Dose

Initial oral dose for anxiety is 1–2mg, once/twice per day; increase the dose gradually as needed. Do not use >10mg/day and monitor for hypotension and excessive sedation.

Diazepam Contraindications

Avoid diazepam (Valium) in the pregnant patient, the obese patient, the elderly patient, patients taking CNS drugs, and patients on H_2 blockers.

LORAZEPAM (ATIVAN)

Reduce the dose by one-third when combining lorazepam with an opioid. Dilute 1:1 in compatible solution immediately before administering IV.

IV Lorazepam (Ativan)

The maximum total dose for IV lorazepam is 0.05mg/kg to 4mg. Onset of action occurs in 5–15 minutes and the duration of action is up to 48 hours. The half-life of lorazepam is 10–20 hours. The long half-life of lorazepam makes midazolam a preferable choice.

Lorazepam (Ativan) Dosages

Oral Lorazepam Adult Dose for Anxiety

1–10mg/day in 2–3 divided doses; usual dose: 2–6mg/day in divided doses.

Healthy Older Patient Oral Lorazepam Antianxiety Dose

0.5–4mg/day; initial dose should not exceed 2mg.

Oral Lorazepam for Insomnia in Adults

2–4mg hs (at bedtime). Oral lorazepam is available as a 0.5mg, 1mg, or 2mg tablet.

Oral Lorazepam Dose for Stress Management

1–2mg hs the previous night and 1–2mg 30–60 minutes prior to the appointment.

Lorazepam Contraindications

Contraindications for lorazepam (Ativan) are the same as those for diazepam (Valium).

MORPHINE
Morphine (IV) Dose

2–5mg. 1–2mg increments are given over a 30-second period every 5–10 minutes. Onset of action is rapid and peak effect occurs in 20 minutes. The half-life of morphine is 2–3 hours.

HYDROMORPHONE (DILAUDID)
IV Hydromorphone Dose

1.5mg. 0.1–0.5mg increments of hydromorphone are given over a 30-second period every 5–10 minutes. Onset of action is rapid and peak effect occurs in 15–30 minutes. The half-life of hydromorphone is 2–4 hours.

PO (Oral) Hydromorphone Dose

2mg, 1 hour prior to procedure.

FENTANYL (SUBLIMAZE)

Fentanyl (Sublimaze) is a synthetic opioid that provides excellent analgesia. It is indicated for its analgesic action, for short procedures. If used alone, start the dosage at 1–2 µg/kg.

Average Adult IV Fentanyl (Sublimaze) Dose

75–150 µg. Use a smaller dose in conjunction with a benzodiazepine. The average patient usually requires 50–100 µg. Fentanyl produces an immediate response. Onset of action occurs in 1–2 minutes and peak effect occurs in 3–5 minutes. The half-life of fentanyl is 2–4 hours. Administer doses very slowly over 2–5 minutes.

Patients should avoid fine motor or cognition skills activity post treatment. Rapid IV administration of fentanyl can cause difficulty breathing. Breathing difficulty can be reversed with naloxone (Narcan), or it may require a muscle relaxant and intubation.

MEPERIDINE (DEMEROL)
Meperidine IV Dose

25–100mg. Administer in 10mg increments over a 30-second period every 5–10 minutes. Inject slowly, as meperidine can be painful on injection. Onset of action is immediate and peak effect occurs in 5–7 minutes. The half-life of meperidine is 3–8 hours. Meperidine metabolites accumulate with kidney disease. Avoid Demerol use in the renal-compromised patient.

Intramuscular (IM) Meperidine (Demerol)

IM meperidine is usually combined with the antihistamine, hydroxyzine (Vitaril).

IM Meperidine + Hydroxyzine Dose

50–75mg meperidine IM and 25mg Vistaril IM. Duration of action is 2–6 hours.

BARBITURATES

Both pentobarbital (Nembutal) and secobarbital (Seconal) are used primarily on the evening before the dental appointment.

Pentobarbital (Nembutal) Dosages

- Pentobarbital adult oral dose: 100–200mg hs
- Pentobarbital adult IM dose: 150–200mg
- Pentobarbital adult IV dose: 100mg q1-3 min
- Maximum IV dose for pentobarbital: 200–500mg

Secobarbital (Seconal) Dosages

- Secobarbital adult oral dose: 100mg hs
- Secobarbital adult IM dose: 100–200mg
- Secobarbital adult IV dose: 50–250mg

CONSCIOUS SEDATION OVERDOSE MANAGEMENT AND REVERSAL DRUGS

When experiencing excessive sedation with just an opioid, the opioid dose must be decreased. Combination of benzodiazepines and opioids may cause sedation and respiratory depression. Initial doses of both should be decreased when used in combination. With excessive sedation, the dose of the benzodiazepine must be decreased **before** decreasing the dose of the opioid. Benzodiazepines have **no** analgesic properties so decreasing the dose of benzodiazepines will not affect pain control.

If the opioid dose is decreased first, pain control can be lost. Opioids provide sedation plus analgesia. A desirable level of sedation and pain control can often be achieved in this type of situation by simply decreasing the dose of benzodiazepine while maintaining the opioid dose.

Conscious Sedation Reversal Drugs

- Benzodiazepines overdose antidote: flumazenil (Romazicon)
- Narcotics overdose antidote: naloxone (Narcan)

FLUMAZENIL (ROMAZICON)

Flumazenil (Romazicon) is a benzodiazepine antagonist that competes for receptor sites, consequently reversing the effects of benzodiazepines. Start by giving 0.1–0.2mg flumazenil IV over 15 seconds. If reversal does not occur (the patient does not become awake), give 0.2mg IV and repeat at one-minute intervals until 1mg is given. The flumazenil effect lasts for one hour. It can cause seizures in patients who have overdosed on barbiturates or TCAs.

Flumazenil Seizure Alert

Flumazenil, when used in patients receiving benzodiazepines chronically, are at risk for grand mal seizures. Patients with a history of seizures should receive flumazenil with extreme caution. Seizures have occurred after the reversal of benzodiazepines even with patients not dependent on benzodiazepines. Flumazenil should not be used as a matter of routine in such cases. If needed, it should be administered slowly and the patient should be carefully and continuously monitored.

NALOXONE (NARCAN)

Naloxone is a pure narcotic antagonist. It competes for the receptor sites reversing effect of the narcotic. All opioid effects are reversed in parallel: An injection of Narcan reverses sedation, respiratory depression, and analgesia. This sudden unmasking of pain may result in significant sympathetic and cardiovascular stimulation. This, in turn, can cause hypertension, stroke, tachycardia and arrhythmias, pulmonary edema, congestive heart failure, and cardiac arrest.

Naloxone Dose

0.1–0.2mg IV. Repeat naloxone (Narcan) after three minutes if the respiratory rate is less than 12 breaths/min and/or the level of consciousness is depressed. Give naloxone until the patient is alert, ventilating, and without significant pain or discomfort. Give no more than 0.5mL over two minutes, up to 0.8mg maximum.

The effects are seen in 1–2 minutes and they last from 1–4 hours. The half-life of naloxone is 60–90 minutes. Due to the short half-life, patients can become narcotized after the effects of naloxone have worn off. Patients should be closely monitored to watch for re-narcotization.

IV

Hematopoietic System

Complete Blood Count: Assessment, Analysis, and Associated Dental Management Guidelines

HEMATOPOIETIC SYSTEM OVERVIEW

The hematopoietic stem cell resides predominantly in the bone marrow and, very particularly, in the pelvis and the long bones. The hematopoietic stem cell differentiates and matures to form the three cell lines found in the blood: the white blood cells (WBCs), red blood cells (RBCs), and platelets (Plts). Discussion in this section centers on disease states associated with these cell lines.

COMPLETE BLOOD COUNT COMPONENTS

The following are components of the complete blood count (CBC):

- The total white blood cell (WBC) and red blood cell (RBC) count
- Hemoglobin (Hb)
- Hematocrit (Hct)
- Mean corpuscular volume (MCV)
- Mean corpuscular hemoglobin (MCH)
- Mean corpuscular hemoglobin concentration (MCHC)
- Red cell distribution width (RDW)
- Platelet count
- WBC differential

The WBC differential count consists of neutrophils plus bands (immature neutrophils), lymphocytes, monocytes, eosinophils, and basophils. The total RBC count, Hb, Hct, MCV, MCH, MCHC, and RDW help analyze some of the common RBC-related conditions encountered such as anemia, polycythemia, and hemochromatosis. The

Dentist's Guide to Medical Conditions, Medications, and Complications, Second Edition. Kanchan M. Ganda.
© 2013 John Wiley & Sons, Inc. Published 2013 by John Wiley & Sons, Inc.

reticulocyte count, which is not part of the CBC, is also evaluated to determine the status of anemia, polycythemia, and hemochromatosis.

The total WBC and the WBC differential counts help analyze infection, inflammation, underlying allergy states, leukemias, lymphomas, and so on. Serial WBC with differential (WBC w/diff.) helps determine the patient's response to treatment. The platelet (Plt) count helps assess the number of platelets available for primary or platelet-associated hemostasis. The Plt count also highlights any platelet-related disorders such as thrombocytopenia (decreased Plt count) or thrombocytosis (increased Plt count).

The bleeding time (BT), which is not a part of the CBC, shows the functioning capacity of the platelets. The function of the platelets is to stick together during primary hemostasis and arrest the bleeding when injury occurs.

The Red Blood Cell (RBC)

The RBC count can be normal or decreased depending on the acuteness of the anemia. A decreased RBC count can occur because of decreased RBC production by the bone marrow or overdestruction of the RBCs, as with hemolysis. The average life span of the normal RBC is 120 days. The normal RBC count for male patients is 4.5–5.9 million/µL; for female patients it is 4.0–5.2 million/µL.

Hemoglobin (Hb)

All mature RBCs contain hemoglobin (Hb). Hemoglobin in the fetus is hemoglobin F, and following birth it changes to hemoglobin A. Hemoglobin A contains two alpha (α) chains and two beta (β) chains. Anemia is associated with a reduction in the hemoglobin content. A reduction in the hemoglobin content results in tissue hypoxia and poor wound healing. The normal hemoglobin value in males is 13.5–17.5 g/dL; in females it is 12.0–16.0 g/dL.

Hematocrit (Hct)

Hematocrit is expressed as a percentage and it reflects the red cell mass divided by the total blood volume. The hematocrit can also be estimated by multiplying the hemoglobin by 3. Anemia is associated with a decreased hematocrit. The hematocrit thus helps establish the extent of anemia. The normal hematocrit value is 37–47%.

Mean Corpuscular Volume (MCV)

MCV measures the size/volume of the **mature** RBC. The red cells are said to be **microcytic** when the MCV is below normal value and **macrocytic** when the MCV is above normal value. Microcytic cells occur when there is a problem with hemoglobin synthesis, affecting either the heme or globin components. Iron deficiency is the leading cause for microcytic cells, followed by thalassemia. Macrocytic cells occur when there are problems associated with DNA synthesis. Common causes for macrocytic cells are pernicious anemia, B_{12} or folic acid deficiency, HIV/AIDS medications, and some cytotoxic drugs. The normal MCV is 80–100 fL/RBC.

Mean Corpuscular Hemoglobin (MCH)

MCH measures the average amount of hemoglobin in each mature RBC. Microcytic anemias are associated with low MCH, and the macrocytic anemias are associated with "increased" MCH. The "increased" MCH in the macrocytic cell is a relative increase caused by an increase in cell size. That the increase is relative is further confirmed by the associated presence of a **normal** mean corpuscular hemoglobin concentration (MCHC). The normal MCH is 26–34 pg/RBC.

Mean Corpuscular Hemoglobin Concentration (MCHC)

MCHC measures the hemoglobin concentration in a given volume of packed RBC. The MCHC is labeled as **hypochromic** when the MCHC is decreased, and this hypochromic pattern is associated with the microcytic anemias. The MCHC is listed as **normochromic** when the MCHC is normal and this pattern is associated with the macrocytic anemias. MCHC is calculated as follows: MCHC = Hemoglobin + Hematocrit. The normal MCHC is 31–37 g/dL.

MCV-MCHC Values and Associated RBC Types

The MCV and MCHC patterns on the CBC help categorize the RBC types as the following:

- Microcytic, hypochromic cells
- Macrocytic, normochromic cells
- Normocytic, normochromic cells

Red Cell Distribution Width (RDW)

RDW measures the anisocytosis (RBCs of unequal size) associated with the RBCs. Increased anisocytosis is associated with an increased RDW. The greater the number of immature RBCs in the circulation, the greater will be the RDW.

Note that the immature RBCs are larger in size when compared to the mature RBCs, and the immature RBCs **do not** carry oxygen. The RDW also helps differentiate between iron deficiency anemia and thalassemia minor. The RDW is **increased** in iron deficiency anemia and **normal** in thalassemia minor. An increased RDW in the presence of a decreased RBC count indicates an **active** bone marrow. This pattern is frequently seen with many of the anemias, indicating that the body is trying to compensate. A decreased RDW along with a decreased RBC count indicates a depressed bone marrow. The normal RDW is 11.5–14.5%.

Reticulocyte Count

The reticulocyte count measures erythropoietic activity and the response of the bone marrow to anemia. Immature nucleated RBCs abound in the circulation when the reticulocyte count is increased. Hemolysis is associated with an increased reticulocyte count. Hemolysis can occur with any inherited or hemolytic anemias: sickle-cell anemia, thalassemia, G6PD deficiency anemia, and hereditary spherocytosis.

A decreased reticulocyte count can be associated with anemia of chronic disease, anemia due to renal failure because of decreased erythropoietin production, or anemia associated with bone marrow failure.

WHITE BLOOD CELL (WBC) COUNT AND WBC DIFFERENTIAL FUNCTION

Neutrophils

Neutrophils engulf bacteria and cellular debris.

Lymphocytes

Lymphocytes produce antibodies and regulate the body's immune response.

Monocytes

Monocytes engulf cellular debris and are involved in the processing of antigen.

Eosinophils

Eosinophils are associated with response to allergens and parasites.

Basophils

Basophils are associated with hypersensitivity response and histamine release. Average WBC count is $4–10 \, k/mm^3$.

White Blood Cell (WBC) Disorders

Following are the WBC disorders:

1. **Leukocytosis (increased WBCs) causes:**
   - Increased production: leukemia, myeloproliferative diseases
   - Reactive leukocytosis: secondary to infection or inflammation
   - Drugs: prednisone-associated leukocytosis
2. **Leukopenia (decreased WBCs) causes:**
   - Decreased WBC production: secondary to aplastic anemia or exhaustion of the bone marrow due to leukemia
   - Drugs: secondary to drugs causing an allergic reaction or chemotherapy drugs
   - Consumption: due to overwhelming bacterial or viral infections
   - Radiation: secondary to radiation therapy

Leukocytosis and WBC Differential Analysis

The WBC differential is used to follow the course of diseases, infections, or neoplastic conditions. When analyzing the WBC count w/diff., always focus on which specific cell line(s) show change, in association with the increased WBC count. You also must check if the CBC shows any "shift" patterns, as discussed in the next section.

Table 11.1. Summary: Increased WBC Count with Associated Differential Patterns

Leukocytosis (Increased WBC Count):

WBC Differential Analysis:

  I. ↑ **WBC count and** ↑ **Neutrophils Pattern:** Seen with acute Bacterial Infection. Treatment: Antibiotics
 II. ↓ **Neutrophils and** ↑ **Lymphocytes Pattern:** Seen with viral Infections. Treatment: Anti-viral drugs.
III. ↑ **WBC count and** ↑ **Monocytes Pattern:** Seen with chronic bacterial infections: SBE; MTB OR with acute exacerbation of inflammation: SLE; RA. Defer routine dental treatment for 4–6 weeks.
 IV. ↑ **WBC count and** ↑ **Eosinophils Pattern:** Seen with allergies; parasites; Hodgkin's lymphoma.
  V. ↑ **WBC count and** ↑ **Basophils Pattern:** Seen with CML; polycythemia.

Immature WBCs

An acute influx of immature cells in the circulation can be from the following causes:

1. The bone marrow's response to severe infection or inflammation
2. Arrest in the development process due to underlying hematologic disease.

The CBC can show a "shift to the left" or a "shift to the right" when immature cells enter the circulation in abundance.

WBC Shift Patterns

A shift to the left, or a myeloid reaction, is associated with an influx of immature bands or granulocytes in the circulation; this occurs in response to an acute bacterial infection, such as pneumonia. A shift to the right, or a lymphoid reaction, is associated with an influx of immature lymphocytes in the circulation; this occurs in response to viral infections.

WBC Differential Patterns and Suggested Dental Guidelines

Suggested guidelines for specific WBC differential-line changes associated with an increased WBC count are listed in the following sections.

Common WBC Total and Differential Patterns

Common WBC total and differential patterns encountered are discussed in the following sections (Table 11.1).

Increased WBC Count + Increased Neutrophil Count Pattern

Increased WBC count plus an increased neutrophil count pattern occurs with an acute bacterial infection. The treatment required with this pattern is antibiotics, in order to ward off the infection.

Increased WBC Count + Decreased Neutrophil Count + Increased Lymphocyte Count Pattern

This pattern is associated with viral infections. Treatment required with this pattern is antiviral drugs—**not antibiotics**—to ward off the viral infection.

Increased WBC Count + Increased Monocyte Count Pattern

This pattern can be seen with chronic bacterial infections or acute exacerbation of chronic inflammation. Examples of chronic bacterial infections include subacute bacterial endocarditis (SBE) or mycobacterium tuberculosum (MTB).

Acute-on-chronic inflammation can be seen with systemic lupus erythematosus (SLE) or rheumatoid arthritis (RA). Treatment guidelines for this pattern: Defer routine dental treatment for 4–6 weeks so the patient can be treated for the acute flare-up of the chronic condition and fully recover from the precipitating cause.

Increased WBC Count + Increased Eosinophil Count Pattern

This pattern is often associated with allergies, parasites, or Hodgkin's lymphoma. Treatment required for this pattern involves treating the underlying cause: allergy, parasites, or Hodgkin's lymphoma.

This patient will benefit from the use of antihistamine diphenhydramine (Benadryl)—
25–50mg qid × 2–3 days—if the history reveals mild-to-moderate allergy. Always inform the patient that drowsiness will occur with Benadryl.

Nondrowsy antihistamines, fexofenadine (Allegra), 60mg bid (twice/day), or loratadine (Claritin), 10mg/day on an empty stomach, can alternatively be prescribed for 2–3 days. The eosinophil count is increased during the active stage of Hodgkin's lymphoma. Routine dental treatment should be deferred during the acute stage. You must, however, provide supportive care for any associated xerostomia or mucositis that may develop, as a consequence to the medical management.

Increased WBC Count + Increased Basophils Pattern

This pattern is usually seen with chronic mylocytic leukemia (CML) or polycythemia. The treatment for this pattern relies on determining the underlying causes, which need immediate medical attention before dentistry is planned for the patient.

LEUKOPENIA AND ABSOLUTE NEUTROPHIL COUNT (ANC)

When a patient presents with leukopenia or a decreased WBC count, it is extremely important that you calculate the absolute neutrophil count (ANC) **before** you proceed with dentistry (Table 11.2). The ANC count helps assess the gravity of the leukopenia.

ANC Calculation Formula

The ANC is calculated as follows: ANC = Total WBC count × (% neutrophils + % bands). **Bands** indicate the percentage of immature neutrophils.

Table 11.2. Summary Absolute Neurophil Count (ANC)

Neutropenia Type:	Suggested Dental Management Guidelines
Mild Neutropenia: 1,000–1,500 Neutrophils/mm³	Have patient use nonalcoholic mouth rinse prior to dentistry. Mild risk of infection exists. Patient can have major or minor dentistry. Premedicate for **major surgery only** with cidal or static **oral** antibiotics **plus** give cidal or static antibiotics for 3 or 5 days, **post major surgery only**.
Moderate Neutropenia: 500–1,000 Neutrophils/mm³	Have patient use nonalcoholic mouth rinse prior to dentistry. Moderate risk of infection exists. Patient can have major or minor dentistry. Premedicate for major **and** minor dentistry using cidal or static antibiotics. Give cidal or static oral antibiotics for 3 or 5 days, post major surgery.
Severe Neutropenia: 0–500 Neutrophils/mm³	Risk of life-threatening infection. Patient is isolated and hospitalized. Masking of oral infection symptoms and signs. Only palliative care is given. **Prior to Palliative Dentistry:** Determine if a WBC transfusion (Neupogen) is needed. Use only systemic cidal antibiotics. Premedicate with systemic antibiotics as per AHA guidelines. Use a nonalcoholic mouth rinse. **Post-palliative Dental Treatment:** Use systemic antibiotics for 5-7-10 days, post-palliative care. Provide systemic pain medication. Maintain nutritional support for adequate T cell function.

The normal ANC count equals **1,500–7,200 cells/mm³**. As long as the ANC count is above 1,500/mm³, the patient has a good capacity to fight acute bacterial infections. The risk for infection increases when the ANC count drops below 1,500/mm³.

Decreased Absolute Neutrophil Count (ANC) Classification

To best analyze the risk for infection and the severity of leukopenia, it is suggested you divide the **low** ANC counts into three categories:

1. **0–500 neutrophils/mm³:** This range identifies severe neutropenia. An increased risk for life-threatening infections exists with this range.
2. **500–1,000 neutrophils/mm³:** This range identifies moderate neutropenia. Moderate risk of infection exists with this range.
3. **1,000–1,500 neutrophils/mm³:** This range identifies mild neutropenia. Mild risk of infection exists with this range.

Severe Neutropenia and Infection Associated Symptoms and Signs

Fever is usually the only symptom present. Minimal or no pus formation occurs and consequently there is no fluctuation and/or exudates associated with any abscess formation in the oral cavity. Pain and erythema may be the **only** signs of infection.

Severe Neutropenia (0–500 Neutrophils/mm^3) Management Protocol

The patient is always hospitalized because of the increased risk of infection. Prior to the initiation of palliative dentistry, determine if a white blood cell transfusion (Neupogen) is needed to improve survival. Provide only palliative treatment (incision and drainage of an abscess, pain medications, and antibiotics) for acute dental problems. The patient is handled with frequent hand washings, and strict infection control procedures are followed. Use a nonalcoholic mouth rinse prior to attending to the oral cavity. Provide **premedication** prophylaxis with **systemic bactericidal** antibiotics (IV/IM) as per AHA antibiotic premedication guidelines, 30 minutes prior to the handling of the oral tissues. Additionally, use systemic antibiotics for 5, 7, or 10days following palliative dentistry. The duration for which antibiotics are given will depend on the extent of the underlying infection. Provide systemic pain medication and maintain nutritional support for adequate T cell function.

Mild (1,000–1,500 Neutrophils/mm^3) or Moderate (500–1,000 Neutrophils/mm^3) Neutropenia Management Protocol

These patients can have major or minor dentistry. **Oral, cidal, or static** antibiotics can be prescribed. The moderately neutropenic patient (500–1,000 neutrophils/mm^3) gets **antibiotic premedication prophylaxis** as per AHA guidelines **for all types of dental procedures**. The mildly neutropenic patient (1,000–1,500 neutrophils/mm^3) gets **antibiotic premedication prophylaxis for major procedures only**. Additionally, prescribe antibiotics for 3–5days in the mild and moderate neutropenic patient **following major dental procedures**. Always have the patient use a nonalcoholic mouth rinse **prior to all** dental visits in the presence of mild or moderate neutropenia.

Red Blood Cells Associated Disorder: Anemia: Assessment, Analysis, and Associated Dental Management Guidelines

NORMAL IRON METABOLISM

Prior to discussing the different types of anemias, it is important to understand normal iron metabolism. Iron is mainly absorbed in the duodenum and upper jejunum into the intestinal epithelial cells. Iron from within the enterocyte is released into the bloodstream via ferroportin. Iron is then bound in the bloodstream by the transport glycoprotein, transferrin.

Normally, about 20–45% of transferrin binding sites are filled and this is the percent saturation. About 0.1% of total body iron is circulating in bound form to transferrin. Most absorbed iron is utilized in the bone marrow for erythropoiesis. About 10–20% of absorbed iron goes into a storage pool in cells, particularly macrophages.

Iron absorption is regulated by:

- Dietary regulation: When the **intestinal** mucosal cells have accumulated **enough** iron, they "block" any additional uptake.
- Stores regulation: As iron stores increase in the liver, the hepatic peptide hepcidin is released. **Hepcidin** diminishes intestinal mucosal **iron ferroportin release**. The enterocytes retain any absorbed iron and are **sloughed off in a few days**. As body iron **stores fall, hepcidin decreases** and the intestinal mucosa is signaled to release their absorbed iron into circulation.

The composition of the diet may also influence iron absorption. Citrate and ascorbate (in citrus fruits, for example) can form complexes with iron that increase absorption, while tannates in tea can decrease absorption. The iron in heme found in meat is more readily absorbed than inorganic iron by an unknown mechanism. Non-heme dietary iron can be found in two forms: most is in the ferric form ($Fe3+$) that must be reduced to the ferrous form ($Fe2+$) before it is absorbed. Duodenal microvilli contain ferric reductase to promote absorption of ferrous iron.

Only a small fraction of the body's iron is gained or lost each day. Most of the iron in the body is recycled when old RBCs are removed from the circulation and

Dentist's Guide to Medical Conditions, Medications, and Complications, Second Edition. Kanchan M. Ganda.
© 2013 John Wiley & Sons, Inc. Published 2013 by John Wiley & Sons, Inc.

destroyed, with their iron scavenged by macrophages in the mononuclear phagocyte system, mainly the spleen, and returned to the storage pool for re-use. Iron homeostasis is closely regulated via intestinal absorption. Increased absorption is signaled via decreased hepcidin by decreasing iron stores, hypoxia, inflammation, and erythropoietic activity.

Iron Storage

Iron is stored in the body in two forms:

- Ferritin
- Hemosiderin

Iron is initially stored as a protein-iron complex ferritin, but ferritin can be incorporated by phagolysosomes to form hemosiderin granules. Iron is found in red blood cells as heme in hemoglobin and as storage iron occurring mainly in bone marrow, spleen, and liver, with the remainder in myoglobin and in enzymes that require iron.

Laboratory Tests

Laboratory testing for iron may include tests for:

- Serum iron
- Serum iron binding capacity
- Serum ferritin
- Complete blood count (CBC)
- Bone marrow biopsy
- Liver biopsy

The simplest tests that indirectly give an idea of the iron stores are the serum iron and the iron binding capacity, with calculation of the percent transferrin saturation. The serum ferritin correlates well with iron stores, but it can also be elevated with liver disease, inflammatory conditions, and malignant neoplasms.

The CBC also gives an indirect measure of iron stores, because the mean corpuscular volume (MCV) can be decreased with iron deficiency. The amount of storage iron for erythropoiesis can be quantified by performing an iron stain on a bone marrow biopsy. Excessive iron stores can be determined by bone marrow and by liver biopsies.

ANEMIA FACTS AND CLASSIFICATION

Anemia is a clinical condition associated with a reduction of the RBCs and/or the hemoglobin in the blood. Hemoglobin consists of two protein molecules, heme and globin. Oxygen binds to heme, thus enabling hemoglobin to transport oxygen to the tissues. Anemia is associated with a reduction in the oxygen-carrying capacity of the blood, resulting in tissue hypoxia. This lack of tissue oxygenation accounts for the poor wound healing in anemic patients. Anemia can occur when RBC production is affected. It can also occur with excessive RBC destruction associated with the hemolytic anemias, and excessive RBC loss associated with acute or chronic bleeding. A thorough medical history and physical examination will help assess the type and severity of anemia. The patient's dietary history, over-the-counter (OTC) and prescribed medications history, ethnicity, and family history will provide additional clues.

The CBC is the basic test used to evaluate anemia. The CBC analyzes various characteristics of the RBCs along with the WBC count, the WBC differential count, and the platelet count.

ANEMIA CLASSIFICATION BY ETIOLOGICAL FACTORS

Congenital/Hereditary/Hemolytic Anemia

Sickle-Cell Anemia

Sickle-cell anemia is associated with sickle-shaped RBCs.

Thalassemia Major/Minor

Major or minor thalassemia is associated with microcytic hypochromic RBCs.

Glucose-6-Phosphate Dehydrogenase (G6PD)–Deficiency Anemia

The MCV and MCHC are normal, and the reticulocyte count is increased.

Hereditary Spherocytosis

Hereditary spherocytosis is associated with large spherical RBCs. The MCV and MCHC are normal, and the reticulocyte count is increased.

Nutritional Anemia

Iron (Fe) Deficiency

Iron deficiency anemia is associated with a hypochromic, microcytic RBC pattern.

Folic Acid Deficiency

Folic acid deficiency anemia is associated with a macrocytic, normochromic pattern.

Vitamin B_{12} Deficiency

Vitamin B_{12} deficiency anemia is also associated with a macrocytic, normochromic RBC pattern.

Celiac or Crohn's Disease

Celiac or Crohn's disease is associated with nutritional malabsorption of iron, folic acid, or vitamin B_{12}, resulting in iron, folic acid, or vitamin B_{12} anemias.

Acquired Iron Deficiency Anemia

Acquired iron deficiency anemia is due to chronic use of aspirin, NSAIDS, or corticosteroids. Chronic use of these drugs can cause gastric mucosal irritation, ulceration, and bleeding. A microcytic, hypochromic RBC pattern is seen on the CBC.

Anemia of Chronic Disease/Malignancy-Related/Early Iron Deficiency/Acute Blood Loss/Chronic Renal Failure

This is the most common anemia in hospitalized persons. It is a condition in which there is impaired utilization of iron, without either a deficiency or an excess of iron. The probable defect is a cytokine-mediated blockage in transfer of iron from the storage pool to the erythroid precursors in the bone marrow. The defect is either inability to free the iron from macrophages or to load it onto transferrin. Inflammatory cytokines also depress erythropoiesis, either from action on erythroid precursors or from erythropoietin levels proportionately too low for the degree of anemia.

Causes of Anemia of Chronic Disease

Causes of anemia of chronic disease can include chronic infections, ongoing inflammatory conditions, autoimmune diseases, and neoplasms. Anemia of chronic disease is addressed by treating the underlying condition.

Anemia of chronic disease is characterized by:

- Normochromic, normocytic RBC pattern is seen on the CBC. The reticulocyte count is decreased. Chronic renal failure (CRF) is associated with low levels of the erythropoietin hormone. Erythropoietin formed in the kidneys is needed for RBC production.
- Total serum iron is decreased.
- Iron-binding capacity is reduced as well, resulting in a normal-to-decreased saturation.

Bone Marrow Infiltration–Associated Anemia

Cancer cell infiltration of the bone marrow (BM) can cause a reduction in any or all of the cell lines: WBC, RBC, and/or platelets. When all cell lines are decreased, the patient is said to have **pancytopenia**, a status of significant concern in the medical and dental setting. During pancytopenia, the low WBC count can increase the patient's susceptibility to infection. The low RBC count can cause tissue hypoxia and poor wound healing. The low platelet count can be associated with an immediate type of bleeding and excessive oozing at the time of surgery if the platelet count is significantly decreased.

CONGENITAL/HEREDITARY ANEMIA

Overview

The congenital types of anemias are associated with alteration in the alpha (α) or beta (β) chains of hemoglobin, or both. The congenital types of anemias occur commonly in the African-American, Middle Eastern, and Mediterranean populations. The anemias appear early on in life. There is often a history of "crisis bouts" starting from childhood that occur through the years. As and when the patient gets exposed to factors that trigger hemolysis, the symptoms and signs of the crisis bouts occur. The patient experiences fever, pain in the long bones, malaise, and worsening of the anemia. Vascular infarction in the long bones causes the bone pains. This classic presentation pattern is most commonly seen with sickle-cell anemia. The spleen is a common site for sequestration of the abnormal red blood cells. With time, this causes the spleen to increase in size. The enlarged spleen causes pain in the upper-left abdominal quadrant, and an enlarged spleen is often the reason for removal of the organ, in severe cases.

Complications Associated with Frequent Hemolysis

Frequent hemolysis increases the incidence of gallstones. Increased RBC breakdown can also increase the serum bilirubin level and the patient can appear jaundiced. Frequent crisis bouts can also cause renal damage. Always **check the serum creatinine** level prior to dentistry in the hemolytic anemia patients. The hemolytic anemia patient is treated with repeat blood transfusions and, in rare circumstances, by bone marrow transplant.

SICKLE-CELL ANEMIA

Sickle-cell patients have a variant of hemoglobin A called **hemoglobin S**. The **S** denotes **sickle**. Hemoglobin S and hemoglobin C are abnormal types of hemoglobin. Sickle-cell disease can present as sickle-cell anemia (SS) or sickle-hemoglobin C disease (SC). Sickle-hemoglobin C disease (SC) is the milder form.

Red blood cells that contain mostly **hemoglobin S** have a very short life span of about **20 days**. The abnormal hemoglobin causes the RBC to become sickle-shaped, and the sickling is exacerbated during the crisis bouts. Sickle cells have difficulty flowing through the lumen of small blood vessels, thus causing obstruction to the flow of blood and resulting damage of the tissues beyond the obstruction. Patients with sickle-cell anemia are more prone to bacterial infections.

Sickle-Cell Anemia Major Manifestations

The major manifestations specific to sickle-cell anemia are:

- Frequently recurring bone pain: Opioid analgesics are the treatment of choice. Opioid analgesics must be used immediately and aggressively during dentistry.
- Avascular necrosis of the bones: This especially involves the hips and shoulder. Joint prosthesis history is not uncommon, but when present, premedication for the joint prosthesis prior to dentistry will be needed.
- Sickle-cell anemia and kidney disease: Always assess the serum creatinine level prior to dentistry in the sickle-cell anemia patient. When the serum creatinine is elevated, modify the use of anesthetics, analgesics, and antibiotics as outlined in Chapter 28.
- Congestive heart failure (CHF) can occur in the presence of severe anemia.
- Retinopathy can occur due to intraocular bleeding or retinal detachment.

Sickle-Cell Anemia Medical Management

Medical support is provided with the following medications:

1. Hydroxyurea (Droxia/Hydrea) is often used in adult patients to decrease the frequency of severe pain and the need for blood transfusions. This drug results in the formation of a different kind of hemoglobin that then prevents sickling of the RBC.
2. Folic acid helps generate new RBC formation.

Sickle-Cell Trait

The patient with sickle-cell trait has hemoglobin A and S, and hemoglobin A is always more prevalent than hemoglobin S. The patient with sickle-cell trait does not have the disease and goes on to live a healthy life. However, the patient does pass the gene on to the children.

THALASSEMIA/COOLEY'S ANEMIA

Thalassemia is an inherited blood disorder wherein the chains of the hemoglobin molecule are decreased. Mutation can occur in the alpha or beta chain. A patient can thus have alpha or beta thalassemia. **Alpha** thalassemia is the **milder form**, and **beta** thalassemia is the **severe form** of the disease.

Thalassemia Minor

The amount of **beta globin** in the cell is **reduced** by half.

Thalassemia Major

No beta globin protein is produced in the cell.

RBC Pattern

Thalassemia patients have hypochromic, microcytic RBC pattern on the CBC.

GLUCOSE-6-PHOSPHATE DEHYDROGENASE (G6PD) DEFICIENCY ANEMIA

G6PD anemia is an inherited condition associated with a reduction or absence of the enzyme G6PD in the red blood cells. The G6PD patient becomes symptomatic when the red blood cells are exposed to oxidant drugs, severe stress, or infections, resulting in immediate hemolysis. The G6PD patients cannot protect their RBCs against buildup of oxygen chemicals, and this causes RBC destruction and consequent anemia.

Oxidant Drugs and Associated Hemolysis

Oxidant drugs that can be associated with hemolysis in the dental setting and should therefore be avoided are acetaminophen (Tylenol), acetyl salicylic acid (ASA), Anacin, APC tablets, aspirin, celecoxib (Celebrex), Exedrin, NSAIDS, phenacetin, propoxyphene

(Darvon), sulfa antimicrobial drugs, plus sulfite, and metabisulfite, present in the local anesthetics.

Oxidant Drugs Contraindicated in the Medical Setting

Oxidant drugs contraindicated with G6PD anemia fall into two general categories: nitrites or aromatic amines. Benzocaines, lidocaine, prilocaine, phenazopyridine (Pyridium) are the local anesthetics that can cause methemoglobinemia. Acetaminophen, acetanilid, celecoxib, phenacetin, dapsone, nitrofurans, P-amino-salicylic acid, and sulfonamides, are the analgesics and antibiotics that can precipitate methemoglobinemia. **Dapsone and benzocaine are the drugs that more commonly cause methemoglobinemia.**

Avoid all sulpha drugs in patients with G6PD deficiency. Be attentive and vigilant when assessing the patient's medical history. G6PD patients could indicate in the medical history that they are "unable to tolerate" trimethoprim-sulphamethoxazole (Bactrim). Bactrim is not an effective antibiotic for oral infections. It is used to treat respiratory and urinary tract infections.

These patients will also tell you that they are not able to eat fava beans. Fava beans are oxidative in action and are a staple dietary item among Middle Eastern and Mediterranean descent populations.

G6PD CBC Pattern

The MCV and MCHC are normal, and the reticulocyte count is increased.

HEREDITARY SPHEROCYTOSIS

This type of anemia is associated with a congenital defect of the RBC membrane. Abnormal permeation of sodium causes the RBCs to be thickened, spherical, and fragile.

Hereditary Spherocytosis RBC Pattern

The MCV and MCHC are normal, and the reticulocyte count is increased.

IRON DEFICIENCY ANEMIA

Iron (Fe) deficiency anemia is the most common type of anemia seen globally. Women and children are more affected than men. A growing child is increasing the RBC mass and needs additional iron. Also, a developing fetus draws iron from the mother, so extra iron is needed in pregnancy. Iron in breast milk is more readily absorbed. Acute or chronic blood loss is the leading cause of iron deficiency anemia and women are more prone to this type of anemia. Women of reproductive age who are menstruating require double the amount of iron that men do, but usually the efficiency of iron absorption from the gastrointestinal tract can increase to meet this demand.

Aside from trauma, the most common form of pathologic blood loss occurs via the gastrointestinal tract. Gastrointestinal lesions that can bleed include: ulcers, carcinomas, hemorrhoids, and inflammatory disorders. Also, ingestion of aspirin will increase occult blood loss in the GI tract. Celiac disease or sprue can impair iron absorption. Therefore, a history of menorrhagia (heavy menstrual cycles); metrorrhagia (frequent menstrual cycles); gastrointestinal bleeding; hemorrhoids; or chronic intake of aspirin, NSAIDS, or corticosteroids should always be explored during patient assessment.

A positive stool **Guiac** test will identify the presence of microscopic gastrointestinal bleeding.

Iron deficiency can also trigger **pica**. Pica is an abnormal craving of nonfood items such as dirt, chalk, ice, and so on. It is postulated that once the low iron level is corrected, it can reverse the pica. Pica is often seen in children with poor dietary intake of iron and in pregnant patients suffering from iron deficiency.

Iron deficiency causes significant cold intolerance and this presents as tingling and numbness of the extremities. Iron deficiency is the leading cause of cracking at the corners of the mouth or angular cheilitis.

Iron deficiency anemia is characterized by:

- Decreased mean corpuscular volume (MCV) or decreased red blood cell size
- Decreased serum iron
- Somewhat increased iron binding capacity
- Much lower than normal percent transferrin saturation

Iron Deficiency Anemia Treatment

Treatment is as follows:

1. **Eliminate the etiological factors and correct the low serum ferritin level.** The serum ferritin level indicates the patient's total iron stores and the serum ferritin levels are decreased in iron deficiency anemia.
2. **Daily iron replacement in the form of ferrous sulfate pills.** Ferrous sulfate is easily absorbed from the upper gut. The pills should be taken with food to decrease abdominal cramping. The ferrous sulfate pills can also cause green or black tarry discoloration of the stool.

Avoid the use of **macrolide antibiotics** erythromycin (no longer used in the dental setting), azithromycin, and clarithromycin in patients with iron deficiency anemia because these drugs can cause abdominal cramping.

B$_{12}$ DEFICIENCY ANEMIA

Macrocytic or megaloblastic pattern on the CBC can be caused by pernicious anemia, B$_{12}$ or folic acid deficiency, HIV/AIDS medications, and some cytotoxic drugs affecting DNA synthesis. B$_{12}$ deficiency anemia is common in older women, ages 55–60. The initial complaint is often **burning** of the tongue. The patient being in the peri-menopausal age range may be labeled as being psychosomatic, because no other symptoms or signs may be present as a cause for the burning upon intraoral examination. As the condition progresses, the patient develops depapillation of the tongue, microglossia, beefy red tongue, angular cheilitis, plus circumoral and peripheral tingling numbness. All symptoms and signs mentioned previously with the **exception** of the **neurological symptoms** also occur with folic acid deficiency anemia. The neurological symptoms are specific for B$_{12}$ deficiency only.

PERNICIOUS ANEMIA

Pernicious anemia is a consequence to an autoimmune destruction of the parietal cells in the stomach. The parietal cells produce the intrinsic factor, which is needed for B_{12} absorption. Pernicious anemia is therefore associated with a poor absorption of vitamin B_{12}. The following conditions are also associated with low levels of vitamin B_{12}, due to low levels of intrinsic factor:

1. Partial gasterectomy (partial removal of stomach).
2. Inadequate absorption due to bowel disease.
3. Bacterial overgrowth in the intestine.
4. Pancreatic insufficiency.

The Schilling's Test

The Shilling's test is performed to evaluate vitamin B_{12} absorption, and it is most commonly used to evaluate patients with pernicious anemia. Vitamin B_{12} deficiency due to any cause is treated with vitamin B_{12} injections in the gluteus muscle, once or twice per month.

FOLIC ACID DEFICIENCY ANEMIA

Folic acid deficiency anemia has the same symptoms and signs as B_{12} deficiency with the exception of the neurological symptoms, as previously noted. Folic acid deficiency anemia can occur at any age.

Folic Acid Deficiency Anemia Etiological Factors

Leading etiological factors for folic acid deficiency are chronic alcoholism, phenytoin sodium (Dilantin) intake for grand mal epilepsy, cytotoxic/cancer drugs, or HIV/AIDS medications. Diagnosis is confirmed by evaluating the serum folic acid level.

Folic Acid Deficiency Anemia Treatment

Treatment consists of daily oral intake of folic acid in tablet form.

DIAGNOSTIC CRITERIA FOR ALL TYPES OF ANEMIAS

It is evident from all the previous discussions that the diagnosis of anemia is best achieved by assessing the medical history, physical examination, and laboratory tests.

Anemia Symptoms and Signs

With anemia from any cause, the general symptoms experienced depend on the severity of the anemia.

Symptoms of Mild Anemia

Symptoms include tiredness, weakness, and fatigue, and shortness of breath **on exertion**. Additionally, the patient experiences general malaise, loss of appetite, palpitations, and chest pain.

Symptoms of Moderate-to-Severe Anemia

The intensity of the symptoms worsens. The patient experiences symptoms not only on exertion, but also at rest. History-taking will demonstrate that a patient who was active in the past, now has decreased the level of activity, spacing the activity over a longer period of time, or performing the activity in fractions to minimize the fatigue. This is a lifestyle modification to minimize the anemia symptoms.

Symptoms of Severe Anemia

Significant worsening of the symptoms and signs at rest occur, leading to cardiac failure. Thus, hospitalization becomes inevitable as the patient experiences the symptoms and signs associated with congestive heart failure (CHF).

Anemia Signs

The following are signs associated with anemia:

1. **Pallor** of the conjunctiva, oral mucosa, and nail beds. Severe cases will also show pallor of the palmar creases.
2. **Nail changes:** Chronic anemia will show brittle nails and clubbing or convexity of the nails. Koilonychia or spooning or concavity of the nails can occur with chronic iron deficiency anemia.
3. **Tachycardia:** The body tries to compensate for the anemia by increasing the cardiac output and consequently the heart rate.
4. **Severe anemia-associated congestive heart failure (CHF) signs**.
5. **Functional systolic murmur:** Severe anemia is associated with a hyperdynamic circulation and gushing of blood through the pulmonic valve, giving rise to a functional systolic murmur. This murmur does not need to be premedicated prior to dentistry.

ANEMIA LABORATORY DIAGNOSIS AND TREATMENTS

The CBC, as discussed, is the gold standard test used to assess anemia.

Anemia Patterns

Look for the following specific patterns:

- ↓ **Hemoglobin (Hb), ↓ hematocrit (Hct), ↓ mean corpuscular volume (MCV), ↓ mean corpuscular hemoglobin concentration (MCHC):** associated with iron deficiency anemia and thalassemia.
- ↓ **Hemoglobin (Hb), ↓ hematocrit (Hct), ↑ MCV, normal MCHC:** associated with folic acid/B_{12} deficiency, pernicious anemia, HIV/AIDS medications, and some cytotoxic drugs that affect DNA synthesis.

↓ **Hemoglobin (Hb),** ↓ **hematocrit (Hct), normal MCV, normal MCHC:** associated with anemia of chronic disease, malignancy-related anemia, **early** iron deficiency anemia, acute blood loss, or chronic renal failure (CRF)–associated anemia.

Anemia Treatments

Treatment guidelines are as follows:

1. **Eliminate the cause:** Eliminate the underlying cause.
2. **Provide replacement therapy:** Iron/folate/B$_{12}$.
3. **Blood transfusion:** Do this especially in the presence of acute hemolysis.
4. **Erythropoietin (Epogen):** Epogen is used to treat anemia of chronic disease or chronic renal failure (CRF)–associated anemia.
5. **Corticosteroids:** In the very occasional type of antibody-associated RBC destruction anemia, corticosteroids sometimes prove to be helpful.

SUGGESTED ANESTHETIC, ANALGESIC, ANTIBIOTIC, AND STRESS MANAGEMENT PROTOCOLS FOR ALL ANEMIAS

During dental management of the anemic patient, it is suggested that chair-side, when reviewing the CBC, you note the percentage drop in the patient's hemoglobin level and mentally categorize the anemia as mild, moderate, or severe. This helps with the decision of whether to treat the patient, and what local anesthetics would be appropriate. Use the following guidelines.

Mild Anemia: Hemoglobin Drop of 25% from Normal

The normal hemoglobin is 13.5–17.5 g/dL in males and 12–16 g/dL in females. A reduction of up to 25% would be 10.12–13.13 g/dL in males and 9–12 g/dL in females. 2% lidocaine (Xylocaine) with 1:100,000 epinephrine; 0.5% bupivacaine marcaine or 2% mepivacaine (Carbocaine) with 1:20,000 levonordefrin (NeoCobefrin), maximum 2 carpules, can be used. Vasoconstriction with epinephrine will minimize bleeding, but it will not cause any worsening of anemia symptoms. **Avoid all** epinephrine-containing LAs with G6PD deficiency anemia.

Moderate Anemia: Hemoglobin Drop of 25–50% from Normal

The upper hemoglobin limit for moderate anemia will be just below the mild anemia range, as previously discussed. The lower hemoglobin limit for moderate anemia will be 6.25–8.25 g/dL in male patients and 6–8 g/dL in female patients. Any value below the lower limit identifies severe anemia, and routine dentistry is contraindicated until the underlying cause is treated or eliminated. For moderate anemia, use local anesthetics without epinephrine because the palpitations and other associated cardiac symptoms can worsen with epinephrine-containing LAs. It is suggested that you use only 3% mepivacaine HCL (Carbocaine). Do not use 4% prilocaine (Citanest Plain) or 4% septocaine (Articaine) because these local anesthetics can precipitate methemoglobinemia in the presence of moderate to severe hypoxia.

Note that in addition to anemia, 4% prilocaine HCL with 1:200,000 epinephrine (Citanest Forte) or 4% prilocaine HCL (Citanest Plain) and 4% septocaine (Articaine) should not be used in all other conditions that can cause moderate-to-severe hypoxia. This guideline is suggested to prevent methemoglobinemia from occurring. Conditions that can be associated with moderate-to-severe hypoxia are chronic cardiac or respiratory disease, cyanotic congenital cardiac defects, chronic renal failure (CRF) due to a lack of erythropoietin, and COPD. Methemoglobinemia is a rare but serious clinical condition in which the amount of oxygen carried through the blood stream is greatly reduced because methemoglobin does not bind to oxygen, leading to functional anemia. Affected patients have greater than the normal 1% level of methemoglobin present in the circulation. Methemoglobin is an oxidative product of hemoglobin. Cyanosis without respiratory distress occurs when the methemoglobin level reaches 10–20%. It is hard to correct or reverse the process once methemoglobin levels rise above 20–30%. Methemoglobin level above 70% is lethal. **Avoid** epinephrine-containing LAs with G6PD deficiency anemia.

Severe Anemia: Hemoglobin Drop of More than 50% from Normal

Routine dental treatment must be deferred in the presence of severe anemia.

Suggested Local Anesthetic for G6PD Anemia

The only LA that can be used in a patient with G6PD anemia is 3% mepivacaine HCL (Carbocaine) without epinephrine. Epinephrine-containing LAs contain bisulfites as preservatives. Bisulfites are oxidant drugs and can cause hemolysis in the G6PD patient.

Suggested Analgesic Protocol for All Anemias Except G6PD Anemia

Aspirin and NSAIDS should not be used in any anemic patient because these drugs promote gastrointestinal bleeding, cause platelet dysfunction, and, being acidic, promote acidosis.

Acetaminophen (Tylenol) or codeine with acetaminophen (Tylenol #1–4), hydrocodone with acetaminophen (Vicodin), or oxycodone with acetaminophen (Percocet), are safe. Avoid aspirin and NSAIDS because these drugs promote bleeding. Immediate and aggressive pain management in the patient with hemolytic anemia will prevent the occurrence of crisis bouts and consequent hemolysis.

Suggested Analgesic Protocol for G6PD Anemia

Do not use acetaminophen (Tylenol) in patients with G6PD anemia because acetaminophen is an oxidant drug. If a narcotic analgesic is needed in the G6PD patient, prescribe codeine phosphate (not sulphate) without acetaminophen (Tylenol) or oxycodone without acetaminophen (Oxycontin).

Codeine phosphate is available as a 30 mg tablet. The dose for codeine phosphate is 15–60 mg/dose q4–6 h, for 2–3 days and the maximum dose per day is 360 mg.

Oxycodone (Oxycontin) is dosed at 20 mg oral, q8–12 h PRN.

Tramadol (Ultram), dosed at 25–50 mg q6 h PRN can also be prescribed if narcotics cannot be prescribed and a non-narcotic analgesic is needed. It is advisable to give pain medications for 2–3 days only to prevent overuse or addiction. If the pain still persists beyond 2–3 days, it is best to have the patient come in so that you can evaluate the cause of the persistent pain.

Complete Blood Count with WBC Differential and Platelets

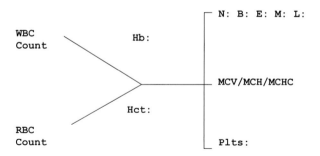

Complete Blood Count Key:

WBC: White Blood Cell; **RBC:** Red Blood Cell; **Hb:** Hemoglobin;

Hct: Hematocrit; N: Neutrophils; **B:** Basophils;

E: Eosinophils; **M:** Monocytes; **L:** Lymphocytes;

MCV: Mean Corpuscular Volume;

MCH: Mean Corpuscular Hemoglobin; **MCHC:** Mean Corpuscular

Hemoglobin Concentration; **Plts:** Platelets

Figure 12.1. Standardized complete blood count lattice recording.

Suggested Antibiotics Protocol for All Anemias

The following antibiotics are safe to use in the anemic patient: penicillins, cephalosporins, macrolides (avoid with iron deficiency anemia, as previously discussed), clindamycin, metronidazole, or doxycycline.

Hypoxia, infection, and acidosis promote crisis bouts in the hemolytic anemia patients. Use antibiotics judiciously and aggressively in these patients to prevent infections, promote healing, or treat infections.

Anemia and Stress Management

As previously stated, hypoxia promotes crisis bouts in the hemolytic anemia patients. These patients benefit when given stress management with $O_2 \square N_2O$. Stress management also decreases undue stress, which by itself can trigger hemolysis. Provide stress management for all anemic patients using $O_2 \square N_2O$. Do not prescribe the benzodiazepines, such as diazepam (Valium), or lorazepam (Ativan), and so on. All these drugs depress the respiratory center and worsen the hypoxia.

The CBC recording by physicians in medical records, is usually a "lattice" pattern recording and is often passed on as such, when the CBC is requested by the dentist. The lattice pattern is shown in Figure 12.1.

Red Blood Cells Associated Disorder: Polycythemia: Assessment, Analysis, and Associated Dental Management Guidelines

Polycythemia is a disease in which too many red blood cells are made in the bone marrow. Polycythemia can present as primary or secondary polycythemia. Polycythemia vera is **primary polycythemia**. It is a myeloproliferative disorder associated with an increased number of circulating RBCs. The white blood cell (WBC) and platelet counts are also increased and the **erythropoietin** level is **low**. These extra blood cells may collect in the spleen and cause it to swell. The increased number of red blood cells or platelets in the blood can cause bleeding problems and make clots form in blood vessels. This can increase the risk of stroke or heart attack. The risk of stroke or heart attack is higher in patients who are older than 65, or who have a history of blood clots. Patients also have an increased risk of acute myeloid leukemia or primary myelofibrosis.

Chronic obstructive pulmonary disease (COPD), smoking, erythropoietin-producing tumors, and other long-standing heart or lung problems can cause chronic hypoxia (low oxygen level), and chronic hypoxia causes secondary polycythemia.

The leading physiological cause for erythrocytosis (increased RBC count) or secondary polycythemia is high altitude. The **erythropoietin production is always increased in secondary polycythemia**.

Polycythemia is mainly a disease of the elderly. Males are affected more than females. An excessive number of RBCs in the circulation causes sluggishness in blood flow, and this increases the incidence of strokes, myocardial infarctions, and deep vein thrombosis (DVTs).

These patients also experience gout and excessive gastrointestinal bleeds. It is not uncommon for these patients to have gout due to the excessive breakdown of RBCs. Increased RBC breakdown increases the serum uric acid level and this, in turn, precipitates gout. Gout can compromise the kidney status. Always check the CBC and serum creatinine prior to dentistry.

Dentist's Guide to Medical Conditions, Medications, and Complications, Second Edition. Kanchan M. Ganda.
© 2013 John Wiley & Sons, Inc. Published 2013 by John Wiley & Sons, Inc.

POLYCYTHEMIA SYMPTOMS AND SIGNS

This condition is often asymptomatic initially. It is sometimes found during a routine blood test. Symptoms may occur as the number of blood cells increases. When symptoms occur, these patients often experience headaches and a feeling of fullness below the ribs on the left side, excessive itching of the skin on exposure to warm water, and severe burning of the hands and feet. The patient has a flushed appearance. Physical examination reveals conjunctival engorgement and hepatosplenomegaly.

ABNORMAL LABORATORY VALUES ASSOCIATED WITH POLYCYTHEMIA

The following are the abnormal lab values associated with polycythemia:

1. **Red blood cells (RBCs):** In addition to a bone marrow aspiration and biopsy including cytogenetic analysis and a serum erythropoietin test, a complete blood count is used to diagnose polycythemia vera. The RBC count is usually elevated to 8–12 million/μL in primary or polycythemia vera. In secondary polycythemia, the RBC count is 6–8 million/μL.
2. **Hemoglobin (Hb):** The hemoglobin is usually increased to 18–24g/dL.
3. **Hematocrit (Hct):** The Hct is usually increased to 55–60% or 70–80%, depending on the type of polycythemia.
4. **MCV and MCH:** The MCV and MCH are normal or decreased.
5. **Platelets:** The platelets are increased to over 400,000/mm^3 but they are often dysfunctional.
6. **White blood cell (WBC) count:** The WBC count is elevated to over 12,000 cells/mm^3, and this elevation occurs is in the **absence** of fever.

TREATMENT OF POLYCYTHEMIA

Polycythemia treatment is as follows:

1. Eliminate the precipitating factors.
2. Symptomatically treat itching, burning of hands and feet, DVTs, stroke, and so on.
3. Give low-dose aspirin to prevent thrombosis.
4. Set up regular hospital-based phlebotomy visits, which is the treatment of choice, to decrease the blood volume. One pint of blood is removed weekly until the hematocrit level is less than 45% in males and under 42% in females. Then the therapy is continued as needed.
5. **Other therapies:** Occasionally, chemotherapy, specifically with hydroxyurea, may be given to reduce the number of red blood cells made by the bone marrow. Interferon may also be given to lower the blood counts. Anagrelide may also be given to lower the platelet counts. Some patients are advised to take aspirin to reduce the risk of blood clots, though it increases the risk for stomach bleeding. Ultraviolet-B light therapy can reduce the severe itching that some patients experience.

SUGGESTED DENTAL CONSIDERATIONS WITH POLYCYTHEMIA

The following are dental alerts and guidelines for polycythemia:

1. Evaluate the CBC. The patient may need local hemostasis due to inadequate platelet function.
2. Determine the dose of aspirin or other blood thinners that the patient could be taking. Always check with the patient's MD before you stop the aspirin or any other blood thinner. In some cases, the MD may not allow aspirin to be stopped because of the increased threat of thrombosis. In such situations you will use local hemostatic materials. When clearance is obtained for aspirin stoppage, it will need to be stopped seven days prior to major surgery only.
3. Evaluate the status of the affected organ systems: brain, kidney, heart, and deep veins. Assessment of the organ systems will dictate the deviations in the use of stress management, anesthetics, analgesics, and antibiotics in the dental setting.
4. Review the appropriate sections in this book to determine a final treatment plan for your patient, with regard to the use of stress management, anesthetics, analgesics, and antibiotics.

Red Blood Cells Associated Disorder: Hemochromatosis: Assessment, Analysis, and Associated Dental Management Guidelines

Hereditary hemochromatosis (HHC), due to mutations in the HFE gene, is an autosomal recessive disorder of iron metabolism. **Human hemochromatosis protein**, also known as the **HFE protein**, is a protein in humans that is encoded by the HFE gene. The primary mode of action of HFE is through the regulation of the iron storage hormone hepcidin. It is thought that this protein functions to regulate iron absorption by regulating the interaction of the transferrin receptor with transferrin. The HFE protein binds to the transferrin receptor and reduces its affinity for iron-bound transferrin.

The exact mechanism for development of HHC is not known, but there appears to be interaction of HFE with transferrin and movement of iron across epithelial surfaces. The mutant HFE does not bind properly to the transferrin receptor. Patients with HHC have very high iron stores because they absorb dietary iron at two to three times the normal rate. HHC patients accumulate iron at a rate of 0.5–1.0gm per year. Eventually, their total iron stores may exceed 50gm. Thus HHC is a disease state associated with an increased uptake of dietary iron in the presence of excessive iron in the body stores.

Symptoms of HHC usually develop after 20g of iron has accumulated in the body. Therefore, men tend to become symptomatic in their 40s, and women, because of increased iron loss from menstruation in reproductive years, become symptomatic after menopause. Alcohol consumption can accelerate the effects of iron overload. Chronic alcoholics can exhibit hepatic fibrosis or cirrhosis almost twice as frequently as nonalcoholic men. About 10% of alcoholics with cirrhosis have extensive iron deposition. The iron deposition associated with chronic alcoholism, however, is typically limited to the liver and not seen extensively in other organs.

Iron deposition in many organs occurs and the excess iron affects organ function, presumably by direct toxic effect. Excessive iron stores exceed the body's capacity to chelate iron, and free iron accumulates. This unbound iron promotes free radical formation in cells, resulting in cellular injury. This increased iron deposition in specific tissues (**hemosiderosis**) and organs, particularly affects tissues and organs. It affects the skin, causing skin pigmentation; the lungs, causing pulmonary hemorrhage; the liver, causing cirrhosis; the pancreas, causing diabetes; the kidney, causing renal failure; the

Dentist's Guide to Medical Conditions, Medications, and Complications, Second Edition. Kanchan M. Ganda.
© 2013 John Wiley & Sons, Inc. Published 2013 by John Wiley & Sons, Inc.

joints, causing polyarthritis; the gonads, causing hypogonadism; and the heart, causing cardiomyopathy. Irreversible multiple organ damage ultimately occurs. Lungs and kidneys are especially affected. Severe pulmonary hemorrhage can deplete the iron levels and cause iron deficiency anemia.

The incidence of HHC is between 1:200 and 1:500 for populations of Northern European and Caucasian descent. However, cases of HHC can be found in other races, and there is considerable variability in expression of the disease. As previously stated, HHC is common in men age 40 and older and in postmenopausal women.

HEMOCHROMATOSIS SYMPTOMS AND SIGNS

Dark bronze pigmentation of the skin, malaise, abdominal pain, and arthritis are common symptoms associated with hemochromatosis. Type 2 diabetes, cirrhosis, cardiac arrhythmias, cardiomyopathy, congestive heart failure (CHF), adrenal cortical dysfunction, pituitary failure, and atrophy of the gonads are common findings associated with hemochromatosis.

HEMOCHROMATOSIS DIAGNOSIS

The following blood tests will establish the diagnosis of hemochromatosis:

1. **Serum iron level:** The serum iron level is markedly increased beyond 200μg/dL and so is the percent of saturation.
2. **Complete blood count (CBC):** CBC can indicate the presence of iron deficiency anemia.
3. **Serum ferritin level:** The serum ferritin level is markedly increased. Serum ferritin indicates the total iron stored by the body.
4. **Transferrin level:** The transferrin level is decreased.
5. **Transferrin saturation:** The transferrin saturation is increased beyond 70%. The transferrin saturation indicates the ratio of the serum iron and total iron-binding capacity × 100. Measurements of ferritin and transferrin saturation are less specific methods of screening.
6. **Liver biopsy:** The liver biopsy confirms the diagnosis of hemochromatosis. The diagnosis of the severity of disease is made by liver biopsy with quantization of the amount of iron. The biopsy shows fibrosis or changes due to cirrhosis.

Additional Tests to Evaluate Affected Organ Systems

The following are additional tests for the evaluation of other organs:

1. The serum creatinine (S.Cr): kidney assessment
2. The liver function tests (LFTs): liver assessment
3. The fasting blood sugar (FBS), postprandial/post-meal blood sugar (PPBS), and hemoglobin A_1C (HbA_1C): diabetes assessment
4. Cortisol levels: adrenal cortical assessment for presence of Addison's disease
5. The electrocardiogram (ECG) and lipid profile: cardiac assessment

HEMOCHROMATOSIS MANAGEMENT

The most common causes of death in individuals with HHC are hepatocellular carcinoma associated with cirrhosis, hepatic failure, and cardiac failure. Some young patients present with severe cardiac involvement and in whom the outcome is poor as a result of congestive heart failure if they remain untreated. Thus, treatment must be started early in the disease process to minimize organ damage. Treatment consists of the following:

1. **Consultation with the dietician:** The goal is to eliminate foods high in iron and increase the intake of calcium to decrease iron absorption.
2. **Weekly phlebotomy:** Weekly phlebotomy is the treatment of choice to remove excess iron, when the ferritin level is markedly increased: 500mL of blood is removed per week until the iron levels reach baseline and the ferritin level is below 50ng/L. Early diagnosis and institution of therapeutic phlebotomy can prevent complications and normalize life expectancy, but once organ damage occurs, many of the manifestations are irreversible.
3. **Treatment of associated organ problems:** Liver, kidney, pancreas, heart, and pituitary.

Hemochromatosis and Suggested Dental Considerations

In addition to the CBC with platelets these are the management considerations for hemochromatosis:

1. Evaluate the status of the affected organ systems: liver, kidney, heart, and adrenal cortex.
2. Assess the PT/INR in the presence of cirrhosis.
3. Coexisting Addison's disease is treated with daily prednisone intake.
4. Determine the daily prednisone dose and provide extra steroids for major dental surgical procedures after confirming with the patient's MD.
5. Evaluate the presence of diabetes and existing diabetes control.
6. Assessment of items 1–5 will dictate the deviations in the use of stress management, anesthetics, analgesics, and antibiotics in the dental setting.

Review the appropriate sections in this book for the associated organ system and/or diseases precipitated by hemochromatosis to determine a final treatment plan for your patient with regard to the use of stress management, anesthetics, analgesics, and antibiotics.

Hemostasis and Associated Bleeding Disorders

Primary and Secondary Hemostasis: Normal Mechanisms, Disease States, and Coagulation Tests: Assessment, Analysis, and Associated Dental Management Guidelines

PRIMARY AND SECONDARY HEMOSTASIS: OVERVIEW, FACTS, AND ASSOCIATED DISEASE STATES

Hemostasis Introduction

Coagulation is now determined to be a complex interaction of procoagulation factors, anticoagulation factors, and the fibrinolytic system. The normal clotting process goes through four phases to achieve optimal clot formation, clot limitation, and clot dissolution. Primary hemostasis and secondary hemostasis relates to clot formation; antithrombin processes in addition to proteins C and S relate to clot limitation; and fibrinolysis relates to clot dissolution.

Thus, to understand bleeding disorders, one needs to have a good understanding of the following:

1. The elements of hemostasis
2. The physiology of hemostasis: primary and secondary hemostasis
3. Problems associated with the elements of hemostasis
4. The congenital and acquired bleeding disorders
5. Drugs that potentiate or cause bleeding or affect bleeding
6. Clot limitation: antithrombin processes plus proteins C and S
7. Clot dissolution: fibrinolysis process

The Elements of Hemostasis

The elements of hemostasis are:

1. **Vascular response:** This refers to the vascular contraction or response that occurs following injury.
2. **Platelet number:** Bleeding time (BT) is prolonged in the presence of thrombocytopenia (decreased platelet number).

Dentist's Guide to Medical Conditions, Medications, and Complications, Second Edition. Kanchan M. Ganda.
© 2013 John Wiley & Sons, Inc. Published 2013 by John Wiley & Sons, Inc.

3. **Platelet function:** Bleeding time (BT) is prolonged when platelet cohesiveness or platelet function is affected.
4. **Adequate von Willebrand's factor (vWF) level:** vWF enhances platelet function/cohesiveness.
5. **Adequate Clotting Factor levels:** PTT and PT/INR assess the functioning status of the intrinsic and extrinsic clotting pathways, respectively.

Physiology of Hemostasis

Primary and secondary hemostasis has to function optimally for a patient to have a negative bleeding history. Additionally, there needs to be a physiologic balance between bleeding and clotting mechanisms. The immediate type of bleeding occurs when there are problems associated with the elements involved with primary hemostasis. The delayed type of bleeding occurs when there are problems associated with the elements involved with secondary hemostasis.

Elements Associated with Primary Hemostasis

The elements associated with primary hemostasis include:

1. Adequate vascular response
2. Adequate platelet number
3. Adequate platelet function
4. Adequate level of the von Willebrand's Factor (vWF)

Elements Associated with Secondary Hemostasis

Good secondary hemostasis is dependent on appropriate and adequate Clotting Factor interactions leading to formation of the fibrin clot.

Primary Hemostasis: Detailed Discussion

Primary hemostasis is a procoagulation clot forming process associated with the initiation and formation of the platelet plug. When injury occurs, within seconds to minutes the blood vessels at the injured site constrict and attract the circulating platelets (out of the circulation), promoting the adhesions of these circulating platelets to the subendothelium at the site of injury. The platelets aggregate in large number and link with one another to form the platelet plug. Von Willebrand's Factor (vWF) enhances the sticking together, or cohesiveness, of the platelets. The surface phospholipids of platelets provide the surface for factor complexes and for the propagation of clot formation. Thus, platelets and vWF protein cooperate to form a loose plug in the lacerated blood vessel. This is primary hemostasis. Primary hemostasis defect is associated with excessive oozing at the time of surgery and oozing that continues beyond 24 hours postoperatively.

Factor VIII gene produces two transcripts of factor VIII. Transcript 1 (VIII-vWF) is the FVIII associated with von Willebrand factor and it helps in platelet aggregation (primary hemostasis). Transcript 2 consists primarily of the phospholipid-binding domain of Factor VIIIc. vWF helps stabilize and transport Factor VIIIc, which participates in the clotting cascade. Thus, von Willebrand Factor (vWF) plays a very important role in both primary and secondary hemostasis.

As you will see in the secondary hemostasis discussion, activated platelets express their cell surface phosphatidylserine (P-serine) that promotes the conversion of Factor II (prothrombin) to thrombin via Factors Xa, Va, and calcium. This is the starting phase of a chain of events that leads to Thrombin generation and the final conversion of fibrinogen to fibrin. Fibrin is stabilized Factor XIII, and fibrinolysis is responsible for degradation of fibrin through a complex mechanism of pro-activators and anti-activators that regulates the generation of plasmin.

Drugs affecting primary hemostasis:

- Aspirin
- NSAIDS
- Aspirin plus dipyridamole (Aggrenox)
- Adenosine diphosphate inhibitors: clopidogrel (Plavix)
- Ticlopidine (Ticlid)

Note that an immediate type of bleeding can also occur from increased vascular fragility due to chronic corticosteroid therapy. Chronic steroid use causes thinning of the vascular connective tissue lining, resulting in increased fragility of the small blood vessels. The bleeding time (BT) and platelet counts are **normal** and not affected with chronic corticosteroid use. During dentistry these patients respond well to local pressure and local hemostats.

Secondary Hemostasis: Detailed Discussion

Secondary hemostasis is also a procoagulation clot forming process and it is associated with the propagation of the clotting process via the intrinsic and extrinsic coagulation cascades. All Clotting Factors, with the exception of Factor VIII, are manufactured in the liver. Factor VIII and vWF are manufactured in the endothelial cells of the blood vessels. Factors II, VII, IX, and X are vitamin K–dependent clotting factors, and they participate in the intrinsic and extrinsic clotting cascades. The clotting factors are present in the circulation in the inactive form. Normal coagulation system is a Y-shaped pathway with separate intrinsic and extrinsic component initiators. Factor XII and Factor VIIa/tissue Factors are initiators of the intrinsic and extrinsic pathways respectively, and both then lead to a common pathway of Factor Xa/Factor Va. The intrinsic and extrinsic clotting cascades demonstrate the sequential order in which the clotting factors activate to promote secondary hemostasis. Tissue factor released from the injured vasculature immediately activates Factor VII in the extrinsic clotting pathway and exposure to collagen from the ruptured vessel wall slowly activates Factor XII in the intrinsic pathway. The chain reaction that follows in the intrinsic and extrinsic clotting cascades (Figure 15.1) results in the formation of the fibrin clot that gets deposited on the platelet plug mesh (from primary hemostasis), and, together, they seal the injured site. The clot starts to stabilize in minutes to less than two hours. This is secondary hemostasis. Patients experiencing problems with secondary hemostasis present with deep-tissue bleeding 4–10days postoperatively. Anticoagulants/blood thinners, heparin or warfarin (Coumadin), affect secondary hemostasis.

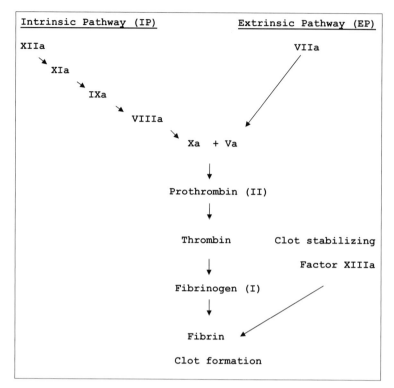

Figure 15.1.   The clotting cascade.

Clot Limitation

Antithrombotic control mechanisms plus proteins C and S are anticoagulation, clot-limiting processes. They bring about cessation of the clotting process.

Clot Dissolution

Fibrinolysis is an anticoagulation clot dissolution process. Fibrinolysis is mediated by the enzyme plasmin, which remodels or dissolves the clot once the bleeding stops. The clot breaks down hours after the initial clot has formed. Fibrinogen and plasmin balance is crucial for optimal hemostasis.

Clotting Factor Facts

Optimal vitamin K absorption from the gut is needed for the manufacture of Factors II, VII, IX, and X in the liver. Low levels of these factors prolong the PT/INR and the PTT. Liver disease, particularly decompensated alcoholic cirrhosis, is the leading cause of Clotting Factor deficiency. It is important to note that not all patients with cirrhosis will have a prolonged PT/INR. Clotting Factor **activity** has to **drop by more than 75%** to cause prolongation of the PT/INR.

Note that platelets are also produced in the liver, and **thrombocytopenia** can occur in the presence of **cirrhosis**. Always determine the PT/INR and the CBC with platelets prior to probing a cirrhotic patient. Chronic small bowel disease affects vitamin K absorption. Thus, Factors II, VII, IX, and X can be low in the presence of significant vitamin K deficiency due to chronic small bowel disease. The deficiency can be corrected by injecting 10mg vitamin K daily, IV for three days. Vitamin K IV promotes reversal in 6–12 hours. Oral vitamin K will be ineffective in the presence of chronic malabsorption.

The liver normally modifies the vitamin K–dependent clotting Factors (II, VII, IX, and X) for proper physiologic function, and this function may be deranged in patients with vitamin K deficiency associated with cirrhosis. Vitamin K deficiency occurs commonly in end-stage liver disease (ESLD) because of poor nutrition, malabsorption of fat-soluble vitamins, biliary tract obstruction, bile salt deficiency, bile salt secretory failure, and with the use of broad-spectrum antibiotics. Additionally, cirrhotic patients develop an acquired unresponsiveness to vitamin K, which is reflected by increased levels of hypocarboxylated vitamin K–dependent clotting factors. Vitamin K deficiency is more likely in primary cholestatic diseases such as primary biliary cirrhosis and primary sclerosing cholangitis.

Providing vitamin K by oral, subcutaneous, or intravenous administration can correct the decline. The **IV** route is **preferred** because of edema and possible gut malabsorption in severely jaundiced patients. 10mg of vitamin K injections for three days is adequate enough to correct the vitamin K deficiency and should be given to patients with **decompensated** liver cirrhosis. **Oral** vitamin K has **no** role in the management of coagulopathy in **decompensated** liver cirrhosis. However, **oral** vitamin K **can be given to** patients with **compensated** liver cirrhosis. **Compensated** liver cirrhosis refers to **early liver damage** in which the body functions well despite the damaged liver tissue, and often times patients with compensated cirrhosis **show no symptoms** of disease.

Clotting Factor Deficiency Causes

The following conditions can or may cause clotting factor deficiency:

1. Hemophilia A (Factor VIII deficiency)
2. Hemophilia B (Factor IX deficiency)
3. Some cases of von Willebrand's Disease (VWD) can present with Factor VIII deficiency
4. Anticoagulants, unfractionated Heparin (affects the intrinsic pathway), and Coumadin (affects the extrinsic pathway in therapeutic doses, and extrinsic plus intrinsic pathways in doses above therapeutic levels)
5. Cirrhosis of the liver

Coagulation Abnormalities Associated with Cirrhosis

Compared to patients with normal coagulation who have an optimal balance of clotting factors, regulatory proteins, and platelets, patients with liver disease have a disturbed balance of procoagulant and anticoagulant factors. The fundamental problem underlying the coagulopathy in patients with liver disease is a lack of protein production by the poorly functioning liver. Thus, hepatic synthetic dysfunction (all of the coagulation factors with the exception of vWF are produced in the liver), malnutrition, and vitamin K malabsorption due to cholestasis, contribute to this abnormality.

In isolated Factor deficiencies like hemophilia, patients present with bleeding, which is in contrast to patients with liver disease who have decreased levels of procoagulants and anticoagulants. This leads to a balance in the hemostasis without increasing the risk of bleeding, but this balance may be disrupted by bleeding or thrombosis by external factors such as infection, renal failure, and so on.

Hemostasis is affected in patients with severe liver disease because of decreased synthesis of Factors II, V, VII, IX, X, XI, XIII, fibrinogen, protein C, protein S, dysfibrinogenemia, enhanced fibrinolysis, diffuse intravascular coagulation, thrombocytopenia, impaired clearance of activated clotting factors, plasminogen activators, fibrinogen degradation products, and vitamin K deficiency due to malabsorption or malnutrition. The liver normally modifies the vitamin K–dependent clotting Factors (II, VII, IX, and X) for proper physiologic function, and this function may also be deranged in patients with vitamin K deficiency associated with cirrhosis. Clinically, all the changes outlined can lead to abnormal bleeding, abnormal bleeding tests, and thrombosis. Measuring the risk of bleeding is one of the most challenging areas in the clinical care of patients with cirrhosis. The provider needs to have a good understanding of all components causing coagulation abnormalities to better provide for these patients.

Coagulation Abnormalities Encountered with Cirrhosis

Hypocoagulation

Hypocoagulation in cirrhosis is caused by thrombocytopenia, which results from:

- Decreased thrombopoietin/TPO levels
- Splenic sequestration
- Auto-antibody destruction of platelets

Bone Marrow Suppression

Bone marrow suppression occurs because of underlying liver disease. All the following contribute to an increased risk of bleeding:

- Platelet-endothelial adhesion dysfunction
- Altered platelet function
- Platelet inhibition by nitric oxide
- Fibrinogen abnormalities
- Decreased Thrombin Activatable Fibrinolysis Inhibitor (TAFI)
- Decreased production of non-endothelial cell-derived coagulation factors, II, V, VII, IX, X, XI, and XIII

Hypercoagulation

Cirrhosis is associated with an increased incidence of thrombosis due to:

- Decreased levels of proteins C and S, which are liver-synthesized natural anticoagulants
- Decreased anti-thrombin levels

- Decreased plasminogen
- Elevated levels of endothelial cell-derived Factor VIII and vWF

Platelet Dysfunction

Platelet dysfunction occurs from associated uremia. Patients with liver disease and coexisting renal insufficiency (hepatorenal syndrome) may have platelet dysfunction because of associated uremia. Platelet dysfunction can also occur from changes in vessel wall endothelial function.

Thrombocytopenia and Associated Thrombin Production

Another important factor in coagulation dysfunction in patients with decompensated liver cirrhosis is platelets. Patients with decompensated liver cirrhosis have thrombocytopenia and thrombocytopathy. This can be due to autoantibodies, low-grade disseminated intravascular coagulation (DIC), platelets sequestration, and thrombopoietin deficiency from myelosuppression, folate deficiency, or alcohol toxicity. Thrombin generation is directly affected by the platelet count in patients with cirrhosis. As previously discussed, platelets potentiate the clotting cascade, leading ultimately to thrombin (Factor IIa) generation, and thrombin then converts fibrinogen to fibrin. Studies have shown that for thrombin production to be adequate in the cirrhotic patient, the platelet count must be around 50,000–60,000/microL. For optimal thrombin production in these patients, the platelet count must be around 100,000/microL.

Infection and Endogenous Heparinoids

The overall incidence of infection in patients with liver disease is high. Overt sepsis in the cirrhotic can affect platelet function, platelet production, and platelet adhesion. Infection is also associated with increased detection of endogenous heparinoids, probably because of endothelial dysfunction. Heparinoids found in the vessel wall are bound by the endothelium and maintain hemostatic balance by preventing clot formation, thus enhancing blood flow within a given vessel.

Hyperfibrinolysis

Cirrhosis is considered a hyperfibrinolytic state. The fibrinolytic system consists of plasminogen that is converted to plasmin via intrinsic activation with Factor XIIa, kallikrein, tissue plasminogen activator (tPA), and urokinase. All these Factors are synthesized by the liver. Research has shown that thrombin-activated fibrinolysis inhibitor (TAFI) is decreased in liver cirrhosis. Hyperfibrinolysis can be detected in nearly half of the patients with cirrhosis.

Hyperfibrinolysis can cause intractable bleeding following dental extractions or puncture wounds, because of premature clot dissolution, consumption of clotting factors, and degradation of vWF with consequent reduction in platelet aggregation. Cirrhotics also have high fibrinolytic activity in the saliva, and this can potentiate bleeding following dental extractions.

Factor VIII and vWF levels in Cirrhosis

Patients with cirrhosis have **increased** levels of factor **VIII** and **decreased** levels of **protein C and antithrombin**. Elevation in Factor VIII levels is due to decreased clearance from the circulation.

Factor VIII and von Willebrand Factor (vWF) are endothelium-derived procoagulant factors. They are both increased in cirrhosis. Factor VIII is an acute phase reactant and is known to be prothrombotic.

Increased levels of vWF result from compensatory increased vWF production, decreased levels of vWF cleaving protein ADAMTS13 (a disintegrin and metalloproteinase with a thromboplastin type 1 motif, member 13), and an increased presence of vWF on endothelial walls due to underlying chronic inflammation. ADAMTS13 is a protein that helps regulate clotting by cutting through vWF, which traps platelets and helps them clot. All these alterations contribute to a new, unstable, rebalanced hemostatic system in cirrhotics, and this can tilt in either direction.

In cirrhotics, vWF plays a key role, along with factor IX and negatively charged phospholipids of activated platelets, in boosting thrombin generation. Protein C activation by thrombin, in complex with its endothelial receptor thrombomodulin, acts as a powerful thrombin-quenching protease by inhibiting the activated form of Factors V and VIII.

CLOTTING FACTOR TESTS PT/INR AND PTT

Prothrombin Time (PT)/International Normalized Ratio (INR)

The PT/INR measures the extrinsic pathway, and the normal range of PT is 10–12 seconds.

The International Normalized Ratio (INR)

The INR is a universal test that is used to effectively monitor the effect of warfarin (Coumadin). INR is the prothrombin time (PT) ratio obtained using the international reference thromboplastin reagent (Figure 15.2).

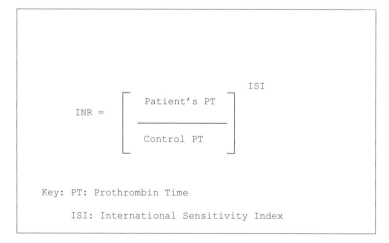

$$INR = \left[\frac{Patient's\ PT}{Control\ PT} \right]^{ISI}$$

Key: PT: Prothrombin Time

ISI: International Sensitivity Index

Figure 15.2. International Normalized Ratio calculation equation.

The normal INR range is 0.9–1.2, and average is 1. Only the PT/INR is affected by therapeutic doses of warfarin (Coumadin).

The Partial Thromboplastin Time (PTT)

The PTT measures the intrinsic pathway. The normal PTT range is 25–38 seconds. PTT is affected by IV/unfractionated heparin and high doses of warfarin (Coumadin). When the patient is anticoagulated with IV heparin, the PTT is maintained at 1.5–2.5 times normal. PTT is not affected by low molecular weight heparins (LMWHs).

Global Coagulation Assessment Tests in Cirrhotics

- The quandaries that exist in patients with liver cirrhosis are which of the humoral or hematological tests can predict risk of bleeding versus the risk of thrombosis, and which of the prophylactic intervention measures can be used effectively from both the bleeding and thrombosis perspective.
- The procoagulant and anticoagulant proteins are diminished in unpredictable ratios and the varying degree of disruption of hypocoagulation and hypercoagulation leads to changing hemostatic activity in patients with cirrhosis. Consequently, predicting the occurrence of bleeding by the conventional coagulation tests such as PT/INR or aPTT is difficult. Additionally, the reduction of procoagulants in cirrhosis (as reflected by a prolonged PT/INR) is offset by decreased levels of anticoagulant factors, proteins C and S, and anti-thrombin, but these components are not measured by conventional tests such as PT/INR or aPTT.
- Consequently, the conventional coagulation tests such as bleeding time (BT), clotting time, prothrombin time (PT), activated partial thromboplastin time (APTT), thrombin time (TT), whole blood clot lysis, plasma fibrinogen, serum fibrinogen degradation product, plasma D-dimer, euglobulin lysis time, Factor assays for F XIII, protein C, protein S, and antithrombin III, are of little value in predicting bleeding risk in patients with cirrhosis. These tests should not be the sole source of information in predicting bleeding events, especially post-procedural/post-treatment complications in patients with cirrhosis.
- Global coagulation assessment tests such as thrombin generation time, thromboelastography, sonorheometry, and national normalized ratio calibrated for cirrhosis (INRliver) are needed to judge the risk of bleeding in cirrhosis. However, these tests have yet to be prospectively evaluated in patients with liver disease.
- **Global thrombin generation time test:** Thrombin plug formation is a dynamic process. Prothrombin time (PT) and activated partial thromboplastin time (aPTT) assess only the early phase of thrombin formation. Typically, they measure the time it takes from the initiation of clotting to the initial generation of trace amounts of thrombin. The tests do not take into account the rate of subsequent blast of thrombin generation, peak thrombin concentration achieved, total amount of thrombin formed, and eventual inhibition of thrombin by the natural anticoagulants. Also, some key factors are not taken into account, such as platelets that support thrombin generation by assembling activated coagulation factors on their surface, and thrombomodulin, a protein situated on vascular endothelial cells (which is the main physiological activator of protein C, a strong inhibitor of thrombin).

Thrombin formation is globally measured by using a thrombin generation assay modified by addition of thrombomodulin. The global thrombin test is not just sensitive to the low plasma level of coagulation factors but it is also sensitive to the reduced levels of naturally occurring coagulation inhibitors in patients with liver disease.

- **Thromboelastography (TEG) and thromboelastometry:** Both assays detect dynamic aspects of clot formation and lysis, such as the initiation time, the rate of rise in clot strength, maximum clot strength, and the rate of clot decline as lysis occurs.

  Thromboelastography (TEG) measures clot formation, clot strength, and clot dissolution but does not measure vascular tone. Thromboelastography thus assesses global heamostasis and is vital during surgical interventions like liver transplantation. Except for thromboelastogram (TEG) clot lysis index, no other commercial test evaluates global fibrinolysis.

- **INR-Liver:** A major drawback in utilizing the PT/INR in patients with cirrhosis is that there is wide inter-laboratory variation in INR values because of the type of thromboplastin used in conducting the test. This variability has significant clinical implications in assessing bleeding risk in these patients and so the "INR-Liver," an INR based on a standard of patients with liver disease, is now being attempted. The INR-liver is prothrombin time (PT/INR) calibrated using plasma from patients with cirrhosis instead of vitamin K antagonists.

  Dental alert: Because of inter-laboratory INR variation, it is difficult to set a specific INR cutoff that demonstrates bleeding risk reduction or intervention in patients with liver disease and active bleeding. A conservative approach is to limit the replacement dose to two units of plasma, because this dose is unlikely to alter coagulation factor levels significantly and it does not cause volume overload.

- **Platelet count:** Standard diagnostic tests of platelet functions are of little value to predict the bleeding risk in patients with liver disease. Decrease in platelet function in cirrhosis is compensated by high plasma levels of vWF, which compensates for platelet capacity to provide surface for thrombin generation. Platelet count beyond 50,000/μL is adequate enough for normal heamostasis. It is well documented that in cirrhotics a specific number of circulating platelets (50,000–60,000/μL) promotes hemostasis and thrombin production. Optimal levels of thrombin occur at platelet levels closer to 100,000/μL.

  Dental alert: The dental provider must aim for platelet counts of at least 55,000/μL during mild-to-moderate risk procedures and platelet counts closer to 100,000/μL in high risk situations or in the presence of active bleeding.

- **Protein C function:** The protein C function test is a standardized laboratory test that can determine the relative risk of clotting versus bleeding in patients with cirrhosis. It is a simple laboratory test that has recently gained importance, and it focuses on the function of protein C deficiency, which can promote clotting in patients with cirrhosis.

Coagulopathy Management in Patients with Decompensated Cirrhosis

- Currently, the use of blood products is one of the only options available for the bleeding cirrhotic patient.

- **Vitamin K therapy:** Vitamin K is a required cofactor for gamma-carboxylation of glutamic acid residues on prothrombin (FII), FVII, FIX, FX, proteins C and S—a modification required for binding to phospholipid surfaces. Vitamin K deficiency occurs commonly in end-stage liver disease (ESLD) because of poor nutrition, malabsorption of fat-soluble vitamins, biliary tract obstruction, bile salt deficiency, bile salt secretory failure, and use of broad-spectrum antibiotics. Cirrhotic patients also develop an acquired unresponsiveness to vitamin K, which is reflected by increased levels of hypocarboxylated vitamin K–dependent clotting factors. Vitamin K deficiency is more likely in primary cholestatic diseases such as primary biliary cirrhosis and primary sclerosing cholangitis.

  Providing vitamin K by oral, subcutaneous, or intravenous administration can correct the decline. The IV route is preferred because of edema and possible gut malabsorption in severely jaundiced patients.

  10mg of vitamin K injections for three days is adequate enough to correct the vitamin K deficiency and should be given to patients with decompensated liver cirrhosis. Oral vitamin K has no role in the management of coagulopathy in decompensated liver cirrhosis. However, oral vitamin K can be given to patients with compensated liver cirrhosis, which refers to early liver damage in which the body functions well despite the damaged liver tissue, and often times patients with compensated cirrhosis show no symptoms of disease.

- **Fresh Frozen Plasma (FFP):** With prolongation of the PT/INR, patients may be treated with fresh frozen plasma (FFP), especially prior to invasive procedures. Traditional blood products like FFP or plasma concentrates only transiently reverse the cirrhosis-associated coagulopathy. The patient may require a significant volume of FFP to correct significantly elevated INR values. This large volume influx can worsen pre-existing edema and cause an increase in the intracranial pressure.

  Additionally, FFP has an unpredictable response in patients with decompensated liver cirrhosis and is associated with significant side effects such as volume overload, exacerbation of portal hypertension, risk of infections, and risk of transfusion-related acute liver injury. Prothrombin times greater than four seconds over control are unlikely to get corrected with FFP. Prophylactic correction of prothrombin time (PT/INR) using FFP is not recommended. Fresh frozen plasma contains all coagulation factors, inhibitors of coagulation, and fibrinolytic factors; however, therapeutic improvement is transient.

- **Recombinant activated Factor VII (rFVIIa):** Recombinant activated Factor VII (rFVIIa) has now become a conventional means of correcting the PT/INR to circumvent volume overload problems associated with FFP. Recombinant Factor VIIa (rFVIIa) is a low volume, safe agent that can rapidly correct prolonged PT/INR, but it is a costly product. rFVIIa is shown to improve prothrombin time and clot formation without enhanced fibrinolysis. The effect is immediate but transient, so repeated dosing is required.

- **Cryoprecipitate:** Cryoprecipitate contains the cold-insoluble residue that remains when FFP is thawed to a temperature of 4°C. It contains fibronectin, fibrinogen, and von Willebrand factor (vWF) in a volume-reduced solution. Recommended dosing is one bag of cryoprecipitate/10kg of body weight. Cryoprecipitate and the treatment are continued until normal fibrinogen levels are reached.

  Dental alert: In high-risk or actively bleeding cases, it is best to measure fibrinogen levels and replace with cryoprecipitate if fibrinogen levels are less than

120–150mg/dL. This avoids the use of large volumes associated with plasma infusion. Raising fibrinogen increases the likelihood that a "rescue" product such as rFVIIa would be effective should there be uncontrollable hemorrhage.

- **Platelet transfusion:** Platelet transfusions cause an immediate increase in the platelet counts, maximal at about one hour after completion of the transfusion. In stable non-refractory patients, a six-pack of pooled platelets or one unit of apheresis/harvested platelets should raise the platelet levels by about 30,000/mL. Platelet transfusion is given if the platelet count is less than 50,000/microL. The goal is to achieve platelet count greater than 70,000/microL.
- **Antifibrinolytic agents:** Antifibrinolytics should be considered in the setting of delayed bleeding following a procedure such as dental extractions. They are effective, safe to use, and they play a major role in treating local bleeding in the cirrhotic patient.
- **Aminocaproic acid:** Loading dose ranging from 1–15g, is given IV at a dose of 4–5g for the first hour followed by 1g/hour for up to 8 hours, with a maximum total dose of 30g. Aminocaproic acid can also be given as a 10mL (4g) oral rinse solution for dental procedures. The patient holds the solution in the mouth for two minutes and then expectorates. This is repeated every six hours for up to two days. It can also be added to a gauze pad as a local compress.
- **Intravenous tranexamic acid:** Tranexamic acid is given as a 10mg/kg loading dose, followed by repeat doses 3–4 times/day for 2–8 days.
- **Prothrombin complex concentrates (PCCs):** PCCs contain vitamin K–derived Factors II, VII, IX and X, plus the natural anticoagulants, proteins C and S. PCCs have the advantage of a lower volume infusion compared to FFP.
- **Desmopressin (DDAVP):** Desmopressin is an analogue of the antidiuretic hormone vasopressin, and it increases levels of factor VIII and vWF. Desmopressin shortens the bleeding time, and peak response is achieved in 30–60 minutes after intravenous (IV) administration. Intravenous doses of 0.3mcg/kg in patients with cirrhosis improves bleeding times with minimal systemic hemodynamic effects. Intranasal DDAVP at 300mcg for dental extractions has been found to have comparable results to infusion with FFP, but is a lot more convenient, is better tolerated, and has fewer side effects. DDAVP administration is not beneficial in patients with major bleeding episodes.
- **Management of superimposed infection:** Patients with bleeding episodes should be assessed for superimposed causes of coagulopathy such as infections, and these insults should be corrected aggressively and immediately.
- **Topical Hemostats:** Bleeding can also be controlled with topical hemostatics such as fibrin glue, thrombin, and sutures.

Platelet Disorders: Thrombocytopenia, Platelet Dysfunction, and Thrombocytosis: Assessment, Analysis, and Associated Dental Management Guidelines

As discussed in previous chapters, platelets play a very important role in primary hemostasis. Platelet deficiency and/or platelet dysfunction can promote excessive oozing during surgery, and the oozing can continue beyond 24 hours postoperatively depending on the extent of the problem. Common platelet disorders are thrombocytopenia/platelet deficiency, platelet dysfunction, and thrombocytosis.

THROMBOCYTOPENIA/PLATELET DEFICIENCY

The average platelet count is 150,000–400,000/mm^3. A patient is said to have thrombocytopenia if the platelet count is under 150,000/mm^3. Spontaneous bleeding can occur when the platelet count is below 20,000/mm^3.

Thrombocytopenia Causes

The following are etiological factors causing of thrombocytopenia:

- Drugs such as heparin, chemotherapeutic agents, and alcohol
- Leukemia, lymphoma, or bone marrow tumors
- HIV, mumps, rubella, or parvovirus infections
- Sequestration of the platelets by an enlarged spleen. Acute or chronic liver disease is the leading cause for an enlarged spleen.
- Autoimmune destruction of the platelets by IgG antibodies, causing Idiopathic Thrombocytopenia Purpura (ITP). ITP is most common in children and young adults.

Thrombocytopenia Symptoms and Signs

Thrombocytopenia and platelet dysfunction causes easy bruising and easy bleeding. Small, superficial bruises; petechiae; and bleeding mucus membranes are common

Dentist's Guide to Medical Conditions, Medications, and Complications, Second Edition. Kanchan M. Ganda.
© 2013 John Wiley & Sons, Inc. Published 2013 by John Wiley & Sons, Inc.

findings. Petechiae are pinpoint hemorrhagic flat lesions that occur in clusters. Petechiae can be seen on the oral mucosa and on the skin of the extremities.

Thrombocytopenia Laboratory Tests

Thrombocytopenia is associated with a **prolonged** bleeding time (BT) and a **decreased** platelet count.

Thrombocytopenia Treatment (Except ITP)

Thrombocytopenia (except ITP) can be treated as follows:

1. Platelet Rich Plasma (PRP) or Platelet Rich Concentrate (PRC) transfusion
2. Desmopressin/Stimate/DDAVP. DDAVP elevates the von Willebrand's Factor level in the blood and stimulates platelet release

Platelet transfusion, when required, is given 20 minutes prior to the planned procedure. One platelet concentrate transfusion increases the platelet count by 10,000/μL.

Thrombocytopenia Dental Alerts

Spontaneous bleeding occurs when the platelet count is below 20,000/mm^3. Routine dental treatment is contraindicated if the platelet count is below 50,000/mm^3.

In the presence of significant thrombocytopenia, the CBC with platelet count should be assessed prior to dentistry. The test obtained should have been done **within the past seven days** and usually confirmed on the day of surgery in very severe cases following replacement therapy. For outpatient oral surgery or periodontal surgery the platelet count must be above 75,000/mm^3, and for major dental surgical procedures done in the operating room (OR) under general anesthesia, it is best to have the platelet count above 100,000/mm^3.

IDIOPATHIC THROMBOCYTOPENIC PURPURA (ITP)

Idiopathic thrombocytopenic purpura (ITP), also called immune thrombocytopenic purpura, affects both children and adults. Children often develop idiopathic thrombocytopenic purpura after a viral infection and usually recover fully without treatment. However, in adults the disorder is often chronic.

Symptoms

Easy or excessive bruising (purpura), petechiae typically on the lower legs, prolonged bleeding from cuts, spontaneous bleeding from gums or nose, blood in urine or stools, unusually heavy menstrual flows, and profuse bleeding during surgery can occur.

Causes

The exact cause of ITP is not known but it is well documented that the immune system malfunctions and begins attacking platelets as if they were foreign substances. Antibodies produced by the immune system attach to the platelets, marking the platelets for destruction. The spleen recognizes the antibodies and removes the platelets from the system.

Adults and children with ITP often have platelet counts below 20,000/μL. As the number of platelets decreases, the risk of bleeding increases. The greatest risk occurs when the platelet count falls below 10,000/μL. At this point, internal bleeding can occur despite a lack of any injury. In most children with ITP, the disorder follows a viral illness, such as the mumps or the flu. It may be that an infection sets off the immune system, triggering it to malfunction.

Risk Factors

Women are approximately twice as likely to develop ITP than are men. Once considered a young person's disease, ITP is actually far more common in people older than 60 than it is in younger adults.

Recent viral infection: Many children with ITP develop the disorder after a viral illness, such as mumps, measles, or a respiratory infection. In most children, ITP clears on its own within **two to eight weeks**.

Complications

The biggest risk associated with idiopathic thrombocytopenic purpura is bleeding, especially bleeding into the brain (intracranial hemorrhage), which can be fatal. However, major bleeding is rare with ITP. Complications are more likely to arise from the treatments, corticosteroids, and surgery that are used for chronic or severe ITP. In fact, many therapies pose more serious potential risks than does the disease itself. Long-term use of corticosteroids can cause serious side effects including osteoporosis, cataracts, loss of muscle mass, increased risk of infection, high blood sugar, and even diabetes. Splenectomy may be performed if corticosteroids are ineffective, but splenectomy also makes the patient permanently more vulnerable to infection.

Pregnant women with mild ITP usually have a normal pregnancy and delivery, though antibodies to platelets can cross the placenta and affect the baby's platelet count. The baby's platelet count will improve without treatment, but if the count is very low, treatment can help speed recovery. With very low platelet count there is a greater risk of heavy bleeding during delivery.

Tests and Diagnosis

Idiopathic thrombocytopenic purpura diagnosis is a diagnosis of exclusion. By excluding other possible causes of bleeding and a low platelet count, such as an underlying illness or medications, a diagnosis of ITP is made.

A physical exam, including a complete medical history, is crucial. You need to look for signs of bleeding under the skin, and you need to ask about previous illnesses that the patient has had and the types of medications and supplements that the patient has recently taken.

Complete blood count: With ITP, white and red blood cell counts are usually normal, but the platelet count is low.

Blood smear: This test is often used to confirm the number of platelets observed in a complete blood count.

Bone marrow examination: Another test that may help identify the cause of a low platelet count is a bone marrow biopsy or aspiration. With ITP, the bone marrow is normal because the low platelet count is caused by the destruction of platelets in the bloodstream and spleen and not from a problem with the bone marrow.

Treatments and Drugs

The goal of treating ITP is to ensure a safe platelet count and to prevent bleeding complications, while minimizing treatment side effects. In children, ITP usually runs its course without the need for treatment. Most children recover completely within six months. Even in children who develop chronic ITP, complete recovery may still occur years later.

Adults with mild cases of ITP may require nothing more than regular monitoring and platelet checks. But if the symptoms are troublesome and the platelet count remains low, treatment with medications, and sometimes splenectomy, is considered. The MD may have the patient discontinue certain drugs that can further inhibit platelet function, such as aspirin, ibuprofen (Advil, Motrin, etc.), or drugs that affect platelet number, such as unfractionated heparin.

Medications

The following are common medications used to treat idiopathic thrombocytopenic purpura.

Corticosteroids: The first line of therapy for ITP is a corticosteroid, usually prednisone, which can help raise the platelet count by decreasing the activity of the immune system. Once the platelet count is back to a safe level, the drug can gradually be decreased and then discontinued by the MD. In general, this takes about **two to six weeks**.

Many adults experience a relapse after discontinuing corticosteroids, in which case a new course of corticosteroids may be pursued, but long-term use of these medications is not recommended because of the risk of serious side effects, including cataracts, high blood sugar, and increased risk of infections and loss of calcium from the bones (osteoporosis). If corticosteroids are taken for longer than three months, calcium and vitamin D supplements are usually recommended to help maintain bone density.

Intravenous immune globulin (IVIG): IVIG is usually given in the presence of critical bleeding or when a quick increase in blood count is needed before surgery. IVIG is quick and effective, but the effect usually wears off in a couple of weeks. Possible side effects include headache, nausea, and vomiting.

Thrombopoietin receptor agonists: The newest medications approved to treat ITP are romiplostim (Nplate) and eltrombopag (Promacta). These drugs help the bone marrow produce more platelets, which helps prevent bruising and bleeding. Possible side effects include headache, joint or muscle pain, dizziness, nausea or vomiting, and an increased risk of blood clot.

Splenectomy: Splenectomy is considered in the presence of severe ITP or when an initial course of prednisone has failed. This eliminates the main source of platelet destruction in the body and improves the platelet count within a few weeks. However, splenectomy for ITP is not as routinely performed as it once was. Serious post-surgical complications sometimes occur, and not having a spleen permanently increases the patient's susceptibility to infection. Splenectomy is rarely performed in children because of the high rate of spontaneous remission.

Emergency treatment/care: Although rare, severe bleeding can occur with ITP, regardless of age or platelet count. Severe or widespread bleeding is life-threatening and demands emergency care. This usually includes transfusions of platelet concentrates, intravenous methylprednisolone, and intravenous immune globulin.

Other ITP treatments: If neither the initial round of corticosteroids nor a splenectomy has helped the patient achieve remission and the symptoms are severe, another course of corticosteroids is recommended, usually at the lowest effective dose.

Immunosuppressant drugs: Medications that suppress the immune system, such as rituximab (Rituxan)—the most commonly used of this group, cyclophosphamide (Cytoxan), and azathioprine (Imuran, Azasan), have been used to treat ITP, but they can cause significant side effects, and their effectiveness has yet to be proven.

H. pylori treatment: Some people with ITP are also infected with Helicobacter pylori, the same bacteria that cause most peptic ulcers. Eliminating the bacteria has helped increase platelet count in some patients, but the results for this therapy are inconsistent and need to be studied further. **Treatment decisions** are usually based on the severity of signs and symptoms (active bleeding is usually an indication for treatment).

Platelet count: Even relatively low counts of less than 30,000/μL of blood may not merit treatment, especially if there is no active bleeding and the patient does not have an active lifestyle. Risk of bleeding based on other medical conditions, such as high blood pressure, infections, alcoholism, chronic liver disease, peptic ulcer, or needed medications, such as aspirin, should be weighed in. No treatment is needed if there are no signs of bleeding and the platelet counts are not too low. More serious cases are treated with steroids or, in critical situations, with surgery/splenectomy.

Thus, the steroid protocol for each ITP patient is designed by the patient's MD. The dose and duration of steroids given will depend on the extent of thrombocytopenia, the gravity of the bleeding, and how affected the patient is with the thrombocytopenia.

Steroid Treatment Protocol

Initial Steroid Treatment Protocol for ITP

Initial steroid treatment protocol for ITP is 1mg/kg/day prednisone, PO for 2–6 weeks.

Subsequent Steroid Treatment Protocol for ITP

Prednisone dose is individualized for every patient. Usually, the dose of prednisone is tapered to less than 10mg per day for 3 months and then withdrawn. Splenectomy is done if discontinuation of prednisone causes a relapse.

Suggested Dental Guidelines for ITP

Always consult with the patient's physician when corticosteroids have been used to treat ITP. If the platelet counts are lower than the required cutoff for dental surgery, the patient could receive additional steroids, per physician's advice. You need to follow the "rule of twos" for major dental treatment and provide extra steroids prior to surgery if the patient is currently on steroids or has been on steroids for two weeks or longer within the past two years.

PLATELET DYSFUNCTION

Platelet function is assessed by the capacity of the platelets to adhere/stick to one another. Antiplatelet drugs minimize platelet aggregation and promote thinning of the blood.

Drugs Associated with Platelet Dysfunction

Drugs associated with platelet dysfunction include NSAIDS, aspirin, dipyridamole (Persantin), clopidogrel (Plavix), and ticlopidine (Ticlid). All these drugs, with the exception of the NSAIDS, irreversibly and permanently affect the entire life span of the platelets, which is about 7–10 days (average 7 days). The affect of NSAIDS is temporary and lasts until the drug clears the system, which is about 24 hours. The platelet count is not affected by any one of these drugs. Platelet dysfunction is confirmed when the bleeding time (BT) is prolonged. The normal BT is 2.4–8 minutes.

Platelet Dysfunction and von Willebrand's Disease (vWD)

Platelet dysfunction can also be due to deficiency of the von Willebrand's Factor (vWF). vWF promotes the sticking of the platelets to the injured vascular endothelium and also sticking to each other to form a mesh on which fibrin gets deposited. The platelet count is normal in all types of von Willebrand's Disease (vWD), except Type 2B (vWD discussion follows).

Antiplatelet Drug Therapy

Conditions Associated with High Risk for Thrombosis

Conditions associated with high risk for thrombosis are transient ischemic attacks (TIAs), cardiovascular accidents (CVA/stroke), unstable angina, myocardial infarction (MI), and history of angioplasty, history of medicated or bare-metal stents, atrial fibrillation, and peripheral vascular disease. Antiplatelet drugs are given to all these patients presenting with a high risk for thrombosis.

Suggested Dental Guidelines for Patients on Antiplatelet Drugs

The following are dental guidelines for patients on antiplatelet drugs:

1. Minor procedures like amalgams, composites, prophys, and SCRP (scaling root planing) can be done without stopping any one of these drugs.
2. Always consult with the patient's MD before you plan to stop any of these drugs prior to dentistry. If allowed by the MD, all drugs except NSAIDS are stopped seven days prior to surgery and restarted one to two days post operation. NSAIDS are stopped 24 hours prior to surgery and restarted in the evening once bleeding has stopped, or the next day.
3. Combination therapy with one daily 81mg/325mg aspirin and one of the other antiplatelet drugs—Plavix, Persantin, or Ticlid—is often given to patients with a higher-than-normal risk for thrombosis. The general trend today is to treat these

patients in the dental setting without interrupting the intake of any of these medications. The risk of thrombosis far outweighs the bleeding associated with dentistry.

4. For major or minor surgery, sustained pressure and/or local hemostats will con-
    trol any excessive bleeding. You can serve these patients best by providing regular
    checkups and treating any oral problem immediately.
5. Aspirin and ibuprofen combination: When given in combination, some studies have
    shown ibuprofen to competitively inhibit the antiplatelet action of aspirin, whereas
    other studies have found thromboxane inhibition by aspirin to be reduced by only
    1% after 10 days of concurrent ibuprofen use. Routine low-dose aspirin intake is
    important for patients at increased risk for thrombosis and this effect of ibupro-
    fen on aspirin is important, no matter how small the risk. It is important to note
    that the antiplatelet action of aspirin occurs within the hepatic portal system after
    absorption. So in situations when you have to prescribe ibuprofen, it is best for the
    patient to take daily aspirin on waking up and delay the intake of ibuprofen by
    1–2 hours, for optimal aspirin effect. Per FDA documents, there is only minimal
    risk that ibuprofen will interfere with the effect of low-dose aspirin, if ibuprofen is
    used occasionally. If you need only a single dose of ibuprofen, the FDA recommends
    that the patient take ibuprofen eight hours before or 30 minutes after taking a reg-
    ular (not enteric-coated) low-dose aspirin. FDA recommendations are only for reg-
    ular, immediate-release low-dose aspirin (81mg). The ability of ibuprofen to inter-
    fere with the anticlotting effects of enteric-coated aspirin or larger doses of aspirin,
    such as an adult aspirin (325mg), is not known. Diclofenac and celecoxib (Celebrex)
    do not have the above interaction with aspirin, and when NSAIDS are needed in
    the presence of low dose aspirin, diclofenac and celecoxib are more appropriate
    to dispense.

THROMBOCYTOSIS

Thrombocytosis is a condition associated with platelet counts greater than 450,000/
mm^3. Thrombocytosis can be from reactive bone marrow stimulation due to the need
for more RBCs, as seen in iron deficiency anemia. It can also occur in the presence of
significant inflammation or certain malignancies.

Thrombocytosis-Associated Symptoms

Thrombocytosis-associated symptoms experienced are thrombosis, strokes, and bleeds.

Suggested Dental Guidelines for Thrombocytosis

The following are dental guidelines for thrombocytosis:

1. Assess the cause.
2. Evaluate the medications: antiplatelet or anticoagulants.
3. Incorporate guidelines discussed for antiplatelet activity or anticoagulants.

Von Willebrand's Disease: Assessment, Analysis, and Associated Dental Management Guidelines

The vWF gene is responsible for the making of von Willebrand factor, which is made within endothelial cells of blood vessels and the bone marrow cells. The factor is made of several identical subunits and mutations in the vWF gene, which results in the different types of von Willebrand Disease (vWD). Von Willebrand Disease (vWD), hemophilia A, and hemophilia B are the three leading inherited bleeding disorders, and vWD is the most common of the three. Von Willebrand's Disease (vWD) affects both males and females.

As discussed in the previous chapter, when injury occurs, the blood vessels at the injured site constrict. This attracts the circulating platelets to the site of injury. The platelets link with each other and form the platelet plug. Von Willebrand's Factor (vWF) thus plays a very important role in primary hemostasis because it enhances platelet cohesiveness. Von Willebrand Factor also helps transport and stabilizes Factor VIIIc (VIII clotting) in the circulation. Factor VIIIc participates in the clotting cascade.

Depending on the severity of the disease in patients with vWD, the half-life and activity of Factor VIIIc is decreased. The PTT will be prolonged in such cases. Therefore, patients with von Willebrand's disease can present with problems associated with either primary or secondary hemostasis, or both.

TYPES OF VON WILLEBRAND'S DISEASE

Type 1 vWD

Type 1 vWD is the most common and mildest form of the disease; 85% of patients diagnosed with vWD have type 1 vWD. It is least symptomatic in most patients, but if symptomatic, it usually presents as nosebleeds, easy bruising, or menorrhagia (heavy menstrual periods). However, some cases may present with significant bleeding.

The quality of the vWF is normal. The amount of von Willebrand's Factor (vWF) in the blood is reduced, but adequate amounts exist in the endothelial stores. Thus, it is a

Dentist's Guide to Medical Conditions, Medications, and Complications, Second Edition. Kanchan M. Ganda.
© 2013 John Wiley & Sons, Inc. Published 2013 by John Wiley & Sons, Inc.

quantitative defect. These patients are usually asymptomatic but can have the immediate type of bleeding and significant oozing beyond 24 hours following an extraction.

Type 2 vWD

Type 2 vWD accounts for about 20–30% of cases. Mutations that disrupt the **function** of the von Willebrand factor cause the four subtypes of type 2 von Willebrand disease. These mutations can disrupt the factor's ability to form a blood clot. There are normal levels of vWF but the multimers are structurally abnormal. **Thus, the quality of the vWF is affected**, both in the blood and at the storage sites. There are four subtypes that exist: 2A, 2B, 2M, and 2N. Type 2B is also associated with a decreased platelet count or thrombocytopenia.

Type 3 vWD

Type 3 is the most severe form of von Willebrand disease. It is associated with a complete absence of production of vWF. **The quality of the vWF is normal**, but the amount of vWF is severely depleted in the blood and in the endothelial stores. As previously discussed, the von Willebrand factor protects Factor VIII from breakdown, thus a total lack of vWF leads to an extremely low Factor VIII level, similar to that seen in severe hemophilia A, along with its clinical manifestations of life-threatening external and internal hemorrhages. All type 3 vWD patients and some cases of type 2 vWD patients are not able to transport Factor VIIIc in the blood. Consequently, in addition to problems with primary hemostasis, these patients have problems with secondary hemostasis when the Factor VIIIc level drops by more than 75%.

Symptoms and Signs of vWD

Excessive bruising at unusual sites, mucous membrane bleeding, heavy nosebleeds, heavy menstrual cycles, and prolonged oozing following extraction(s) are some of the common symptoms experienced with vWD. All these symptoms relate to problems with primary hemostasis. vWD patients with associated low levels of Factor VIIIc activity will complain of deep tissue bleeding in the muscles and bleeding in the joints (hemarthrosis).

Diagnosis of vWD

VWD diagnosis is confirmed by the following:

1. **The platelet count:** The platelet count is normal in all types of vWD except type 2B. Type 2B VWD is associated with thrombocytopenia.
2. **The bleeding time (BT):** The BT is prolonged in all types of vWD.
3. **The Ristocetin Induced Platelet Aggregation (RIPA) test:** The RIPA test shows decreased platelet aggregation in all types, except type 2B, where the aggregation is increased.
4. **The Ristocetin cofactor activity test:** This test measures the amount of vWF activity. The test shows reduced cofactor activity.

5. **Factor VIII activity:** The Factor VIII activity can be normal or decreased depending on the type of vWD.
6. **The PT/INR:** The PT/INR is normal.
7. **The PTT:** The PTT can be normal or prolonged, depending on the Factor VIIIc activity level. The test will be normal if there is more than 25% Factor VIIIc activity.

VWD TREATMENT

Treatment of Type 1 and Type 2A vWD

Primary Therapy

Primary therapy consists of giving desmopressin (DDAVP), IV, intranasal, or PO (oral). Desmopressin (DDAVP) is a vasopressin analog and it is only effective in type I or type 2A vWD. Some type 2A vWD patients have such a minor qualitative defect, that one can easily compensate by increasing the release of vWF from the stores. When used, it is typically given a half-hour before the procedure.

Secondary Therapy

Secondary therapy is provided with factor concentrate or cryoprecipitate. Humate-P is a concentrate of vWF and Factor VIII. You need to calculate the amount of factor needed to replete to 50–100% activity, preferably 100%. It is available as an IV formulation only and is dosed every 8–12 hours. Cryoprecipitate contains Factor VIII, vWF, and fibrinogen.

Treatment of Type 2B and Type 3 vWD

Primary Therapy

Primary therapy is provided with factor concentrate.

Secondary Therapy for Type 2B vWD

Secondary therapy for type 2B vWD is provided with cryoprecipitate.

Secondary Therapy for Type 3 vWD

Secondary therapy for type 3 vWD is provided with cryoprecipitate or platelet transfusions.

DDAVP is contraindicated in the type 2B vWD patient because more of the abnormal vWF will get released causing aggregation of the dysfunctional platelets and thrombosis. DDAVP is of no use in type 3 vWD because the factor levels are depleted in the blood and in the endothelial stores.

Additional Therapies

Epsilon aminocaproic acid (Amicar) prevents clot lysis by preserving the fibrin mesh for a little longer. It is available as oral or IV formulations and can be used with all vWD types.

Suggested Dental Guidelines for vWD

The following are dental guidelines for vWD:

1. Consult with the patient's MD and determine the type and extent of vWD in the patient.
2. Relay to the MD the type of procedures planned for both major and minor dentistry.
3. Confirm with the MD the DDAVP or Factor concentrate (Humate-P) or cryoprecipitate or platelet transfusion protocol.
4. With IV DDAVP, the surgery can begin in 30–60 minutes.
5. With oral or intranasal DDAVP, the surgery can begin 60–90 minutes later.
6. With platelet transfusion, the surgery can begin in 20 minutes.
7. Surgery can begin immediately after Humate-P cryoprecipitate (CPP) transfusion. Cryoprecipitate contains ten times the amount of Factor VIII compared to fresh frozen plasma (FFP). One bag of cryoprecipitate contains 100 units of Factor VIII. Cryoprecipitate has the highest concentration of vWF. Ten bags of CPP, when given immediately before the procedure, decrease the bleeding time for up to 12 hours.
8. The local anesthetic, analgesic, and antibiotic (AAAs) guidelines for vWD are similar to the guidelines for hemophilia.s

18

Coagulation Disorders: Common Clotting Factor Deficiency Disease States, Associated Systemic and/or Local Hemostasis Adjuncts, and Dental Management Guidelines

HEMOPHILIA A AND HEMOPHILIA B: OVERVIEW, FACTS, AND MANAGEMENT

Hemophilia A and Hemophilia B

Hemophilia A, hemophilia B, and von Willebrand Disease (vWD) are the three most common inherited bleeding disorders. Hemophilia A and hemophilia B (Christmas disease) are x-linked recessive traits that affect only males. Females are often carriers unless both parents carry the hemophilia gene. Either hemophilia is often diagnosed in childhood, though mild hemophiliacs may remain undiagnosed until adulthood. Clinical history is often positive for joint hemorrhage (hemarthroses) with joint deformities, gingival hemorrhage, persistent oral bleeding, and bleeding into soft tissues.

Hemophilia A is associated with Factor VIII deficiency, and hemophilia B is associated with Factor IX deficiency. Factor VIII has a half-life activity of 8–12 hours. Factor IX has a half-life activity of 12–24 hours. Factor VIII and Factor IX are part of the "intrinsic" pathway, and patients with hemophilia will present with a prolonged APTT test. The PT is normal because the extrinsic pathway is not affected; the bleeding time (BT) and the platelet count are also normal because platelets are not affected with either hemophilia. It is important to remember that patients with hemophilia A and B can have mild, moderate, or severe disease depending on the factor activity levels of Factors VIII or IX, respectively.

Hemophilia Severity Classification

Hemophilia can be of mild, moderate, or severe intensity:

1. **Mild hemophilia:** The specific Factor (VIII or IX) activity level is 5–25% normal. The mild hemophiliac bleeds minimally. Bleeding is usually associated with surgery, and the patient's past history may reveal bleeding after a dental extraction.

Dentist's Guide to Medical Conditions, Medications, and Complications, Second Edition. Kanchan M. Ganda.
© 2013 John Wiley & Sons, Inc. Published 2013 by John Wiley & Sons, Inc.

2. **Moderate hemophilia:** The specific Factor (VIII or IX) activity level is 1–5% normal. A moderate hemophiliac bleeds after minor injury and requires immediate attention.
3. **Severe hemophilia:** The specific Factor (VIII or IX) activity level is less than 1% normal. A severe hemophiliac bleeds very often, with or without provocation.

Hemophilia A and B Treatment

Factor replacement therapy with the specific clotting factor is the treatment of choice for hemophilias A and B. Most patients with mild hemophilia A can be treated with desmopressin (DDAVP/Stimate). DDAVP/Stimate is a synthetic analogue of vasopressin. It stimulates the release of Factor VIII, von Willebrand's Factor (vWF), and tissue plasminogen activator from the endothelial storage sites. There is a two- to threefold increase of Factor VIII from baseline level. At least 25–30% Factor VIII activity is needed for adequate hemostasis.

DDAVP/Stimate Therapy for Hemophilia A

DDAVP/Stimate is given orally, intravenously, or intranasally prior to a planned dental procedure to prevent bleeding. DDAVP should not be used too frequently because it can deplete the storage pools. Do not use DDAVP more than twice or three times over a 48-hour period.

DDAVP Dosing

1. **DDAVP IV dose:**
   Rx: Give 0.3 µg/kg of DDAVP in 50 cc saline IV slowly over 15–30 min. With IV DDAVP, Factor VIII and von Willebrand's Factor (vWF) levels peak in 30–60 min.
2. **DDAVP intranasal dose:**
   Rx: Desmopressin/DDAVP, 1.5 mg/mL.
   0.1 mL is pumped with each spray, giving a 150 µg dose.
   Adult dose: 300 µg.
   Child's dose: 150 µg. The intranasal absorption is slow and the effect lasts for 5–21 h. With intranasal DDAVP, Factor VIII and von Willebrand's Factor levels peak in 60–90 min.
3. **DDAVP Oral Dose:**
   Rx: DDAVP, 0.1 or 0.2 mg/tablet.
   Sig: 0.05 mg twice daily.
   Total Daily Oral Dose: 0.1–1.2 mg. Onset of action occurs in 0.9–1.5 h following oral intake.

   Note that DDAVP is not used in the management of hemophilia B because it does not stimulate the release of Factor IX.

Hemophilia A and B Clotting Factor Replacement Therapy

The moderate and severe hemophilia A or B patient will always need specific Factor replacement prior to any major or minor dental procedure, and this includes probing or local anesthesia injection. One unit of Factor VIII/kg provides a 2% rise in Factor VIII level. To provide recombinant Factor VIII replacement, the clinician needs to obtain baseline Factor VIII activity and then correct to the desired percentage of factor activity. The factor activity level must be rechecked to confirm adequate replacement. The replacement formula for Factor VIII is as follows: $\{(\%\ \text{Desired} - \%\ \text{Actual})/2\%\} \times \text{Wt}$ (kg) = # units. One unit Factor IX/kg provides a 1% rise in Factor IX level. Here, too, the clinician needs to obtain baseline Factor IX activity and correct to desired percentage factor activity. Recheck factor activity to confirm adequate replacement. Factor IX replacement formula is as follows: $(\%\ \text{Desired} - \%\ \text{Actual}) \times \text{Wt}$ (kg) = # units. Clearly, in both cases, the clotting Factor dose prior to surgery will depend on the severity of bleeding expected and is decided by the patient's physician: **50%** Factor **activity** is a must for block anesthesia.

The commercial Factors are powders that need to be dissolved in sterile water prior to use. Often it is the patient who injects the factor intravenously (IV), approximately 15 minutes prior to a planned procedure.

Repeat infusions every 8–12 hours for Factor VIII and every 12–24 hours for Factor IX; this will depend on the planned dental procedure, the extent of postop bleeding, and if antifibrinolytic drugs tranexamic acid (Cyklokapron) or epsilon aminocaproic acid (Amicar) have been prescribed. The antifibrinolytic drugs prevent fibrinolysis/clot breakdown by inhibiting the activation of plasminogen to plasmin.

Factors VIII and IX Sources

Factors VIII and IX are obtained from two sources:

1. Clotting Factor concentrate from plasma
2. Commercially produced Recombinant Factor

Factor VIII Products for Hemophilia A

The Factor VIII products available for hemophilia A are:

1. **Recombinant products:** Bioclate, Helixate, Kogenate, and Recombinate
2. **Plasma-derived product:** Hyate derived from pork plasma

Factor IX Products for Hemophilia B

The Factor IX products available for hemophilia B are:

1. Recombinant product: BeneFIX
2. Plasma-derived products: AlphaNine SD, Konyne 80, Mononine, Proplex T, and Profilnine

Note that inhibitors or antibodies to clotting factors can develop in some cases of hemophilia A and hemophilia B. In these situations the patient is infused with the anti-inhibitor and the specific clotting factor.

ANTIFIBRINOLYTIC DRUGS: EPSILON AMINOCAPROIC ACID (AMICAR) AND TRANEXAMIC ACID (CYKLOKAPRON)

Before you prescribe these drugs, always confirm that the patient has no prior history of moderate or severe headaches, acute vision problems, transient ischemic attacks (TIAs), cardiovascular accidents (CVAs/strokes), blood clots, or any other indicators for thrombosis. Confirm that the liver and kidneys are optimally functioning.

The antifibrinolytic drugs can be ingested by mouth (PO), used as a mouth rinse, or injected IV. Always alert and advise the patient to discontinue the oral or IV antifibrinolytic drug and proceed to the nearest emergency room should symptoms and signs of thrombosis develop. Sudden, severe headaches; acute vision loss; sudden severe pains in the chest, calves, or abdomen; or sudden motor/sensory deficits in the extremities should be cause for immediate action and attention.

Epsilon Aminocaproic Acid (Amicar) Oral (PO) and Mouthwash Prescriptions

1. **Rx:** Epsilon aminocaproic acid **(Amicar)**, 500 mg/tablet.
    Sig: First dose: 5 g (10 tablets) orally, 1 hour post surgery, followed by 2 g (4 tablets) q6h, postoperatively until the bleeding stops, or prescribe for 5–7 days. **Maximum dose:** 30 g/day.
2. **Rx: Amicar syrup**, 250 mg/mL or 1.25 g/tsp (5 mL).
    Sig: 5–10 mL qid × 5–7 days, starting 6 h prior to surgery, if needed. Use as **mouthwash** for 2 min and **expectorate**.
    The mouthwash decreases recurrent bleeding and the need for factor replacement after surgery. Amicar prevents clot breakdown by the enzymes in the saliva. This allows healing of the tissues beneath the clot.
    Disp: 240 mL/480 mL bottle.

Tranexamic Acid/Cyklokapron Oral (PO) and Mouthwash Prescriptions

1. **Rx:** Tranexamic acid (**Cyklokapron**), 500 mg/tablet.
    Sig: 25 mg/kg orally tid/qid × 2–8 days, starting one day prior to surgery.
2. **Rx:** 4.8% **Cyklokapron** oral rinse solution.
    Sig: Use 10 mL as **mouthwash** for 2 min and **expectorate** qid × 5–7 days.
    Disp: 280 mL.

Cyklokapron is ten times more potent than Amicar and it has a longer half-life. The Cyklokapron oral rinse is **not** FDA-approved. It is important to remember that the saliva and the oral mucosa contain plasminogen activators that can trigger fibrinolysis. Therefore, use of Amicar or Cyklokapron mouthwash is very beneficial to prevent clot lysis.

Excessive postsurgical oozing can also be controlled by sustained pressure and the use of local hemostatic materials. Review Table 18.1 for a summary of hemostatic adjuncts.

Table 18.1.   Hemostatic Adjuncts: DDAVP, Amicar, and Tranexamic Acid

Therapy	Prescription
Desmopressin or Vasopressin or DDAVP or Stimate therapy: Therapy for Hemophilia A or Von Willebrands Disease Type 1; 2A	1. **DDAVP IV dose:** Give $0.3\mu g/kg$ DDAVP in 50cc saline IV slowly over 15–30 minutes. Levels peak in 30–60 minutes. 2. **DDAVP Intranasal Dose:** Available as 1.5mg/mL spray. Each spray pumps 0.1mL, giving a $150\mu g$ dose. Levels peak in 60–90 minutes. Dose lasts for 5–21 hours. **Adult intranasal Dose:** $300\mu g$ **Child intranasal Dose:** $150\mu g$ 3. **DDAVP Oral Dose:** Rx: DDAVP, 0.1 or 0.2mg/tablet Sig: 0.05mg twice daily. Total daily Dose: 0.1–1.2mg.
Anti-Fibrinolytic drug: Epsilon Aminocaproic acid (Amicar)	1. **Oral Amicar Prescription:** Rx: Amicar, 500mg/tablet Sig: Start dose 5g (10 tabs) PO 1hr post surgery, **then** 2g (4 tabs) q6h until the bleeding stops **or** for 5-7 days. Maximum oral Dose: 30g/day. 2. **Amicar Mouthwash:** Rx: Amicar syrup, 250mg/ml or 1.25g/teaspoon (5ml) Sig: 5–10mL qid x 5–7 days, starting 6 hours prior to surgery, if needed. Use as mouthwash for 2 minutes and **expectorate**. Disp: 240mL/480mL bottle
Anti-Fibrinolytic drug: Tranexamic acid (Cyklokapron)	1. **Oral Cyklokapron:** Rx: Cyklokapron, 500mg/tablet Sig: 25mg/kg PO tid/qid x 2-8 days, starting one day prior to surgery. 2. **Cyklokapron Mouthwash:** Not FDA approved. Has a longer half-life than Amicar and is also 10 times more potent. Rx: 4.8% Cyklokapron rinse Sig: Use 10mL as mouthwash for 2 minutes and **expectorate**, qid x 5-7 days. Disp: 280mL

LOCAL HEMOSTATIC AGENTS

Microfibrillar Collagen (Avitene or Helistat)

Avitene or Helistat is a mesh-like hemostat that attracts and triggers platelet aggregation plus fibrin formation. It can be applied to the bleeding site to control moderate-to-severe bleeding in two to five minutes. It does not inhibit healing. It can be used in patients taking aspirin or heparin.

Gelfoam

Gelfoam is an absorbable gelatin sponge that is made from purified gelatin solution. It stimulates thromboplastin release and thrombin formation. It gets absorbed in 3–5 days and works best in patients on blood thinners.

Thrombostat

Thrombostat is topical thrombin and it directly converts fibrinogen to fibrin. It works extremely well for severe bleeding.

Fibrin Glues

Fibrin glues contain fibrinogen and thrombin. Rapid hemostasis occurs when used at the bleeding surgical site.

Surgicel

Surgicel is oxidized regenerated cellulose. It swells immediately on contact with blood and forms a sticky mass. On doing so, it presses down on the bleeding site causing hemostasis. It can be kept in place indefinitely or removed after bleeding has stopped. Surgicel works when all other local hemostats have failed.

Amicar or Cyklokapron Mouthwashes

These mouthwashes prevent the conversion of plasminogen to plasmin. Gauze soaked with either mouthwash can be held in place for about 10–30 minutes to stop the bleed. Additionally, you can prescribe the mouthwash for 5–7 days, post surgery.

Calcium Sulfate

An absorbable biocompatible hemostatic agent, calcium sulfate gets resorbed in 2–4 weeks.

Moist Tea Bag

Biting down on a moist tea bag for 10–30 minutes can also decrease bleeding because of the tannic acid present in the tea bag.

SUGGESTED DENTAL GUIDELINES FOR HEMOPHILIAS A AND B

The following are dental guidelines for hemophilia:

1. Consult with the MD and understand the type and extent of the hemophilia.
2. How you treat will depend on severity of disease as well as type of procedure. Major surgeries may require 100% correction, whereas in some minor surgeries in mild hemophiliacs, DDAVP or Amicar may be sufficient: DDAVP will work because vWF is able to capture factor VIII in circulation. Therefore, it is important that you inform the patient's MD of the dental procedures planned and categorize them as major or minor surgical procedures.

3. Confirm with the MD if preoperative DDAVP (Stimate) use will suffice. Confirm route and time of administration for preoperative use. Surgery will begin in 30–60 minutes with IV use, in 60–90 minutes with intranasal use, and in 0.9–1.5 hours with oral use. DDAVP can minimize the need for Factor VIII use in some patients.

4. Confirm with the MD when Factor replacement should be done. When needed, it is usually done 15 minutes prior to most surgical procedures.

5. Factor VIII activity level must be increased to 50% of normal for block anesthesia.

6. Plan on doing more than one procedure at a given time to optimize the factor transfusion.

7. Keep a two-week interval if several procedures are planned for the patient. This will ensure optimal postoperative hemostasis and healing.

8. Assess the CBC with platelets and WBC differential to confirm the level of tissue oxygenation (by reviewing the RBC count), primary hemostasis and immediate bleeding (by reviewing the platelet count), and healing status (by reviewing the WBC total and differential count).

9. **Anesthetics:** There are no contraindications to any local anesthetics, but make appropriate changes per anemia guidelines if the patient has associated anemia. Also, any other existing systemic condition status will need to be factored in when deciding on the local anesthetic.

10. Use local hemostats, when needed.

11. Use reabsorbable sutures because they retain less plaque and therefore cause less inflammation at the surgical site.

12. **Analgesics:** Provide adequate pain management for 2–3 days with acetaminophen (Tylenol), acetaminophen with codeine, acetaminophen with oxycodone (Percocet), or hydrocodone (Vicodin). Do **not** prescribe aspirin or NSAIDS.

13. **Antibiotics:** Provide antibiotic coverage postoperatively with penicillin VK 250–500 mg qid or clindamycin 150–300 mg tid/qid (in the presence of penicillin allergy) for five days. This will promote the healing process and prevent infection and inflammation. Local infection and/or inflammation can cause secondary hemorrhage.

14. Advise the patient to consume cold liquids and soft foods until the bleeding stops, and to avoid using a straw because it promotes sucking and consequent clot displacement.

15. Depending on the procedures done and the gravity of the hemophilia, postsurgical Factor replacement should be planned and the protocol communicated to the patient. Factor VIII is given q12h and Factor IX is given q24h.

16. Prescribe Amicar or Cyklokapron orally or as mouthwash to minimize postoperative Factor transfusion.

17. Communicate with the patient for the next 2–3 days to confirm excellent recovery.

18. Last but not least, maintain good oral status by implementing four-to-six-month checkups to prevent major dental problems from developing.

HEMOPHILIA INHIBITORS

Patients may develop antibodies against Factors.

- Severe hemophilia is often associated with a truncated protein formed by large gene deletions. The patient's immune system sees this truncated protein as normal. This

is immune-mediated destruction of normal protein. Consequently, these patients develop antibodies to the normal protein that is seen as foreign. These antibodies that develop are inhibitors. The patient is no longer able to respond to the normal protein.
- An inhibitor is identified in a mixing study when there is a failure to correct APTT.

Mixing Study

- Mix one part patient plasma with one part normal plasma and repeat APTT.
- Mixture should be incubated at 37°C for at least 1 hour, as inhibition is dependent on time and temperature.
- Test value (APTT) corrects to normal range in presence of factor deficiency.
- If APTT is prolonged, then the patient has an inhibitor that will destroy the factor in the normal plasma.

ADDITIONAL FACTOR DEFICIENCIES

Factor XII Deficiency

The patient with Factor XII deficiency does not bleed in the presence of a very prolonged PTT.

Factor XIII Deficiency

Factor XIII deficiency can be associated with excessive bleeding in the presence of normal PT/INR and PTT.

Anticoagulants: Assessment, Analysis, and Associated Dental Management Guidelines

ANTICOAGULATION THERAPY OVERVIEW

Anticoagulation therapy is indicated in the presence of thrombosis formation or when there is a risk of thrombosis. Because of its immediate action, intravenous (IV) heparin (standard heparin/unfractionated heparin) is the anticoagulant of choice, and it is used in a hospitalized setting to stabilize a patient experiencing an acute thrombotic episode. Once the acute state is brought under control, warfarin (Coumadin) is started orally. Coumadin cannot be used at the start of an acute thrombotic episode because of its slow onset of action and slow achievement of optimal action. IV heparin is withdrawn when the therapeutic level of Coumadin is reached and blood thinning can be completely maintained using warfarin (Coumadin). At the time of discharge, the patient is sent home taking only warfarin (Coumadin) to continue with the blood-thinning process.

Common indications for anticoagulation: Anticoagulation is needed to prevent pathologic clot formation or thrombus, which may lead to stroke or death. It is also needed in conditions in which you want to inhibit clotting, as in the case of protein defects that compromise hemostasis. The most common indications for anticoagulation include transient ischemic attacks (TIAs) or strokes, atrial fibrillation, low ejection fraction causing stasis/pooling of blood, which promotes thrombus formation, pulmonary embolism, deep vein thrombosis (DVT), and hypercoagulation states: proteins C/S deficiency, Factor V Lieden mutation, lupus anticoagulant, antiphospholipid antibody syndrome, and antithrombin III deficiency.

WARFARIN (COUMADIN)

Warfarin (Coumadin) antagonizes the synthesis of the vitamin K–dependent clotting factors II, VII, IX, and X. Deficiency of vitamin K can thus affect the intrinsic and extrinsic clotting pathways causing a prolongation of the activated partial thromboplastin time (APTT) and the prothrombin time (PT), respectively.

Dentist's Guide to Medical Conditions, Medications, and Complications, Second Edition. Kanchan M. Ganda.
© 2013 John Wiley & Sons, Inc. Published 2013 by John Wiley & Sons, Inc.

Coumadin is given PO (oral) and it peaks in 60–90 minutes after oral administration. Once ingested, Coumadin gets highly bound to albumin. It takes 9–16 hours for Coumadin to be effective and 36–48 hours for therapeutic levels to be established. The plasma half-life of warfarin (Coumadin) is about 37 hours. Warfarin is a racemic mixture of R- and S-warfarin, with the S-form being two-to-five times more potent. Both forms are metabolized by cytochrome P450 with predominant involvement of CYP1A1, CYP1A2, CYP2C9, CYP2C19, and CYP3A4. S-warfarin is metabolized primarily by CYP2C9, whereas CYP1A2 and CYP3A4 account for most of the metabolism of R-warfarin.

At the therapeutic level, Coumadin affects only Factor VII, which is part of the extrinsic pathway. This accounts for why PT/INR is the only test monitored to assess warfarin (Coumadin) response. The half-life of Factor VII is **eight hours**, so when the Coumadin intake is temporarily stopped prior to major dental surgery, it takes **48 hours** (**six half-lives**) for the PT/INR to normalize.

The warfarin (Coumadin) level can be affected by certain dietary foods that are high in vitamin K. Dark green leafy vegetables, avocados, turnips, beets, and liver are the food items that **decrease** the effectiveness of warfarin (Coumadin), thus increasing the risk for thrombosis.

Warfarin (Coumadin) Reversal

During dire situations when emergency dental surgery is needed in a patient on Coumadin, the effect of Coumadin can immediately be reversed with Fresh Frozen Plasma (FFP). The PT/INR is always checked post FFP transfusion to confirm the reversal. Post-surgery FFP transfusion does not negatively affect the future doses of Coumadin. Vitamin K can also be used to reverse the effects of Coumadin. However, a significantly large dose of vitamin K is needed for the reversal process to be quick. Large doses of vitamin K (oral or IV) used for reversal have a negative impact on the future doses of Coumadin. Higher doses of Coumadin will be needed, post emergency surgery. Therefore, as a preventive measure, only low-dose vitamin K is used to reverse the effects of Coumadin in semi-urgent situations. It can take almost 24 hours for Coumadin action reversal to occur. Low-dose vitamin K, as stated previously, does not affect the future doses of Coumadin. In most patients with a history of Coumadin intake, the INR is maintained at a therapeutic range of 2.0–3.0. Patients maintained at this range can tolerate a physician-approved, temporary interruption of Coumadin for major surgical procedures, as they are not at high risk for thrombosis. It is always best to communicate with the patient's M.D. for advice when the patient is on Coumadin. Indicate the type of major and/or minor procedures planned and the amount of bleeding expected.

Patients with a high risk for thrombosis need higher doses of Coumadin. **The PT/INR in such cases is maintained between 3.0–4.5 or greater.** In the presence of higher Coumadin doses, the PTT will also be affected. Nevertheless, the PT/INR is the only test evaluated when monitoring even the high-risk patients.

Conditions Associated with Increased Risk of Thrombosis

The following are conditions associated with increased risk of thrombosis:

1. Mechanical prosthetic heart valves
2. Recent/within the past 6 months, deep vein thrombosis (DVT)

3. Recent/within the past 6 months, massive myocardial infarction (MI)
4. Atrial fibrillation (AF) associated with stroke/MI
5. Recent or multiple episodes of pulmonary embolism (PE)

Presence of any documented end-organ thrombosis-associated condition with AF places the patient at a high risk for thrombosis. The end-organ conditions can be TIA/CVA/MI. Therefore, high-risk patients cannot afford to have their blood-thinning process stopped at any time, and for all surgical procedures these patients will have to be switched from Coumadin to heparin. Depending upon the dental procedure planned, the patient's M.D. could switch the patient to either low molecular weight heparin (LMWH) or standard/unfractionated/IV heparin.

The PT/INR is monitored every 4–6 weeks when the patient is on Coumadin. The dentist must always request and evaluate the latest PT/INR from the physician's office before starting any dental treatment. In a patient who has always been in the therapeutic range, a PT/INR done no earlier than one week prior is most reliable and helpful.

STANDARD/UNFRACTIONATED HEPARIN (UFH)/INTRAVENOUS HEPARIN AND LOW MOLECULAR WEIGHT HEPARINS (LMWHS)

Mechanism of Action of IV and Low Molecular Weight Heparins

The anticoagulant effect of heparin is directly related to its activation of antithrombin III, which rapidly inactivates thrombin and Factor Xa in the coagulation process. Unfractionated heparin (UFH) or IV heparin potentiates the action of antithrombin III, and this rapidly inactivates thrombin and Factor Xa in the coagulation process. Intravenous (IV) heparin also inactivates Factors IX, X, XI, XII, and plasmin, plus IV heparin inhibits the conversion of fibrinogen to fibrin. LMWHs have less anti–Factor IIa activity and more Factor Xa activity. LMWHs bind to antithrombin III and this instantly inactivates Factor Xa and Factor II (prothrombin).

IV or standard heparin **inhibits** thrombin-induced platelet activation, thus causing IV heparin-induced **thrombocytopenia**. This effect is more pronounced if the patient has had several past exposures to IV heparin. This accounts for why it is important to check the platelet count at one, three, and seven days postoperatively after the use of IV heparin. LMWHs have decreased platelet-activation action and affinity and are less likely to cause thrombocytopenia.

IV heparin is extensively bound to plasma proteins and has a short half-life (60–90 minutes). LMWHs have a longer plasma half-life. LMWHs are minimally bound to plasma proteins and the proteins released from activated platelets and endothelial cells. Thus the anticoagulation action of LMWH is more consistent and predictable.

IV heparin does not cross the placental barrier, so it can be safely given to pregnant patients when needed. Heparin clearance from the plasma is **reduced** in patients with cirrhosis or severe kidney disease.

The plasma half-life of IV heparin or unfractionated heparin is approximately one hour. It is injected intravenously (IV). The onset of action is immediate following an IV injection and the total clearance time is six hours.

Standard heparin effectiveness is judged by monitoring the PTT. Standard heparin is **the** drug used in the hospitalized setting when any acute thromboembolic state needs immediate attention. Once stable, warfarin (Coumadin) is added orally. When the anticoagulation is completely supported by Coumadin in about 2–4 days, standard heparin is then totally withdrawn.

Massive myocardial infarction (MI), stroke, atrial fibrillation (AF) associated with stroke/MI (end-organ problems), heart valve surgery, deep vein thrombosis (DVT), or pulmonary embolism (PE) are examples of acute thromboembolic states. LMWHs are prepared by depolymerization of unfractionated heparin chains. They are injected subcutaneously (SC) by the patient. This is a huge advantage because the patient can be ambulatory and does not need hospitalization. LMWHs are widely used in pregnant patients. They do not cross the placenta and have a fetal safety profile similar to UFH.

The onset of action of LMWH occurs in 30–60 minutes. The plasma half-life of LMWHs is 2–4 hours. The amount of LMWH given is determined by the patient's height and weight. LMWH is usually given q12h.

LMWHs, as previously discussed, have better bioavailability, longer half-lives, more predictable dose response, and less negative effect on the platelets, compared to standard heparin. LMWHs are the preferred choice in the dental setting when blood thinning has to be continued for high-risk patients (after Coumadin withdrawal) for major procedures.

LMWH Preparations

The LMWHs preparations available are enoxaparine (Lovenox), ardeparin (Normiflo), dalteparin (Fragmin), nadroparin (Fraxiparine), reviparin (Clivarin), and tinzaparin (Innohep). Enoxaparin (Lovenox) is the most commonly prescribed LMWH.

DDIs Associated with Heparin

The following drugs enhance heparin action and should not be prescribed in the dental setting in conjunction with heparin: aspirin, NSAIDS, cephalosporins, tetracyclines, and antihistamines.

Heparin Antidote

Excessive bleeding associated with heparin can be reversed by protamine sulphate: 1mg protamine sulphate neutralizes 100 units of heparin, dose for dose.

WARFARIN AND HEPARIN PROTOCOLS AND SUGGESTED DENTAL GUIDELINES

The following are protocols and dental guidelines:

1. Always consult with the patient's M.D. to determine whether warfarin (Coumadin) can be stopped prior to the surgical procedure.
2. Most physicians will feel comfortable advising when you let them know the extent of surgery planned and the bleeding expected. State whether you plan on doing a major or minor dental procedure, or both.
3. Amalgams, composites, cleanings, scaling root planing, and endodontic or prosthodontic procedures are considered "minor procedures" because the bleeding is minimal or easy to control.

4. Gum surgery, extractions, sinus lifts, and so on are considered "major procedures" because of the increased risk for bleeding, tissue trauma, associated local inflammation, and/or infection.

5. In most patients, when the PT/INR is in the therapeutic range, amalgams, composites, cleanings, and endodontic and prosthodontic procedures can be done without stopping the Coumadin. The bleeding is minimal and can be controlled by adequate pressure or local hemostats.

6. For some of the planned major procedures, when warfarin (Coumadin) can be temporarily stopped without a risk to thrombosis per M.D., it is usually stopped 48 hours (two days) prior to the surgical procedure. Occasionally, some physicians may want you to stop the Coumadin five days prior to the planned surgical procedure. The Coumadin in such cases is restarted the evening of the surgical procedure or the next day, depending on when the patient typically takes the Coumadin. So always confirm through patient communication if warfarin (Coumadin) intake is occurring in the evening or morning hours.

7. If the patient's PT/INR has always been in the therapeutic range in the past, you can proceed without confirming the PT/INR prior to surgery. You will, however, need to confirm the PT/INR prior to major surgery for those patients with a pretreatment PT/INR above the therapeutic range.

8. Trauma should be kept to a minimum in all cases, and the INR should ideally be checked on the day of the treatment.

9. Follow the sutures and local-hemostat use guidelines discussed in Chapter 18.

10. For patients with an increased risk for thrombosis, heparin is the bridging blood-thinning medication used during the period prior to and immediately following the dental procedure. You need to let the M.D. know whether you plan on doing major or minor dentistry. The M.D. will then decide whether IV heparin or low molecular weight heparin (LMWH) will be used. For anticoagulation conversion from Coumadin to IV heparin, the patient is **hospitalized**. On the day of admission, the Coumadin intake is stopped and the PT/INR plus APTT are constantly monitored. IV heparin is started q6h when the INR drops below 2. The IV heparin dose is progressively increased to compensate for the Coumadin washout and maintain adequate blood thinning. Heparin ultimately takes over the anticoagulation process from Coumadin. When complete, Coumadin washout has been achieved and the PT/INR attains baseline level (1.0). At this point, IV heparin is the only anticoagulant that supports the blood thinning. Always confirm that the PT/INR is normal before you begin the surgical procedure. The major surgical procedure is done **6 hours after** the last IV heparin dose. Once adequate hemostasis is achieved post surgery, IV heparin is restarted. The APTT is monitored to regulate the IV heparin dose.

   When the patient is stable postoperatively, Coumadin is restarted by mouth on the evening of the procedure or the next day. The PT/INR and the APTT are now monitored. As the PT/INR rises, the IV heparin dose is progressively decreased. The dropping APTT will reflect the heparin washout. The entire process from start to finish takes approximately seven days.

11. For anticoagulation conversion from warfarin (Coumadin) to LMWH, no hospitalization is needed. The patient injects the LMWH subcutaneously (SC). The APTT is **not** monitored with LMWH use. The M.D. will decide the Coumadin washout and LMWH protocols, prior to the surgery.

12. 12. Enoxaprine (Lovenox) is the most common LMWH preparation prescribed and it is injected twice daily. Planned major surgical procedures in patients on Lovenox should be done 18–24 hours (six half-lives) **after the last intake** of the drug. The patient usually **skips** the Lovenox subcutaneous injection on the evening prior to **and** the morning of the surgery.

    Lovenox is restarted the **evening of or the next day**, depending on the thrombosis risk status of the patient. Patients with a higher risk will restart the Lovenox on the evening following the procedure, once hemostasis has occurred.

    Once the patient is stable with the LMWH, Coumadin is restarted by mouth and then the PT/INR is monitored. When the PT/INR is in the therapeutic range of 2–3, the LMWH is withdrawn.

13. Aspirin, NSAIDS, alcohol, liver disease, kidney disease, and other bleeding disorders can increase the risk of bleeding in patients on Coumadin and heparin.

14. Uncomplicated oral surgical procedures can be performed without altering the Coumadin dose in patients with an INR less than 3. Minimal trauma during surgery, absorbable sutures, and local hemostats will additionally help. Amicar or tranexamic acid mouthwash can also provide hemostatic support.

15. For emergency dental surgery it is best to rely on an INR test that is no more than one-week old.

16. Intrapapillary and intraligamentary injections are far safer than regional block anesthesia in patients with an INR above the therapeutic range. Regional block anesthesia can cause bleeding into the facial spaces, which can precipitate airway obstruction.

17. Intramuscular injections are administered very cautiously in the following populations: patients on anticoagulants, cirrhosis patients, and patients with Crohn's or Celiac disease–associated malabsorption of vitamin K. It is best to avoid.

DDIs Associated with Warfarin (Coumadin)

Antibiotics

The more potent antibiotics such as amoxicillin plus clavulanic acid (Augmentin), cephalexin (Keflex), cephadroxyl (Duricef), doxycycline (Vibramycin), and metronidazole (Flagyl) should be **avoided** because they deplete the intestinal flora bacteria, impairing vitamin K absorption, thereby promoting bleeding by increasing the INR. Penicillin VK and clindamycin are **safe** to use with Coumadin.

Analgesics

Recent studies have shown that excessive use of acetaminophen (Tylenol), particularly Extra-Strength Tylenol with Coumadin, can cause a 4–9 times increase in the INR within 18–48 hours. It is best to use regular-strength Tylenol, Tylenol with codeine, Tylenol with hydrocodone (Vicodin), or oxycodone (Percocet) for 2–3 days only. Stress adequate hydration (6–8 glasses of water/day) and no alcohol use while on the pain medications. Avoid using morphine analogues, dihydrocodeine, acetaminophen-propoxyphene (Darvocet), and pethidine because they raise the INR. Excessive pain may prevent the patient from eating, **so start the pain medication just prior to major surgery or soon after**. Fasting raises the INR, so prompt and proper analgesic use will prevent this from happening.

Antifungals

The **systemic** azole antifungals, fluconazole (Diflucan), ketoconazole (Nizoral), and griseofulvin (Fulvicin) **promote** bleeding in the presence of Coumadin. Use the topical antifungals, clotrimazole (Mycelex) or nystatin (Mycostatin) instead, when needed.

NEWER ANTICOAGULANTS

Introduction

Warfarin (Coumadin) is the oldest oral vitamin K antagonist (VKA), indicated to reduce the risk of death, recurrent myocardial infarctions (MI), and thromboembolic events such as stroke, systemic embolism, and post MI. The newer anticoagulants discussed further on, target either Factor IIa or Factor Xa.

Factor IIa/direct thrombin inhibitors (DTI), act by binding to thrombin, inhibiting the conversion of Fibrinogen to Fibrin. The DTIs not only inhibit free thrombin, but they also inhibit thrombin bound to fibrin. Dabigatran (Pradaxa) is the only drug in this class currently approved to reduce the risk of stroke and systemic embolism in patients with nonvalvular atrial fibrillation (NVAF).

Apixaban (Eliquis), rivaroxaban (Xarelto), and edoxaban (Lixiana) are the direct Factor Xa inhibitors approved by the FDA for stroke prevention in nonvalvular atrial fibrillation patients. Rivaroxaban and apixaban have additionally been approved for the prevention of recurrent ischemia in acute coronary syndromes. Potential advantages to these agents include oral administration, dose titration, and minimal monitoring requirements. Furthermore, due to their specificity, fewer clinical drug interactions occur. See Figure 19.1.

These drugs are proving to be better than warfarin (Coumadin) for stroke prevention in nonvalvular atrial fibrillation (NVAF) and for secondary prevention after acute coronary syndromes. Unlike warfarin, these anticoagulants are given in **fixed doses** and **do not need coagulation monitoring**. Clinical trials have shown that all these drugs decrease the incidence of stroke, embolism, bleeding, and mortality.

New Anticoagulants General Pharmacology

Dabigatran Etexilate (Pradaxa)

Dabigatran etexilate is an oral anticoagulant, given to prevent and treat venous thromboembolism and nonvalvular atrial fibrillation. The drug binds directly and reversibly to thrombin. It is a **prodrug**, given by mouth. Once absorbed, the drug is rapidly activated by esterase-mediated hydrolysis. Peak plasma levels occur 2–3 hours after intake and the **half-life is approximately 12–14 hours**. Dabigatran is excreted unchanged by the kidneys. Drug clearance of dabigatran is affected in the presence of moderate kidney disease (CrCl 50mL/min), and dose adjustment is required when the renal function is compromised. Dabigatran does not affect the liver. **There is no antidote for dabigatran, and fresh frozen plasma is not effective in reversing its effects**. In the presence of uncontrolled bleeding, activated or unactivated prothrombin complex concentrates or recombinant activated FVII may be helpful.

Dabigatran (Pradaxa) prescribing information has recently been updated to support that Pradaxa 150mg twice daily was superior in reducing ischemic and hemorrhagic strokes relative to warfarin (Coumadin). The label update was based on the results of

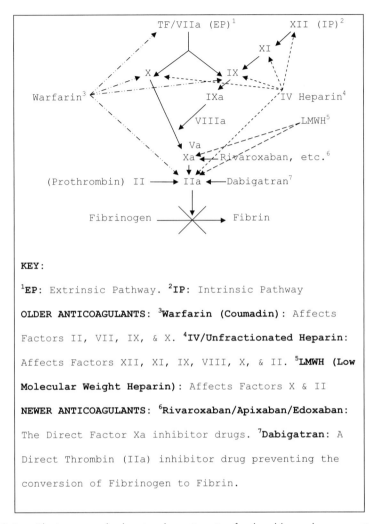

Figure 19.1. Clotting cascade showing the action sites for the older and newer anticoagulants.

the Randomized Evaluation of Long-Term Anticoagulation Therapy (RE-LY) trial conducted in 18,000 patients with nonvalvular atrial fibrillation (NVAF). Results showed that dabigatran (Pradaxa) 150mg taken twice daily significantly reduced stroke and systemic embolism by 35% beyond the reduction achieved with warfarin (Coumadin) in patients with atrial fibrillation. In addition, dabigatran (Pradaxa) 150mg taken twice daily also significantly reduced both ischemic and hemorrhagic strokes, compared to warfarin.

Rivaroxaban (Xarelto)

Rivaroxaban is a reversible direct oral F-Xa inhibitor. Rivaroxaban is given once daily for nonvalvular atrial fibrillation and twice daily for acute coronary syndromes in combination with antiplatelet drugs. Peak plasma levels occur 2–4 hours after intake and the

half-life of the drug is 5–13 hours. Some of the drug is excreted through the kidneys and a large part is metabolized in the liver by CYP3A4 and CYP2J2.

It is important to note that rivaroxaban is a substrate of P-gp and should not be combined with potent CYP3A4 and P-gp inhibitor drugs, such as azole-antifungals and HIV-protease inhibitors. Potent CYP3A4 and P-gp inducers, rifampicin, phenytoin, carbamazepine, and phenobarbital should also be avoided, as they will decrease rivaroxaban levels. **There is no antidote for rivaroxaban.**

Studies have shown Rivaroxaban to be better than warfarin in preventing the risk of stroke or systemic embolism without significantly increasing the risk of major bleeding in patients with nonvalvular atrial fibrillation having a high risk of stroke. Rivaroxaban has the advantage of a convenient once-daily regimen, which may improve adherence.

Most recently, rivaroxaban (Xarelto) has been approved by the FDA for the treatment of deep vein thrombosis (DVT) and/or pulmonary embolism (PE), and also to reduce the risk of recurrence of DVT and PE following initial treatment, especially in patients undergoing knee or hip replacement surgery.

Apixaban (Eliquis)

Apixaban is an oral, reversible, and selective active-site inhibitor of FXa. Apixaban inhibits free and clot-bound FXa and prothrombinase activity. Apixaban has no direct effect on platelet aggregation, but it indirectly inhibits platelet aggregation induced by thrombin. By inhibiting FXa, apixaban decreases thrombin generation and thrombus development.

As a result of FXa inhibition, apixaban prolongs clotting tests such as PT/INR, and activated partial thromboplastin time (aPTT). Changes observed in these clotting tests at the expected therapeutic dose, however, are small, subject to a high degree of variability, and not useful in monitoring the anticoagulation effect of apixaban.

Apixaban Pharmacokinetics

Apixaban displays prolonged absorption. Thus, despite a short clearance half-life of about 6 hours, the apparent half-life during repeat dosing is about 12 hours, which allows twice-daily dosing to provide effective anticoagulation, but it also means that when the drug is stopped for surgery, anticoagulation persists for at least a day.

Discontinuing apixaban places patients at an increased risk of thrombotic events. An increased rate of stroke has been observed following discontinuation of apixaban in clinical trials in patients with nonvalvular atrial fibrillation.

Apixaban DDIs

Apixaban is a substrate of both CYP3A4 and P-glycoprotein (P-gp). CYP3A4 and P-gp inhibitors increase blood levels of apixaban and increase the risk of bleeding. Inducers of CYP3A4 and P-gp, such as rifampin, carbamazepine, phenytoin, St. John's wort, decrease apixaban blood levels and increase the risk of stroke. CYP3A4 and P-gp inhibitors, such as clotrimazole, ketoconazole, itraconazole, ritonavir, and clarithromycin, should be avoided because these drugs increase blood levels of apixaban.

Concomitant use of drugs affecting hemostasis increases the risk of bleeding. These include aspirin and other antiplatelet agents, other anticoagulants, heparin, thrombolytic agents, selective serotonin reuptake inhibitors, serotonin norepinephrine reuptake inhibitor, and nonsteroidal anti-inflammatory drugs (NSAIDS).

Edoxaban (Lixiana)

Edoxaban is also an oral selective direct FXa inhibitor. Peak plasma levels occur 1–3 hours after oral intake, and the **half-life is 7–10 hours**. About half the drug is excreted unchanged in the urine. The drug is partly metabolized in the liver by CYP3A4. The drug is very affected by P-gp inhibitors or inducers. Potent P-gp inhibitors, verapamil, quinidine, or dronedarone will increase drug levels. **There is no antidote for edoxaban**. In case of an overdose, follow the same guidelines as for rivaroxaban.

Conclusions and Dental Alerts

Based on the results obtained from current individual trials, it is evident that both the oral direct thrombin inhibitor dabigatran etexilate and the oral F-Xa inhibitors apixaban and rivaroxaban are good alternatives to warfarin or aspirin in patients with nonvalvular atrial fibrillation and with an increased risk of stroke.

Compared with warfarin, the newer anticoagulants have important advantages, with their lower risk of intracranial bleeding, no clear interactions with food, fewer interactions with medications, and no need for frequent laboratory monitoring and dose adjustments. The new oral anticoagulants are a lot more convenient to use than VKAs in patients with acute coronary syndromes.

Therefore, these new oral anticoagulants are going to be preferred over VKAs for many patients with nonvalvular atrial fibrillation and an increased risk of stroke. Patients stable on VKAs should not be switched to the newer drugs. VKAs are still needed for patients unable to tolerate the new anticoagulants or in patients with very poor renal function.

All of the newer drugs are excreted through the kidneys and a large part of each drug is metabolized in the liver by CYP3A4 and CYP2J2. The newer anticoagulants should not be combined with potent CYP3A4 and P-gp inhibitor drugs, such as erythromycin, clarithromycin, azole-antifungals and HIV-protease inhibitors. Additionally, potent CYP3A4 and P-gp inducers, rifampicin, phenytoin, carbamazepine, and phenobarbital should be avoided, as they will decrease drug levels. Nephrotoxic drugs are also avoided in the presence of dabigatran, rivaroxaban, apixaban, and endoxan.

Discontinuation of Newer Anticoagulants for Surgery

If anticoagulation with any one of the drugs must be discontinued for a reason other than pathological bleeding, coverage with another, older anticoagulant must be strongly considered. When cleared by the physician, the given drug is discontinued for at least 24 hours prior to elective surgery or procedures with a low risk of bleeding or where the bleeding can be easily controlled. The drug is discontinued for at least 48 hours prior to elective surgery or procedures with a moderate or high risk of clinically significant bleeding.

Converting from or to the Newer Anticoagulants

- **Switching from warfarin (Coumadin) to newer anticoagulant:** Warfarin should be discontinued first, and when the international normalized ratio (INR) drops below 2.0, the newer anticoagulant is started.
- **Switching from newer anticoagulant to warfarin:** The Xa inhibitors rivaroxaban, apixaban, and endoxan affect INR, so INR measurements during co-administration with warfarin may not be useful for determining the appropriate dose of warfarin. If continuous anticoagulation is necessary, the Xa or IIa inhibitor drug is discontinued and both a parenteral older anticoagulant such as IV heparin or LMWH and warfarin are begun at the time the next dose of the Xa/IIa inhibitor would have been taken. The parenteral older anticoagulant is discontinued when the INR reaches an acceptable range.
- **Switching between any one of the Xa/IIa inhibitors and anticoagulants other than warfarin:** Discontinue one being taken and begin the other at the next scheduled dose.

Reversal

There is no established way to reverse the anticoagulant effect of the newer anticoagulants, which can be expected to persist for about 24 hours after the last dose, that is, for about two half-lives. A specific antidote for any one of the drugs is not available. Protamine sulfate and vitamin K would not be expected to affect the anticoagulant activity, and there is no experience with the antifibrinolytic agents (tranexamic acid, aminocaproic acid) in individuals receiving the newer anticoagulants.

Cardiology and Renal Disease

VI

Rheumatic Fever: Assessment, Analysis, and Associated Dental Management Guidelines

RHEUMATIC FEVER FACTS AND OVERVIEW

Rheumatic fever (RF) is a nonsuppurative acute inflammatory response to a previously untreated or partially treated Group A, β hemolytic streptococcus infection.

Patients with a diagnosis of RF will give a history of having had strep throat or scarlet fever a few weeks prior to the start of the symptoms and signs associated with RF. RF can occur within three to four weeks of an infection with β hemolytic streptococcus. The prevalence rate of RF following an untreated or incompletely treated β hemolytic infection is 3%.

RF is thought to be an abnormal immune-system response to the streptococcal antigens, streptolysin O and streptolysin S. Streptolysin O is strongly antigenic and triggers the production of antistreptolysin-O antibody (ASLO). The presence of high levels of ASLO during the acute phase of RF confirms the likelihood of the condition. The RF-triggered antigen–antibody cross-reactivity affects the periarteriolar connective tissue, targeting the heart, joints, skin, and neurological tissues.

Note that acute RF is associated with a negative throat culture because it occurs a few weeks **after** a β hemolytic streptococcus infection.

The Major and Minor Jones Criteria

The Major and Minor Jones Criteria, established in 1944, help with the diagnosis of RF.

Major Jones Criteria

The Major Jones Criteria for RF are polyarthritis, carditis, rheumatic chorea, erythema marginatum, and erythema nodosum.

Arthritis

Major joints, when affected, are involved bilaterally with an aseptic arthritis. The joints swell and become extremely painful. Recovery of one set of joints is associated with

---

Dentist's Guide to Medical Conditions, Medications, and Complications, Second Edition. Kanchan M. Ganda.
© 2013 John Wiley & Sons, Inc. Published 2013 by John Wiley & Sons, Inc.

involvement of another set of joints. Once recovery occurs, there is no residual joint deformity.

This type of arthritis is called **fleeting polyarthritis** because of the moving pattern of joint involvement. The polyarthritis is aggressively treated with pain medications until resolution occurs within a few weeks. Rheumatic arthritis is commonly seen in children.

Carditis

RF can affect all three layers of the heart. The endocardium is the most frequently affected layer. Fibrosis of the valves can lead to stenosis (narrowing) or incompetence (widening).

When the blood passes through a stenosed valve, it causes turbulence in blood flow, resulting in a heart murmur. With valvular incompetence, the blood regurgitates back into the heart chamber above and this is also associated with turbulence and a heart murmur.

Mitral stenosis (MS) and mitral incompetence (MI) are common RF-associated valvular lesions in children. Aortic stenosis (AS) and aortic incompetence (AI) are common lesions in adults. The most affected heart valve is the mitral valve and the least affected heart valve is the pulmonic valve. As per the **new 2007** American Heart Association (AHA) guidelines, RF-associated heart valve damage/lesions **no longer** need premedication with antibiotics prior to dentistry. However, premedication **is needed** if any of the damaged heart valves are replaced with **prosthetic valves**. Premedication may occasionally be needed in the presence of diseased valves affecting cardiac output. Patients with low ejection fractions causing blood turbulence may need prophylaxis in spite of the new guidelines stating otherwise. Premedication antibiotic use is directed against bacteria from the surface of tissues around the teeth that have a tendency to spread into the blood and settle on the valves and then cause serious infections.

Involvement of the myocardium is rare, but if it occurs, it presents as cardiomyopathy. Patients with cardiomyopathy also do not need to be premedicated any more, per the new 2007 AHA guidelines.

Pericardial involvement occurs more frequently in children than in adults, and pericardial effusion (fluid collection in the pericardial sac) is the most common form of presentation. Pericardial involvement also no longer needs premedication prior to invasive dental treatments, per the 2007 AHA guidelines.

Rheumatic Chorea/Sydenham's Chorea/St. Vitus's Dance

Rheumatic chorea occurs exclusively in children. It causes involuntary, jerky movements involving the face and the upper extremities. These movements are absent when the child sleeps but are exacerbated with emotional disturbance. Rheumatic chorea affects females more frequently and the condition improves as the child grows. **Stress management** during dentistry is extremely **helpful** for these patients.

Erythema Marginatum

Erythema marginatum is a rash that is found to occur in only 10% of patients affected with RF. Erythema Marginatum is characterized by a doughnut-shaped (pale center, dark margins) serpigineous rash that occurs on the trunk and upper limbs. As the rash migrates upward from the lower trunk area, the lower rash starts to disappear. This rash, which is more frequently seen on light-skinned than dark-skinned individuals, is diagnostic of RF.

Erythema Nodosum/Subcutaneous Nodules/Aschoff's Bodies

Erythema nodosum/subcutaneous nodules are pea-sized, painless nodules. They recur periodically on bony areas of the elbows, wrist, and shins.

Minor Jones Criteria

Minor Jones Criteria are presented in the following sections.

Fever

Moderately high fever is common.

Arthralgia

Patients experience recurrent joint pains but there is no joint swelling or deformity.

Pain in the Right Upper Quadrant (RUQ) of the Abdomen

Liver enlargement/engorgement occurs when RF precipitates congestive heart failure (CHF). This causes pain in the RUQ of the abdomen.

Elevated ESR

Elevated erythrocyte sedimentation rate (ESR) is seen commonly with RF and it indicates acute inflammation. ESR measures the levels of globulin and fibrinogen in the blood. A decreasing ESR during the management phase indicates that the patient is responding to the treatment and that the inflammation is resolving.

Increased WBC Count

Leukocytosis occurs in response to the acute inflammation associated with RF.

Increased C-Reactive Protein

Increased C-reactive protein titer is a marker that identifies a recent β hemolytic streptococcal infection.

Elevated Antistreptolysin-O (ALSO) Titer

Rising ASLO titer is a strong marker for RF.

EKG Changes

RF-associated myocardial involvement is associated with EKG changes. Cardiac conduction can be affected with RF.

RHEUMATIC FEVER (RF) DIAGNOSIS

To confirm the diagnosis of RF, the patient must have at least two Major Jones Criteria present, or one Major Criterion plus two Minor Criteria.

RF Treatment

RF treatment is a two-phase treatment.

RF Acute Phase Treatment

Pain medications and steroids are aggressively used to counteract the intense pain and inflammation associated with acute RF.

RF Secondary Prevention Treatment

Once the primary RF attack has resolved, future attacks of RF are prevented by maintaining uninterrupted low-dose antibiotic levels in the patient for the next five years. This prevents invasion of the β hemolytic streptococcus. The non-penicillin allergic patient gets 1.2 million units benzathine penicillin G IM (intramuscularly), once per month for five years. Each injection provides a low concentration of the antibiotic for four weeks. Penicillin-allergic patients are given erythromycin or azithromycin (Zithromax), 250 mg/day × 5 years.

Infective Endocarditis and Current Premedication Prophylaxis Guidelines

INFECTIVE ENDOCARDITIS

Overview

Infective endocarditis is associated with microbial infection of the endocardial surface of the heart. The valves are particularly affected with vegetation that contains bacteria, platelets, and inflammatory cells. Infective endocarditis can present as acute bacterial endocarditis (ABE) or subacute bacterial endocarditis (SBE).

Premedicating the patient prior to dentistry, when premedication is called for or required, can prevent infective endocarditis. Premedication provides a high level of a recommended antibiotic in the blood **prior** to the dental procedure, and this helps destroy any bacterium that enters the bloodstream during invasive dentistry.

Acute Bacterial Endocarditis (ABE)

ABE is an aggressive type of endocarditis with galloping symptoms. It occurs within approximately seven days of an invasive dental procedure done without premedication, when premedication is required. ABE is common in the elderly and in IV drug users. Staphylococcus aureus, viruses, and fungi are the most common offending organisms causing ABE.

Subacute Bacterial Endocarditis (SBE)

SBE is the most common form of infective endocarditis, and streptococcus viridans is the most common offending organism. Symptoms and signs usually present insidiously within 2–3 weeks after an invasive dental procedure done without premedication, when premedication is required. SBE presentation can also occur 2–3 months later.

Dentist's Guide to Medical Conditions, Medications, and Complications, Second Edition. Kanchan M. Ganda.
© 2013 John Wiley & Sons, Inc. Published 2013 by John Wiley & Sons, Inc.

Infective Endocarditis Clinical Features

It is quite common for patients to experience "flu-like" symptoms at the start of the endocarditis. The symptoms associated with ABE are rapidly progressive; those associated with SBE are gradual in onset. Fever, anorexia, malaise, weight loss, night sweats, salmon-colored urine or hematuria, conduction abnormalities, new valvular regurgitation, and CHF are common findings associated with infective endocarditis.

Splinter hemorrhage of the fingernails, Roth's spots (retinal hemorrhages), Osler's nodes (painful red bumps on the fingertips), and Janeway lesions (nontender hemorrhagic nodules on the palms and soles) are common peripheral signs associated with infective endocarditis.

Infective Endocarditis Treatment

Any patient presenting with ABE or SBE is immediately hospitalized for treatment of the systemic infection and associated vital organ involvements. A maximum of three blood cultures are obtained to determine the offending organism (bacterial/viral/fungus), and the specific infection is then aggressively treated for 2–3 weeks with intravenous (IV) antibiotics (penicillin plus gentamycin, or vancomycin in the penicillin-allergic patient), antivirals, or antifungals, depending on the outcome of the blood cultures.

Symptomatic care is additionally provided for the associated symptoms and vital organ involvements (heart and kidneys). Post recovery, all patients with a past history of infective endocarditis (ABE or SBE), with or without valvular problems, must be premedicated prior to all invasive dental procedures, per the 2007 American Heart Association (AHA) guidelines. Any antibiotic listed in the AHA premedication guideline protocol can be used, depending on the patient's allergy status and DDI with the patient's routine medication list (Table 21.1).

PREMEDICATION PROPHYLAXIS

Conditions That Require AHA Premedication Prophylaxis

- Prosthetic heart valves
- Past history of infective endocarditis
- Unrepaired or incompletely repaired cyanotic congenital heart disease, including those with palliative shunts or conduits
- A completely repaired congenital heart defect with prosthetic material or device, during the first 6 months after the repair procedure. This is because epithelial overgrowth of the graft material usually occurs within the first 6 months of repair.
- Any repaired congenital heart defect with persistent residual defect at the site or adjacent to the site of a prosthetic patch or a prosthetic device. This defect is usually confirmed with an echocardiogram.
- Cardiac transplant patients who develop heart valve–associated problems.

In addition to the aforementioned conditions outlined by AHA as needing antibiotic premedication prophylaxis some non-cardiac conditions also require antibiotic premedication prophylaxis:

- Systemic intracranial hydrocephalic shunt: ventriculoatrial (VA) or ventriculovenous (VV).

Table 21.1. 2007 American Heart Association (AHA) Recommended Antibiotic Prophylaxis Regimen

Recommended Regimens for Dental Procedures

Standard Regimen:
Amoxicillin (Amoxil, Trimox, Wymox, etc.):
Adults: 2g PO (oral), 1hr before procedure
Children*: 50mg/kg PO, 1hr before procedure

Patients unable to take Oral Medications:
Ampicillin:
Adults: 2g intramuscular (IM) or intravenous (IV) 30 minutes before the procedure
Children: 50mg/kg IM or IV 30 minutes before the procedure

OR
Cefazolin (Ancef) or Ceftriaxone (Rocephin):
Adults: 1g IM or IV 30 minutes before the procedure
Children: 50mg/kg IM or IV 30 minutes before the procedure

Amoxicillin/Penicillin–allergic Patients:
Clindamycin (Cleocin):
Adults: 600mg PO (oral), 1hr before the procedure
Children: 20mg/kg PO 1hr before the procedure

Cephalexin (Keflex)**
Adults: 2g oral 1hr before the procedure
Children: 50mg/kg oral 1hr before the procedure

Azithromycin (Zithromax) or Clarithromycin (Biaxin):
Adults: 500mg oral 1hr before the procedure
Children: 15mg/kg oral 1hr before the procedure

Penicillin allergic patient unable to take oral medications:
Cefazolin (Ancef) or Ceftiaxone (Rocephin)**
Adults: 1g IV or IM 30 minutes before the procedure
Children: 50mg/kg IM or IV 30 minutes before procedure

Systemic Clindamycin:
Adults: 600mg IV 30 minutes before the procedure
Children: 20mg/kg IV 30 minutes before the procedure

*Total children's dose should **not** exceed adult dose.
**Avoid Cephalosporins in patients with immediate-type hypersensitivity/acute anaphylaxis reaction to Penicillin.

- Systemic hemodialysis shunts (arteriovenous catheter or arteriovenous synthetic graft shunt): Do not monitor the blood pressure or draw blood from the arm with the shunt.
- Peritoneal dialysis: Only if the patient has an indwelling catheter.
- Synthetic graft materials (Dacron, Teflon, etc.) when used for **extracardiac** vascular repairs, as with aortic aneurysm and so on. Epithelial overgrowth of the graft material is never 100%, and some areas may stay denuded and promote infective endocarditis.
- Patients receiving cancer drugs through an infuse port or a Hickman catheter line.

- Patients with a history of cirrhosis and associated **ascites** need to be premedicated per AHA guidelines. The ascitic fluid is a good medium that can promote bacterial growth and increase the risk of infective endocarditis.
- **Prosthetic joints:** Per the December 2012 joint evidence-based clinical practice guideline (CPG) statement issued by the American Dental Association (ADA) and the American Academy of Orthopedic Surgeons (AAOS), there is "limited" evidence for joint prosthesis premedication prophylaxis in **non-high-risk** patients. "Limited" or "weak" evidence means that there is no real advantage in providing or not providing joint prosthesis prophylaxis. The dental provider should use his or her judgment for limited recommendations and independently decide on a case-by-case basis whether to follow the suggestion. Clearly, the provider can opt to treat without premedication prophylaxis only those patients that have **no** associated potentially high-risk states that can increase the risk of joint prosthesis infection. The provider should, of course, be reviewing the current literature and evidence on this subject as it unfolds. The provider should inform the patient about this limited evidence, because of the CPG-issued statement that, ultimately, the "patient preference should have a substantially influencing role" in whether to premedicate.

Premedication prophylaxis of joint prosthesis **should be considered/required** for patients with the following high-risk states (see the detailed discussion in the latter part of the chapter):

1. Congenital or acquired immunocompromised states: Type 1 diabetes, or uncontrolled Type 1 or Type 2 diabetes, HIV/AIDS, chemotherapy, radiotherapy, malignancy, or chronic corticosteroid therapy.
2. Chronic inflammatory joint diseases: rheumatoid arthritis, lupus arthritis.
3. History of recent joint prosthesis: within six months of surgery.
4. Multiple joint prosthesis history.
5. Past history of joint prosthesis infection.
6. Congenital bleeding disorders: hemophilias, vWD.
7. Malnutrition.
8. Chronic skin conditions associated with large, open sores (psoriasis/eczema: this is a distant source of infection propagation).
9. Severe periodontal disease and/or the presence of one or more odontogenic abscesses: this is a local source of infection propagation.

Conditions That Do Not Require AHA Premedication Prophylaxis

- All types of atrial septal defects: primum or secundum atrial septal defect (ASD)
- Ventricular septal defect (VSD)
- Hypertrophic cardiomyopathy
- Mitral valve prolapse, with or without regurgitation
- Rheumatic heart disease
- Bicuspid valve disease
- Calcified aortic stenosis
- No premedication is required **after** the first six months for atrial septal defect (ASD), ventricular septal defect (VSD), or patent ductus arteriosus (PDA) repairs
- Coronary artery bypass surgery
- Extracranial hydrocephalic shunt: ventriculoperitoneal (VP) shunt

- Severe anemia, hyperthyroidism, or functional systolic murmur associated with multiple pregnancies
- Cardiac pacemakers or defibrillators
- Phen-fen–associated heart valve damage
- Arteriovenous fistula for hemodialysis
- Beyond six months of joint prosthesis surgery in a normal, healthy, non-immune-compromised patient

As is evident from the 2007 AHA guidelines and the 2012 joint clinical practice guideline (CPG) statement issued by AAOS and ADA, many patients who were previously premedicated now **do not** need the antibiotic coverage. It is suggested that you always confirm the cessation of antibiotic premedication with the patient's physician, prior to initiation of dentistry without antibiotic coverage.

Note that there will be an occasional patient for whom the physician may want to continue with the premedication to prevent infective endocarditis, in spite of the new guidelines.

PROSTHETIC CARDIAC VALVES

There are two types of prosthetic/artificial valves: bioprosthetic valves and mechanical/metal valves. Both of these valves require endocarditis prophylaxis prior to invasive dentistry as per the 2007 AHA guidelines.

Bioprosthetic Valves

Bioprosthetic valves come from three sources: pig, bovine, or human cryopreserved heart valves. The pig valves have a shorter lifespan compared to the bovine valves and in comparison the human cryopreserved heart valves have the longest lifespan. In general, the bioprosthetic valves have a low risk for clot formation.

When compared to the mechanical valves, calcium deposition and consequent calcification and hardening of the valves accounts for the decreased longevity of the bioprosthetic valves. The average life span of the pig and bovine bioprosthetic valves is approximately ten years; it is longer than ten years for the human valves. All bioprosthetic valves require **uninterrupted** blood thinning with warfarin (Coumadin) in the initial 3–6 months, and then the patient with pig or bovine valve prosthesis is switched to daily aspirin. The human prosthetic valves **do not** require any blood thinning with aspirin beyond the initial 3–6-month postoperative period.

It is best to **delay** routine dental treatment for the time the patient has to be on the **uninterrupted** anticoagulation. If treatment has to be done during the first 3–6 months, either be conservative or consult with the patient's physician, who may then decide to switch the patient to IV or low molecular weight heparin. Premedication is needed prior to invasive dentistry for **all types** of bioprosthetic valves.

Mechanical Valves

Mechanical valves last about 20 years and have a high risk for clot formation. Lifetime anticoagulation with warfarin (Coumadin) is standard with the mechanical valves. Accordingly, when major or minor surgery is needed, the patient will have to be switched from Coumadin to heparin. It is best to plan one or two procedures at a given time to minimize the need for frequent switches.

JOINT PROSTHESIS

Joint Prosthesis Overview and Facts

The December 2012 joint evidence-based clinical practice guideline (CPG) statement issued by the American Dental Association (ADA) and the American Academy of Orthopedic Surgeons (AAOS) titled, "Prevention of Orthopedic Implant Infection in Patients Undergoing Dental Procedures," reports that there is limited evidence for joint prosthesis premedication prophylaxis in **non-high-risk** patients who have no associated, potentially high-risk states that might increase the risk of joint prosthesis infection. Per the statement, limited or weak evidence is data that "suggested that invasive dental procedures, with or without antibiotics, had no effect on the likelihood of developing a periprosthetic joint infection (PJI)."

The CPG statement clearly states that, "subgroup analysis for patients at potentially higher risk was not performed." The CPG also states that, "the provider of care should utilize his or her experience and clinical decision-making skills to identify those high-risk patients (e.g., immunocompromised) and determine the best care choices for those patients." Also, "The interaction between patient and clinician is critical to determining the applicability."

The dental provider should use his or her judgment for limited recommendations and independently decide on a case-by-case basis whether to follow the statement suggestion. Clearly, the provider **can opt** to treat **without** premedication prophylaxis only those patients that have **no** associated high-risk states that can increase the risk of joint prosthesis infection. Always consult with the patient's orthopedic surgeon before you plan to implement the guideline for no premedication in the patient that is not high risk. The provider should inform the patient that the CPG statement is based on the existence of limited/weak evidence for prophylaxis and also discuss his or her assessment of the patient's risk status. It is crucial that the provider review all future literature reporting evidence on this subject, in order to continue to make sound, evidence-based choices for the patient.

The **high-risk states** for which premedication prophylaxis should continue include:

- Patients with systemic diseases associated with decreased immunity due to HIV/AIDS, Type 1 diabetes, or uncontrolled Type 1 or Type 2 diabetes, malignancy, radiotherapy, chemotherapy, or chronic corticosteroid therapy.
- Patients with a history of chronic inflammatory joint diseases such as rheumatoid arthritis or systemic lupus erythematosus.
- Patients with a history of multiple prosthesis or prosthesis implanted less than six months ago, or those with a past history of prosthetic joint infection.
- Patients with a history of hemophilia A/B, vWD, and other congenital bleeding disorders.
- History of malnourishment.
- Patients presenting with a peripheral site of chronic skin infection (oozing eczema/bleeding dermatitis) or patients presenting with moderate-to-severe periodontal disease and/or oral abscesses.

Bacteremias can infect the artificial joint in the high-risk patients and cause rejection. The consequence of joint prostheses infection far outweighs the risk for antibiotic prophylaxis. Always consult with the orthopedic surgeon regarding prophylaxis so you can optimally protect your patient. Extractions, periodontal surgery, implants, endodontic surgery beyond the apex, cleaning, placement of orthodontic bands, and intraligamentary or intraosseous injections are dental procedures linked to a high risk of bacteremia. The taking of impressions in a partially edentulous patient should also be added to this list because the impression material can often lodge between the teeth and cause mucosal tears as the impression is removed.

Joint Prosthesis Premedication Antibiotic Selection Criteria

Studies have shown staphylococcus aureus to be the most common offending organism involved with infections of the prosthetic joint. Streptococci have been isolated on occasion. Staphylococcus aureus is often resistant to penicillin. Amoxicillin may be used for joint prophylaxis; however, it is **not** as effective against staphylococcus aureus, nor as penetrative of bone tissue, when compared with the oral penicillinase-resistant penicillin (Dicloxacillin), Augmentin, cephalosporins (Cephalexin/Keflex, Cephadroxyl/Duricef, or Cephazolin/Ancef), the newer macrolides (azithromycin, clarithromycin), or clindamycin. The AHA-recommended dose of cephalosporins, macrolides, and clindamycin should be used for premedication of patients with joint prostheses.

Some orthopedic surgeons may occasionally recommend the use of Augmentin, Dicloxacillin, or Keflex/Cephalexin for an extended 2–3 days period of prophylaxis, before and after the procedure. Communicate with the surgeon in such cases to understand why this altered guideline is needed for the patient. The patient may have multiple joint prostheses or may have some additional underlying factors known to the surgeon that make such a patient a high risk that requires an altered regimen.

Patients with pins and plates do not need to be premedicated. However, some orthopedic surgeons premedicate a patient with multiple pins and plates. In this case, as well, confirm the need by directly communicating with the surgeon.

SUGGESTED DENTAL GUIDELINES IN THE PRESENCE OF PREMEDICATION PROPHYLAXIS

The following are dental guidelines for premedication prophylaxis:

1. When successive appointments are planned for a patient needing premedication with one specific antibiotic for all visits, the appointments must be spaced **seven days apart** to allow for the regrowth of antibiotic-susceptible flora and to prevent any bacterial resistance to the premedication antibiotic. The streptococcus viridans can get resistant when the same antibiotic is given more frequently or when given less than seven days apart.
2. Plan more than one procedure to minimize antibiotic use.
3. Patients who need premedication prophylaxis should have good, daily oral hygiene practices at home. Prior to any dental appointment, have the patient **gently rinse for 30 seconds** with any mouthwash or use non-alcoholic chlorhexidine.

Rinsing the mouth prior to treatment will de-germ the oral cavity and minimize the bacteremia.

4. Avoid aggressive gingival irritation and avoid repeat, prolonged use of alcoholic chlorhexidine during visits, because this will increase the population of resistant bacteria.

5. Acutely infected teeth must be extracted 10–14 days prior to any planned cardiac/major surgery to prevent SBE. The 10–14 days provide adequate time for healing to occur.

6. Use amoxicillin/azithromycin/clindamycin alternatively if appointments are necessary at intervals shorter than seven days. Always make certain that the required gap of seven days is maintained for each class of antibiotic. As an example, use amoxicillin on day 1, switch to azithromycin on day 3, switch to clindamycin on day 6, and go back to amoxicillin again on day 9. This protocol will effectively maintain the required interval. Use this protocol **only** when you think you really need it.

   Try scheduling the patient no more than twice per week because there is always the risk of intestinal flora washout with the high premedication dosages or frequent use of premedication antibiotics.

7. Recommend simultaneous use of probiotics or acidophilus/yogurt drinks when prescribing antibiotics, because this will help maintain the intestinal flora.

8. For patients who want to come in once per week for dental care and who do not mind longer appointments for the day, you can schedule using the following protocol:

   a. In a dental school setting you can have the patient for a morning, 9:00AM, and an afternoon, 1:00PM, appointment. If you schedule a subgingival procedure associated with bleeding in the morning and a supragingival procedure in the afternoon, you need to premedicate the patient only **once**, one hour prior to the start of the first appointment. If both the procedures are going to be associated with bleeding, you need to give an additional **half-dose** of the premedication antibiotic prior to the 1:00pm appointment and proceed without waiting for an hour. There is no need to wait after the second dose because the second dose provides merely a boost for the morning dose of the antibiotic.

   b. In a private practice setting, one single dose of premedication can provide sufficient antibiotic coverage for 5–6 hours and that would be sufficient time for more than one procedure!

9. Co-infection in a premedicated patient can be treated in one of two ways:

   a. Use the **same antibiotic** for premedication and the treatment of infection. **Using the same antibiotic** is greatly preferred and less confusing to the patient. **For example**, give amoxicillin as premedication, 2.0g PO one hour prior to treatment, **followed** by amoxicillin 250/500mg tid × 5 days, **starting** six hours after the 2.0g amoxicillin intake. With this protocol, you have to **change** the premedication antibiotic for the visits planned in the next 2–3 weeks because the streptococcus viridans will become resistant with the five-day intake of amoxicillin. It takes about 2–3 weeks for a responsive oral flora to be reestablished and become sensitive to the same antibiotic. Thus amoxicillin can be used again for premedication in 2–3 weeks. It is important to remember that in this protocol, using amoxicillin for treatment of infection can be implemented only if the patient has been symptomatic with the infection for **less** than three days. If the symptoms have lasted longer than three days, clindamycin is **the** antibiotic of choice for treatment of the infection.

b. Another option is to use a different antibiotic for premedication and treatment of infection: **For example**, give amoxicillin for premedication and clindamycin for treatment of the infection; 6 hours after the intake of 2.0g amoxicillin, start clindamycin 150–300mg tid/qid × 5 days to treat the infection. No change in the premedication antibiotic is needed for subsequent dental visits with this protocol.

10. Before starting any dental treatment, always confirm with the patient that he/she has taken the premedication antibiotic. Occasionally, the patient forgets to take the antibiotic. You might also forget to ask the patient whether the antibiotic was taken. You could complete a procedure associated with bleeding and realize this error subsequently. Giving the premedication antibiotic **within two hours** after the procedure will provide effective prophylaxis. Any prophylaxis after two hours will not be beneficial.

11. As discussed in Chapter 20, immediately after recovering from an acute RF attack, the patient is given **secondary prevention treatment** with penicillin, erythromycin, or azithromycin. The streptococcus viridans or α-hemolytic streptococcus is constantly exposed to the antibiotic during this secondary prevention treatment phase and thus becomes resistant to the specific antibiotic. If premedication is needed during dentistry in this phase for reasons specified under conditions that call for premedication, always select an antibiotic that belongs to **another** family.

Because penicillin is bactericidal you will need to select a bactericidal premedication antibiotic. Due to the possibility of cross-resistance with the cephalosporins, it is best to select 600mg clindamycin (bactericidal dose) for premedication. In the patient getting erythromycin/azithromycin for secondary prevention treatment, the only premedication antibiotic that can be used is 600mg clindamycin. Always keep an interval of **six hours** between the bacteriostatic erythromycin/azithromycin and the bactericidal dosed 600mg clindamycin, because cidal and static drugs cannot be combined.

Hypertension and Target Organ Disease States: Assessment, Analysis, and Associated Dental Management Guidelines

AUTONOMIC NERVOUS SYSTEM

This chapter will begin with a discussion of the autonomic nervous system, which is part of the peripheral nervous system and responsible for regulating involuntary functions such as heartbeat, blood flow, breathing, and digestion. This system has two branches, the sympathetic system and the parasympathetic system. The sympathetic division of the autonomic nervous system regulates the "flight or fight" defense responses: urinary bladder relaxation, increase in heart rate, and dilation of the pupils. The parasympathetic division of the autonomic nervous system helps maintain normal body functions and conserve physical resources.

The heart is innervated by sympathetic and parasympathetic fibers. The sympathetic adrenergic system innervates the SA node, AV node, cardiac conduction pathways, and myocytes in the heart. The parasympathetic cholinergic nerve fibers that come to the heart come from the vagus nerves. Acetylcholine (ACh) released by the vagus nerve fibers binds to the M_2 muscarinic receptors in the cardiac muscle, particularly at the SA and AV nodes, which have strong vagal innervations. This produces bradycardia, decreased cardiac conduction, decreased cardiac contractility, and decreased myocyte relaxation in the atria.

Epinephrine and norepinephrine are neurotransmitters associated with the adrenergic system. Epinephrine released by the adrenal medulla in response to the body's "flight or fight" defense mechanism binds to the alpha and beta-adrenergic receptors on the heart and on the myocytes, causing tachycardia and blood sugar elevation. Norepinephrine (NE) is secreted by most postganglionic neurons and once released binds to specific receptors in the target tissues, producing physiological responses and changes in cardiac function.

The adrenergic system has two types of receptors, alpha and beta-receptors, with each having two subtypes: 1 and 2. The alpha 1 (α-1) and beta 1 (β-1) receptors are stimulatory in action and the alpha 2 (α-2) and beta 2 (β-2) receptors are inhibitory in action. β1- and

---

Dentist's Guide to Medical Conditions, Medications, and Complications, Second Edition. Kanchan M. Ganda.
© 2013 John Wiley & Sons, Inc. Published 2013 by John Wiley & Sons, Inc.

β2-adrenergic receptors often coexist in the same tissue, sometimes mediating the same physiological effect.

Alpha-adrenergic receptors respond to norepinephrine. The alpha 1 (α-1) receptors are densely located in the vascular smooth muscles of the oral and nasal mucosa; sparsely in the coronary vasculature smooth muscles; around urinary and GI sphincters; in arrector pili muscles of the hair follicles; on apocrine sweat glands of the palms, armpits, and groin; and on dilator muscles of the iris. Contraction of the smooth muscle fibers located in these areas from alpha-1 stimulation causes vasoconstriction, constriction of sphincters, "goose bumps," nervous sweating, and pupillary dilation. Norepinephrine additionally binds to α1-adrenergic receptors found on myocytes, producing small increases in cardiac contractility.

Alpha-2 receptors are abundantly located in the brain, peripheral smooth muscles of veins, platelets, nerve termini, and pancreatic islets. Alpha-2 receptor stimulation is the negative feedback component that inhibits further secretion of norepinephrine, causing platelet aggregation, vasoconstriction, and inhibition of insulin secretion.

Beta-1 receptors are located in the heart, conduction system, ventricular muscles, cerebral cortex, and eccrine salivary and sweat glands. When β1-receptors are activated by epinephrine or NE tachycardia, increased cardiac conduction, increased cardiac contractility, increased myocyte relaxation, and lipolysis occurs.

Beta-2 receptors are located on the circular smooth muscles of the lungs and some arterioles, the visceral smooth muscles of the GI tract, the urinary bladder, the cerebellum, and the liver. Beta-2 receptors are affected by epinephrine only and the action is inhibitory. Beta-2 receptor stimulation causes bronchodilation, vasodilatation, and an increase in cell energy production and utilization. The β2-adrenergic receptors become functionally more important in heart failure because β1-adrenergic receptors become down regulated. The brain contains both β1 and β2 receptors.

The autonomic nerve terminals also possess prejunctional adrenergic and cholinergic receptors that function to regulate the release of NE. Prejunctional α2-adrenergic receptors inhibit NE release, whereas prejunctional β2-adrenergic receptors increase NE release. Prejunctional M_2 receptors inhibit NE release, which is one mechanism by which vagal stimulation overrides sympathetic stimulation in the heart.

Certain diseases can be managed by using drugs that block adrenergic and cholinergic receptors. For example, beta-blockers are used in the treatment of angina, hypertension, arrhythmias, and heart failure. Muscarinic receptor blockers such as atropine are used to treat electrical disturbances (e.g., bradycardia and conduction blocks) associated with excessive vagal stimulation of the heart. Many of these adrenergic and cholinergic blockers are relatively selective for a specific receptor subtype.

HYPERTENSION

Hypertension Classification

Hypertension (Htn) is classified as primary/essential hypertension or secondary hypertension.

Primary/Essential Hypertension

Primary/essential hypertension is the most common type of hypertension and it accounts for 95% of all cases presenting with high blood pressure. This type of hypertension has a genetic link and is often associated with cardiovascular risk factors, such as cigarette smoking, obesity (body mass index $\geq$30 kg/m^2), lipid problems, age (>55 years for men, >65 years for women), family history of premature cardiovascular disease (<55 years for men, >65 years for women), hypertension, microalbuminuria, estimated GFR <60mL/min, physical inactivity, and diabetes. It is insidious in onset and is often asymptomatic in the early stages.

Secondary Hypertension

Secondary hypertension is always due to an underlying cause. Renovascular disease, renal artery stenosis, coarctation of the aorta, pheochromocytoma, Cushing's syndrome, thyroid or parathyroid disease, heavy alcohol consumption, chronic corticosteroid therapy, chronic NSAIDS therapy, or long-term oral contraceptive use can lead to secondary hypertension. The secondary hypertension patient experiences symptoms relatively early on in the disease process compared to the primary/essential hypertension patient, and the symptoms are also more severe compared with the patient with essential hypertension.

2003 VII JOINT NATIONAL COMMISSION'S HIGH BLOOD PRESSURE GUIDELINES

The following are high blood pressure guidelines from the 2003 VII Joint National Commission (JNC) Report (Table 22.1).

1. Classification of blood pressure for adults ages 18 years and older
2. List of major risk factors for hypertension
3. List of target organ damage/clinical cardiovascular disease
4. Recommendations for follow-up based on initial set of BP readings for adults

Table 22.1.   VII Joint National Commission (JNC-2003) Blood Pressure Classification for Adults Aged 18 Years and Older*

Blood Pressure Classification		
Category/BP Staging	Systolic, mmHg	Diastolic, mmHg
Normal	<120	<80
Pre-Hypertension	120–139	80–89
Stage I	140–159	90–99
Stage II	$\geq$160	$\geq$100
Stage III: Defer Dental Treatment	$\geq$180	$\geq$110

*Based on the average of two or more readings taken at **each** of two or more visits after an initial screening, not taking BP medications and not acutely ill.
When systolic and diastolic pressures fall into different categories, the higher category should be selected to classify the individual's blood pressure status. For instance, 154/82mmHg should be classified as stage I, and 164/95mmHg should be classified as stage II.
Isolated sys-tolic hypertension is defined as a systolic blood pressure of 140mmHg or more and a diastolic blood pressure of less than 90mmHg plus it is staged appropriately (e.g., 154/82mmHg is defined as stage I isolated systolic hypertension). In addition to staging hypertension on the basis of average blood pressure levels, the clinician should specify presence or absence of target-organ dis-ease and additional risk factors. This specificity is important for risk classification and treatment.

```
* Smoking

* Dyslipidemia

* Diabetes Mellitus

* Age >60 years

* Sex: men and postmenopausal women

* Family history of cardiovascular disease: women <65

years or men <55 years
```

Figure 22.1.   Major risk factors for hypertension.

MAJOR RISK FACTORS FOR HYPERTENSION

Major risk factors for hypertension are listed in Figure 22.1.

Target Organ Damage/Clinical Cardiovascular Diseases

The target organ damage or clinical cardiovascular diseases that result from hypertension are listed in Figure 22.2.

Blood Pressure Measurement Follow-Up Guidelines

Recommendations for follow-up based on the initial set of BP readings for adults are listed in Table 22.2.

Blood Pressure Monitoring and Hypertension-Related Facts

When monitoring the BP make sure that the patient has not smoked or had a caffeinated drink 30 minutes prior to measuring the BP, because this will erroneously **raise** the BP. If the patient has just consumed a heavy meal, it will erroneously **lower** the BP reading.

```
* Heart diseases

* Left ventricular hypertrophy

* Angina or prior myocardial infarction

* Prior coronary revascularization

* Heart failure

* Stroke or transient ischemic attack

* Nephropathy

* Peripheral arterial disease

* Retinopathy
```

Figure 22.2.   Target organ damage/clinical cardiovascular diseases.

Table 22.2.   Blood Pressure Monitoring Follow-Up Guidelines

Systolic	Diastolic	BP Monitoring Follow-Up Guidelines
<120mmHg	**<80mmHg**	Recheck in two years.
120–139	**80–89**	Recheck in one year.
140–159	**90–99**	Confirm within two months.
≥160	**≥100**	Assess or refer to MD in one month.
≥180	**≥110**	Refer symptomatic patient to MD/ER immediately. Refer asymptomatic patient to MD within one week.

Use an appropriate-sized cuff when recording the patient's BP. Use a pediatric/adult/thigh cuff to match the patient's arm size. When monitoring the BP, the patient's arm should be relaxed and supported over your arm or it should be resting on the arm of the dental chair. The arm should be positioned such that the cuff is at the cardiac level. Allow a five-minute interval between BP measurements. Take an average of two to four readings to diagnose hypertension.

Elevated systolic blood pressure (SBP) and widened pulse pressure are associated with greater cardiovascular risk compared with the diastolic blood pressure (DBP). The pulse pressure (PP) is the difference between the SBP and the DBP. The normal PP is 40 mmHg.

Each increment of 20 mmHg SBP/10 mmHg DBP **doubles** the cardiovascular risk for the patient. Currently, more than two-thirds of elderly patients are hypertensive. The high prevalence of obesity is largely responsible for the increased incidence of hypertension in both children and adults. Hypertension should be suspected during pregnancy if the patient presents with either an elevation of the SBP by 30 mmHg or an elevation of the DBP by 15 mmHg when compared to the average BP reading obtained pre-pregnancy or prior to 20 weeks of pregnancy. It should also be suspected when you detect a BP reading **greater** than 140/90 mmHg, when no previous reading for the patient is known. Routine dental treatment **must be deferred** in patients presenting with Stage III hypertension. Refer immediately to the emergency room (ER) if the patient is experiencing new onset target organ disease (TOD): stroke, angina, MI, and so on. For the Stage III asymptomatic patient contact the patient's physician and refer for immediate care **within 1 week**.

Postural/Orthostatic Hypotension

Prior to dentistry, always monitor the BP in the upright and lying-down positions in patients reporting a history of postural hypotension, and assist these patients out of the chair following completion of dental treatment. Refer to Chapter 9 for a discussion of etiology, prevention, and management of orthostatic hypotension.

Hypertension Treatment

Lifestyle modification to eliminate risk factors, weight loss, diet modification, and drugs are the main tools for treatment of hypertension (Table 22.3). The clinician's goal should always be to maintain the BP below 140/90 mmHg in all patients **except** the patient with

Table 22.3.   Drug Therapy for Hypertension

Drug Class and Side Effects (SE)	Generic Name	Trade Name
Ia: ANGIOTENSIN CONVERTING ENZYME INHIBITORS (ACEIs):	Captopril	Lotensin
	Enalapril Maleate	Capoten
	Fosinopril Sodium	Vasotec
Frequent SE:	Lisinopril	Monopril
Rash,loss of taste or metallic	Moexipril	Prinivil/Zestril
taste, and dry hacking cough.	Perindopril Erbumine	Univasc
ACEIs are contraindicated in	Quinapril HCL	Aceon
pregnancy.	Ramipril	Accupril
Rare SE:	Trandolapril	Altace
Leukopenia		Mavik
Proteinuria		
Angioneurotic edema		
ACEIs + CCBs:		
	Benazepril + Amlodipine	Lotrel
	Trandolapril + Verapamil	Tarka
ACEIs + DIURETICS:		
	Benazepril + HCTZ	Lotensin HCT
	Captopril + HCTZ	Capozide
	Enalapril + HCTZ	Vaseretic
	Lisinopril + HCTZ	Prinzide/Zestoretic
	Moexipril + HCTZ	Uniretic
	Quinapril + HCTZ	Accuretic
Ib: ANGIOTENSIN II RECEPTOR BLOCKERS (ARBs):	Azilsartan Medoxomil	Edarbi
	Candesartan Cilexetil	Atacand
	Eprosartan	Teveten
SE:	Irbesartan	Avapro
May cause stomach upset and	Losartan	Cozaar
dizziness.	Olmesartan medoxomil	Benicar
No metallic taste or dry hacking	Telmisartan	Micardis
cough with ARBs.	Valsartan	Diovan
ARBs are contraindicated in		Benicar
pregnancy.		Micardis
		Diovan
ARBs + CCBs + DIURETICS:		
	Olmesartan/Amlodipine/HCTZ	Tribenzor
ARBs + DIURETICS:		
	Azilsartan/Chlorthalidone	Edarbyclor
	Candesartan Cilexetil/HCTZ	Atacand
	Eprosartan/HCTZ	Teveten HCT
	Irbesartan/HCTZ	Avalide
	Losartan/HCTZ	Hyzaar
	Olmesartan Medoxomil/HCTZ	Benicar HCT
	Telmisartan/HCTZ	Micardis HCT
	Valsartan/HCTZ	Diovan HCT
ARBs + CCBs:		
	Olmesartan Medoxomil/Amlodipine	Azor
	Telmisartan/ Amlodipine	Twynsta
	Valsartan/Amlodipine	Exforge

(continued)

Table 22.3. Drug Therapy for Hypertension (*Continued*)

Drug Class and Side Effects (SE)	Generic Name	Trade Name
ARB + DIRECT RENIN INHIBITORS:		
	Valsartan/Aliskiren	Valturna
IIa. ADRENERGICS:	Acebutolol (cardioselective)	Sectral
BETA BLOCKERS (BB):		
Serious SE:	Atenolol (cardioselective)	Tenormin
Bronchospasm, especially with the	Betaxolol (cardioselective)	Kerlone
non-selective BBs.	Bisoprolol (cardioselective)	Ziac
CHF	Metoprolol (cardioselective)	Lopressor/Toprol-XL
Masking of insulin-induced	Nadolol (nonselective BB)	Corgard
hypoglycemia Depression	Nebivolol (cardioselective)	Bystolic
Less Serious SE:	Penbutolol (nonselective BB)	Levatol
Poor peripheral circulation	Pindolol (nonselective BB)	Visken
Insomnia	Propranolol (nonselective BB)	Inderal/Inderal LA
Bradycardia	Sotalol (nonselective BB)	Betapace
Fatigue	Timolol (nonselective BB)	Blocadren
Increased triglycerides		
Decreased HDL-cholesterol		
IIb: ALPHA-1 BLOCKERS:	Doxazocin	Cardura
SE:	Prazocin	Minipress
Postural hypotension mainly with	Terazocin	Hytrin
first dose; Lassitude		
IIc: ALPHA AND BETA BLOCKERS:	Carvedilol (α and β-blocker)	Coreg
SE:	Labetalol (α and β-blocker)	Trandate
Postural hypotension		
Upset stomach		
Beta-blocking side effects; Masking of hypoglycemic symptoms		
IId: CENTRALLY ACTING DRUGS:	Clonidine	Catapres
	Methyldopa	Aldomet
SE:		
Sedation		
Liver dysfunction Fever		
Autoimmune disorders		
Sedation		
Dry mouth		
Withdrawal hypertension		
IIe: PERIPHERAL NERVE ACTING DRUGS:	Guanethidine	Ismelin
	Reserpine	Serpalan
SE:		
Sedation		
Nasal congestion Depression Orthostatic hypotension		
Diarrhea		
BBs + HCTZ:		
	Atenolol + Chlorthalidone	Tenoretic
	Bisoprolol + HCTZ	Ziac
	Metoprolol + HCTZ	Lopresor HCT
	Metoprolol ER + HCTZ	Dutoprol
	Nadolol + Bendrflumethiazide	Corzide
	Propranolol + HCTZ	Inderide

Table 22.3. Drug Therapy for Hypertension (*Continued*)

Drug Class and Side Effects (SE)	Generic Name	Trade Name
III. DIRECT ACTING VASODILATORS:	Hydralazine	Apresoline
SE:	Minoxidil	Loniten
Fluid retention Tachycardia Headaches		
IV. CALCIUM CHANNEL BLOCKERS (CCBs):	Amlodipine	Norvasc
	Diltiazem	Cardizem/Dilacor
SE:	Felodipine	Plendil
Flushing	Isradipine	DynaCirc CR
Headache	Nicardipine	Nicardipine/Cardene
Gingival hyperplasia (seen mostly with Nifedipine)	Nifedipine	Adalat/Procardia
	Nisoldipine	Sular
Constipation	Verapamil	Calan/Isoptin
Upset stomach Conduction defects		
CCBs + ACEI:		
	Amlodipine + Benazepril	Lotrel
	Verapamil + Trandolapril	Tarka
CCBs + ARBs:		
	Amlodipine + Olmesartan	Azor
	Amlodipine + Valsartan	Exforge
CCBs + DIRECT RENIN INHIBITORS (RIs):		
	Amlodipine + Aliskiren	Tekamlo
CCBs + DIRECT RIs + HCTZ:		
	Amlodipine + Aliskiren + HCTZ	Amturnide
V. DIURETICS:	Amiloride (K+ sparing)	Midamor
SE:	Chlorothiazide (Thiazide-like)	Diuril
Hypokalemia	Chlorthalidone (Thiazide-like)	Thalitone
Hypercholesterolemia	Eplerenone (K+ sparing MRA*)	Inspra
Glucose intolerance	Furosemide (Loop diuretic)	Lasix
Hhyperglycemia	Hydrochlorothiazide (Thiazide-like)	HCTZ
Hyperurecemia	Indapamide	Lozol
Muscle spasms	Metolazone (Thiazide-like)	Zaroxolyn
Hypomagnesemia	Spironolactone (K+ sparing MRA)	Aldactone
	Torsemide (Loop diuretic)	Demadex
	*Mineralocorticoid receptor antagonist (MRA)	
DIURETIC COMBINATIONS:		
	HCTZ + Amiloride	
	HCTZ + Spironolactone	Aldactazide
	HCTZ + Triamterene	Dyazide/Maxide
CENTRAL α-AGONISTS + THIAZIDE DIURETICS:		
	Methyldopa + HCTZ	Aldoril/Aldoril D
THIAZIDE DIURETICS + DIRECT RIs:		
	HCTZ + Aliskiren	Tekturna HCT
VI. DIRECT RENIN INHIBITORS:		
	Aliskiren	Tekturna

chronic kidney disease and in some cases of diabetes. In patients with chronic kidney disease, the goal is to maintain the BP below 130/80 mmHg.

Per the 2012 American Diabetes Association (ADA) guidelines, the current goal is to maintain the BP below 140/80 mmHg. The new ADA recommendation raises the target for systolic blood pressure from below 130mmHg to below 140mmHg, on the basis of evidence that there is no substantial additional value and there is an increased risk in pushing systolic pressure much lower than 140mmHg. Meta-analysis studies have shown that although the use of intensive versus standard blood pressure targets in patients with type 2 diabetes was associated with a small reduction in the risk for stroke, there was no evidence for decreased mortality or myocardial infarction but, rather, there was an increased risk for hypotension and other adverse events. The new recommendations do state that a target below 130mmHg should be appropriate for patients with a history of coronary artery disease or patients with multiple risk factors, as long as the target can be achieved safely.

HYPERTENSION AND TARGET ORGAN DISEASE

Hypertension can cause target organ disease (TOD) and affect the major circulations. Atherosclerosis, thrombosis, or arterial spasm due to long-standing hypertension can affect any one of the following circulations: cerebral, coronary, renal, or peripheral. Transient ischemic attack (TIA) or cerebrovascular accident (CVA) can occur with involvement of cerebral circulation. Involvement of coronary circulation can cause angina (stable, unstable) or myocardial infarction (MI). Involvement of the renal circulation can lead to chronic renal failure (CRF). Involvement of the peripheral circulation affecting the medium-sized arteries of the legs can cause intermittent claudication, which is associated with severe pain in the calves when walking briskly or walking uphill.

Presence or absence of TOD determines how the patient is faring with hypertension control. The patient's current BP readings and the current status of **each** major circulation must be **collectively** evaluated to ultimately decide **when** to proceed with dentistry and **what** anesthetics, analgesics, and antibiotics (AAAs) to use during dental care.

ANTIHYPERTENSIVE MEDICATIONS

Some of the antihypertension drugs discussed in this section include:

- Peripheral adrenergic-receptor blockers: alpha and beta-blocker drugs
- Centrally acting adrenergic blockers
- Peripheral nerve-acting adrenergic blockers
- Direct renin inhibitors
- Mineralocorticoid receptor antagonists (MRAs)

Peripheral Adrenergic Receptor Blockers

The two major groups of peripheral adrenergic receptor blockers are beta-blockers and alpha-blockers. Beta-blockers block the beta-receptors and prevent epinephrine from stimulating the heart, thereby causing a reduction in the heart rate and blood pressure.

Beta-Blockers

Beta-blockers are classified as:

- Cardioselective
- Noncardioselective

The cardioselective beta-blockers primarily attach to beta-1 receptors in the heart. The noncardioselective beta-blockers attach to beta-1 receptors in the heart and to beta-2 receptors in the lungs, blood vessels, and other tissues. Even though both types of beta-blockers can worsen asthma or other chronic pulmonary disorders, the noncardioselective blockers are more dangerous for patients with respiratory disease. Beta-blockers mask hypoglycemia symptoms in patients with diabetes; fatigue, depression, shortness of breath, and reduced exercise tolerance are common side effects associated with beta-blockers.

Alpha-Blockers

Alpha-blockers act on the alpha-receptors, primarily affecting norepinephrine that works on peripheral vessels causing vasoconstriction. Alpha-1 blockers reduce blood pressure by blocking alpha-receptors in the heart and blood vessels. Additionally, alpha-1 blockers reduce LDL cholesterol and increase HDL cholesterol. By relaxing the smooth muscles surrounding the prostate, alpha-1 blockers relieve urethral constriction and ease urine flow in patients with benign prostatic hypertrophy. Side effects of alpha-blockers include orthostatic hypotension, palpitations, dizziness, headaches, and dry mouth. The drugs labetalol (Normodyne) and carvedilol (Coreg) have both alpha- and beta-blocking effects.

Centrally Acting Adrenergic Blockers

Clonidine (Catapres) and methyldopa (Aldomet) are drugs that block sympathetic nervous system activity.

Common side effects include orthostatic hypotension, dry mouth, depression, and sedation.

Peripheral-Nerve Acting Adrenergic Blockers

Peripheral-nerve acting adrenergic blockers reserpine (Serpalan) and guanethidine (Ismelin) block the action of norepinephrine, causing the blood vessels to relax, thus lowering the blood pressure. Side effects include depression, nasal stuffiness, and orthostatic hypotension.

DIRECT RENIN INHIBITORS

Aliskiren (Tekturna) belongs to a newer blood pressure medication category that inhibits renin activity, thus preventing the conversion of angiotensin I to angiotensin II.

Mineralocorticoid Receptor Antagonists

Aldosterone contributes significantly to cardiovascular disease by targeting changes at the level of the heart, blood vessels, and kidney. It causes fluid retention by affecting the transport of Na and K at the level of the collecting tubules in the kidney, and it induces inflammation at the level of the heart and blood vessels.

Spironolactone (Aldactone) is a mineralocorticoid receptor antagonist (MRA) that acts as a competitive inhibitor of the mineralocorticoid (aldosterone) receptor. Unwanted progestational and antiandrogenic side effects limit the use of spironolactone in the chronic treatment of disease.

Eplerenone (Inspra), a new MRA, has excellent selectivity for the mineralocorticoid receptor over other steroid receptors, thus proving to be more selective and more effective than spironolactone.

Spironolactone (Aldactone) and eplerenone (Inspra) are the MRAs currently available for the treatment of hypertension. They have similar safety and antihypertensive efficacy. Eplerenone has a lower incidence of antiandrogenic and progestational side effects.

Here are the reasons why MR blockade works well in the treatment of hypertension:

- Significant evidence showing antihypertensive efficacy.
- The phenomenon of "aldosterone escape" occurring with angiotensin-converting enzyme inhibitor and angiotensin-receptor blockade therapy.
- MR antagonism reduces target-organ damage in hypertensive patients and improves survival in patients with cardiovascular disease.
- Blockade of the MR may be very useful in many patients with hypertension, particularly those at risk for or having evidence of target-organ damage.

HYPERTENSION-ASSOCIATED SUGGESTED DENTAL GUIDELINES

Anesthetics and Hypertension

The following are dental guidelines for anesthetics and hypertension:

1. The decision about the type of LA that can be used in the hypertensive patient depends on the **average BP reading** obtained **and** the presence or absence of **end organ disease**.
2. Use xylocaine with epinephrine or the 4% local anesthetics or 2% mepivacaine (Carbocaine) with 1:20,000 levonordefrin (NeoCobefrin), maximum two carpules if the patient is well controlled, has an ASA status I/II, and there is **no** underlying history of arrhythmias, TIA, CVA, unstable angina, or renal disease. Also, the patient should not be taking digoxin (Lanoxin).
3. As specified under the end organ circulation's discussions in the following chapters, epinephrine is contraindicated in any patient with a history of arrhythmias, unstable angina, chronic renal failure (CRF), TIA, recent CVA, intermittent claudication, digoxin, and ASA III/IV.
4. 4% prilocaine HCL with 1:200,000 epinephrine (Citanest Forte) or 0.5% bupivacaine (Marcaine) with 1:200,000 epinephrine should be used in the mild hypertension patient with **no** end organ problems. Restrict the use of 4% septocaine (articaine)

with epinephrine in the presence of elevated blood pressure readings and/or in the presence of arrhythmias, as the local anesthetic is known to trigger tachycardia.

5. 3% mepivacaine HCL (Carbocaine) with no epinephrine should be used in the moderately hypertensive patient with **no** end organ problems.

6. 4% prilocaine HCL (Citanest Plain) should be the *only* **LA** used in the hypertensive pregnant patient, if the obstetrician allows dental treatment to proceed.

7. Routine dental treatment is deferred if the patient has severe hypertension, so the blood pressure elevation can be addressed immediately.

Cerebral Circulation Diseases TIAs and CVAs: Assessment, Analysis, and Associated Dental Management Guidelines

TRANSIENT ISCHEMIC ATTACKS (TIAS)

TIA is associated with temporary cerebral ischemia due to cerebral vascular spasm. No permanent brain damage occurs. Once the spasm is released, the symptoms disappear. The symptoms last for a few seconds to a few minutes, but occasionally they can last for a few hours. Resolution of symptoms occurs within 24 hours. Patients with a history of TIA have a 50–60% chance of progressing to CVA/stroke.

Acute TIA Attack Management

Please refer to Chapter 9 for a discussion on the etiology, clinical features, and management of an acute TIA attack.

TIA-Associated Suggested Dental Management Guidelines

The following are dental guidelines for TIA:

1. TIA patients could be on any one of the following blood thinners: aspirin, dipyridamole (Persantine), clopidogrel (Plavix), or warfarin (Coumadin). Always consult with the MD to determine whether the drug or drugs can be temporarily discontinued prior to major surgery. When possible, Coumadin is usually stopped 48 hours prior to treatment and restarted the evening of the surgery or the next day. The restart time depends on when the patient typically takes the warfarin (Coumadin). Aspirin, dipyridamole (Persantine), and clopidogrel (Plavix), when approved for stopping, can be typically stopped seven days prior to treatment and restarted 1–2 days post operatively. Currently, most physicians are reluctant to stop blood thinners or may stop them for a shorter duration compared to routine. In such cases, the provider should rely on local hemostatic material to control the bleeding.

2. **TIAs and LAs:** 3% mepivacaine HCL (Carbocaine) or 4% prilocaine HCL (Citanest Plain) are the only LAs that can be used. No epinephrine-containing LAs should be

Dentist's Guide to Medical Conditions, Medications, and Complications, Second Edition. Kanchan M. Ganda.
© 2013 John Wiley & Sons, Inc. Published 2013 by John Wiley & Sons, Inc.

used at any time during dentistry, particularly if the TIAs are frequently recurring, because epinephrine promotes vasoconstriction and this can trigger more TIAs and consequent cerebral hypoxia.

3. **TIAs and analgesics:** Regular or extra-strength acetaminophen (Tylenol) is safe. Tylenol with codeine, Tylenol with hydrocodone (Vicodin), or Tylenol with oxycodone (Percocet) can also be used as long as you use them judiciously and dispense them for only 2–3 days.

4. **TIAs and antibiotics:** No antibiotics are contraindicated with TIAs.

5. **TIAs and stress management:** The benzodiazepines—lorazepam (Ativan) or diazepam (Valium)—should be avoided because these drugs depress the respiratory center and can promote TIAs.

STROKE/CEREBROVASCULAR ACCIDENTS (CVA)

Obstruction of the cerebral circulation by a thrombus, embolus, or ruptured intracranial aneurysm can precipitate stroke. Stroke causes permanent neurological damage that usually affects the contralateral side of the body.

Acute CVA Attack Management

Please refer to Chapter 9 for discussion of etiology, clinical features, and management of CVA.

CVA-Associated Suggested Dental Management Guidelines

The following are dental guidelines for CVA:

1. Stroke patients could be on blood thinners, such as aspirin, dipyradamole (Persantine), clopidogrol (Plavix), or warfarin (Coumadin), post recovery. Prior to major surgery, always consult with the patient's physician to determine whether and when the blood thinners can be stopped and subsequently restarted.

2. Following a CVA that required significant hospitalization, routine dental treatment must be **delayed by six months**.

3. Routine dental treatment should be **delayed by three months** if the post-CVA recovery was uneventful and the patient was admitted overnight solely for observation. These patients experience Transient Intermittent Neurological Deficits (TINDs), or the so-called mini-stroke, and they recover during the overnight hospitalization and are subsequently discharged.

4. **CVA and LAs:** Avoid epinephrine-containing LAs during the **first six months** of dental treatment. Subsequent use of epinephrine depends on the patient's prognosis. Epinephrine-containing LAs can be used starting one year after the stroke, when the patient demonstrates progressive improvement of the CVA and absence of TIAs.

5. **CVA analgesics, antibiotics, and stress management:** The guidelines are the same as those listed with TIAs.

Coronary Circulation Diseases, Classic Angina, and Myocardial Infarction: Assessment, Analysis, and Associated Dental Management Guidelines

Angina and myocardial infarction (MI) can occur with involvement of the coronary circulation. Hypertension causes narrowing of the coronary arteries, and when the patient is involved in an activity, these narrowed arteries are unable to supply adequate nutrition and oxygenation to the heart, thus leading to angina. Hypertension-associated angina is classic angina and it can be stable or unstable.

PREVENTION AND TREATMENT OF ANGINA

Stable Angina

Stable angina is always brought on by activity; it happens infrequently and it is always controlled immediately with 1–3 nitroglycerine (NTG) pills. Patients with stable angina have a good prognosis but the patient can deteriorate progressively in proportion to the severity of symptoms. The most recent evidence-based clinical guidelines on the management of stable angina are detailed in the following sections.

Angina Treatment and Prevention: Short-Acting Drugs

Glyceryl trinitrate/nitroglycerine and nifedipine capsules can be used to treat or prevent episodes of angina. Sublingual glyceryl trinitrate relieves episodes of angina more effectively than sublingual nifedipine. Glyceryl trinitrate spray is easy to use and can be stored over long periods without loss of effectiveness. Glyceryl trinitrate tablets lose efficacy after exposure to air and should be discarded after eight weeks of use. Short-acting nitrates should also be used for prophylaxis before planned exercise or exertion.

Optimal Prevention Treatments

Per new evidence-based guidelines, all patients with stable angina should get optimal medical treatment for angina prevention with one or two anti-anginal drugs, in addition to drugs for secondary prevention of cardiovascular disease.

Dentist's Guide to Medical Conditions, Medications, and Complications, Second Edition. Kanchan M. Ganda.
© 2013 John Wiley & Sons, Inc. Published 2013 by John Wiley & Sons, Inc.

First-Line Anti-Anginal Drugs

β Blockers and Calcium Channel Blockers

- These anti-anginal drugs prevent angina by decreasing myocardial oxygen demand by lowering heart rate, blood pressure, myocardial contractility, and/or by increasing myocardial oxygen supply through increased coronary blood flow. Monotherapy with a β blocker or with a calcium channel blocker is effective in the treatment of stable angina, but a β blocker is the preferred first-line treatment.
- β blocker members include propanolol, atenolol, and metoprolol. Calcium channel blocker members include nifedipine, diltiazem, and verapamil. The choice of drug used is determined by comorbidities, contraindications, and patient preference. If the first drug is not tolerated or does not control the symptoms, the patient is switched to the other drug class, or combination therapy with both drug classes is offered. A dihydropyridine calcium channel blocker is used when a calcium channel blocker is combined with a β blocker.

Additional Anti-Anginal Drugs

Long-Acting Nitrates

Long-acting organic nitrates are used widely in the treatment of patients with stable angina. Isosorbide mononitrate (Imdur) or felodipine (Plendil) is added to a β blocker and is effective short-term. Long-term nitrate use is limited due to the development of tolerance.

Ivabradine

Ivabradine lowers the heart rate by selectively inhibiting the I_f ion current, which is significantly expressed in the sinoatrial node. Short-term trials of ivabradine versus atenolol or amlodipine in patients with stable angina demonstrated similar increases in exercise time and reductions in angina frequency.

Nicorandil

Nicorandil is a nitrate derivative of nicotinamide that dilates epicardial and systemic venous capacitance vessels, but it also opens ATP-sensitive potassium channels in vascular smooth muscle cells, thereby dilating arterial resistance vessels in the peripheral and coronary circulations. Short-term trials of nicorandil versus monotherapy with another anti-anginal drug (diltiazem, amlodipine, propanolol) showed similar reductions in the frequency of episodes of angina and similar increases in total exercise capacity in both treatment groups.

Ranolazine (Ranexa)

- Ranolazine is the most recent first-line, FDA-approved drug for the medical management of angina. It works by blocking the "late sodium channel" in heart cells that are experiencing ischemia. Blocking this sodium channel improves the metabolism in ischemic heart cells, thereby reducing damage to the heart muscle and reducing angina symptoms.

- Ranolazine (Ranexa) has been shown to significantly improve the amount of time patients with stable angina are able to exercise before developing symptoms. The drug has been shown to actually reduce the risk of developing ventricular arrhythmias and atrial fibrillation; plus, QT interval prolongation risk is minimal or nonexistent with ranolazine.
- Headache, constipation, and nausea are the most common side effects associated with ranolazine.

Choice of Second-Line Drug

- Evidence suggests that long-acting nitrate and the newer anti-anginal agents (ivabradine, nicorandil, and ranolazine) are effective in the short term.
- A long-acting nitrate or one of the newer anti-anginal drugs (ivabradine, nicorandil, or ranolazine) can be used as monotherapy, or in combination with another anti-anginal agent, if first-line treatment is not tolerated or is contraindicated.
- Triple anti-anginal therapy should only be considered when patients have persisting symptoms and are being considered for revascularization, or when revascularization is not appropriate.

Angina: Secondary Prevention

The objectives of treatment in patients with stable angina are to relieve symptoms and improve outcomes, and secondary prevention measures are important to reduce the long-term risk of adverse cardiovascular events.

- The benefits of lipid-lowering therapy in people with coronary artery disease are established and a statin is recommended for all adult patients with clinical evidence of cardiovascular disease, including patients with stable angina.
- Aspirin in patients with stable angina reduces the risk of non-fatal myocardial infarction, taking into account the bleeding risk and comorbidity.
- ACE inhibitors may be indicated for the treatment of concomitant hypertension or heart failure, or after myocardial infarction.

Coronary Angiography and Revascularization

Randomized trials support myocardial revascularization by coronary artery bypass grafting (CABG) or by coronary angioplasty/percutaneous coronary intervention (PCI) to improve symptoms of angina relative to continued medical treatment. The main indication for revascularization in patients with stable angina is relief of symptoms. CABG provides slightly more effective relief of angina than PCI, but the absolute difference is small and decreases over time.

UNSTABLE ANGINA

Progressive worsening of stable angina over time can lead to the development of unstable angina. A change occurs in the ASA status from ASA II to ASA III. The patient does not need much activity at this stage to trigger an attack. The coronary arteries are narrowed quite significantly. The patient could be on daily isosorbide (Isordil), or the patient uses a daily nitroglycerine patch to control the unstable angina. NTG pills are additionally used during an attack. Isosorbide (Isordil) is a long-acting nitrate and a very potent vasodilator. In addition to the previously mentioned medical medication for unstable angina, other therapies are also now in use.

Initial Medical Management of Unstable Angina

Medications used in the initial management of unstable angina include: aspirin, beta-adrenergic blocking agents, thienopyridines clopidogrel or prasugrel, glycoprotein IIb/IIIa antagonists, heparin, direct thrombin inhibitors, and nitrates.

Aspirin

- Platelet aggregation is central to acute coronary syndrome; death or myocardial infarction is significantly reduced with aspirin in cases of unstable angina.
- With the peak effect of aspirin occurring within 30 minutes of administration, chewable aspirin 162–325mg should be given promptly to patients who are not at high risk for bleeding.
- In the event of angioplasty or percutaneous coronary intervention (PCI), aspirin 162–325mg is given uninterrupted, along with clopidogrel, for at least **1 month** after **bare metal stent** implantation and uninterrupted for at least **12 months** after **drug-eluting stent** implantation. Thereafter, aspirin 75–162mg is continued indefinitely. Bleeding associated with any dental treatment during the uninterrupted periods is controlled with local hemostats, and no premedication antibiotic prophylaxis is required during or after the uninterrupted time lines.

Beta-Blockers

Oral beta-blockers decrease ischemic symptoms and the occurrence of myocardial infarctions in unstable angina patients who are hemodynamically stable.

Thienopyridines

- Clopidogrel (Plavix) and prasugrel are the two approved thienopyridine antiplatelet agents for the management of patients with unstable angina/non-ST-elevation myocardial infarction (UA/NSTEMI).
- Maintenance dose of a thienopyridine is then given for at least 12 months.
- Clopidogrel is given to patients intolerant to aspirin, and it is given along with aspirin when dual antiplatelet therapy is required to reduce the incidence of cardiovascular death, myocardial infarction, or stroke.
- Patients who are clinically unstable are given clopidogrel or are taken immediately for coronary angiography.
- Prasugrel is used as an alternate to clopidogrel but is not recommended in patients 75 years or older.

Dual and Triple Antiplatelet Therapies

Current guidelines recommend dual-antiplatelet therapy with aspirin and a second antiplatelet agent for medium-risk to high-risk patients for whom an initial invasive procedure is chosen.

Glycoprotein IIb/IIIa Antagonists

- Low molecular weight heparin (LMWH) or unfractionated heparin (IV heparin) and early cardiac catheterization are options considered for patients at high risk for myocardial infarction.
- All glycoprotein IIb/IIIa inhibitors increase the safety of acute PCI.
- Low molecular weight heparin (LMWH) and intravenous unfractionated heparin (UH) are comparable anticoagulants in the treatment of unstable angina.
- LMWH is preferred initially, because anticoagulation activity cannot be measured during PCI.
- Direct thrombin inhibitors are potential alternatives to heparin, particularly in the presence of heparin-induced thrombocytopenia.
- Direct thrombin inhibitors are associated with higher rates of bleeding, but they are slightly better at reducing myocardial infarction when compared to heparin.

Nitrates

Intravenous nitrates may be used in the treatment of ischemic chest pain, symptoms of heart failure, or hypertension, but they are not associated with appreciable long-term clinical benefit.

Acute Angina Attack

Refer to Chapter 9 for a discussion of etiology, clinical features, and management of stable and unstable angina attacks.

Angina Pectoris–Associated Suggested Dental Guidelines

Anesthetics for Stable Angina

Local anesthetics with or without epinephrine can be used. Use maximum 2 carpules of 2% lidocaine (Xylocaine), 0.5% bupivacaine (Marcaine), 4% prilocaine HCL (Citanest Forte), 3% mepivacaine (Carbocaine), 4% prilocaine HCL (Citanest Plain), 4% septocaine (Articaine), or 2% mepivacaine (Carbocaine) with 1:20,000 levonordefrin (NeoCobefrin).

Anesthetics for Unstable Angina

Avoid LAs with epinephrine.

Analgesics and Antibiotics for Angina Pectoris

There are no analgesics or antibiotics contraindicated per se with stable or unstable angina; however, be discreet in prescribing narcotic analgesics in the unstable angina patient.

Angina Stress Management

Benzodiazepines or O_2 + N_2O can be used for stress management in the stable angina patient. Benzodiazepines are contraindicated in the unstable angina patient, and you should use only $O_2 + N_2O$ in these patients. Prophylactic use of NTG/Isordil is advised in anticipation of stress for the unstable angina patient.

Prinzmetal's Angina

Prinzmetal's angina is due to coronary artery spasm. This angina is more common in females, often affecting the type-A personality woman. Prinzmetal's angina occurs mostly at rest and is often cyclical. It can occur continuously for a period of time and then disappear.

Prinzmetal's Angina Symptoms and Signs

Symptoms and signs are similar to stable angina.

Prinzmetal's Angina Medical Management

Nifedipine (Procardia), a Ca^{+2} channel blocker is the treatment of choice; 10 or 20 mg Procardia SL (sublingual) helps relieve the spasm.

Prinzmetal's Angina Anesthetics, Analgesics, Antibiotics, and Stress Management

Determine the severity of Prinzmetal's angina along with the ASA status of the patient, and then follow the guidelines as outlined for classic angina.

MYOCARDIAL INFARCTION

Myocardial infarction (MI) is a consequence of complete obstruction in the coronary artery blood supply to the heart resulting in death of the myocardium beyond the obstruction.

Acute Myocardial Infarction Attack

Refer to Chapter 9 for discussion of etiology, clinical features, and management of MI.

MI Diagnosis Confirmation in a Hospital Setting

In the hospital setting, the diagnosis of a suspect case of MI is confirmed with analyses of the clinical presentation, specific EKG findings (most commonly ST segment elevation, T wave inversion, new bundle-branch blocks), and specific laboratory test results indicating myocardial injury: elevated SGOT, LDH, creatine kinase (CK), troponin I and T.

In-Hospital MI Reperfusion Management

The confirmed MI cases are immediately triaged for reperfusion with thrombolytic drugs and/or surgical reperfusion options.

MI Management with Thrombolytic Drugs

Thrombolytic drugs, streptokinase, or recombinant tissue plasminogen activator (rTPA) are most effective when given in the first two hours of the MI. IV heparin, LMWH, aspirin, and clopidogrel (Plavix) are additional blood thinners used for the care of MI.

Surgical Reperfusion Options Post MI

Percutaneous coronary interventions (PCI) via cardiac catheterization (formerly called **angioplasty, percutaneous transluminal coronary angioplasty [PTCA], or balloon angioplasty**), laser angioplasty, stents, or coronary artery bypass graft (CABG) surgery are invasive surgical treatment options commonly used to reperfuse the myocardium.

Stents Post MI

Two kinds of stents are used during angioplasty: bare metal stents and drug-eluting stents (DES). Bare metal stents require **uninterrupted** antiplatelet activity with aspirin and Plavix for a minimum period of **4–6 weeks** and drug-eluting stents (DES) require Plavix and aspirin **uninterrupted** for a minimum period of **12 months**. Patients with stents do not need antibiotic premedication prophylaxis.

Coronary Artery Bypass Post MI

Bypass rates have gone down because of the high success rates of PCI. The internal mammary artery or the long saphenous vein grafts are used for bypass surgery. Bypass surgery patients do not need premedication prior to dentistry.

MI Management Post Acute-Phase Recovery

Once recovered, in addition to being maintained on aspirin and/or clopidogrel (Plavix), beta-blockers, ACE inhibitors, and cholesterol-lowering drugs to prevent future myocardial infarction attacks, the patient may also be maintained on additional newer drugs, if heart failure is an ongoing issue. Refer to the 2012 guidelines for heart failure (HF) management that are discussed in Chapter 25.

MI-Associated Complication: CHF and Cardiac Arrhythmias

Complications associated with MI are congestive heart failure (CHF) and cardiac arrhythmias. MI causes structural changes that affect the proper filling and pumping of the heart, leading to CHF. CHF can also be due to worsening severe anemia, anorexia, or thyrotoxicosis where the failure occurs because of a hyperdynamic circulation caused by the underlying disease state. Worsening cardiac disease or worsening pulmonary disease can also lead to CHF.

Dental Disease and MI Link

Periodontal inflammation is associated with increased levels of fibrinogen, C-reactive protein (CRP), and cytokines. Extensive research has shown that inflammation is an

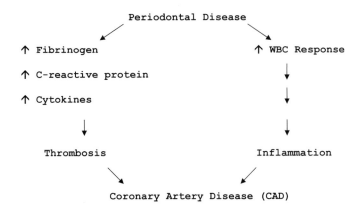

Figure 24.1. Postulated periodontal disease and coronary artery disease link.

important step in the formation of atherosclerotic plaques. The link between periodontal disease and coronary artery disease (CAD) has long been discussed in the literature. The link that was hypothesized is schematically illustrated in Figure 24.1.

So, even though age, diabetes, and smoking are common risk factors associated with both periodontal disease (PD) and atherosclerotic vascular disease (ASVD), and treating PD does decrease disease burden by reducing systemic inflammation and endothelial dysfunction, research analysis has shown that there is no evidence for any association, nor is there a cause and effect between the two conditions. Additionally, treating PD does not affect the outcome of existing ASVD nor does it prevent AVSD.

MI-ASSOCIATED SUGGESTED DENTAL GUIDELINES

The following are dental guidelines for MI:

1. It is worth scheduling frequent hygiene recalls every 3–4 months for patients with severe periodontal disease and/or coronary artery disease.
2. In patients with significant cardiac disease (ASA III/IV; patients on lanoxin/digoxin, isosorbide/isordil, or nitroglycerine patch; or patients being managed for heart failure), minimize stress and avoid the use of vasoconstrictors in the local anesthetics.
3. Delay routine dental treatment post MI, by **6 months** if the patient has had a massive MI that required significant hospitalization.
4. Delay dental treatment post MI, by **3 months** for a patient with minimal MI that might have needed overnight or short-term hospitalization for observation.
5. After stent placement, angioplasty, or CABG, the patient can be scheduled for routine dental procedure once daily activities have begun. This resumption of activity usually occurs within 2–4 weeks of the procedure.
6. As indicated previously, bare metal stents require **uninterrupted** antiplatelet activity with aspirin and Plavix for a minimum period of **4–6 weeks** and drug-eluting stents (DES) require Plavix and aspirin **uninterrupted** for a minimum period of **12 months**. Planned or routine dentistry has to accommodate the uninterrupted antiplatelet activity period.

A way to arrange this is to schedule minor procedures (amalgams, composites, or cleanings) causing minimal or no bleeding during the uninterrupted antiplatelet activity period; this care will not be affected with the aspirin and Plavix.

For major procedures you can incorporate one of two options. One is to schedule major procedures that can be done with the use of local hemostats to control the bleeding in the presence of aspirin and Plavix. Another way is to delay the major dental treatment needing the temporary interruption of aspirin and/or Plavix for a time **beyond** the specified time periods.

7. Drug-eluting stents (DES) have been associated with an increased risk of thrombosis, compared to the bare metal stents, because they have been found to prevent the regrowth of normal arterial tissue lining in immediate or close proximity to the stents, thus causing an increased incidence of thrombosis. In spite of this untoward side effect, the drug-eluting stents are preferred because they are superior compared to bare-metal stents. Many cardiologists, for this reason, prefer using aspirin and Plavix for 1–2 years or indefinitely, depending on the patient's current medical status and bleeding history.

8. A dental practitioner should always consult with the patient's MD to determine whether the antiplatelet medications can be temporarily interrupted and **when** in relation to the time of angioplasty or stents.

    Dependent on the patient's current cardiac status and risk for thrombosis, the MD could **extend** the specified time lines for **uninterrupted** aspirin and Plavix intake. In such situations when major surgery is needed, local hemostats and appropriate suturing should be utilized to minimize bleeding.

9. Stents **do not** require premedication. However, with the recent focus on the higher threat for thrombosis with stents, some cardiologists may want an occasional patient to receive antibiotic premedication prophylaxis prior to dentistry, if the underlying cardiac status is still associated with a **poor ejection fraction** (EF).

10. During the early recovery period, patients with MI do best with shorter appointments that are scheduled in the morning.

11. **Anesthetics and MI:** Use 3% mepivacaine HCL (Carbocaine) without epinephrine, or 4% prilocaine HCL (Citanest Plain) during the **first 6 months** of dental care. 0.5% bupivacaine (Marcaine) or 4% prilocaine HCL (Citanest Forte), both with 1:200,000 epinephrine, can be used subsequently if the patient has been stable during the first six months of dental care. Remember, however, that this switch to local anesthetics with epinephrine is moot if the patient is on digoxin (Lanoxin) following recovery from MI. According to the suggested guidelines set for digoxin, epinephrine is contraindicated.

12. High-risk patients should have questionable teeth extracted and removable prosthetic management provided.

13. Advanced periodontal surgery and complex fixed prosthetics are generally contraindicated in the unstable cardiac patient.

Congestive Heart Failure: Assessment, Analysis, and Associated Dental Management Guidelines

CONGESTIVE HEART FAILURE (CHF) SYMPTOMS AND SIGNS

CHF Symptoms

The following are CHF symptoms:

1. **Orthopnea:** Orthopnea is shortness of breath experienced on lying down. Therefore, the patient should always be propped up in bed.
2. **Paroxysmal nocturnal dyspnea or "cardiac asthma":** Shortness of breath is experienced hours or minutes after lying in bed.
3. **Cough with frothy sputum:** Severe CHF compromises cardiac output and this leads to pulmonary congestion or edema. Significant pulmonary congestion causes cough with a frothy sputum expectoration.

CHF Signs

The following are CHF signs:

1. **Distended neck veins:** The forward flow of blood is compromised with CHF, causing a backup and consequent distention of the neck veins.
2. **Rales on auscultation:** Rales, or coarse crackles, on auscultation are heard in the base of both lungs and indicate the presence of fluid in the lungs.
3. **Functional systolic murmur:** CHF can be associated with a functional systolic murmur, and this murmur is corrected following treatment and recovery. This murmur is heard in the second left intercostal or pulmonic space upon physical examination of the chest.
4. **Ankle edema:** The compromised cardiac status causes fluid collection in the peripheral tissues and **pitting** edema. Pitting edema can be confirmed by applying transient pressure with your thumb on the patient's edematous tissue, particularly on the feet, near the ankles. Transient pressure leaves a dent, indicating fluid collection.

Dentist's Guide to Medical Conditions, Medications, and Complications, Second Edition. Kanchan M. Ganda.
© 2013 John Wiley & Sons, Inc. Published 2013 by John Wiley & Sons, Inc.

CONGESTIVE HEART FAILURE MEDICAL MANAGEMENT

The type of CHF treatment implemented is dictated by the cause of CHF. In addition to the common drugs that have been used in the management of CHF, such as diuretics, vasodilators, ACE inhibitors, beta-blockers, and digoxin, there are newer drugs for heart failure (HF) management, per the 2012 guidelines. These are the highlighted changes in the guidelines for the Diagnosis and Treatment of Acute and Chronic Heart Failure (HF):

- The new 2012 guidelines call for an expanded indication for mineralocorticoid receptor antagonists (MRA).
- There is a new indication for ivabradine, a sinus node inhibitor.
- There is a focus on decreasing not only mortality but also the rate of hospitalizations.
- Using the following three drug categories is crucial in first-line therapy for HF management: ACE inhibitor or ARB (angiotensin receptor blocker), beta-blocker, and mineralocorticoid receptor antagonist.
- Diuretics and disease-modifying drugs are used as concomitant or adjunct therapy.

SYSTOLIC HEART FAILURE NEW TREATMENT GUIDELINES

Beta-Blockers and Angiotensin-Converting Enzyme Inhibitors (ACEI)

A beta-blocker and an ACE inhibitor/ARB (if ACEI is not tolerated) is started immediately following diagnosis of heart failure (HF) with an ejection fraction (EF) $\leq$40%.

Mineralocorticoid Receptor Antagonists (MRA)

MRAs are recommended for patients with persisting symptoms and an EF $\leq$35% despite therapy with an ACEIs/ARBs and a beta-blocker.

Diuretics

Diuretics are given to relieve dyspnea and edema in patients with symptoms and signs of congestion, irrespective of EF. Loop diuretics produce more intense, shorter diuresis than thiazide diuretics and are preferred in heart failure with reduced ejection fraction. Thiazides are usually less effective in reduced kidney function.

Ivabradine (Procoralan)

Ivabradine is a selective sinus node if channel inhibitor is approved for the treatment of stable angina. It is the first drug that lowers the heart rate without negatively affecting any other cardiac ionic currents. It decreases myocardial oxygen demand and simultaneously increases myocardial oxygen supply. The drug is given to non-responder HF patients with a heart rate $\geq$70 bpm, or to patients who are unable to tolerate a beta-blocker.

Digoxin

Digoxin is given to patients who are non-responders to above therapy or for patients who are unable to tolerate a beta-blocker. Ivabradine is an alternative in patients with a heart rate ≥ 70 bpm. In addition to Digoxin, patients get an ACEI/ARB and an MRA/ARB.

Hydralazine and Isosorbide Dinitrate

Hydralazine and isosorbide dinitrate are considered for non-responders of conventional therapy or for those patients unable to tolerate ACEI/ARB. The patient continues to get a beta-blocker and a MRA.

ADDITIONAL CHF DRUG FACTS OF DENTAL IMPORTANCE

Diuretics

Diuretics help deplete the excess fluid collection and correct the peripheral and pulmonary edema associated with CHF. Hypokalemia, hypocalcemia (muscle spasm), hypomagnesemia, hyperglycemia, hyperuricemia, and hypercholesterolemia are major side effects associated with the thiazide diuretics.

Vasodilators

Dry cough and metallic taste in the mouth are frequent side effects associated with the ACE inhibitors. Hydralazine/Apresoline is another vasodilator that is used to treat moderate-to-severe CHF. Orthostatic hypotension, dizziness, light-headedness, or fainting spells may occur with the vasodilators.

Lanoxin (Digoxin)

Lanoxin (digoxin) is a cardiac glycoside that helps a diseased heart function well. Lanoxin (digoxin) is used to treat CHF, atrial fibrillation (AF), or supraventricular arrhythmias. Lanoxin (digoxin) has significant DDIs with the anesthetics, analgesics, and antibiotics (AAAs) used in dentistry. To determine what AAAs are safe to use with lanoxin (digoxin), it is important to know the drug's mechanism of action and the specific AAAs that negatively interact with it. Refer to Chapter 2 and Table 2.1 for information on Lanoxin (digoxin) and associated DDIs with the AAAs.

Digoxin and Hypokalemia

In addition to the medications listed in Table 2.1, digoxin toxicity can also be precipitated by hypokalemia. Always look for the symptoms and signs of hypokalemia in patients taking digoxin or thiazide diuretics. Hypokalemia may also be seen with prolonged and severe vomiting, diarrhea, or laxative abuse. The normal Serum K^+ level range is 3.5–5.5 mEq/L.

Hypokalemia Symptoms

Hypokalemia can be associated with muscle weakness, muscle fatigue, severe muscle pain, muscle cramps, and irregular heartbeat due to abnormal cardiac contraction.

Hypokalemia Treatment

A symptomatic hypokalemia patient may feel better drinking a cup of orange juice or eating a banana. If this does not prove to be effective the patient must seek medical care. Avoid dental treatment in the presence of symptomatic hypokalemia and refer the patient to the MD.

Lanoxin (Digoxin) Toxicity

Lanoxin (digoxin) overdose can cause nausea, vomiting, anorexia, blurring of vision, green or yellow halos, or green/yellow tinting of images and arrhythmias. Hypokalemia markedly increases the incidence of arrhythmias during lanoxin (digoxin) toxicity.

Cardiac Arrhythmias: Assessment, Analysis, and Associated Dental Management Guidelines

CARDIAC ARRHYTHMIAS OVERVIEW

Cardiac arrhythmias can be an increase in heart rate, a decrease in heart rate, or an irregularity in heart rate, when compared with normal states. An increased heart rate can be associated with sinus tachycardia, atrial or supraventricular arrhythmias, and ventricular arrhythmias. When the heart rate is decreased, the patient is said to have bradycardia.

Sinus Tachycardia

Sinus tachycardia is associated with a pulse rate greater than 100 beats/min and it occurs in response to stress, anxiety, excitement, or exercise. The patient experiences no prolonged symptoms and no further treatment is required.

Atrial or Supraventricular Arrhythmias

Atrial arrhythmias are seldom life threatening. The symptoms experienced with AF will depend on the severity of the arrhythmia. Common symptoms experienced are palpitations, light-headedness, dizziness, chest pain, shortness of breath (SOB), hypotension, CHF, syncope, or thrombosis-associated TIAs or CVAs. Thrombosis is often a complication of AF due to the chaotic beating of the heart. Drugs like the newer anticoagulants rivaroxaban or dabigatran, or the older anticoagulants such as warfarin (Coumadin), aspirin, or clopidogrel (Plavix), are often included in the management of AF for this reason—to prevent complications from emboli.

AF is frequently treated with cardiac glycosides (digoxin), calcium channel blockers (Diltiazam/Cardizam), or beta-blockers (Metaprolol or Propranolol) that help slow

Dentist's Guide to Medical Conditions, Medications, and Complications, Second Edition. Kanchan M. Ganda.
© 2013 John Wiley & Sons, Inc. Published 2013 by John Wiley & Sons, Inc.

down the heart rate. Quinidine or amiodarone are used to treat refractory cases of atrial fibrillation (AF).

Atrial Fibrillation (AF) and Ablation Therapy

The most recent advances in the management of atrial fibrillation are ablation therapy of the ectopic foci in the atrial wall around the pulmonary vein, or ablation of the AV node. The patient is up and about within a few days following the ablation therapy, which corrects the arrhythmia and allows for the discontinuation of the anti-arrhythmia medications. Routine dental treatment can continue once the patient resumes normal activity in a few days.

Ventricular Arrhythmias

Ventricular arrhythmia and ventricular tachycardia (VT) are potentially life-threatening complications of MI. Electrical cardioversion, defibrillators, quinidine, procainamide, lidocaine, and propranolol are often used to manage ventricular arrhythmias. Patients on procainamide may occasionally develop a lupus-like syndrome. An implantable defibrillator is often the choice to help restore normal sinus rhythm in patients with a high risk for ventricular fibrillation. Do not use any electrical appliances in the dental setting in the presence of an implantable defibrillator.

SUGGESTED DENTAL GUIDELINES FOR ARRHYTHMIAS

Suggested Dental Guidelines for Tachyarrhythmias

Consult with the MD and understand the nature of the arrhythmia. Provide stress management because it helps reduce the occurrence of exacerbation of arrhythmias. These patients do best with shorter appointments. Avoid epinephrine because it can precipitate life-threatening arrhythmias.

Bradycardia

Bradycardia is associated with a pulse rate of less than 60 beats/min. A pulse rate of less than 60 beats/min at rest can be physiological or pathological. Physically active individuals can have a slow heart rate or physiological sinus bradycardia due to daily exercise. Certain medications with increased parasympathetic effects similar to phenothiazines or digoxin can cause bradycardia. Beta-blockers like propranolol and metaprolol decrease cardiac excitability and also cause bradycardia. Pathologically, cardiac conduction problems can be associated with bradycardia, and this is treated with an implanted pacemaker.

Bradycardia Symptoms

With significant bradycardia the patient can experience light-headedness, dizziness, and fainting spells due to poor blood flow in the cerebral circulation. Diagnosis is confirmed with a Holter monitor.

Suggested Dental Guidelines for Patients with Bradycardia

The following are dental guidelines for bradycardia:

1. Consult with the MD and understand the severity of the bradycardia.
2. Provide stress management and have the patient in for shorter appointments.
3. Do not use a pulp tester, cavitron, or any other electrical device on patients with pacemakers. Electrical devices, when used in an adjacent operatory, must be at a distance beyond the pacemaker patient's outstretched arm span.

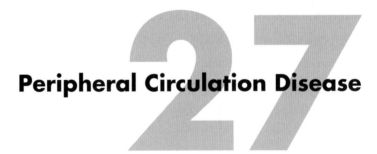

Peripheral Circulation Disease

Long-standing, hypertension-associated involvement of the peripheral vascular circulation causes narrowing of the medium-sized arteries of the leg due to severe atherosclerosis.

SYMPTOMS OF PERIPHERAL CIRCULATION DISEASE

While walking a few blocks or uphill the patient experiences intermittent claudication, or pain, in the legs, calves, or feet. The narrowed vessels are not able to meet the tissue oxygen demand associated with activity, which prompts the patient to stop walking. The patient often experiences relief of symptoms with rest.

SIGNS OF PERIPHERAL CIRCULATION DISEASE

The patient's skin on the lower extremities will be shiny and show hair loss.

SUGGESTED DENTAL GUIDELINE

The atherosclerosis is significant, causing a narrowing of the medium-sized arteries, and it is best to avoid epinephrine-containing local anesthetics in symptomatic patients.

Dentist's Guide to Medical Conditions, Medications, and Complications, Second Edition. Kanchan M. Ganda.
© 2013 John Wiley & Sons, Inc. Published 2013 by John Wiley & Sons, Inc.

Renal Function Tests, Renal Disease, and Dialysis: Assessment, Analysis, and Associated Dental Management Guidelines

KIDNEY FUNCTION TESTS

Tests evaluated to assess kidney function are:

1. The serum creatinine
2. The creatinine clearance
3. The extent of proteinurea
4. The blood urea nitrogen (BUN)
5. The glomerular filtration rate (GFR)
6. Renal imaging

Serum Creatinine (S.Cr)

Creatinine is a waste product generated from muscle cell breakdown, and it is filtered out in the urine by the kidneys. As kidney function decreases, the serum creatinine (s.Cr) levels rise. Muscle mass and diet can affect serum creatinine values, so it is best to estimate renal function by calculating the GFR. The normal s. creatinine in most labs is 0.4–1.2 mg/dL. In general and oversimplified terms (given the variability of s. creatinine based on muscle mass), a patient is said to have a 50% **reduction** of kidney function when the serum creatinine is ≥1.7 mg/dL in men and ≥1.4 mg/dL in women.

It is safe to assume that individuals with a serum creatinine of 2.0 mg/dL have moderate-to-severe decrease in GFR, regardless of the equation used to estimate GFR.

Creatinine Clearance (CrCl)

The creatinine clearance shows how well the kidneys are functioning. This test indicates **how efficiently** the kidneys can remove creatinine from the blood and pass it into the urine. The test compares the amount of urine creatinine in a 24-hour collection with the level of serum creatinine.

Dentist's Guide to Medical Conditions, Medications, and Complications, Second Edition. Kanchan M. Ganda.
© 2013 John Wiley & Sons, Inc. Published 2013 by John Wiley & Sons, Inc.

Cockcroft-Gault (C-G) Creatinine Clearance Equation

$$\text{Estimated creatinine clearance, or GFR} = [(140 - \text{Patient's Age})$$
$$\times \text{ Mass or Patient's weight (in kg)}] \div [72 \times \text{Serum creatinine (in mg/dL)}]$$

If the patient is female, the clinician must multiply the resulting value by 0.85. Creatinine clearance is measured as mL/min. The normal creatinine clearance is 80–130 mL/min.

Proteinuria

Another marker of kidney function is the presence of protein in the urine. Protein normally **does not** filter out of the kidneys. Healthy kidneys remove all wastes from the blood but do not remove protein. Diseased kidneys may fail to separate albumin from the wastes. Initially, only small amounts of albumin leak into the urine. This **microalbuminuria** is an indication of deteriorating kidney function. As kidney function worsens, the amount of albumin and other proteins in the urine increases, resulting in proteinuria. A 24-hour urine collection measures the total amount of protein lost in the urine.

Blood Urea Nitrogen (BUN)

Urea is formed in the liver as a waste product when protein is broken down in the body. The urea is then eliminated in the urine. Blood urea nitrogen (BUN) measures the amount of **nitrogen** in the blood. The nitrogen comes from urea. BUN thus gives an estimate of how effectively the kidneys are in removing urea from the blood. The normal BUN in most labs is 7–20 mg/dL.

Glomerular Filtration Rate (GFR)

The GFR shows how efficiently the kidneys are filtering wastes from the blood in normal and diseased patients. GFR is estimated by using the modification of diet in renal disease study group (MDRD) equation, which is based on the patient's age, weight, gender, race, and serum creatinine. Use the following site to calculate your patient's GFR: www.kidney.org/professionals/kdoqi/gfr_calculator.cfm

Serum creatinine-based estimation of GFR provides a basis for the classification of chronic kidney disease.

Glomerular Filtration Rate and Staging of Chronic Renal Disease

The Kidney Disease Outcomes Quality Initiative (K/DOQI) of the National Kidney Foundation (NKF) defines chronic kidney disease (CKD) as either kidney damage or a decreased glomerular filtration rate (GFR) of less than 60mL/min/1.73m^2 for three or more months. Kidney damage is defined as pathologic abnormalities or markers of damage, including abnormalities in blood or urine tests or imaging studies. Per K/DOQI, these are the classification stages of CKD:

Stage 1 (Kidney damage with normal or increased GFR): GFR $\geq$90 mL/min/1.73 m^2
Stage 2 (Kidney damage with mild reduction in GFR): GFR 60–89 mL/min/1.73 m^2

Stage 3 (Moderate reduction in GFR): GFR 30–59 mL/min/1.73 m^2
Stage 4 (Severe reduction in GFR): GFR 15–29 mL/min/1.73 m^2
Stage 5 (Kidney failure): GFR <15 mL/min/1.73 m^2

Patients with CKD stages 1–3 may be asymptomatic. Clinical manifestations typically appear in stages 4–5, but may appear as early as stage 3. A patient is said to have CKD when the GFR is <60 mL/min/1.73 m^2 for three months. As a conscientious provider, you must help prevent the progression of kidney disease by **using the appropriate AAAs** and insist that the patient control associated diseases, such as hypertension and diabetes, which commonly cause CKD.

Renal Imaging

Ultrasound, computed tomography (CT scan), and magnetic resonance imaging (MRI) are tools used to detect unusual changes in the kidney structure or impairment in urinary flow.

CHRONIC KIDNEY DISEASE

Sound knowledge of normal renal physiology is needed to better understand the changes associated with renal dysfunction. The dental provider has to address these alterations before proceeding with dentistry. Additionally, the provider needs to modify the use of anesthetics, analgesics, antibiotics, and antivirals in the dental setting, so the renal-compromised patient can be optimally treated.

Chronic Kidney Disease Pathophysiology

Introduction

The kidney has an innate ability to maintain GFR, even in the presence of injury, via hyperfiltration and compensatory hypertrophy of the remaining healthy nephrons. This nephron adaptability allows for continued normal clearance of plasma solutes. Plasma levels of urea and creatinine start to show significant increases only after total GFR has decreased to 50% when the renal reserve has been exhausted. The plasma creatinine value approximately doubles with a 50% reduction in GFR. **A rise in plasma creatinine from a baseline value of 0.6–1.2mg/dL in a patient, although still within the reference range, actually represents a loss of 50% of functioning nephron mass.**

Hyperkalemia

CKD patients are able to maintain potassium (K) excretion at near-normal levels as long as both aldosterone secretion and distal renal flow are maintained. Through the effect of aldosterone, the body is also able to increase potassium excretion in the gastrointestinal (GI) tract. Hyperkalemia usually develops when the GFR falls below 20–25mL/min, when the renal **excretion** of potassium **decreases**. It can occur sooner in patients who ingest NSAIDS.

Metabolic Acidosis

It is necessary to discuss the normal acid-base balance first and then discuss metabolic acidosis associated with CKD. It is important to note that in the presence of acid-base abnormality, the system that is not primarily responsible for the acid-base imbalance assumes the responsibility for returning the pH to the normal range. Acid-base imbalance can be from multiple causes but **the two main systems that can affect the acid-base status are the respiratory system and the renal system**. In primary respiratory disorders, the pH and $PaCO_2$ go in opposite directions; in metabolic disorders the pH and $PaCO_2$ go in the same direction.

ABG pattern in metabolic acidosis: pH: <7.35; $PaCO_2$: normal; HCO_3: $<22mEq/L$. The acidosis is less likely to be of respiratory origin and very likely to be of non-respiratory or metabolic origin. A low pH (<7.35) and a low HCO_3 ($<22mEq/L$), which are consistent with acidosis, are very likely due to non-respiratory causes. Common causes of metabolic acidosis include diabetes, shock, and renal failure.

Metabolic alkalosis is not associated with kidney disease, but if the reader is wondering what metabolic alkalosis is, here is a synopsis: Metabolic alkalosis is characterized by an increased pH and increased HCO_3 and is seen with hypokalemia, chronic vomiting or diarrhea, or sodium bicarbonate overdose.

Metabolic Acidosis Associated with CKD

In CKD patients, the kidneys are unable to produce enough ammonia in the proximal tubules to excrete the endogenous acid into the urine in the form of ammonium. This accounts for the accumulation of phosphates, sulfates, and other organic anions causing an increase in the anion gap in the stage-5 CKD patient. Metabolic acidosis is associated with protein-energy malnutrition, loss of lean body mass, and muscle weakness.

Metabolic acidosis plays a role in the development of renal osteodystrophy, as bone acts as a buffer for excess acid, resulting in mineral loss. Acidosis interferes with vitamin D metabolism, and patients who are persistently more acidotic are more likely to have osteomalacia or low-turnover bone disease.

Refer to Chapter 29 for a discussion on respiratory acidosis-alkalosis, and refer to Chapter 41 for a detailed discussion outlining the role of parathyroid glands, vitamin D, kidney, and gut in normal calcium metabolism.

Salt and Water Retention

Failure of sodium and free water excretion by the diseased kidney generally becomes clinically evident when the GFR falls below $10–15mL/min$. This leads to peripheral edema, pulmonary edema, and hypertension.

Anemia

Normochromic normocytic anemia develops from decreased renal synthesis of erythropoietin, the hormone responsible for bone marrow stimulation for red blood cell (RBC) production. It starts early and becomes more severe as the GFR progressively decreases. In the presence of less viable renal mass, no reticulocyte response occurs. RBC survival is decreased, and tendency of bleeding is increased from the uremia-induced platelet dysfunction.

CKD and Calcium Metabolism

CKD results in a fundamental disruption of the normal regulation of extracellular calcium, bone calcium, and vascular calcification. Vitamin D absorbed from sunlight and dietary vitamin D are converted in the liver to calcidiol or 25-hydroxyvitamin D, [25(OH)D]. 25(OH)D is the specific vitamin D metabolite that is measured in the serum to determine a patient's vitamin D status. Part of 25(OH)D is converted to 1,25-dihydroxyvitamin D3, [1,25(OH)2D/calcitriol], by the kidneys. This hormone then circulates in the blood, regulating the concentration of calcium and phosphate in the bloodstream, promoting the healthy growth and remodeling of bone.

Calcium absorption occurs through two mechanisms in the gut. There is an active mechanism that results in transcellular movement of calcium. The active transport is regulated, and the primary regulator is 1,25(OH)2D, which is saturable. This regulated active transport of calcium is critically important when dietary calcium is very low. Most calcium is absorbed in the small intestine. There is also a paracellular calcium movement in the gut that is not highly regulated, and it is not particularly 1,25(OH)2D dependent, nor is it saturable.

When there is no 1,25(OH)2D/calcitriol, active calcium absorption is essentially zero and passive absorption is actually negative because there is calcium excretion into the gut. As 1,25(OH)2D levels increase in the gut, active calcium absorption increases, and one can absorb up to 80% of the calcium in the meal if one has enough 1,25(OH)2D. But when calcium intake with the meal is very low, you can actually lose calcium through the gut. Even if there is no active absorption, there is enough passive absorption with the meal of 300mg that one can be in positive calcium balance with the positive calcium absorption from that meal. This is the reason why patients with normal 1,25(OH)2D levels can be in neutral calcium balance on very low calcium intakes, because of the role 1,25(OH)2D plays in increasing gut calcium absorption. Adequate calcium absorption can occur with passive absorption of calcium that is not D-dependent. Patients on dialysis absorb a significant percentage of dietary calcium given as a meal or as a binder even if they do not have high circulating calcitriol and the mean gut calcium absorption stays around 15–25%.

In summary, kidney disease is associated with a decrease in the production of active vitamin D3, causing hypocalcemia, secondary hyperparathyroidism, hyperphosphatemia, and renal osteodystrophy. Secondary hyperparathyroidism develops in chronic kidney disease because of hyperphosphatemia, hypocalcemia, decreased renal synthesis of 1,25-dihydroxycholecalciferol (1,25-dihydroxyvitamin D, or calcitriol), intrinsic alteration in the parathyroid gland (which gives rise to increased PTH secretion as well as increased parathyroid growth), and skeletal resistance to PTH.

Hyperphospatemia

Calcium and calcitriol are primary feedback inhibitors for PTH; hyperphosphatemia is a stimulus to PTH synthesis and secretion. Phosphate retention begins in early chronic kidney disease: When the GFR falls, less phosphate is filtered and excreted, but serum levels do not rise initially because of increased PTH secretion, which increases renal excretion. As the GFR falls toward chronic kidney disease stages 4–5, hyperphosphatemia develops from the inability of the kidneys to excrete the excess dietary intake. Hyperphosphatemia suppresses the renal hydroxylation of inactive 25-hydroxyvitamin

D to calcitriol, so serum calcitriol levels are low when the GFR is less than 30mL/min. Increased phosphate concentration also effects PTH concentration by its direct effect on parathyroid gland. Hypocalcemia develops primarily from decreased intestinal calcium absorption because of low plasma calcitriol levels and possibly from calcium binding to elevated serum levels of phosphate.

Low serum calcitriol levels, hypocalcemia, and hyperphosphatemia are all independent triggers of PTH synthesis and secretion. With persistent effect, the parathyroid glands become hyperplastic. With the persistently elevated PTH levels, high-turnover bone disease or renal osteodystrophy occurs.

DECREASED RENAL FUNCTION AND ASSOCIATED HEMATOLOGICAL CHANGES SIGNIFICANT IN DENTISTRY

Every dental provider must be aware of the following hematological changes associated with decreased renal function:

1. **Anemia:** Anemia that is caused by decreased erythropoietin production associated with kidney disease.
2. **Increased Potassium:** Reduction in acid, potassium, salt, and water excretion causes acidosis, hyperkalemia, hypertension, and edema.
3. **Sodium:** The serum sodium level is **unchanged** with kidney disease but it could get altered with water retention.
4. **Increased phosphate:** Increased phosphate level is a consequence of low level of 1,25 dihydroxy-D (active vitamin D).
5. **Decreased calcium:** Decrease in production of active vitamin D3, causes hypocalcemia, secondary hyperparathyroidism, hyperphosphatemia, and renal osteodystrophy.
6. **Decreased magnesium:** Kidney disease can decrease the magnesium level, and low magnesium often causes skeletal muscle soreness, tingling, and TMJ dysfunction.
7. **Prolonged bleeding time (BT):** Uremia from kidney disease causes decreased platelet cohesiveness and a prolongation of the bleeding time (BT).
8. **Increased BUN and serum creatinine:** Impairment of the excretory function of the kidney especially results in an elevation of blood urea nitrogen (BUN) and serum creatinine levels.

HEMODIALYSIS AND PERITONEAL DIALYSIS

Dialysis Overview

Dialysis is a means to removing waste products and excess fluid from the blood on a regular basis, when the patient's kidneys have failed and have become nonfunctional. There are two main types of dialysis: hemodialysis and peritoneal dialysis. Patients with end-stage renal disease (ESRD) may be on peritoneal dialysis or hemodialysis.

Hemodialysis

Hemodialysis treatments are typically done at a dialysis center through a permanent **hemodialysis access** created in the patient's arm or leg. It is important that every provider know some important facts about the various forms of hemodialysis access so these patients can be treated optimally and correctly in the dental setting.

Hemodialysis Accesses

Hemodialysis access can be attained through an intravenous catheter (internal jugular vein or femoral vein), an arteriovenous (AV) fistula, or a synthetic graft. These accesses help connect the patient to the dialysis machine. These accesses are usually **not removed** when the kidney failure patient gets a renal transplant. Thus, the premedication requirements indicated for specific accesses before transplant, **must be followed** post transplant as well.

Intravenous Catheter Access

Intravenous catheter access is a **temporary, short-term access** and is typically reserved for immediate or sudden dialysis. This form of access (placed either in the neck or groin) can be associated with catheter-induced infection and stenosis of the vasculature because of the indwelling IV catheter. A patient with an **indwelling catheter** should be **premedicated** prior to invasive dentistry.

Arteriovenous (AV) Fistula or Arteriovenous Synthetic Graft

The AV fistula and the synthetic graft are the **more permanent and preferable** forms of hemodialysis accesses. Both forms, however, have to **mature** before becoming available for hemodialysis.

The AV Fistula

The AV fistula is the **most opted** for type of access. An artery and a vein are joined together and an anastomosis is created using the patient's own vasculature. It takes an average of 4–6 weeks for the fistula to mature; consequently, this procedure is planned in advance of anticipated dialysis. Fistulas are usually created in the arm and it is extremely important that the provider **not** use that arm for BP monitoring or IV/IM injections. The AV fistula infection rate is low compared with the synthetic graft or the intravenous catheter because no foreign material is used in its formation. The potential for thrombosis is also low with the AV fistulas. A patient with an AV fistula **does not** require premedication for invasive dental procedures. However, always confirm with the patient's physician before you proceed with dentistry without premedication, because, occasionally, the MD may want premedication for a "young" or newly forming fistula, or if the patient has severe periodontal disease/infection.

Arteriovenous Synthetic Graft

An arteriovenous graft using synthetic (PTFE, Goretex®) or bovine graft material is almost like a fistula, except that synthetic material is used to join or link the artery and vein. An AV graft is created when the patient's blood vessels are not optimal and so do not allow the creation of a fistula. An AV graft matures faster than a fistula and it can be placed in the thigh or even in the neck. Grafts are associated with a higher risk of thrombosis and infection because synthetic material is used. The patient with an **AV graft** should always be **premedicated** prior to invasive dentistry. Some clinicians prefer to use intravenous (IV) vancomycin during dialysis because it provides prophylaxis up to seven days.

Hemodialysis

The patient gets dialyzed three times per week, and each dialysis session lasts four hours. IV heparin is administered during the first three hours of hemodialysis, so 50% of the IV heparin is cleared at the end of the fourth hour of hemodialysis. Total heparin clearance occurs five hours after the **end** of the hemodialysis. Consequently, you need to wait five hours post hemodialysis if you plan on treating the patient on the day of hemodialysis. It is always best to treat these patients on the "off days" of dialysis.

Peritoneal Dialysis

Peritoneal dialysis is less efficient than hemodialysis and it can be in the form of continuous ambulatory peritoneal dialysis (CAPD) or continuous cycling peritoneal dialysis (CCPD). The patient carries it out at home using a portable peritoneal dialysis machine. This accounts for the peritoneal dialysis patient being a lot more mobile compared with the patient undergoing hemodialysis. As previously stated, the hemodialysis patient has to visit a dialysis center for dialysis to occur.

In peritoneal dialysis, the peritoneal membrane acts as a semipermeable membrane through which dialysis or exchange occurs. Premedication prophylaxis per se is **not** needed with peritoneal dialysis. However, in some cases, the patient will need to be premedicated prior to invasive dentistry if there is an **indwelling catheter** for anticipated long-term peritoneal dialysis. So always confirm!

The dialysate consists of a sterile solution of minerals and glucose. It is run through a tube into the peritoneal cavity where it is left for some time so the waste products can be absorbed. This fluid containing waste product is then drained out through the tube and discarded. This exchange cycle is repeated 4–5 times during the day and/or overnight with an automated dialysis machine.

ANESTHETICS, ANALGESICS, ANTIBIOTICS, AND KIDNEY DISEASE

Long-standing daily use of painkillers composed of two or more analgesics (particularly acetaminophen and NSAIDS), together with caffeine or codeine, are most likely to damage the kidneys (Table 28.1).

NSAIDS block prostaglandin (PG) formation. Vasodilator PG inhibition can impair glomerular filtration, especially in volume-depleted states. Acetaminophen has reactive metabolites that are neutralized by glutathione. Significant nephrotoxicity can occur when the neutralizing capacity of glutathione is taxed. Long-term use of NSAIDS and acetaminophen has been linked with an increased risk of end-stage renal disease (ESRD).

Impairment of drug clearance: Drugs normally excreted by the kidney can accumulate to toxic levels in CKD patients. It is best to adjust dosages or avoid using such

Table 28.1. Renal Disease and Dental Drugs Guidelines

Drugs: Generic/Trade	Suggestion(s)
ANESTHETICS:	
2% Lidocaine (Xylocaine)	Use maximum 2 carpules Use with Serum Creatinine <2mg/dL
2% Mepivacaine (Carbocaine) with 1:20,000 Levonordefrin (NeoCobefrin)	Use maximum 2 carpules Use with Serum (S.) Creatinine (Cr) <2mg/dL
3% Mepivacaine HCL (Carbocaine)	**The** LA with S.Cr >2mg/dL
4% Prilocaine HCL (Citanest Forte or Citanest Plain)	**Avoid Citanest** in the presence of **hypoxia** due to low Erythropoeitin
4% Septocaine (Articaine)	**Avoid Articaine** in the presence of **hypoxia** due to low Erythropoeitin
ANALGESICS:	
Aspirin	**Predialysis:** Use normal dose **Dialysis:** Avoid **Best to avoid**
NSAIDS	**Avoid NSAIDS**
Acetaminophen (Tylenol)	1. **CrCl >50mL/minute or S.Cr <2mg/dL:** Dose normally: 325mg q6h OR 1000mg q6-8h/day 2. **CrCl 10–50mL/minute or S.Cr >2mg/dL to Pre-dialysis:** Give 325–650mg **q6-8h** 3. **CrCl <10mL/minute or Dialysis:** Use 325–650mg **q8h** **Avoid extra strength Tylenol with S.Cr >2mg/dL**
Codeine + Acetaminophen: Tylenol #1–4	1. **CrCl >50mL/minute or S.Cr <2mg/dL:** Normal Codeine dose, 30–60mg. Give 1–2 Tylenol #3 **q4-6h** PRN 2. **CrCl 10–50mL/minute or S.Cr >2mg/dL to Predialysis:** Use 50% dose of Codeine (15–30mg). Dispense 1–2 Tylenol #2 **q6h** PRN 3. **CrCl <10mL/minute or Dialysis:** Use 75% dose of Codeine (7.5–15mg): 1–2 Tylenol #1 **q8h** PRN
Propoxyphene (Darvon)	**Contraindicated.** Metabolites accumulate in ESRD (end stage renal disease)
Meperidine (Demerol)	**Contraindicated** as metabolites accumulate in ESRD
Hydrocodone + Acetaminophen: (Vicodin)	**Predialysis:** Vicodin, 1 tab **q6h** PRN **Dialysis:** Vicodin, 1 tab **q8h** PRN
Oxycodone + Acetaminophen: (Percocet)	**Predialysis:** One 2.5/325 tab **q6h** PRN **Dialysis:** One 2.5/325 tab **q8h** PRN
Methadone:	**Dose:** Give 50–75% of normal Methadone dose in the presence of CrCl <10mL/min.

(continued)

Table 28.1. Renal Disease and Dental Drugs Guidelines (*Continued*)

Drugs: Generic/Trade	Suggestion (s)
ANTIBIOTICS:	
Penicillin VK	1. **S.Cr <2.0mg/dL:** Normal dose
	2. **S.Cr >2.0mg/dL to Pre-dialysis:** Pen VK 250–500mg **q8-12h**
	3. **Dialysis:** Pen VK 250–500 **q12-16h**
Amoxicillin	1. **S.Cr <3.3mg/dL:** Normal dose
	2. **S.Cr >3.3mg/dL to Predialysis:** 250–500mg **q12h**
	3. **Dialysis:** 250–500 **q24h**
Other Penicillins	Decrease the dose by 50%
Cephalosporins	Decrease dose by 50%
Erythromycin	Safe but no longer used in dentistry
Azithromycin (Zithromax)	Safe to use
Clarithromycin (Biaxin): Best to **avoid**, but if needed, use the scripts listed	1. **S.Cr <3.3mg/dL:** 250mg **q12h.**
	2. **S.Cr >3.3mg/dL to predialysis:** Give 125mg **q12h**
	3. **Dialysis:** 125mg **q24h**
Clindamycin (Cleocin)	No dose adjustment for renal failure
Tetracycline HCl: Best to **avoid** with kidney disease. If absolutely needed **then** use the listed scripts	1. **S.Cr 1.25–2mg/dL:** 250–500mg **q8-12h**
	2. **S.Cr 2mg/dL to Predialysis:** 250–500mg **q12-24h**
	3. **Dialysis:** 250–500mg **q24h**
Doxycycline (Vibramycin)	No dose change
Diazepam (Valium)	Safe to use if the patient is on Erythropoeitin replacement therapy
Lorazepam (Ativan)	

drugs. Avoid meperidine (Demerol) in patients with CKD or ESRD because the active metabolite (normeperidine) can accumulate and cause seizures.

Additional concerns associated with the CKD Patient:

- The provider must always be concerned with excess surgical morbidity in CKD patients, especially because surgery can lead to acute renal failure, hyperkalemia, volume overload, and infection.
- Hyperkalemia can be precipitated in the major surgical setting by tissue breakdown, transfusions, acidosis, and the use of Ringer lactate solution as a replacement fluid. Ringer lactate solution contains potassium, which is often disregarded but can cause hyperkalemia.
- Diarrhea, and/or vomiting can result in both volume contraction and hypokalemia. Hypokalemia is sometimes associated with hypomagnesemia.
- Most patients with CKD have chronic acidosis; major surgical disease can further complicate the acidemia. Such patients are at a higher risk for hyperkalemia, myocardial depression, and cardiac arrhythmia.
- Patients on hemodialysis usually require preoperative dialysis within 24 hours before major surgery to reduce the risk of volume overload, hyperkalemia, and excessive bleeding.
- Patients on peritoneal dialysis should continue with the dialysis when undergoing major surgery in the dental setting.

- Consult with the patient's nephrologist, for preoperative evaluation of patients with CKD who have received kidney transplantation. Cyclosporine or tacrolimus taken by renal transplant recipients for immunosuppression are metabolized by the CYP450 system in the liver and thus interact with a wide variety of drugs. Diltiazem, statins, macrolides, and antifungal drugs inhibit the 3A4 system, elevate levels, and can precipitate nephrotoxicity. Carbamazepine (Tegretol), barbiturates, and theophylline, induce the 3A4 system, reduce levels, and can precipitate rejection.
- Establish the level of renal function impairment by calculating the GFR and assessing the BUN and creatinine levels.
- Determine if the patient has preexisting diabetes, edema, CHF, or pulmonary congestion or other cardiovascular concerns prior to surgery.
- Avoid using potential nephrotoxic drugs such as aminoglycosides, acyclovir, amphotericin, sedatives, muscle relaxants, and NSAIDS.

VII

Pulmonary Diseases

Pulmonary Function Tests and Sedation with Pulmonary Diseases: Assessment, Analysis, and Associated Dental Management Guidelines

Pulmonary disease can involve the upper airway or the lower airway. Rhinitis, sinusitis, and pharyngitis are common upper airway diseases. Asthma, bronchitis, emphysema, and chronic obstructive pulmonary disease (COPD) are conditions that affect the lower airways.

The dentist should not only be familiar with disease states but should also be knowledgeable about the diagnostic tools used to detect and assess the control statuses of pulmonary diseases. This becomes particularly important with the conditions causing significant changes in the patient's ASA status.

THE DIAGNOSTIC TOOLS TO DETECT PULMONARY DISEASE

The diagnostic tools used to detect pulmonary disease are presented in the following sections.

History and Physical Examination

History can reveal the presence of symptoms and/or etiological factors such as smoking, specific allergens, or genetic predisposition, which are responsible for the pulmonary disease(s). Sinus congestion, headaches, cough, dyspnea, wheezing, hemoptysis (coughing up blood), sleepiness, snoring, and morning headaches are some of the more common symptoms experienced with pulmonary disease. Physical examination can reveal nasal congestion, nasal inflammation, and cobblestoning of the pharynx from constant postnasal dripping, macroglossia, nasal polyps, and cervical lymphadenopathy, in addition to findings detected through the classic inspection, palpation, percussion, and auscultation findings in the lungs.

Dentist's Guide to Medical Conditions, Medications, and Complications, Second Edition. Kanchan M. Ganda.
© 2013 John Wiley & Sons, Inc. Published 2013 by John Wiley & Sons, Inc.

Laboratory Tests

Pulmonary Function Tests (PFTs)

Pulmonary function is measured by spirometry. The tests detect how efficiently the oxygen from the lungs is transferred into the blood and how well the carbon dioxide is removed from the blood. The following list details terminologies and facts associated with spirometry.

Common Spirometry Associated Terminologies, Definitions, and Disease Types

- **Forced vital capacity (FVC):** FVC measures the amount of air exhaled forcefully after deep inspiration.
- **Forced expiratory volume (FEV):** FEV measures the amount of air exhaled forcefully in one breath. FEV_1 is the amount of exhaled air measured at 1 second. FEV_1/FVC can then be determined.
- **Forced expiratory flow 25–75%:** This measures the air flow halfway through an exhale.
- **Peak expiratory flow (PEF):** PEF measures how quickly one can exhale. It is usually measured at the same time as forced vital capacity (FVC).
- **Total lung capacity (TLC):** TLC measures the amount of air in the lungs following deep inspiration.
- **Residual volume (RV):** RV measures the amount of air in the lungs after complete expiration.

It is important to note that staging of COPD is generally done by spirometry. This is discussed in detail in Chapter 34.

Lung Disease Types

There are two main types of lung disease that can be found with lung function tests: obstructive lung disease and restrictive lung disease.

Obstructive lung disease is associated with narrowed airways and it takes a long time for the patient to empty the lungs. Asthma, chronic bronchitis, emphysema, bronchiectasis, bronchiolitis, and chronic obstructive pulmonary disease (COPD) are conditions listed as obstructive lung diseases, and of these disease states, asthma, chronic bronchitis, emphysema, and chronic obstructive pulmonary disease (COPD) are the most common obstructive lung diseases encountered. The narrowed airways in these states are associated with increased airway resistance. **Obstructive lung disease is associated with** FVC that could be normal or lower than predicted value; low FEV_1, FEV_1/FVC, forced expiratory flow 25–75%, and PEF; and high RV. The FEV_1 often increases after bronchodilator use, especially with reversible obstructive disease like asthma. The severity of obstruction is defined as the absolute value of the FEV_1. The lower the FEV_1 the worse is the obstruction.

Restrictive lung disease is associated with decreased distensibility of the lungs, pleura, or chest wall during inhalation; thus, increased pressure is required to distend the lungs. A diseased, thickened interstitium can be associated with diffusion problems. Therefore, scarring of lung tissues, chest wall deformity, or problems with the chest wall muscles can also cause inability to inhale a normal volume.

Restrictive lung disease can be due to:

- Lung parenchymal disease: pulmonary fibrosis, sarcoidosis
- Pleural disease: pleural effusion, pneumothorax
- Inadequate filling from acute lung disease: pneumonia or CHF
- Neuromuscular conditions: muscular dystrophy, myasthenia gravis
- Chest wall anomalies: obesity-related chest deformity, kyphosis, or scoliosis

Restrictive lung diseases are best assessed by measuring the lung volume. A normal FEV_1/FVC ratio occurs in a normal patient or a patient with restrictive lung disease. The difference is that the FVC is low in the patient with restrictive lung disease and is normal in a healthy patient.

Restricted lung disease findings: Low FVC; FEV_1, FEV_1/FVC, and forced expiratory flow 25–75% are all normal/lower; and RV is normal/lower/higher.

With asthma, there is no reduction in lung volumes and there is no impairment in the gas transportation from the alveoli to the blood. Therefore, the PFTs in asthma show a low FEV_1/FVC ratio, normal total lung capacity (TLC), and normal gases diffusion. The obstruction typically improves with a bronchodilator challenge.

Emphysema is associated with obstruction, hyperinflation, air trapping, and impairment in gas transportation from the air to the blood. Therefore, the PFTs in emphysema show a low FEV_1/FVC ratio, an elevated total lung capacity (TLC) and a reduced diffusion of gases. The obstruction is not reversible in emphysema.

In interstitial lung disease, the lung volume becomes progressively smaller and impairment of gas exchange occurs. The PFTs show a normal FEV_1/FVC ratio, a low TLC, and a low diffusion of gases.

Arterial Blood Gases

- Arterial blood gas (ABG) analysis provides information on the oxygenation of blood through gas exchange in the lungs; the carbon dioxide (CO_2) elimination through respiration; and the acid-base balance or imbalance in the extra-cellular fluid (ECF).
- ABG analysis also provides information on the oxygen saturation of arterial blood (SaO_2). SaO_2 measures the amount of oxygen bound to hemoglobin and is expressed as a percentage. Oxygen saturation **below 94%** indicates a decrease in respiratory function.
- The ABG analysis is an indicator of pulmonary function and can be used along with spirometry and chest x-rays to diagnose COPD and other pulmonary diseases compromising gas exchange.
- The following are normal values identified with normal respiratory function for the partial pressure of oxygen (PaO_2), the partial pressure of carbon dioxide ($PaCO_2$), the pH or the acid-base balance, the bicarbonate (HCO_3) concentration, and the oxygen saturation (SaO_2) in the arterial blood: **PaO_2:** 75–100mmHg; **$PaCO_2$:** 35-45mmHg, **pH:** 7.35–7.45; **HCO_3:** 22–26mEq/L (milliequivalents/liter); and **SaO_2:** 95–100%.
- It is important to note that in the presence of acid-base abnormality, the system that is **not** primarily responsible for the acid-base imbalance assumes the responsibility for returning the pH to the normal range. Acid-base imbalance can be from

multiple causes, but **the two main systems that can affect the acid-base status are the respiratory system and the renal system.**

- In primary respiratory disorders, the pH and $PaCO_2$ go in opposite directions; in metabolic disorders the pH and $PaCO_2$ go in the same direction.

Respiratory Acidosis

- **ABG Pattern:** pH <7.35; $PaCO_2$ >45mmHg; HCO_3: normal.
- A high $PaCO_2$ will cause a low pH, so the respiratory system is quite likely responsible for the acidosis. Always keep in mind that the lungs control the level of CO_2 in the arterial blood. When the HCO_3 is normal in the presence of acidosis, the acidosis is most likely of respiratory origin.
- In respiratory acidosis the patient does not get enough oxygen in and enough carbon dioxide out. Common causes include chronic obstructive pulmonary disease (COPD), pneumonia, and oversedation from narcotics. A COPD patient may also display low levels of dissolved oxygen and oxygen saturation.

Respiratory Alkalosis

- Respiratory alkalosis, characterized by an increased pH and a decreased PCO_2, is due to overventilation caused by hyperventilating, pain, emotional distress, or specific lung conditions that interfere with oxygen exchange.

GENERAL ANESTHESIA OR CONSCIOUS SEDATION CONSIDERATIONS WITH PULMONARY DISEASES

An increase in adverse outcomes can occur with outpatient general anesthesia or conscious sedation in patients with pulmonary disease, and complications are more common in the ASA III/IV patient. Hypoxemia and drug overdose are the most frequent problems encountered. When conscious sedation or general anesthesia is used, it is best to increase the dose slowly, especially in the elderly patient.

Conscious Sedation

Benzodiazepines and opioids suppress the respiratory drive and this is a significant problem in obstructive sleep apnea (OSA).

Oxygen Plus Nitrous Oxide

Oxygen plus nitrous oxide has the advantage of rapid onset and recovery. The disadvantage is that it can expand and rupture the bullae. Thus it is contraindicated if the patient cannot tolerate an increase in the PO_2.

Upper Airway Disease: Allergic Rhinitis, Sinusitis, and Streptococcal Pharyngitis: Assessment, Analysis, and Associated Dental Management Guidelines

ALLERGIC RHINITIS

Allergic rhinitis can be seasonal or constant. Most patients have associated allergies of some sort.

Allergic Rhinitis Symptoms

Nasal discharge, sneezing, and itchy eyes are the most common symptoms experienced.

Allergic Rhinitis Treatment

The patient should avoid exposure to known allergens. Additionally, the patient should be evaluated for underlying allergies and receive appropriate allergy shots when possible. Nasal or oral antihistamines are often prescribed along with nasal or systemic steroids to gain relief.

SINUSITIS

Sinusitis could be bacterial or viral in origin. S. aureus is a common pathogen in sphenoid sinusitis. The most common pathogens isolated from maxillary sinus cultures in patients with acute bacterial rhinosinusitis include Streptococcus pneumoniae, Haemophilus influenzae, and Moraxella catarrhalis. Streptococcus pyogenes, Staphylococcus aureus, and anaerobes are less commonly associated with acute bacterial rhinosinusitis. The vast majority of sinusitis episodes are caused by viral infection. Most viral upper respiratory tract infections are caused by rhinovirus, but coronavirus, influenza A and B, parainfluenza, respiratory syncytial virus, adenovirus, and enterovirus are also causative agents. Patients can sometimes present with unilateral sinusitis, and, in such

Dentist's Guide to Medical Conditions, Medications, and Complications, Second Edition. Kanchan M. Ganda.
© 2013 John Wiley & Sons, Inc. Published 2013 by John Wiley & Sons, Inc.

cases, it is always important to rule out a dental-related cause or an underlying neoplasm cause.

Sinusitis Symptoms

The patient experiences mild, moderate, or severe pain over the sinuses affecting the cheeks, forehead, and eyes, in addition to the top and back of the head. Additionally, the patient experiences malaise, nasal obstruction, headaches, purulent rhinorrhea, and, at times, thick nasal discharge.

Sinusitis Treatment

Medical Management

Acute sinusitis typically presents with nasal congestion, purulent nasal discharge, and facial pain. **In the immunocompetent host, antibiotics are initially unnecessary**. Initial treatment should consist of topical decongestants used every four hours, steam inhalations, saline flushes, and sleeping in a semi-upright position to facilitate drainage – especially when the maxillary sinuses are involved. Antibiotics should be used in toxic-appearing patients, those in whom initial therapy fails, and in patients with comorbid conditions.

Amoxicillin 500mg tid × 10–14 days; clarithromycin 250mg or 500mg bid × 10–14 days; or azithromycin 500mg on day 1 followed by 250mg for the next 4 days are first-line antibiotics for bacterial sinusitis. Trimethoprim-sulfamethoxazole (TMP-SMZ) for 3 days is as effective as a traditional 10-day course of the antibiotic. Treatment also consists of dispensing decongestants such as Afrin spray for **less than** 4 days. Afrin spray, when used for more than 4 days, will cause rebound congestion and consequent worsening of symptoms.

Surgical Intervention

Surgery sometimes becomes necessary in refractory cases.

STREPTOCOCCAL THROAT INFECTION/BACTERIAL PHARYNGITIS

Most cases of acute pharyngitis are commonly caused by viruses, but bacteria, when involved, need to be eradicated quickly with antibiotics. The normal oral flora contains α-hemolytic streptococcus, also called **streptococcus viridans**. Group A β-hemolytic streptococcus (GABHS), an invading bacterium, is the organism associated with causing streptococcal infection of the throat, or streptococcal pharyngitis, and it should be recognized and treated immediately.

Symptoms and Signs of Streptococcal Throat Infection

Symptoms and signs of streptococcal throat infection include fever, muscle aches and pains (myalgia), dysphagia (difficulty swallowing), lack of cough, swollen and painful anterior cervical lymph nodes in the neck, and tonsillar exudates. The watery eyes and runny nose that typically occur with viral pharyngitis do not occur with bacterial pharyngitis.

Streptococcal Pharyngitis Diagnosis

Streptococcal pharyngitis diagnosis is confirmed with a rapid antigen detection test (RADT) and/or a throat culture.

The Rapid Antigen Detection Test (RADT)

The RADT detects the presence of group A streptococcal carbohydrate on a throat swab, and the result is obtained in 5–10 minutes. A positive RADT confirms the presence of streptococcal pharyngitis. The validity of a negative RADT must be confirmed with a follow-up throat culture when there is a high suspicion of streptococcal pharyngitis, because the RADT is less sensitive than the throat culture test. It is important to note that even in the presence of the rapid streptococcal antigen detection test, which is highly specific but lacking sensitivity, a throat culture should always be sent and the patient followed-up with 48-hours later. Be advised that immediate antibiotic therapy is warranted when GABHS acute pharyngitis is highly suspected and the patient has **no** cough.

Throat Culture Test

The culture of a throat swab on a sheep-blood agar plate is the standard test to document the presence of acute streptococcal pharyngitis. The throat culture provides results in 24–48 hours and it is 90–95% sensitive.

Streptococcal Pharyngitis Treatment

Treatment in the emergency room setting: Single-dose benzathine penicillin is recommended for GABHS pharyngitis or tonsillitis in the acute care/emergency room setting, clearly for compliance reasons. The recommended dosage is 600,000 units intramuscularly (IM) for patients weighing 27kg or less and 1,200,000 units for patients weighing more than 27kg.

    Treatment in practice setting:

1. **Non-penicillin sensitive patients:**
   a. **Pen VK or amoxicillin** adult dose: 500 mg bid × 10 days.
      Adolescent dose: 250 mg tid/qid × 10 days.
      Child dose: 250 mg bid/tid × 10 days.
      Treatment with Pen VK or amoxicillin must be given for **10 days.** The twice-daily dosing is as effective as the four-time daily dosing when oral penicillin is used, and it is given for a full 10-day course, which is necessary for eradication of the infection.
   b. **Amoxicillin extended-release tablets (Moxatag)**
      Adult dose: 775 mg Moxatag, once daily × 10 days with meal. Do not chew or crush the tablet.
      Note that Moxatag contains three formulations, one immediate-release and two delayed-release amoxicillin formulations.

2. **Penicillin allergy patients:** azythromycin (Zithromax), 500 mg on the first day, followed by 250 mg per day for the next 4 days. Treatment with azithromycin is provided for **5 days** only.

   Adjunct therapy: Steroids like dexamethasone, betamethasone, or prednisone have been shown in studies to shorten the clinical course of pharyngitis when co-administered with antibiotics as adjuvant therapy to prevent overwhelming bacteremia. Steroids are not recommended in patients who are pregnant or have a history of HIV, oral candidiasis, or ulcerative pharyngitis.

31

Asthma and Airway Emergencies: Assessment, Analysis, and Associated Dental Management Guidelines

ASTHMA

Asthma is a condition that is a consequence of an immune response. The airways become sensitive to allergens causing bronchial hyper-responsiveness and narrowing. Increased inflammation and increased mucus production during an asthma attack causes further narrowing of the airways. Wheezing, coughing, shortness of breath, chest tightness, and increased respiratory rate are the hallmark features of asthma. Patients with allergies and eczema have a higher predilection for asthma. IgE is produced in excess in these patients and IgE blocks the β_2 receptors, causing asthma.

Extrinsic Asthma

Allergy-associated asthma is labeled as **extrinsic asthma**. This type of asthma is more common in childhood and improves with age or disappears completely in adulthood. Extrinsic asthma can persist in adulthood, but it rarely progresses to COPD. COPD is less often associated with familial allergies or eczema and is more often associated with intrinsic asthma and smoking.

Intrinsic Asthma

Intrinsic asthma occurs in adulthood and it is often triggered by pulmonary infections. Intrinsic asthma often leads to COPD, and compared to asthma, COPD, in general, is less responsive to brochodilators.

Asthma Symptoms and Signs

Patients are usually symptomatic with asthma at night or during the early morning hours, but an anxious patient can have an asthma attack at any time when faced with stressful situations that act as triggers for the attack. During an asthma attack the

Dentist's Guide to Medical Conditions, Medications, and Complications, Second Edition. Kanchan M. Ganda.
© 2013 John Wiley & Sons, Inc. Published 2013 by John Wiley & Sons, Inc.

respiratory rate is increased, the expiration is prolonged, and the patient experiences tachycardia. Ronchi and wheezing are primarily heard on expiration initially, but with progressive worsening of the asthma, the ronchi and wheezing can be heard by auscultation in both the inspiration and expiration phases. The patient uses the accessory muscles of respiration and the sternocleidomastoid and scalene muscles of the neck to assist with the breathing and oxygenation. Asthma is also associated with a paradoxical pulse, wherein the pulse increases during expiration and decreases during inspiration.

Asthma can be intermittent or it can result in chronic respiratory impairment. The range of severity of asthma is determined by the frequency of asthma attacks and the number of attacks that occur at night or in the early hours of the morning.

Asthma Classification per the US National Heart, Lung, and Blood Institute

The four categories of asthma identified by the US National Heart, Lung, and Blood Institute (NHLBI) are mild intermittent, mild persistent, moderate persistent, and severe persistent. A severe asthma attack is a true emergency needing immediate attention because it can be associated with near closure of the airways and decreased oxygen supply to the vital organs. This is of particular concern in the patient with severe persistent asthma where the FEV_1 is <60%.

Asthma Etiological Factors

Common etiological factors causing asthma are:

- Viral infections, which are the leading cause for asthma attacks in children.
- Irritants, such as cigarette smoke and cold air.
- Allergens, such as dust and pollen.
- Exercise.
- Medications, such as β-blockers, aspirin, sulfites, penicillin, glaucoma medications, and NSAIDS.

Asthmatic patients often have allergies, and allergy-associated asthma most often begins in childhood.

ASTHMA DIAGNOSIS

Diagnosis of asthma is made as follows:

1. **History of asthma attack presentation features:** Presenting symptoms of asthma attacks are adequate in many cases where the presenting features are classic, as with extrinsic asthma starting in childhood and intrinsic asthma starting in adulthood.
2. **Spirometry:** Spirometry, as stated in Chapter 29, demonstrates the amount of air that the patient's lungs can take in and the rapidity with which the inhaled air can be thrown out by the patient. Narrowed, inflamed airways will show lower results. Spirometry can also be used to determine the extent of improvement in the airway status with medications, once treatment is instituted.
3. **Allergy testing:** Because allergens frequently cause asthma, patients are often subjected to allergy testing to determine the cause of asthma.
4. **Chest x-ray:** The chest x-rays determine if there is any other associated lung disease.

ASTHMA TREATMENT

The goal of asthma management should be such that the patient has good exercise capacity, has fewer attacks, and is less dependent on immediate-relief drugs, as much as possible. Asthma management is best achieved by:

- Elimination of the precipitating factors where possible, especially with allergens.
- Implementation of care by the patient immediately on recognizing the signs and symptoms of asthma.
- Medications.

The medications for the management of asthma can be categorized as:

- Immediate-relief medications.
- Medications for long-term control and prevention of asthma attacks.
- Asthma emergency treatment drugs.

Immediate-Relief Medications

Short-acting, inhaled β_2 agonist bronchodilators (metaproterenol, albuterol, terbutaline, and pirbutrol) are the preferred quick-relief medications that open up the airways and bring relief within minutes of using the inhaler.

Patients should always carry their bronchodilator with them and use it immediately when becoming symptomatic. An early addition of corticosteroid inhalants with the β_2 agonist can often show an arrest in the progression of asthma.

Occasionally, the β_2 agonist bronchodilators can cause an increased heart rate or an increased BP at higher doses. When this happens, ipratropium bromide, an anticholinergic medication, can be used instead because the drug has no cardiac side effects. The disadvantage, however, is that ipratropium bromide is not immediate in action and is not as effective as the β_2 agonist.

Medications for Long-Term Control and Prevention of Asthma Attacks

Medications for long-term control and prevention of asthma are taken daily (Table 31.1). To become optimally effective they need to be taken for weeks. Be aware that the long-acting inhalers are slow in action, so the short-acting inhalers may have to be used during an asthma attack.

Inhaled glucocorticoids (beclomethasone, triamcinolone), long-acting β_2 agonists (salmeterol, albuteral SR), mast-cell stabilizers (cromolyn), leukotreine modifiers (zafirlukast), anticholinergics (ipratropium bromide), and methylxanthines (theophylline, aminophylline) provide long-term control and prevention of asthma attacks. Methylxanthines are often added when inhaled steroids and the other long-acting β agonists have not provided adequate control.

Asthma Emergency Treatment Drugs

When the patient's own medications are not as effective during an asthma attack, other medications or measures such as short-acting β_2 agonists, systemic steroids, methylxanthines, and oxygen are used.

Table 31.1. Asthma Medications

Drug Class:	Drug Name: Generic (Trade)	Comments:
Inhaled selective β₂ adrenergic agonists:	– Metaproterenol (Alupent) – Albuterol (Ventolin or Proventil) – Terbutaline (Brethaire) – Pirbutrol (Maxair) – Salmeterol (Serevent)	• Serevent is a much better B₂ selective agent. It is a long-acting drug that has a slow onset of action. • However, Serevent is **not** advised for the management of an acute asthma attack.
Anti-inflammatory drugs: Corticosteroids	**Inhaled steroids:** – Triamcinolone (Azmacort) – Beclomethasone (Beclovent or Vanceril) – Flunisolide (Aerobid or Nasalide) – Budesonide (Rhinocort) – Fluticasone (Flonase)	• Inhaled steroids are not systemically absorbed and you **do not** need to follow the "rule of twos" with inhaled steroids. • Inhaled steroids can cause candida infection affecting the palate.
Oral Steroids	– Prednisone – Prednisolone – Dexamethasone	• Prednisone is most often used. • Dexamethasone is the longest acting steroid with frequent systemic side effects.
Injectible Steroids:	– Hydrocortisone sodium succinate (Solucortef)	• Reserved for very severe attacks.
Methyl-Xanthines:	– Theophylline (Theodur/Theobid) – Aminophylline – Oxtriphylline (Choledyl)	• Theodur has a very narrow therapeutic index. Toxicity occurs with caffeine, chocolate, epinephrine, macrolides, quinolones, or cimetidine. • Signs and symptoms of Theophylline toxicity: The patient is agitated and the pulse becomes very rapid and fluttery. • Aminophylline is the injectible form of Theophylline.
Mast Cell Stabilizers:	– Cromolyn sodium (Intal) – Nidocromil (Tilade)	• Prevent allergic rhinitis and asthma by decreasing histamine release from mast cells. • **Not** used for acute asthma attack.
Leukotriene Receptor Antagonists:	– Zafirlucast (Accolate) – Monteleukast sodium (Singulair)	• Prevent Leukotriene release from mast cells, eosinophils, and basophils. • Leukotrienes cause bronchial smooth muscle contraction. • Avoid Macrolides because they decrease drug bioavailability.
Lipoxygenase Inhibitors:	– Zileuton (Zyflo)	• These drugs inhibit Leukotriene formation • Used for asthma prevention, **not** to treat an acute attack.
Muscarinic Antagonists:	– Ipratropium bromide (Atrovent) – Tiotropium (Spireva)	• They inhibit acetylcholine released from parasympathetic nerve terminals. Acetylcholine causes bronchial smooth muscle contraction.
Combination Drugs:	– Salbutamol + – Beclomethasone (Aerocort) – A steroid, Fluticasone + Salmeterol, a selective β₂ Agonist (Advair)	

Asthma Management

Asthma management is a two-tiered process: pharmacologic and nonpharmacologic.

Pharmacological Management of Asthma

- Inhaled corticosteroids (ICS), alone or in combination with long-acting β_2 agonists (LABAs), are the first-choice drugs for the management of asthma.
- Leukotriene receptor antagonists (LTRA), theophylline, oral corticosteroids (OCS), or omalizumab are second-choice drugs.

Nonpharmacological Management of Asthma

- **Patient education:** Educational activities have reduced asthma-associated disability.
- **Self-management:** Assessment of control by the patient and single-inhaled maintenance and reliever therapy (SMART) has been clearly beneficial.

Other Treatment Facts

- The newest drugs for asthma are the leukotriene receptor antagonists (LTRA), and they have a complementary effect to the ICS.
- The anti-IgE monoclonal antibody drug omalizumab is prescribed to patients with severe allergies who are not responding adequately to the currently available therapies.
- Asthma exacerbations are commonly treated with a short course of systemic corticosteroids along with an increase in bronchodilators.
- In patients with uncontrolled asthma due to the high inflammatory "drive" not controlled by high-dose ICS and a combination of bronchodilators (LABA, theophylline, and tiotropium), continuous or intermittent short bursts of oral corticosteroids are required. In these patients, omalizumab may be used, but omalizumab's prescription is limited by the allergic component and the serum IgE level.
- Theophylline is metabolized by N-demethylation and 8-hydroxylation. CYP1A2 is involved with the N-demethylation and 8-hydroxylation of theophylline, whereas CYP3A4 only plays a role in 8-hydroxylation process. The well-known interaction of macrolide antibiotics with theophylline occurs due to the inhibition of CYP1A2 and CYP3A4 by macrolides.
- Interactions of macrolides with theophylline are fairly well documented. In most studies, erythromycin and clarithromycin decreased theophylline clearance by 20–25% after 7 days of concomitant administration. The interaction is most likely to occur in patients receiving relatively high dosages and in patients receiving prolonged therapy.

Biological Treatments for Asthma

- Two cytokines are showing great promise in asthma management: IL-5, which is involved in eosinophil maturation, recruitment, and activation; and IL-13, which is strongly involved in many cellular responses relevant to asthma.

- Mepolizumab is a very specific monoclonal antibody directed toward IL-5. It has shown excellent results in asthmatic patients with severe eosinophilic uncontrolled asthma.
- The anti-IL-13 monoclonal antibody lebrikizumab has been found to attenuate both the early and the late airway response to allergens. It is effective in improving pulmonary function in severe asthmatics, particularly in patients with a high serum osteopontin level.

Recent Advances in Inhaled Corticosteroids (ICS)

- ICS have shown to be superior to any other new drug category, as far as disease control is concerned. Several major advances in the use of ICS in asthma have occurred.
- The first advance is the availability of the new ICS ciclesonide, which is activated locally in the lower airways with very low systemic absorption. Thus, there is negligible risk of local or systemic side effects, even for long-term, high-dose treatment.
- The second advance is the improvement in drug delivery. ICS are now delivered as metered dose inhalers, which reach the smaller airways more effectively; this is especially important in the more severe asthmatics.
- The third advance is the development of the "single-inhaler maintenance and reliever therapy." The idea is the "as-needed" use of a single inhaler containing a rapid-onset bronchodilator (e.g., formoterol) and an ICS (e.g., budesonide) at the time of the occurrence of asthma symptoms. This allows the delivery of higher doses of ICS at the very start of an asthma attack, thus preventing the need for oral corticosteroids or hospitalization. The single-inhaler maintenance and reliever therapy strategy has been shown to significantly reduce the number and the severity of acute asthma exacerbations in addition to maintaining good asthma control.

Additional Asthma Facts

As previously discussed, inhaled corticosteroids are the most common long-term control medications that decrease inflammation and airway swelling, especially in the mild, moderate, or severe persistent asthma patients. They are generally safe when used as directed but can cause **oral candidiasis** in the area of the roof of the mouth. This can be prevented by having the patient **rinse** the mouth after inhaler use.

Short-acting inhalants **are needed** to control an attack in patients using the long-acting inhalers. Patients suffering from severe asthma often use handheld peak flow meters to estimate the effectiveness of their medications.

Combinations of inhaled steroids and the long-acting β_2 agonists (Fluticasone + Salmeterol/Advair) have recently become available and are often being prescribed.

ASTHMA-ASSOCIATED SUGGESTED DENTAL GUIDELINES

The following are dental guidelines for asthma:

1. Question the patient about what triggers the asthma attacks and be aware that 95% of attacks are stress-related. Provide stress management if needed.
2. Have the patient use a puff of their bronchodilator prior to treatment as an alternate to stress management, particularly in the ASA III and IV patient.

3. Confirm the medications used for asthma management and have the patient bring the inhalers to the dental office.
4. Evaluate the severity of the asthma and determine how quickly the medications are effective during an attack.
5. Avoid using antihistamines **during** an asthma attack because antihistamines cause mucus thickening, thereby worsening the asthma attack.
6. Aspirin, Indocin, NSAIDS (ibuprofen, Anaprox), penicillin, codeine, and morphine can frequently precipitate allergies and/or asthma attacks. Check if the patient has used these medications before without any adverse reactions. Use these drugs **only** if they have caused no reactions.
7. Determine if the patient has used oral or injectable corticosteroids for two weeks or longer in the past two years. You will have to follow "the rule of twos" for major dental surgery in such patients.
8. Treat the ASA III and IV patient in a semi-sitting position.

Local Anesthetics and Asthma

The following are local anesthetics used with asthma:

- **A well-controlled asthmatic (ASA I/II):** Use 2% lidocaine with epinephrine (Xylocaine) or 2% mepivacaine (Carbocaine) with 1:20,000 levonordefrin (NeoCobefrin), but use no more than 2 carpules.
- **Severe asthma (ASA III/IV):** Use 3% mepivacaine (Carbocaine) or 4% prilocaine HCL (Citanest plain) because epinephrine is contraindicated.

Analgesics and Asthma

Avoid narcotic analgesics in the ASA III and IV patient.

Oral Antibiotics and Asthma

Macrolides are contraindicated with the following:

1. **The β_2 adrenergic agonists:** Alupent, Proventil, Brethaire, Maxair, and Serevent
2. **The methylxanthines:** theophylline and aminophylline
3. **The leukotriene receptor antagonists:** Accolate and Singulair

Acute Airway Emergencies

See Chapter 9 for discussions on clinical features and management of acute asthma, hyperventilation syndrome, and foreign body obstruction.

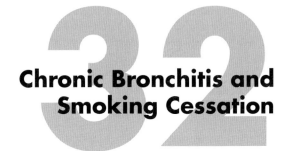

Chronic Bronchitis and Smoking Cessation

CHRONIC BRONCHITIS

Chronic bronchitis is a disease state wherein the patient has had cough with expectoration for **two to three months** of the year, for at least **two** successive years. This patient will give a history of using bronchodilators, antibiotics during flare-ups, and oral or injectable corticosteroids during exacerbation of the chronic bronchitis.

Chronic Bronchitis Treatment

Chronic bronchitis management consists of quitting smoking, using bronchodilators, and using corticosteroids to control or attenuate a flare-up.

Chronic Bronchitis Suggested Dental Guidelines

The following are dental guidelines for chronic bronchitis:

1. Follow the suggested dental and AAA guidelines as outlined for asthma, focusing on the specific bronchodilators used by the patient.
2. Follow "the rule of twos" if steroids were used for two weeks or longer within the past two years.

SMOKING CESSATION

Smoking Cessation treatment helps smokers overcome their nicotine addiction by providing tools, information, and support for people who want to quit smoking. Further outlined are smoking cessation facts, local and national smoking cessation efforts, the 5A cessation-counseling model, and smoking cessation prescription medications.

Dentist's Guide to Medical Conditions, Medications, and Complications, Second Edition. Kanchan M. Ganda.
© 2013 John Wiley & Sons, Inc. Published 2013 by John Wiley & Sons, Inc.

Smoking Cessation Facts

- According to analysis from the Centers for Disease Control and Prevention (CDC), tobacco use causes more deaths each year the world over compared with deaths resulting from human immunodeficiency virus (HIV), illicit drug or alcohol use, motor vehicle accidents, suicides, and murders combined.
- Most smokers have a difficult time quitting because they are addicted to nicotine. A smoker will often give a history of making several attempts to quit before achieving long-term success.
- Young adults are better served with e-health, Internet cessation interventions, because young adults are least likely to use cessation counseling and medications.
- The provider must show genuine interest in helping the patient to quit and must periodically remember to discuss cessation progress with the patient.
- Counseling and medication are each effective in increasing the incidence of smoking cessation, but when they are used together they are even more effective.
- FDA analysis recently concluded that menthol cigarette use results in lower rates of smoking cessation compared with nonmenthol cigarette use.
- The FDA also issued a warning against e-cigarettes (electronic cigarettes), stating that they "may contain ingredients that are known to be toxic to humans, and may contain other ingredients that may not be safe." Electronic cigarettes are handheld nicotine-delivery devices that use a rechargeable battery-operated heating element to vaporize nicotine that comes in a replaceable cartridge.

Local and National Smoking Cessation Efforts

- There is a site (http://www.cdc.gov/tobacco/quit_smoking/) that provides resources such as quit tips, quit plans, and educational materials that support efforts to quit smoking.
- All states now have a cessation quit-line that can be accessed through a national toll-free number (1-800-QUIT NOW). Providers should refer their patients to the quit-lines so the patients can have access to all steps in the recommended 5A cessation-counseling model. Quit-lines are an effective cessation tool with diverse populations.

The recommended 5A cessation-counseling model:

1. 1. Ask about tobacco use.
2. Advise the patient to quit.
3. Assess willingness of the patient to quit.
4. Assist in the quit attempt.
5. Arrange for a follow-up.

- State health departments are offering nicotine patches for smoking cessation.
- Many establishments are now implementing tobacco-free campus policies in health-care settings and workplaces.
- Medicaid and Medicare now cover smoking cessation counseling for all members.
- National initiatives have been implemented in the United States to quit smoking and more will be implemented soon. The 2010 Patient Protection and Affordable Care Act requires state Medicaid programs to provide cessation coverage to pregnant

Medicaid enrollees at no cost. Per legislation effective January 1, 2014, state Medicaid programs will not be allowed to exclude from Medicaid drug coverage FDA-approved smoking-cessation medications, including the OTC medications. The legislation has already required private health plans to offer cessation coverage at no cost, and health plans are now providing coverage for smoking cessation treatments.

- Under the Centers for Medicare and Medicaid Services electronic health record (EHR) incentive program, participating providers and hospitals must identify a patient's smoking status, and health-care providers also must implement clinical quality measures on tobacco use assessment and intervention.
- The Million Hearts initiative of the US Department of Health and Human Services is another initiative that has made smoking prevention and cessation in communities and health-care systems a priority.

Smoking Risks

- Smoking causes an increased risk of stroke, is responsible for 85% of all lung cancers and cases of chronic obstructive lung disease (COPD), and increases the risk of a number of other cancers and medical disorders. The risk for heart disease is cut by half one year after quitting, and the risk of developing lung cancer also decreases by almost 50% ten years after smoking cessation.
- Secondhand smoke also increases the risk of cancers, heart disease, and lung disease. Secondhand smoke or smoking while pregnant can lead to children with low birth weight, sudden infant death syndrome (SIDS), and serious childhood respiratory diseases, including childhood asthma.

Smoking Cessation Benefits

- The patient feels less fatigued and the extreme shortness of breath previously experienced while exercising disappears once the patient quits smoking.
- With quitting, the levels of carbon monoxide in the blood decrease, the level of oxygen increases toward normal, and the chronic smoker's cough starts to dissipate.
- Smoking cessation causes a drop in blood pressure, the heart rate decreases, and there is a decrease in the risk for myocardial infarction.
- Smokers with comorbidities who quit smoking recover better and live longer than those who continue to smoke.
- Other benefits of quitting smoking include being able to taste and smell food better, having better breath, having younger-looking skin, and not smelling smoke in your surroundings.

Smoking Cessation Steps

Smoking cessation is a process that involves an action plan, counseling, and medication.

Action Plan

The patient should develop an action plan and do the following:

- Draw up a list of the benefits of quitting and read it throughout the process and beyond.

- Identify "triggers" for smoking and activities that bring joy, so the patient can indulge in joyful activities to replace smoking, especially when the urge to smoke arises.
- Avoid smoking triggers or activities that promoted smoking and find ways to face the triggers without smoking.
- Avoid carrying matches, a lighter, pipe, or cigarettes.
- Each day, delay lighting the first cigarette by one hour. By delaying each cigarette, the patient takes control.
- Instead of smoking, start exercising to relax and feel good.
- Enlist the help of a friend or family member, a provider, or someone who wants to quit smoking alongside the patient.
- The patient may quit "cold turkey" or gradually. It takes several attempts for the patient to quit. The patient who has made several attempts to quit is more likely to eventually succeed.
- Alert the patient that during treatment, he or she may experience withdrawal symptoms, such as an increase in appetite; irritability, restlessness, mild depression, or anxiety; difficulty concentrating and falling asleep; and coughing frequently. The withdrawal symptoms gradually subside in 3-4 days, and the more times the patient has attempted to quit, the more the patient knows what to expect during the first few days of quitting.

Counseling

- Research has shown that the most effective quitting strategies are ones that address both the physical and psychological aspects of nicotine dependence. Therefore, using support groups or counseling and smoking cessation medications definitely improves the chances of quitting forever.
- Individual counseling programs can range from brief advice and counseling offered by a health-care professional, to intensive individual counseling available through specialty clinics for smoking cessation or through telephone help-lines.
- Group support programs led by qualified health professionals tend to be more effective and are one of the most successful methods for quitting smoking. Support groups run by national or state voluntary health agencies, public health departments, community health centers, hospitals, or licensed health-care providers are credible and are based on sound scientific and medical recommendations.
- Individual, group, and telephone counseling are effective in helping smokers quit.

Medications

- Advice from a health-care professional increases the amount of quit attempts and the use of effective medications, which can then increase the rates of successful cessation.
- The majority of smoking cessation medications are easily available over the counter. Their use increases long-term smoking abstinence rates, and medications are more often advised by providers compared with counseling.
- Medications can help reduce withdrawal symptoms associated with smoking cessation.

- The provider must assess the patient for associated health issues prior to recommending nicotine replacement therapy, particularly when evaluating the patient for any associated cardiac issues.

SMOKING CESSATION NONPRESCRIPTION MEDICATIONS

Nicotine replacement therapy in the form of patch, gum, lozenge, or inhaler is the most common type of medication used and is easily available over the counter. Nicotine gum, patches, inhalers, or lozenges decrease cravings and ease withdrawal symptoms by providing the body with nicotine.

Nicotine Patches (Nicoderm CQ®/Habitrol)

- As an aid to nicotine replacement therapy (NRT), the patch allows nicotine to enter the bloodstream slowly through the skin.
- Patches are usually available in different strengths. The patient begins with a high dose of nicotine and gradually decreases to lower concentrations as the body adapts.
- **The recommended initial nicotine patch dosage for patients who smoke more than ten cigarettes per day:** Start with one 21mg patch/day for weeks 1–6, followed by one 14mg patch/day for weeks 7 and 8, and, finally, one 7mg patch/day for weeks 9 and 10.
- **The recommended initial nicotine patch dosage for patients who smoke ten or fewer cigarettes per day, or for patients who weight less than 100lb:** Start with one 14mg patch/day for six weeks and then step down to one 7mg patch/day for two more weeks. **Treatment duration is only 8 weeks as opposed to 12 weeks for the heavier smoker.**
- The patch is applied firmly to a clean, dry, hairless part of the upper arm, and a new patch should be applied at the same time each day, but on a different site on the arm. Do not use a patch for more than 24 hours because it will cause irritation at the local site. If a dose is missed, a patch should be applied as soon as possible. If patch use causes insomnia, the patient can remove the patch before bedtime. Nicotine patches should not be used for more than eight weeks at a stretch.
- The patient should not use tobacco products in any form while on the patch, and the patch use is contraindicated during pregnancy and breast-feeding.

Nicotine Gum (Nicorette)

- Nicotine gum works differently compared to nicotine patches, which deliver nicotine slowly and steadily throughout the day. The patient can chew the gum whenever the urge to smoke arises and the nicotine is absorbed through the buccal mucosa. Patients find it convenient because it gives them something to do, and this act takes their minds off smoking. Over time, the patient chews fewer pieces of the gum as the craving for nicotine begins to decline. Nicotine gum is used for 12 weeks maximum.
- **The 4mg nicotine gum is recommended if the patient smokes more than 25 cigarettes per day, and the 2mg nicotine gum is recommended if the patient smokes fewer than 25 cigarettes per day.** The patient chews the gum until tingling begins and then the patient stops chewing and holds the gum between the cheek

and gum until the tingling effect disappears. Then the chewing process should begin again to trigger tingling; this stop-and-start process can continue for 30 minutes. The patient uses 1 piece every 1–2 hours during weeks 1–6; 1 piece every 2–4 hours during weeks 7–9; and 1 piece every 4–8 hours during weeks 10–12. Do not use more than 24 pieces in one day and do not eat or drink 15 minutes prior to chewing and during chewing because the chances of quitting are otherwise decreased.

Nicotine Lozenge (Commit)

- Studies show that the nicotine lozenge is as effective as other NRTs when used as directed and absorption occurs through the oral mucosa. Nicotine lozenges are similar to nicotine gum and can be used by patients that are unable to chew or those who prefer not to chew.
- The nicotine lozenge delivers nicotine to the brain more quickly than the patch, making it easier to match the dosage according to need. The lozenge comes in two strengths, 2mg and 4mg. **The 2mg strength is advised if the patient smokes the first cigarette more then 30 minutes after waking up and the 4mg strength is advised if the patient smokes the first cigarette within 30 minutes after waking up.**
- The patient has to let the lozenge dissolve in the mouth. The patient chooses when to use the lozenge and the number of lozenges used gradually declines as the craving for nicotine decreases.
- One lozenge is a single "dose," and the patient should not use more than 20 lozenges per day. Typically, the patient uses 9 lozenges per day for the first 6 weeks, and the patient should not use the lozenge for more than 12 weeks total. The patient should not eat or drink 15 minutes before using the lozenge or during use.
- The most common side effects of lozenge use are soreness of the teeth and gums, indigestion, and irritated throat. These side effects are usually short-lived. The patient should not bite into or chew the lozenge, as this will cause more nicotine to be swallowed quickly, which will result in indigestion and/or heartburn.

Nicotine Inhalers (Nicotrol)

- A nicotine metered-dose inhaler allows the patient to continue the hand-to-mouth smoking action until needed. Breathing through the inhaler provides the patient with the nicotine but without all the other harmful chemicals that come with cigarette smoking. The patient should stop smoking completely prior to using the nicotine inhaler.
- **The patient self-titrates according to needs and should not use more than 1 cartridge per hour.** Most patients typically use 6–16 cartridges/day via continuous, gentle puffing – similar to cigar or pipe smoking – for 20 minutes for a period of 12 weeks, followed by gradual reduction in the daily dose over the following 6–12 weeks. Advise the patient that the inhaler should not be puffed like a cigarette.

Nicotine Nasal Spray (Nicotrol NS)

- Nicotine nasal spray is also self-titrated by the patient. One squirt per nostril is equivalent to one dose, and the patient can use a maximum of 40 doses per day.

- The patient starts to taper the dose gradually in about 12 weeks and the maximum total duration of therapy is 6 months.
- Nasal irritation, coughing, sneezing, and teary eyes are common side effects.

SMOKING CESSATION PRESCRIPTION MEDICATIONS

Prescription medications help reduce withdrawal symptoms and may not be appropriate for all smokers.

Varenicline (Chantix)

- Varenicline is used along with education and counseling for smoking cessation.
- It should be avoided in patients with a history of allergies, as the drug can cause angioedema.
- It is also contraindicated in patients with a history of any form of mental illness because it has been known to cause agitation, hostility, and depressed mood; changes in behavior; and suicidal ideation. It has been associated with suicidal behavior in patients with or without a past history of psychiatric disease. The patient should stop taking the medication if such changes occur during therapy.
- It is also contraindicated in patients with a history of end-stage kidney disease because the drug is cleared through the kidneys, and 50% daily dose reduction is recommended in the presence of mild or moderate kidney disease. No dose adjustment is needed in the presence of liver disease.
- It is a partial agonist selective for $\alpha 4\beta 2$ nicotinic acetylcholine receptor subtypes and works by blocking the nicotine-associated pleasant effects in the brain. Varenicline also helps with cravings and withdrawal symptoms.
- Unlike nicotine replacement therapy, Varenicline is started while the patient is still smoking and has set a quit date to occur 1–2 weeks after the start of the medication; alternately, the patient can begin the drug and quit within 1–4 weeks of treatment. **Treatment is provided for 12 weeks.** It is best not to combine varenicline with other smoking-cessation therapies.
- **Varenicline prescription:** Varenicline is dispensed as a 0.5mg and 1mg tablet in three monthly packs/box/bottles. Recommended dose during the first week of therapy is as follows: days 1–3, 0.5mg once daily; and days 4–7, 0.5mg twice daily. Then, 1mg should be taken twice daily, from day 8 to the end of treatment at 12 weeks, with no tapering needed. An additional 12-week course is prescribed to successful quitters, to solidify long-term cessation. Unsuccessful patients should be encouraged to try again after relapse triggers have been eliminated.
- **Varenicline side effects:** Advise the patient that driving may be hazardous, as the drug causes drowsiness. Frequently, the drug can cause nausea, diarrhea, insomnia, and abnormal dreams, and, infrequently, xerostomia, oral ulcerations, anemia, thrombocytopenia, and leukocytosis.

Bupropion (Zyban or Wellbutrin)

- Sustained release bupropion as Zyban or Wellbutrin formulation is used for smoking cessation. The long-acting bupropion that is used to treat depression is not recommended for assistance with quitting.

- Bupropion, an antidepressant of the aminoketone class, is chemically unrelated to tricyclic, tetracyclic, selective serotonin reuptake inhibitors or other known antidepressant agents. Bupropion works by helping to control cravings and withdrawal symptoms.
- It is extensively metabolized by the CYP2B6 enzyme and is contraindicated in combination with drugs that are substrates, inducers, or inhibitors of the CYP2B6 enzyme. Bupropion is a potent CYP2D6 inhibitor and should not be used in combination with oxycodone or the prodrug analgesics codeine, hydrocodone, and tramadol.
- Bupropion is contraindicated in patients with a history of seizures, eating disorders, or any form of mental illness because it has been known to cause depression, hostility, agitation, suicidal ideation, or suicidal behavior in patients taking the drug for smoking cessation. The patient should stop taking the medication if these changes occur during therapy and contact the provider immediately.
- Bupropion is also started while the patient is still smoking and it should be used in combination with counseling.
- It can also be used in combination with nicotine replacement therapy to increase chances of success.
- **Bupropion prescription:** Bupropion is dispensed in 75mg- and 100mg-strength tablets. Bupropion can be dispensed in one of three ways:
  - Ideally, the patient should take bupropion 150mg each morning for up to 12 weeks, and an additional 12 weeks can be added, if needed. This option is better tolerated, has fewer side effects, and works well in the older patient wanting to quit.
  - Start with 150mg/day for three days and then switch to 150mg bid (with doses at least 8 hours apart).
  - Start with 100mg, bid (doses at least 8 hours apart) for the first three days, followed by 100mg tid. No dose tapering is needed with bupropion.
- Bupropion should be used with caution and dosed at 75mg/day in patients with mild or moderate liver/kidney disease. Bupropion is contraindicated in the presence of severe liver or kidney disease.
- **Bupropion side effects:** Bupropion causes stomatitis, bruxism, glossitis, dry mouth, constipation, insomnia, and seizures.

Emphysema: Assessment, Analysis, and Associated Dental Management Guidelines

EMPHYSEMA FACTS

Emphysema is a disease state associated with abnormal and permanent enlargement of the airspaces distal to the terminal bronchioles. There is destruction of the walls with or without fibrosis and loss of elastic recoil of the lungs.

The long-standing history of smoking, cough with expectoration, and progressive dyspnea are quite suggestive of emphysema, and spirometry clinches the diagnosis. Emphysema and chronic bronchitis, when present together, constitute COPD.

EMPHYSEMA TREATMENT

Treatment options for emphysema are:

- Quit smoking.
- Use bronchodilators.
- Oxygen therapy: intermittent or continuous low-flow oxygen is prescribed.
- Bronchodilators, oxygen, and theophylline form the mainstay of treatment for emphysema.
- Antibiotics are used to control and treat bouts of pulmonary infection.
- Pulmonary rehabilitation is used to improve breathing and oxygenation.
- Lung reduction surgery provides relief to some patients.
- Lung transplant is the ultimate choice when all else fails.

Note that inhaled corticosteroids do not work well in emphysema but they work extremely well in asthmatics.

Dentist's Guide to Medical Conditions, Medications, and Complications, Second Edition. Kanchan M. Ganda.
© 2013 John Wiley & Sons, Inc. Published 2013 by John Wiley & Sons, Inc.

EMPHYSEMA-ASSOCIATED SUGGESTED DENTAL GUIDELINES

The following are dental guidelines for emphysema:

1. Evaluate the PFTs to determine the severity of the disease and treat the patient in a semi-sitting position.
2. Follow the suggested dental and AAA guidelines as outlined for asthma, focusing on the specific bronchodilators used by the patient.
3. Follow "the rule of twos" to assess if steroids were used for two weeks or longer within the past two years.

Chronic Obstructive Pulmonary Disease: Assessment, Analysis, and Associated Dental Management Guidelines

Chronic obstructive pulmonary disease (COPD) is a disease state associated with irreversible pulmonary damage, progressive airflow limitation, partially obstructed airways, breathing difficulty, and an abnormal inflammatory response. In COPD, the alveoli lose their elasticity, which results in some areas with collapsed airways and some areas with hyperinflated airways. Alveolar damage causes poor air exchange. Additionally, excess mucus production by the mucus-producing cells causes thickening of the airways and the airway blockade. COPD is most prevalent in the elderly.

COPD is a disease state associated with emphysema and chronic bronchitis. Emphysema is associated with hyperinflated alveoli interspersed with alveoli that have been destroyed. Chronic bronchitis is associated with thickened inflamed airways. Therefore, frequent lung infections result in rapid progression toward COPD in such patients.

COPD ETIOLOGY

The etiological factors associated with COPD:

1. Smoking tobacco is the leading cause.
2. Inhaled irritants.
3. Genetic predisposition.

Familial COPD is often associated with α_1 antitrypsin deficiency. Alpha-1 antitrypsin inactivates destructive proteins, so lack of α_1 antitrypsin leads to destruction of the lungs and COPD.

Prevalence rates for COPD are directly related to tobacco smoking and indoor air pollution. COPD is characterized by progressive decline in respiratory function and health-related quality of life, with substantial risk for premature death. COPD affects the proximal and peripheral airways, lung parenchyma, and vasculature. Comorbidities, such as cardiovascular disease, diabetes mellitus, and depression, as well as associated systemic consequences including weight loss and muscle disease, increase the overall burden of disease.

Dentist's Guide to Medical Conditions, Medications, and Complications, Second Edition. Kanchan M. Ganda.
© 2013 John Wiley & Sons, Inc. Published 2013 by John Wiley & Sons, Inc.

The clinical course of COPD is viewed as a progressive decline in lung function over time, as assessed by forced expiratory volume in one-second (FEV_1) measurement. Recently, however, it has been suggested that disease progression depends on contributing phenotypes. Acute exacerbation of COPD is what leads to deterioration in lung function, particularly when this is complicated with acute respiratory failure. The frequency of exacerbations increases with decline in lung function. The patients with the most severe disease, especially the one with many comorbidities, is at risk of more severe attacks and is more likely to need hospital admission. With COPD, a progressive decline in airflow is associated with an abnormal inflammatory response of the lung to noxious particles or gases.

COPD SYMPTOMS AND SIGNS

COPD patients frequently experience shortness of breath on exertion and at rest, in addition to persistent cough with excessive expectoration, wheezing, and chest tightness.

COPD DIAGNOSIS

Diagnosis of COPD is made with the following information:

1. History: Typical history of presentation helps with the diagnosis.
2. Spirometry breathing tests: The spirometry test demonstrates the amount of air that the patient's lungs can take in and the rapidity with which the inhaled air can be thrown out by the patient. The FEV_1 is markedly decreased in these patients.
3. Chest x-ray: The chest x-ray shows the classic changes associated with chronic bronchitis and emphysema.
4. Arterial blood gases: Arterial blood gases show a decreased PO_2 and a normal/increased PCO_2.

COPD CLASSIFICATION

COPD can be classified as:

- Mild
- Moderate
- Severe
- Very Severe

Mild COPD

The patient may not yet be aware of the airway limitation, and it is detected only by spirometry, which shows mild airflow limitation. The PO_2 is close to 75 mmHg and the PCO_2 is normal at 35–45 mmHg.

Moderate COPD

Symptoms occur on exertion and this prompts the patient to seek help. Spirometry shows worsening of airflow. A moderate COPD patient has a PO_2 close to 60mmHg and the PCO_2 is normal.

Severe COPD

Symptoms and signs associated with COPD are present at rest. Spirometry shows severe airflow limitation. Heart or respiratory failure could occur in these patients. In severe COPD, the PO_2 is ≤ 50 mmHg and the PCO_2 is ≥ 50 mmHg.

Very Severe COPD

Very severe COPD is associated with highly significant airflow limitation associated with chronic respiratory failure, cor pulmonale, and/or eventual death. In very severe COPD the PO_2 is ≤ 50 mmHg and the PCO_2 is ≥ 50 mmHg.

COPD TREATMENT GOALS

Relief of the symptoms and signs, improvement in exercise tolerance, and slowing of the progression of the disease are the prime treatment goals. Treatment options include the following:

- **Smoking cessation**
- **Bronchodilators:** The short-acting bronchodilators are used for immediate effect that lasts for 4–6 hours. The long-acting bronchodilator effect lasts for 12 hours.
- **Inhaled steroids:** Steroids work by decreasing the airway inflammation.
- **Oral or injectable steroids:** These steroids provide additional support to decrease airway inflammation.
- **Oxygen**
- **Pulmonary Rehabilitation**

In asthma, inhaled corticosteroids are used up front as first-line therapy; however, this is not the case in COPD. In COPD, a LABA (long-acting beta-agonist) is used initially, and an inhaled corticosteroid is added to reduce the exacerbation rate in patients who are at increased risk, based on a history of two or more exacerbations in the past year.

The management of COPD as outlined includes pharmacologic therapy with new and old drugs, nonpharmacologic strategies that utilize pulmonary rehabilitation (PR), mechanical ventilation, and surgery.

Pharmacological Management of COPD

Medication choices for routine and management of chronic obstructive pulmonary disease (COPD):

First choice: long-acting β_2 agonists (LABA)/ long-acting antimuscarinic antagonists (LAMA).
Second choice: inhaled corticosteroids (ICS), theophylline, or roflumilast.

Nonpharmacological Management of COPD

- **Pulmonary rehabilitation (PR):** PR has a beneficial effect on symptoms and on quality of life. PR is recommended for symptomatic patients with an FEV_1 <50% predicted.
- **Oxygen therapy:** Continuous (more than 15 hours per day) long-term oxygen therapy (LTOT) increases hypoxemic COPD patient survival. LTOT is recommended in

patients with severe resting hypoxaemia (arterial oxygen tension and partial pressure of oxygen in the blood ≤55mmHg).

- Noninvasive positive-pressure ventilation (NPPV) or noninvasive mechanical ventilation (NIMV) are used in acute and chronic respiratory failure; NPPV assists ventilation by improving inspiratory flow rate, correcting hypoventilation, resting respiratory muscles, and resetting the central respiratory drive.
- **Surgery and transplantation:** During lung-volume reduction surgery in COPD patients with emphysema, selected areas of hyperinflated lungs are resected, and this improves exercise tolerance and prolongs life in selected patients.

Additional COPD Facts and Pharmacologic Treatment of Stable COPD

- Spirometry is a critical step in the accurate diagnosis of COPD, along with the collection/assessment of patient-reported outcomes and health status, including smoking history, occupation (past and present), daily symptoms (e.g., breathlessness, cough, and sputum production), activity limitation, and other disease manifestations.
- Regular treatment with bronchodilators and ICS induces significant and persistent improvement in airway quality, especially in patients with moderate severity of disease. Intermittent COPD symptoms can be treated with short-acting bronchodilators.
- **COPD maintenance drugs:** Inhaled anticholinergics (long-acting antimuscarinic antagonists – LAMAs), LABAs, inhaled LABA–ICS combinations, methylxanthines (e.g., theophylline), and short-acting bronchodilators and their combinations.
- Salbutamol, either alone or in combination with ipratropium, is usually reserved for use as rescue medication.
- For stable patients with respiratory symptoms and FEV$_1$ of between 60–80% predicted, inhaled bronchodilators may be used.
- For stable patients with respiratory symptoms and a FEV$_1$ <60% predicted, inhaled bronchodilators are recommended.
- For symptomatic patients with FEV$_1$ <60% predicted, monotherapy with either LAMAs or LABAs are prescribed. Specific monotherapy or combination inhaled therapies (LAMAs, LABAs, or ICS) for symptomatic patients with FEV1 <60% predicted may be prescribed.
- **Ultra-LABA drugs:** Indacaterol is a β_2 agonist with a very long duration of action (more than 24 hours) and it belongs to a new category of drugs called the ultra-LABA drugs. When compared to salbutamol, indacaterol induces rapid-onset and intense bronchodilation for up to 24 hours. Studies have shown it to be better than salmeterol or formoterol. This positive effect on FEV$_1$ results in a significant improvement in dyspnea, exercise capacity, quality of life, and a significant reduction in number of exacerbations, which is greater or similar to that seen with other long-acting bronchodilators. Indacaterol has the potential for being considered first choice among bronchodilators for the long-term pharmacologic treatment of COPD.

COPD Staging, Tests, Symptoms, and Treatment

- The Global Initiative for Obstructive Lung Disease (GOLD) divides the severity of COPD into four stages that are classified by spirometric measurement: mild, moderate, severe, and very severe.

- Using the GOLD criteria, a post-bronchodilator ratio of FEV_1/FVC less than 0.7 is currently the accepted diagnostic criterion for COPD.
- Once the diagnosis is confirmed, COPD severity is then based on the post-bronchodilator FEV_1. Severity of COPD-associated airflow obstruction is thus classified per GOLD spirometry criteria, as detailed in the next section.

Chronic Obstructive Pulmonary Disease (COPD) Staging

Stage I: Mild

FEV_1/FVC: <70%; FEV_1 ≥80% of predicted: 1,200mL (normal FEV_1: 1,500mL).

- The patient has mild airflow limitation and the forced expiratory volume in one second (FEV_1) is >80% of the predicted normal values, with an FEV_1/FVC <70%.
- The patient may not have COPD-related symptoms, or there could be a history of chronic cough and excessive mucus.
- The patient is on **short-acting** bronchodilators **only** at this stage.
- **Mild COPD blood gases:** The partial pressure of oxygen (PaO_2) is close to 75mmHg (normal PaO_2: 75–100mmHg), and the partial pressure of carbon dioxide ($PaCO_2$) is normal (normal $PaCO_2$: 38–42 mmHg).

Stage II: Moderate

FEV_1/FVC: <70%; FEV_1 50–79% of predicted: 750–1,200mL.

- During this stage, the patient starts to experience shortness of breath on exertion plus cough with expectoration.
- The FEV_1 is between 50–79% of the predicted normal values and the FEV_1/FVC is <70%. Most patients seek medical help during this stage.
- The patient is now on **short- and long-acting** bronchodilators.
- **Moderate COPD blood gases:** The PO_2 is <60mmHg and the PCO_2 is normal.

Stage III: Severe

FEV_1/FVC: <70%; FEV_1 30–49% of predicted: 450–750mL.

- Severe COPD is associated with severely impaired quality of life, significantly worsening airflow limitation, easy fatigue, and shortness of breath at rest.
- The FEV_1 is between 30–49% of the predicted normal value and the FEV_1/FVC is <70%.
- The patient is on **short- and long-acting** bronchodilators, **plus** inhaled and/or systemic **corticosteroids** during exacerbations.
- **Severe COPD blood gases:** The PO_2 is ≤50mmHg and the PCO_2 is ≥50mmHg.

Stage IV: Very Severe

FEV_1/FVC: <70%; FEV_1 <30% of predicted: <450mL, or FEV_1 <50% of predicted (<750mL), with chronic respiratory failure.

- Very severe COPD is associated with highly significant airflow limitation.
- The FEV_1 is less than 30% of predicted and the FEV_1/FVC is <70%.

- Stage IV is often associated with chronic respiratory failure, cor pulmonale, and/or eventual death.
- The patient is on short- and long-acting bronchodilators plus inhaled and/or systemic corticosteroid during exacerbations. Roflumilast, an oral, once-daily phosphodiesterase 4 (PDE 4) inhibitor, has also been shown to improve lung function during exacerbations in Stage III and IV patients. In the presence of respiratory failure, O_2 is added. Oxygen is given to counteract resting hypoxemia.

  Additionally, it is not uncommon for severe and very severe patients to be on daily 250mg azithromycin for one year to decrease exacerbations. **Dental alert:** Take this into consideration when prescribing an antibiotic to treat a dental infection. Match the static azithromycin with, for example, static clindamycin for management of the dental infection.
- **Very severe COPD blood gases:** The PO_2 is $\leq$50mmHg and the PCO_2 is at 50mmHg.

  The mainstay of COPD staging, tests, symptoms, and treatment are summarized in Table 34.1.

Table 34.1. COPD Staging, Tests, Symptoms, and Treatment

COPD Severity	$FEV_1 \div FVC$	FEV_1	Symptoms	Treatment
Mild or Stage I COPD Gases: **PO₂:** Close to 75mmHg **PCO₂:** Normal	<70%	>80% of predicted: 1,200mL (normal FEV_1: 1,500mL)	The patient may or may not be symptomatic	Stop smoking; short-acting broncho-dilators and flu vaccine
Moderate or Stage II COPD Gases: **PO₂:** <60mmHg **PCO₂:** Normal	<70%	50–79% of predicted: 750–1,200mL	The patient may or may not be symptomatic	Stop smoking; short- and long-acting β2-agonists (LABA)/ antimuscarinic antagonists (LAMA) bronchodilators; rehabilitation and flu vaccine
Severe or Stage III COPD Gases: **PO₂:** ≤50mmHg **PCO₂:** ≥50mmHg	<70%	30–49% of predicted: 450–750mL	The patient may or may not be symptomatic	Same as Stage II **plus** steroids in the presence of frequent infections, Theophylline or Roflumilast
Very Severe or Stage IV COPD Gases: **PO₂:** ≤50mmHg **PCO₂:** ≥50mmHg	<70%	<30% of predicted: <450mL or FEV1 <50% of predicted (<750mL), with chronic respiratory failure.	Respiratory and right heart failure are common	Same as Stage III **plus** oxygen for respiratory failure. It is not uncommon for severe and very severe patients to be on daily 250mg Azithromycin for one year, to decrease exacerbations

COPD Dental Alerts and Suggested Dental Guidelines

The following are dental alerts and guidelines for COPD:

1. The normal FEV_1 is 1.5 L. Patients with 50% reduction in FEV_1 experience shortness of breath (SOB) on exertion and patients with 75% reduction in FEV_1 experience SOB at rest.
2. In the COPD patient, hypoxia triggers the respiratory drive by stimulating the carotid chemoreceptors, which helps the patient breathe.
3. O_2 administered **during nonemergency** states can cause problems in the COPD patient's breathing because this will eliminate the hypoxic drive. Hypoventilation and CO_2 retention will occur.
4. However, during acute respiratory distress (ARD) when the PO_2 is further decreased and PCO_2 is elevated, O_2 should be given at a flow rate of 5–6 L/min to treat the worsening hypoxia. This is a true emergency and the oxygen is supplied until the emergency is corrected.
5. $O_2 + N_2O$ **cannot** be used for stress management in the COPD patient. If stress management becomes necessary, cautiously give low-dose lorazepam (Ativan) or diazepam (Valium) to a mild COPD patient only.
6. **Never** put the Stage II–IV COPD patient in a horizontal position, because the patient will experience significant orthopnea.
7. **Do not** use epinephrine or epinephrine cords in the COPD patient.
8. Often, the patients are using theophylline, aminophylline, and inhaled and/or oral steroids. Use the guidelines previously discussed.
9. Avoid aspirin, Indocin, NSAIDS, and penicillin if these drugs have caused allergies.
10. Check if the patient needs steroid supplementation for major dentistry when oral or injectable steroids have been used in the past two years.
11. Codeine, morphine, and other sedatives/hypnotics are contraindicated in the COPD patient because these drugs depress the respiratory center and will worsen the patient's breathing status.
12. Follow the antibiotic guidelines as outlined for asthma medications, depending on which anti-asthma drugs are being used in the COPD patient.

Obstructive Sleep Apnea: Assessment, Analysis, and Associated Dental Management Guidelines

OBSTRUCTIVE SLEEP APNEA FACTS

The patient with obstructive sleep apnea (OSA) experiences repetitive episodes of upper airway obstruction associated with a reduction in blood oxygen saturation and arousal from sleep. Apnea may occur hundreds of times nightly—one to two times per minute, especially in patients with severe OSA—and it is often accompanied by wide swings in heart rate and a precipitous decrease in oxygen saturation. The cardinal symptoms of sleep apnea include the "three S's": snoring, sleepiness, and a significant other's reports of sleep apnea. Additionally, morning headaches, excessive daytime sleepiness, and mood swings occur. OSA is more prevalent in men than women.

OSA is a very important diagnosis to consider because of its strong association with and potential cause of the most debilitating medical conditions: hypertension, cardiovascular disease, coronary artery disease, diabetes, depression, and sleepiness-related accidents.

OSA RISK FACTORS

Research indicates that both anatomic and neuromuscular factors are responsible for OSA. Obesity, male patient, snoring, craniofacial abnormalities, nasal obstruction, redundant soft palate, endocrine abnormalities, and family history are some of the common risk factors associated with OSA.

OSA TREATMENT

OSA treatment consists of the following:

- The patient must avoid alcohol or sedating medications and reduce weight.
- A dentally prepared mandibular advancement device can help with the management of OSA.
- Nasal continuous positive airway pressure (CPAP) helps keep the airway open.

Dentist's Guide to Medical Conditions, Medications, and Complications, Second Edition. Kanchan M. Ganda.
© 2013 John Wiley & Sons, Inc. Published 2013 by John Wiley & Sons, Inc.

OSA DENTAL ALERTS

- Thoroughly assess the health history for associated medical conditions and review laboratory tests to determine the control status of underlying disease states.
- Do a complete physical examination of the head and neck region to establish if the patient should be referred to temporomandibular dysfunction (TMD) and/or sleep specialists.
- Restrict the use of a rubber dam in significantly symptomatic OSA patients.
- Treat the patient in a semi-sitting position in the dental chair.
- Avoid the use of narcotics, sedatives, and hypnotics in significantly symptomatic OSA patients.

Tuberculosis: Assessment, Analysis, and Associated Dental Management Guidelines

TUBERCULOSIS EPIDEMIOLOGY

Mycobacterium tuberculosis (MTB) is an aerobic, acid-fast bacillus that usually affects the lungs. There has been an increased incidence of MTB secondary to HIV, homelessness, and emigration. Ninety percent of the adult cases of tuberculosis (TB) are due to reactivation of a dormant infection.

RISK FACTORS

Risk factors for TB are HIV; diabetes; prolonged steroid use; alcoholism; immunosuppressive treatment; and being a prisoner, nursing-home resident, or healthcare worker; and close contact with infectious patients, underweight patients, and persons from countries with a high TB prevalence.

TRANSMISSION

TB is spread from person to person through the air via coughed-infected droplets. Coughed-up, aerosolized particles stay around for a long time and infect susceptible individuals.

SYMPTOMS AND SIGNS

Symptoms and signs frequently associated with TB are fever, chest pain, chills, cough, weight loss, hemoptysis, night fever, night sweats, and fatigue.

Dentist's Guide to Medical Conditions, Medications, and Complications, Second Edition. Kanchan M. Ganda.
© 2013 John Wiley & Sons, Inc. Published 2013 by John Wiley & Sons, Inc.

Table 36.1.   Interpretation of a Positive TST PPD Reaction

Induration Size	At-Risk Populations
5mm induration:	**A 5mm reaction is positive in:** • An immune-compromised patient • A close contact of a patient with TB
10mm induration:	**A 10mm reaction is positive in:** • Recent migrant to the Unites States • An IV drug user • A patient less than 4 years old
15mm induration:	**A 15mm reaction is positive in**: • One with no known TB risk factors

DIAGNOSIS

The diagnosis of TB is made with:

1. **The Tuberculin skin test (TST):** The TST is done using purified protein derivative (PPD) from Mycobacterium tuberculosis. The PPD skin test is a delayed hypersensitivity reaction that shows response in 48–72 hours. The response is indicated by an induration or thickening at the site of the inoculum that is measured to identify if the reaction is positive or negative (Table 36.1).
2. **QuantiFERON TB Gold test (QFT-G):** The QFT-G is a new test for diagnosing latent M. tuberculosis infection. It is an in vitro diagnostic test that measures a component of cell-mediated immune reactivity to M. tuberculosis.

    The test is based on the quantification of interferon-gamma (IFN-γ) released from sensitized lymphocytes in whole blood incubated overnight with purified protein derivative (PPD) obtained from M. tuberculosis. The QFT-G can be used in place of the TST.
3. **Sputum smear and culture:** The bacteria, when cultured, can take 3–6 weeks to grow.
4. **Chest x-ray:** The chest x-ray can show hilar adenopathy, upper-lobe infiltrates, pleural effusion (especially in young patients), and calcifications. The chest x-ray is done if the PPD is positive. If the chest x-ray is abnormal, the patient is evaluated for active TB.

WHEN TO INITIATE TB TREATMENT

Treatment for TB should be initiated with the presence of a positive AFB smear or when there is a high clinical suspicion.

TYPES/FORMS OF TB

The three forms of TB are:

• Latent TB
• Active TB/Pulmonary TB
• Multidrug-Resistant (MDR) and Extensively Drug-Resistant (XDR) TB

Latent TB

With latent TB the patient has a positive skin test; negative chest x-ray; and no symptoms, signs, or physical findings of TB. The patient is treated to prevent future reactivation to the active form of TB.

Active TB/Pulmonary TB

A patient is said to have active/pulmonary TB when the patient has a positive skin test; the chest x-ray may be abnormal; the patient experiences fever, cough, night sweats, hemopytosis, anorexia, and weight loss; and the respiratory specimen smear test is positive.

Multidrug Resistant (MDR) and Extensively Drug-Resistant (XDR) TB

The four-drug standard regimen, or the first-line, anti-TB drugs, when used correctly can successfully treat TB. When these drugs are used incompletely, incorrectly, or not at all, multidrug-resistant TB (MDR-TB) can develop. Drug-resistant TB is a dangerous form of TB caused by the TB bacillus becoming resistant to at least isoniazid and rifampicin, the two most powerful anti-TB drugs. MDR-TB takes longer to treat with second-line drugs and the care is often expensive. Extensively drug-resistant tuberculosis (XDR-TB) develops when the second-line drugs are also incompletely or inappropriately used, such that they become ineffective. Treatment options for XDR-TB are even more restrictive and expensive because the patient has severe resistance to the first **and** second line of TB treatment.

Latent TB Treatment

New CDC guidelines for managing latent tuberculosis infection (LTBI): Tuberculosis can be prevented by treating latent Mycobacterium tuberculosis infection (LTBI). Studies have shown that a new combination of isoniazid (INH) and rifapentine (RPT) given once-per-week for 12 weeks, as directly observed therapy (DOT) to otherwise healthy people ages 12 and older who are at high risk for developing TB, is very effective in preventing TB. The new INH-RPT DOT regimen is beneficial for use in correctional institutions and homeless shelters.

Also, because the INH-RPT combination is given for a shorter duration, patients are more likely to complete this regimen than the nine months daily INH therapy without DOT. It should be noted that previous regimens recommended for treating LTBI are unchanged, and the rifampin-pyrazinamide (RIF-PZA) regimen is **not** recommended any more.

Healthy individuals who are at high risk for developing TB include anyone recently exposed to contagious TB; conversion from negative to positive TB skin test or a chest x-ray showing prior TB disease; and an otherwise healthy HIV patient not taking antiretrovirals if TB preventive treatment is indicated.

It is **not** recommended for children under age 2; pregnant patients or women planning to become pregnant; HIV-infected people taking antiretrovirals; and patients that have been exposed to TB disease that is resistant to isoniazide or rifapentine. The preferred regimen for children aged 2–11 years is the nine months of daily INH. If the patient is HIV-positive and has fibrotic lesions on the chest x-ray, INH is given for nine months.

Active TB/Pulmonary TB Treatment Regimens

Initial Phase

The initial phase therapy consists of rifampin, isoniazide, pyrazinamide, and ethambutol (RIPE) for two months.

Continuation Phase

The continuation phase therapy consists of four months INH/rifampin daily or twice/week of INH/rifampin for seven months. The multidrug approach is needed because of the high incidence of resistance.

PRECAUTIONS

Transmission of TB can be curtailed by using the following precautions: wash hands, sterilize instruments, disinfect surfaces, minimize splash/aerosols, and use approved masks.

TREATMENT GUIDELINES: DETAILED DISCUSSION

The United States Public Health Service (USPHS) and the Infectious Diseases Society of America (IDSA) develop treatment regimens.

Directly observed therapy (DOT) involves monitoring ingestion of each antituberculosis dose to maximize the completion of treatment. This is of particular benefit in the homeless, the drug-abusing population, or individuals with a poor drug-compliance history.

Each antituberculosis regimen has an initial phase of two months of treatment followed by a continuation phase of four or seven months. Isoniazide (INH), rifampin (RIF), ethambutol (EMB), and pyrazinamide (PZA) are considered the first-line drugs in the treatment of tuberculosis. The second-line drugs consist of cycloserine, ethionamide, streptomycin, and capromycin.

All *asymptomatic* patients with positive TST/PPD skin reactions (latent TB) should get preventive therapy with INH and pyridoxine (vitamin B_6) supplementation for six to nine months. As previously stated in the latent TB treatment discussion, the CDC now recommends a new combination of isoniazid (INH) and rifapentine (RPT) given once-per-week for 12 weeks, as directly observed therapy (DOT), to adults and children above age 12.

BCG vaccine is given to all newborns in developing countries where tuberculosis is endemic. It is given to attenuate an actual attack. A PPD skin test with an induration of ≥ 15 mm in a vaccinated individual warrants anti-TB treatment.

Without interruption, six months is the minimum duration of TB treatment. When interruption occurs because of missed doses or drug toxicity, the treatment should be completed in nine months.

In the **initial phase** of two months, the symptomatic patient (active TB) is treated with all four drugs: isoniazide (INH), rifampin (RIF), ethambutol (EMB), and pyrazinamide (PZA). Once the organism shows susceptibility on testing, EMB is discontinued. The **initial phase** may be given in one of three ways: daily for two months, daily for two weeks followed by twice weekly for six weeks, or thrice weekly for two months.

In the **continuation phase** there are three treatment options: daily, twice weekly, or three times weekly, by DOT. The four-months continuation phase is used for most patients.

INH and RIF are given for four months if the initial chest x-ray was positive **or** the sputum smear was positive at two months. If the initial cultures were negative and treatment with the four drugs was initiated for two months (resulting in improvement of the symptoms and signs or improvement of the chest x-ray at two months), INH and RIF can be given for two additional months to complete treatment as an alternate option. If the initial chest x-ray was positive **along with** a positive smear at two months, the patient is given an extended treatment for seven months. Therefore, extended treatment is recommended for patients with drug-susceptible tuberculosis who have cavitation on the chest x-ray and positive sputum cultures, after completion of two months of treatment.

The seven-month phase treatment is **also used** in those patients where PZA could not be used for the initial treatment because of liver problems or gout.

INH, RIF, and PZA can cause hepatitis. If hepatitis occurs, the drugs are stopped immediately for a short period. The medications are restarted once the hepatitis resolves. The physician routinely monitors liver, kidney, and platelet functions during anti-TB treatment. The dental practitioner **must always evaluate** these results **prior** to the start of dental treatment. If the patient has preexisting hepatitis, INH is avoided and the patient is given RIF, EMB, and PZA for six months. In the presence of severe liver disease, only one hepatotoxic anti-TB drug is used along with EMB. This patient is given RIF plus EMB for 12 months.

Gastrointestinal upsets are **common in the first few weeks** of treatment and they resolve progressively. The drugs can, however, be taken with food to minimize the gastrointestinal side effects.

Two drug combinations are approved in the United States:

1.   INH and RIF (Rifamate®)
2.   INH, RIF, and PZA (Rifater®)

Isoniazide (INH) Side Effects

Hepatotoxicity

Hepatotoxicity with enzyme elevations occurs in 10–20% of the patients. The hepatotoxicity is the worst in males around 40 years of age.

Peripheral Neuropathy

The neuropathy is dose-related and is uncommon at conventional doses. It is more common in the presence of conditions that predispose to neuropathy – for example, diabetes, HIV, renal failure, alcoholism, pregnancy, and breast-feeding. Pyridoxine (vitamin B_6)

supplementation is given to prevent this neuropathy. It typically causes circumoral tingling numbness and tingling numbness in the hands and feet.

Rifampin (RIF) Side Effects

The following are RIF side effects:

- Body-fluid discoloration: Orange discoloration of bodily fluids such as saliva, tears, sweat, and urine occurs.
- Cutaneous reactions: Pruritis with or without a rash can occur.
- Transient hepatotoxicity: Liver toxicity can occur and monitoring of LFTs is a requirement with anti-TB treatment.

Ethambutol (EMB) Side Effects

The following are EMB side effects:

- **Retrobulbar neuritis:** Retrobulbar neuritis that occurs is irreversible. It is dose-related and the risk is minimal with routine dose.
- **Peripheral neuritis:** Peripheral neuritis with ethambutol and INH are similar in presentation.

Pyrazinamide (PZA) Side Effects

PZA is associated with the following:

- Hepatotoxicity
- Gastrointestinal side effects: nausea and vomiting
- Non-gouty polyarthritis

DDIs Among Anti-TB Medications and AAAs Used in Dentistry

The following are DDIs among anti-TB medications and anesthetics, analgesics, and antibiotics:

- **Antibiotics:** The concentrations of clarithromycin, erythromycin, and doxycycline are **decreased** (thus becoming ineffective) by RIF because of the effect on the P4503A4 enzyme system. Rifampin is a CYP3A4 inducer drug.
- **Azole antifungals:** Rifampin appears to increase the metabolism of the azole antifungal. Fluconozole, however, can be used with increased doses.
- **Methadone:** Methadone levels are also negatively affected by the anti-TB medications.

SUGGESTED DENTAL GUIDELINES FOR TUBERCULOSIS

The following are dental guidelines for TB:

1. The nonsymptomatic TST/PPD skin test–positive patient does not transmit the disease. This patient needs preventative anti-TB treatment to prevent any **future**

reactivation with decreased immunity or when exposed to a symptomatic coughing patient or "open" case of tuberculosis. This patient can have routine dental treatment without any delay because the patient is not infective.

2. The **noncoughing symptomatic patient:** Within 2–4 weeks of the initial phase of anti-TB treatment, the bacterial count is negligible in the sputum **in most of the non-coughing symptomatic cases.** The patient can be treated in the dental setting subsequent to this time period, after obtaining clearance from the patient's physician.

3. **The symptomatic coughing patient:** The **symptomatic coughing patient** must complete the first **two months** of the initial phase treatment, start the continuation phase treatment, obtain a clearance from the physician, **and then** be scheduled for routine dentistry. Avoid the use of a high-speed hand-piece in the first month of dentistry in such patients, to avoid aerosolization of droplets into the environment.

4. Always consult and confirm with the patient's MD regarding the type of drug therapy recommended for your patient and the status of the disease.

5. Evaluate the liver function tests (LFTs), serum creatinine, complete blood count (CBC) with platelets, and WBC differential before initiating dental treatment.

6. Always use strict universal precautions when treating **all** patients and not just the TB patient.

7. Avoid all drugs metabolized by the liver to minimize added hepatotoxicity.

8. **TB and local anesthetics:** Use no more than two carpules of local anesthetics.

9. **TB and analgesics:** Avoid aspirin, NSAIDS, extra-strength acetaminophen (Tylenol), meperidine (Demerol), and propoxyphene (Darvon). Use regular-strength Tylenol or Tylenol #1–3 or Vicodin or Percocet for 2–3 days only.

10. **TB and antibiotics:** Avoid macrolides, ampicillin, tetracycline HCL, and metronidazole. Use penicillins, cephalosporins, and clindamycin when needed. Clindamycin can be used without dose alteration in the presence of a normal liver or hepatitis. Decrease the total daily dose by 50% in the presence of cirrhosis.

11. Mycobacterium avium intracellulare (MAI) and/or Mycobacterium kansassi (MK) occurs only in the HIV patient due to a dramatic reduction in immunity. The T_4 cell count is usually <200 cells/mm^3 when MK occurs. MAI is frequently seen with a T_4 count of 50cells/mm^3. Anti-TB management protocol for MAI and MK is the same as with MTB, as previously stated.

12. Aerosols pose a threat because of their ability to remain airborne and because they are small enough to reach the lower respiratory tract. Droplet nuclei, however, have been associated with transmission of Mycobacterium tuberculosis (TB). Patients who are known to have an active infection should not receive routine dental care in the dental office, because a higher level of respiratory protection is required during patient care. In treating the patient with active TB, among other precautions, the staff must participate in a respiratory protection program, receive annual training, and wear fit-tested N95 respirators because standard, surgical face masks do not protect against TB transmission.

VIII

Clinical Pharmacology

Prescribed and Nonprescribed Medications: Assessment, Analysis, and Associated Dental Management Guidelines

The following are medications that should be evaluated during patient assessment:

- Prescribed medications
- Over-the-counter (OTC) medications
- Drugs associated with or causing allergic reactions
- Corticosteroids (discussed in Chapter 40)
- Recreational drugs
- Herbal medications

PRESCRIBED MEDICATIONS

As discussed in Chapter 1, you must obtain a complete list of medications prescribed by the patient's physician and determine the DDIs with the anesthetics, analgesics, and antibiotics (AAAs) used in dentistry. The ideal way to assess prescribed medications is presented in Chapter 2, where digoxin (Lanoxin) and theophylline (TheoDur) are discussed.

OVER-THE-COUNTER MEDICATIONS

Review the history and determine the over-the-counter (OTC) medications the patient is taking.

Aspirin or NSAIDS

Aspirin permanently affects the platelet cyclo-oxygenase system causing decreased platelet cohesiveness. Always determine if the patient is taking the 81mg or the 325mg strength aspirin. Check with the patient's physician if either aspirin strength can be stopped temporarily prior to major dentistry. Physicians prefer not to stop aspirin intake in high risk for thrombosis patients, and in such situations, the dental provider must

Dentist's Guide to Medical Conditions, Medications, and Complications, Second Edition. Kanchan M. Ganda.
© 2013 John Wiley & Sons, Inc. Published 2013 by John Wiley & Sons, Inc.

control bleeding using local hemostatic materials. NSAIDS also affect the same system but the effect is temporary. The platelet function returns to normal once the NSAID has cleared the system.

Nasal Decongestants, Cough or Cold Preparations, and Appetite Suppressants

All these preparations contain sympathomimetic agents, epinephrine or neosynephrine. The epinephrine in local anesthetics can synergize with the sympathomimetic agents in these preparations and cause an epinephrine overdose-type reaction resulting in blood pressure elevation, especially if the patient is using the cough/cold preparations multiple times during the day. Obviously it is best to avoid routine dental treatment for the short term if the patient is too sick. However, if you have to treat the patient for a dental emergency, use 3% mepivacaine (Carbocaine) or 4% prilocaine HCL (Citanest Plain) instead.

Laxatives

Check for laxative use. Laxatives do not interfere with dental treatment when used in therapeutic doses. Do not prescribe codeine or other narcotic analgesics that cause constipation to a patient who is habitually on laxatives. Laxative overuse is not uncommon in patients with eating disorders, such as anorexia and bulimia. Laxative overuse or abuse can cause significant hypokalemia or low potassium level.

The normal serum potassium is 3.5–5.5 mEq/dL, and the patient becomes symptomatic in the presence of hypokalemia. Muscle cramps, muscle weakness, tingling numbness in the hands and feet, and irregular pulse can occur with hypokalemia. Do not give any local anesthetic during the hypokalemia state because cardiac arrhythmias could occur. Be aware that hypokalemia can also occur in a patient with a history of severe vomiting and/or diarrhea.

DRUGS CAUSING OR ASSOCIATED WITH ALLERGIES

Sulfites, bisulfites, sulpha antimicrobials, aspirin, NSAIDS, penicillins, cephalosporins, codeine, or morphine can all cause allergies, and you must determine the presence of an allergy history to these medications, before you begin any dental treatment.

Anaphylactic reactions can be mild, moderate, or severe. The longer it takes for reactions to occur, the better the prognosis. Acute reactions occur within the **first hour** of taking the drug. Most frequently, however, the reaction occurs within minutes after taking the drug.

Acute Anaphylactic Reaction

Anaphylaxis Diagnosis and Treatment

Anaphylaxis is highly likely when one of the following three criteria is fulfilled:

1. Sudden onset of an illness (within minutes to several hours), with involvement of the skin, mucosal tissue, or both. The patient can present with hives, itching, flushed feeling, and swollen lips, tongue, uvula, or floor of the mouth. The patient can have

a rash, sudden respiratory symptoms and signs, a sudden drop in the blood pressure, collapse, and incontinence. So in addition to the rash, the patient has to have either respiratory symptoms (SOB, wheezing, stridor, respiratory distress) or a sudden drop in the BP and associated collapse.

2. Two or more of the following symptoms and signs, as previously outlined, occurring suddenly within minutes to hours following exposure to a known or unknown allergen: sudden skin or mucosal symptoms and signs, sudden respiratory symptoms and signs, sudden drop in the BP, and sudden gastrointestinal symptoms resulting in abdominal cramping, abdominal pain, and/or vomiting.

3. The adult patient experiences a drop in the systolic blood pressure below 90mmHg or greater than 30% reduction of BP from baseline, within minutes to several hours, on exposure to a known/unknown allergen. Respiratory collapse is more common in infants and children than hypotension or shock, but when shock occurs, tachycardia precedes a drop in BP/hypotension.

Anaphylaxis Treatment Protocol

1. Assess the patient's ABCs, mental status, and skin.
2. Promptly call for help.
3. Place the patient in a lying down position, with the feet elevated. Do not allow the patient to suddenly sit or stand, as this will cause a sudden BP drop and collapse.
4. In the adult patient, inject 0.01mg/kg of 1:1,000 (1mg/mL) solution epinephrine intramuscularly in the middle of the thigh, anteriorly. The maximum dose for an adult is 0.5mg and the maximum dose for a child is 0.3mg. The dose can be repeated in 5–15 minutes and most patients respond to 1 or 2 doses. Epinephrine can also be injected IM by auto-injector.
   - **Auto-injector dosing:** for weight 10–25kg: inject 0.15mg epinephrine by auto-injector, IM in the anterior-lateral aspect of the thigh; for weight >25kg: inject 0.3mg epinephrine by auto-injector, IM in the anterior-lateral aspect of the thigh.
5. Provide 6–8L/minute oxygen by face mask or oropharyngeal airway.
6. When needed in the presence of sudden collapse, place the patient in recumbent position, with the lower extremities elevated. Establish an IV line and give 1–2 liters of 0.9% isotonic saline rapidly if patient presents with orthostatic hypotension, or there is incomplete response to IM epinephrine. Vasopressors other than epinephrine are given for treatment of refractory hypotension. Also when needed, perform CPR, following the C-A-B protocol for resuscitation.
7. Once stabilized with epinephrine, the patient is given the following medications for two to three days:
   - H_1 **antihistamine diphenhydramine (Benadryl):** 1–2mg/kg per dose; maximum 50mg IV or PO/oral. Be advised that the oral liquid is more readily absorbed than tablets. Alternative dosing may be used with a less sedating, second-generation antihistamine.
   - H_2 **antihistamine ranitidine (Zantac):** dosed at 1–2mg/kg per dose; maximum 75–150mg, PO/oral and IV.
   - **Prednisone:** 1mg/kg; maximum 60–80mg PO/oral or methylprednisolone: 1mg/kg; maximum 60–80mg IV.
8. β_2 **agonist albuterol:** Albuterol is used at the following metered-dose inhaler (MDI) dose; Children: 4–8 puffs; Adults: 8 puffs as adjuvant therapy.

Post-Anaphylaxis Treatment Guidelines

1. Identify and alert the patient about the allergen causing the acute anaphylaxis and make them aware of presenting features of an allergic reaction, how to avoid future exposure, and how to treat a reaction as soon as possible, should one occur.
2. Optimally manage any underlying asthma or allergy promoting diseases.
3. Have the patient see an allergist for desensitization, if possible.
4. The patient should wear an emergency alert bracelet or carry a wallet card.
5. Advise the patient about self-injection with epinephrine and to always carry an auto-injector EpiPen.
6. Should the patient have frequent episodes of allergic reaction to an unknown allergen, the physician may prescribe glucocorticoids and non-sedating H_1-antihistamine prophylaxis for two to three months. These drugs, alone or in combination, can be used as "premedication" drugs to prevent the risk of an acute reaction, especially if the patient has had non-specific symptoms thought to be allergy-related, or if the patient is unsure of the allergen or source of allergy.

Additional discussion of the clinical features and management of an acute anaphylactic reaction can be found in Chapter 9.

Mild or Moderate Anaphylaxis Reaction Management

When a patient experiences a milder form of anaphylactic reaction, the drug or preparation that caused a reaction is first discontinued. Then the patient is given diphenhydramine (Benadryl), 25–50 mg/tablet PO q6h for 48–72 hours.

For a mild reaction, 25 mg per dose is best, and for a moderate reaction 50 mg per dose is best. Warn the patient not to drive while on Benadryl because it causes drowsiness. Write a case note in the record that you have informed the patient about the drowsiness caused by Benadryl. Fexofenatidine (Allegra), loratadine (Claritin), and cetirizine (Zyrtec) are H_1 blockers that do not cause drowsiness. As an alternative, any one of these drugs can be used, and all these drugs are now available OTC.

Fexofenatidine (Allegra) dose: 60mg bid or 180mg once daily for two to three days. Fexofenatidine (Allegra) 60mg once daily for two to three days is recommended in patients with decreased renal function.

Loratidine (Claritin) dose: One 10mg tablet or 2tsp (10mg) of syrup, once daily for two to three days. Loratidine 10mg every other day for two to three days is recommended in patients with liver or renal insufficiency.

Cetirizine (Zyrtec) dose: One 10mg tablet once daily, for two to three days. Cetirizine (Zyrtec), 5mg once daily is recommended in patients with liver or renal insufficiency.

RECREATIONAL DRUGS

The patient could be using or abusing upper (stimulant) or downer (depressant) drugs that can interfere with dental treatment. Delay dental treatment in an intoxicated patient because this patient will not be cooperative during dentistry and the needle-stick; percutaneous injury with grave consequences can occur.

Uppers

Cocaine and amphetamines are considered uppers, or stimulant drugs. Their stimulant effects will synergize with the stimulant effect of epinephrine in local anesthetics.

Downers

Alcohol and marijuana are downers, or depressant drugs. They alter the potency of anti-seizure drugs and antidepressants. Alcohol hastens the utilization of local anesthetics. Ideally, the patient must be drug-free for 24 hours before you use a local anesthetic containing epinephrine.

HERBAL MEDICATIONS

Herbals can have harmful side effects that can interfere with surgery and anesthesia (Table 37.1). Herbal medications can act as powerful blood thinners that can inhibit

Table 37.1.   Common Herbals and Their Side Effects

Herbal Preparation	Side Effects and Drug-Drug Interactions (DDIs) with Anesthetics, Analgesics, and Antibiotics (AAAs)
Chamomile: **Garlic:** **Ginger:** **Gingko:**	• All these interfere with blood clotting and may cause pre/post-op. bleeding. Have the patient stop the herbals 7 days prior to surgery.
Echinacea:	• Inhibits wound healing by interfering with the immune function. Increases the risk of post-surgical infection. • Patient using this herbal may need antibiotics post-op. to promote healing. • Can alter the effectiveness of post-transplant immunosuppressant drugs.
Ephedra:	• Can cause abnormal heartbeat, extreme BP elevation, and coma when combined with some antidepressants and anesthesia. • Stop intake 7 days prior to surgery.
Ginseng:	• Can cause arrhythmias and can interact with epinephrine in the local anesthesia to trigger arrhythmias. • Can cause bleeding during and after surgery but no interference with clotting or local anesthetics with epinephrine, if stopped 7 days prior to surgery.
Kava:	• Interacts with sedatives, causing excessive drowsiness. Can interfere with anesthesia. • Must be stopped 7 days before surgery.
Licorice Herb: (not the candy)	• Can interfere with BP medications. • Stop intake 7 days prior to surgery.
St. John's Wort:	• Has DDIs with blood thinners and several cardiac and blood pressure medications. • Stopped 7 days prior to surgery.
Valerian Root:	• Causes excessive drowsiness with sedatives, can interfere with anesthesia. • Stop 7 days prior to surgery.

clotting. **All** herbal medications cause platelet dysfunction. Thus, it is important to stop all herbal medications at least seven days prior to major surgery.

Specific herbals that promote bleeding or drowsiness or cause cardiovascular side effects are of concern in any surgical setting. Ginkgo biloba, ginseng, and garlic are the "3 G" herbals, which, alone or in combination, have a potential antiplatelet effect and are problematic with prescription antiplatelet medications. St. John's wort is a potent CYP450 3A4 inducer, and there is potential for serotonin syndrome when St. John's wort is taken in combination with SSRIs.

IX

Endocrinology

Introduction to Endocrinology and Diabetes: Assessment, Analysis, and Associated Dental Management Guidelines

INTRODUCTION TO ENDOCRINOLOGY

The Endocrine System: Facts and Function

The endocrine system regulates and maintains responses to:

- Stress and injury
- Growth and development
- Absorption of nutrients
- Energy metabolism
- Water and electrolyte balance
- Reproduction, birth, and lactation

The glands associated with the endocrine system include the pituitary gland, the pineal gland, the hypothalamus, the thyroid gland, the parathyroid glands, the thymus, the adrenal glands, the gonads (the ovaries and testes), and the pancreas. The endocrine glands release hormones into the bloodstream that are meant to alter the metabolism of respective target organs by increasing or decreasing their activity.

The neuro-endocrine system is controlled by the hypothalamus. The hypothalamus sends messages to the pituitary gland. In turn, the pituitary gland releases hormones that regulate body functions through affects on the other endocrine glands.

The hypothalamic nuclei control endocrine function through three mechanisms: (1) direct neural connections, as in the case of the adrenal medulla; (2) **the release of hypothalamic hormones** (ADH and oxytocin are prime examples); and (3) **the production of releasing or inhibiting regulatory factors**. Releasing or inhibiting factors control secretory activities in the pituitary gland.

Releasing factors promote the release of TSH, ACTH, and the gonadotrophic hormones (LH and FSH). The factors involved are called thyroid hormone-releasing factor (TRF), corticotrophin-releasing factor (CRF), and gonadotrophin-releasing factor (GnRF).

Dentist's Guide to Medical Conditions, Medications, and Complications, Second Edition. Kanchan M. Ganda.
© 2013 John Wiley & Sons, Inc. Published 2013 by John Wiley & Sons, Inc.

Inhibiting factors control the release of prolactin and MSH. A releasing factor (GH-RF) and an inhibiting factor (GH-IF) regulate growth hormone secretion. A single releasing or inhibiting factor may have secondary effects on other endocrine cells in the pituitary.

Endocrine Hormone Categories

The hormones released fall into three basic categories:

- Amino acid derivatives (such as catecholamines, thyroid hormones, and melatonin)
- Peptides
- Steroids, which are derivatives of cholesterol

Homeostatic Feedback Mechanisms

Many of the endocrine glands are linked to the hypothalamus by positive or negative homeostatic feedback mechanisms. Most endocrine glands are under the control of negative feedback mechanisms, which decrease the deviation from an ideal normal value and are important in maintaining homeostasis. Regulation of the blood calcium level is a good negative feedback example. In positive feedback mechanisms, the original stimulus is promoted rather than negated. Oxytocin released during childbirth promotes uterine contractions and is a good example of a positive feedback mechanism.

Pituitary Gland

The pituitary gland has two lobes, an anterior lobe and a posterior lobe. The anterior lobe produces and secretes seven hormones in response to stimulation from the hypothalamus.

Anterior Pituitary Hormones

The anterior pituitary secretes the following hormones:

- **Thyroid-stimulating hormone (TSH):** TSH stimulates the release of thyroid hormones.
- **Adrenocorticotrophic hormone (ACTH):** ACTH stimulates the release of glucocorticoids.
- **Follicle-stimulating hormone (FSH):** FSH stimulates estrogen secretion and ova/egg development in females and sperm production in males.
- **Luteinizing hormone (interstitial cell-stimulating hormone; LH/ICSH):** LH/ICSH causes ovulation and progesterone production in women and androgen production in men.
- **Prolactin (PRL):** PRL stimulates the development of the mammary glands and the production of milk, mitosis, and the growth of body tissues.
- **Growth hormone (GH/somatotrophin):** GH stimulates cell growth and protein synthesis via the release of somatomedins by the liver. This stimulation occurs almost immediately, at a time when glucose and amino acid concentrations in the blood are elevated. A second effect appears hours later, as glucose and amino acid levels are declining. Under these conditions, GH causes the breakdown of glycogen and lipid

reserves and directs peripheral tissues to begin using lipids, instead of glucose, as an energy source. As a result, blood glucose concentrations rise. These effects appear through an interaction between growth hormone and somatomedins.

- **Melanocyte-stimulating hormone (MSH):** MSH stimulates the production of melanin in the skin.

TSH, ACTH, FSH, and LH hormones are tropic hormones that simulate other endocrine glands, and, in response, the other endocrine glands produce hormones that affect metabolism. For example, TSH from the pituitary gland stimulates the thyroid gland to produce thyroid hormones; in turn, thyroid hormones inhibit the release of calcium in the blood. ACTH acts on the cortex of the adrenal gland to produce steroid hormones. FSH and LH act in women and men by regulating various sexual characteristics. Prolactin acts on the breast tissue glands of nursing mothers, causing milk production.

Growth hormone (GH) stimulates protein synthesis and cell division in cartilage and bone tissue. Gigantism results when excessive amounts of growth hormone are produced during childhood. Pituitary dwarfism occurs when too little growth hormone is produced, and acromegaly occurs when too much GH is produced during adulthood.

Posterior Pituitary Hormones

The supraoptic and paraventricular nuclei of the hypothalamus produce antidiuretic hormone (ADH) and oxytocin. These hormones are released into the vasculature surrounding the posterior pituitary gland. ADH release occurs when the electrolyte concentration in the blood rises and when blood pressure or blood volume declines. ADH reduces the amount of water lost at the kidneys.

During the birthing process, oxytocin stimulates smooth muscle contractions in the uterus and mammary glands. The uterine action helps with labor, and mammary gland stimulation helps with milk production.

Patterns of Hormonal Interactions

The endocrine system functions as an integrated unit and hormones often interact. Two hormones may have antagonistic, synergistic, permissive, or integrative effects.

Hormones and Growth

Normal growth requires GH, TX, insulin, PTH, and gonadal steroids. As the hormonal concentrations change, so do growth patterns.

Hormones and Stress

Stresses of many different kinds can produce a characteristic response involving both the nervous and endocrine systems. This response is known as the general adaptation syndrome (GAS). There are three phases to the GAS: the alarm phase, the resistance phase, and the exhaustion phase.

The Alarm Phase

The alarm phase is predominately neural in origin and results from sympathetic activation. Epinephrine is the dominant hormone of the alarm phase. During the alarm phase, ADH and CRF are also released by the pituitary gland.

The Resistance Phase

During the resistance phase energy consumption remains elevated due to the production of glucocorticoids, epinephrine, growth hormone, glucagon, and thyroid hormones.

Glucocorticoids are the dominant hormones of the resistance phase. The goals of the resistance phase include mobilization of lipid and protein reserves, elevation and stabilization of blood glucose levels, and conservation of glucose for neural tissues.

The Exhaustion Phase

Exhaustion may result from a depletion of energy reserves, failure to produce the required hormones, or the collapse of one or more vital systems.

Hormones and Behavior

Many hormones affect the functional state of the nervous system producing alterations in mood, emotional states, and various other behaviors.

DIABETES OVERVIEW, FACTS, AND TESTS

Diabetes Overview

The pancreas, gut, and kidneys regularly play significant roles in glucose homeostasis. Consequently, dysfunction at all these levels occurs with diabetes. It is important to review the mechanisms involved to better understand the newer therapies that are targeting these specific areas in the management of diabetes.

The Pancreas

The pancreas contains exocrine and endocrine cell populations. The endocrine cells are found within the pancreatic islets, the islets of Langerhans. Alpha cells secrete glucagon, and β cells of the pancreas produce the anabolic storage hormone insulin. These hormones affect glucose metabolism in the body. Insulin lowers blood glucose by increasing the rates of glucose uptake and utilization in peripheral cells. Insulin plays a very important role in the metabolism of carbohydrates, proteins, and fats. Protein synthesis, fat deposition, and glycogen formation increase under insulin stimulation. Insulin enhances the conversion of glucose to glycogen, amino acids to proteins, and fatty acids to triglycerides. Absence of insulin causes elevated glucagon levels, muscle wasting, and high levels of acetoacetic acid and β hydroxybutyricacid in the blood. Excessive glucose (hyperglycemia) in the blood causes it to spill into the urine resulting in glycosuria and frequent urination.

Total lack of insulin leads to ketoacidosis. Insulin is produced and released in response to eating, in order to utilize the sugars and store excess amounts for use during starvation. Thus, in the fed state, insulin levels are high after eating.

Glucagon action is opposite to that of insulin. It elevates blood glucose by increasing the rates of glycogen breakdown and glucose production in the liver. Glucagon stimulates the release of fatty acids from adipose tissues and amino acids from skeletal muscles. It is important to know that the brain always gets glucose at all times, and it does not matter if the individual is in a fed state or is starving. In the extreme fasting state, glucagon levels rise and elevate blood glucose thus making it available to the brain. Therefore, alpha and beta cells monitor the glucose concentrations of the circulating blood.

Gut and Glucose Homeostasis

The gastrointestinal tract has a crucial role in the control of energy homeostasis through its role in the digestion, absorption, and assimilation of ingested nutrients. Enteroendocrine cells have important roles in regulating energy intake and glucose homeostasis through their actions on peripheral target organs, including the endocrine pancreas. After food ingestion, the digestion and absorption of nutrients is associated with increased secretion of multiple gut peptides that act on distant target sites to promote the efficient uptake and storage of energy. These peptide hormones are synthesized by specialized enteroendocrine cells located in the epithelium of the stomach, small bowel, and large bowel, and are secreted at low basal levels in the fasting state.

Plasma levels of most gut hormones rise rapidly within minutes of nutrient intake and fall quickly thereafter, mainly because they are cleared by the kidney and are enzymatically inactivated. Gut hormones activate neural circuits that communicate with peripheral organs, including the liver, muscle tissue, adipose tissue, and islets of Langerhans in the pancreas, to coordinate overall energy intake and assimilation. Gastrointestinal/incretin hormones such as glucose-dependent insulinotropic polypeptide (GIP) and glucagon-like peptide-1 (GLP1), which cause an increase in the amount of insulin released from the β cells of the islets, augment the magnitude of meal-stimulated insulin secretion from islet β cells in a glucose-dependent manner. Incretin action facilitates the uptake of glucose by muscle tissue and the liver while simultaneously suppressing glucagon secretion by the α cells of the islets, leading to reduced endogenous production of glucose from hepatic sources.

Kidneys and Glucose Homeostasis

The kidney also plays a significant role in maintaining glucose homeostasis. This includes functions such as release of glucose into the circulation via gluconeogenesis, uptake of glucose from the circulation for its own energy needs, and reabsorption of glucose at the level of the proximal tubule. Renal release of glucose into the circulation is the result of glycogenolysis and gluconeogenesis, respectively, involving the breaking down and formation of glucose-6-phosphate from precursors (for example, lactate, glycerol, and amino acids). With regard to renal reabsorption of glucose, the kidneys normally retrieve as much glucose as possible, rendering the urine virtually glucose free.

The glomeruli filter approximately 180g of D-glucose per day from plasma, all of which is reabsorbed through glucose transporter proteins that are present in cell membranes within the proximal tubules. If the capacity of these transporters is exceeded, glucose appears in the urine. Transporters that are active (sodium-coupled glucose co-transporters) and passive (glucose transporters) mediate the process of renal glucose reabsorption. In hyperglycemia, the kidneys may play an exacerbating role by reabsorbing excess glucose, ultimately contributing to chronic hyperglycemia, which in turn contributes to chronic glycemic burden and the risk of microvascular consequences.

Type 1 Diabetes

The exact etiology of type 1 diabetes is not known. Autoimmune attack on the β cells of the pancreas is thought to cause destruction of the cells and consequent lack of insulin production. An environmental stimulus, however, is the cause in most cases. The patients are usually younger, thin, and prone to ketosis, weight loss, and blackouts. Adults can get type I diabetes, as well.

Type 2 Diabetes

These patients have a combination of insulin resistance and insulin deficiency. Of diabetics encountered, 90% suffer from type 2 diabetes. Type 2 diabetes has a higher genetic predisposition compared to type 1 diabetes.

The patients are usually obese and older at the time of disease onset. However, this fact has changed with the obesity epidemic affecting populations globally. It is not uncommon now to encounter obese patients in their preteens, teens, or twenties who are suffering from type 2 diabetes.

Diabetes Symptoms and Signs

The following are symptoms and signs of diabetes:

- Polyuria (excessive urination), polydipsia (excessive thirst), and polyphagia (excessive appetite) are the hallmark symptoms associated with diabetes. Patients with type 1 experience these symptoms a lot more frequently compared to patients with type 2.
- It is not uncommon for these patients to experience weight loss, fatigue, and blurred vision due to elevated blood sugar levels.
- A history of weight loss is a lot more common in the type 1 patient than in the type 2 patient. The blurred vision is caused by adherence of sugar to the optic lens and changes in glycosylation of cornea and lens when sugars go rapidly up or down. The blurring of vision improves when sugar levels improve, with treatment.
- Poor wound healing and opportunistic infections occur with chronic elevation of the blood sugar values.

Diabetes Diagnostic Tests

Fasting Blood Sugar (FBS)

A diagnosis of diabetes is made when the fasting blood sugar (FBS) is $\geq$126 mg/dL. With treatment, the FBS should be maintained between 70–120 mg/dL. The FBS should be maintained >70 mg/dL to avoid severe hypoglycemia.

Impaired FBS

A patient is said to have **pre-diabetes** or impaired fasting glucose when the FBS is 100–125 mg/dL. The patient can normalize the impaired FBS sugar levels with stringent implementation of proper diet control and exercise.

Postprandial Blood Sugar (PPBS)

For optimal control, the PPBS, or the two-hour post-meal blood sugar, should be maintained between 120–160 mg/dL.

Random Blood Sugar

A diagnosis of diabetes is made when a random blood sugar is ≥200 mg/dL.

Oral Glucose Tolerance Test (OGTT)

The OGTT measures the patient's ability to utilize glucose in a laboratory setting. The patient's FBS is checked, and the patient is made to drink 75 g of glucose. The blood sugar levels are then monitored at half-hour intervals for two hours. The patient is said to be pre-diabetic if the blood sugar at two hours ranges between 140–199 mg/dL. Values >200 mg/dL definitely indicate diabetes.

HemoglobinA$_1$C (HbA$_1$C)

The normal reference range of HbA$_1$C is **4–5.9%**. Hemoglobin A in the RBCs combines with glucose, forming a glycated hemoglobin molecule, HbA$_1$C. The percentage of HbA that turns into HbA$_1$C increases as the blood glucose concentration increases. The HbA$_1$C percentage indicates the blood glucose level averaged over the half-life of red blood cells, which is typically 50–60 days. Poor diabetes control is associated with an elevated HbA$_1$C level, and effective treatment is associated with a declining HbA$_1$C level toward normal.

The American Diabetes Association states that for optimal control it is best to maintain the HbA$_1$C below 7%. The International Diabetes Federation and American College of Endocrinology, however, suggest that for optimal control the HbA$_1$C should be maintained below 6.5%.

Table 38.1 shows the American Diabetes Association recommended comparison list of the HbA$_1$C and the corresponding average blood sugar value. **Note** that all patients over age 45 should get screened for diabetes. Latinos, Native Americans, Asian Americans, Alaskans, and gestational diabetes patients should get screened earlier in life because they are all high-risk populations.

Table 38.1.   Comparison: HbA$_1$C and Average Blood Sugar Level

HbA$_1$C	Comparison to average blood sugar level
6% HbA$_1$C	Reflects an average blood sugar level of 120mg/dL
7% HbA$_1$C	Reflects an average blood sugar level of 150mg/dL
8% HbA$_1$C	Reflects an average blood sugar level of 180mg/dL
9% HbA$_1$C	Reflects an average blood sugar level of 210mg/dL

ACUTE MEDICAL EMERGENCIES ASSOCIATED WITH DIABETES

Hypoglycemia and hyperglycemic coma are the two acute complications associated with diabetes.

Hypoglycemia

Acute hypoglycemia reaction can occur in both the diabetic and the non-diabetic patient. The brain is completely dependent on the glucose supply for its energy requirements. When hypoglycemia occurs and the patient collapses, the brain can sustain itself for less than only three minutes. Hence treatment with juice, crackers, or glucola; IV D5, D10, or D50; or IM glucagon, has to be immediate in order to avoid brain damage or other negative consequences. Refer to Chapter 9 for a complete discussion on predisposing factors, clinical features, and the management of hypoglycemia.

Hyperglycemia

Diabetic ketoacidosis (DKA) and coma can occur because of infection, poor intake of medications, and other factors. Severe volume depletion and acetone breath is very apparent, along with the underlying precipitating factors. The patient must be sent to the emergency room where treatment is provided with fluids and insulin. Refer to Chapter 9 for a complete discussion on predisposing factors, clinical features, and the management of hyperglycemia.

CHRONIC MEDICAL COMPLICATIONS OF DIABETES

Microvascular Disease

Microvascular disease associated with retinopathy and nephropathy is specific for diabetes. Retinopathy is the leading cause of blindness and should be differentiated from the blurring of vision caused by excessive sugar attaching to the lens in the eyes. Diabetes accounts for 25% of all kidney failure and is the leading cause for dialysis, with many of these patients needing kidney transplants.

Retinopathy

High blood sugar increases the risk of eye problems, and diabetes is the leading cause of blindness in adults who are 20–74 years old. Elevated blood sugar in diabetes causes the lens of the eye to swell, causing vision impairment from early cataract formation. The three major eye problems that people with diabetes may develop are cataracts, glaucoma, and retinopathy. Symptoms experienced with eye problems include black spots in one's vision, flashes of light, "holes" in one's vision, and blurred vision.

Cataracts and Diabetes

Patients with diabetes get these eye problems at an earlier age and the conditions progress more rapidly than in people without diabetes. The diabetic patient experiences progressively blurring vision.

Glaucoma Overview: Open-Angle Versus Narrow-Angle

Diabetic or non-diabetic patients may present with a diagnosis of "open-angle" or "narrow-angle" glaucoma. The "angle" referenced is the angle between the iris and the cornea. In a normal-sized eye, the angle is "open" and the aqueous humor has uninterrupted access to the drainage pores of the trabecular meshwork at the outer periphery of the cornea.

Patients with open angles develop glaucoma because the trabecular meshwork pores become narrowed or plugged, and the exact etiology for this narrowing is unknown. This "open-angle" glaucoma accounts for about 90% of all glaucoma cases and it is treated with eye drops, laser, or microsurgery.

With open-angle glaucoma, there may be no symptoms until the disease is very advanced and there is significant vision loss. In the less-common form of this eye problem, symptoms can include headaches, eye aches, pain, blurred vision, watering eyes, halos around lights, and loss of vision.

A very small number of patients have eyes that are smaller than normal, resulting in farsightedness or hyperopia. In early life, the patient may need only glasses, but with the natural lens growing throughout life, it progressively pushes the iris forward. Thus, over time, there is less space between the iris and the cornea, and the angle becomes "narrow." When the angle narrows to the point where the iris actually touches the peripheral cornea, the iris then covers the trabecular meshwork like a drawn curtain. This causes the intraocular pressure to increase dramatically, resulting in an acute, angle-closure attack.

Hence dilating the pupil in patients with narrow-angle glaucoma can trigger an acute, angle-closure attack. The aqueous humor is produced behind the iris, so the pressure behind the iris is always slightly higher than it is in front of the iris. When the pupil is small, the iris is more stretched and flatter, but when the pupil is in mid-position, it is more flaccid and the aqueous produced behind the pupil pushes the iris forward, closing the angle. Narrow-angle glaucoma attacks typically occur when the pupil is in mid-position.

Glaucoma and Diabetes

Open-angle glaucoma treatment in diabetes can include eye drops, laser procedures, medications, or surgery. Surgery and laser treatments are directed at improving the aqueous drainage.

People with diabetes are also more likely to get an uncommon type of glaucoma, called neovascular glaucoma. In this form of glaucoma, new blood vessels grow on the iris. These blood vessels block the normal flow of fluid out of the eye, raising the intraoccular pressure. This type of glaucoma is difficult to treat. One option is laser surgery, which reduces the vessels.

Laser Iridotomy

When a hole is made in the iris by laser iridotomy, it equalizes the pressure, thus preventing the iris from ballooning forward. Most patients agree to the procedure to prevent the occurrence of severe pain and potential vision loss associated with an acute, angle-closure attack. Once the iridotomy is done, the eye can be safely dilated. Once a patient is diagnosed with narrow-angle glaucoma, laser iridotomy is immediately advised. This procedure is curative and the morbidity associated with it is extremely low. Dilating the pupil following the laser treatment has no effect on intraocular pressure.

Drugs that Dilate the Pupil

Drugs that potentially dilate the pupil are anticholinergics, antihistamines, anti-Parkinson's drugs, antipsychotics, anti-spasmolytics, monoamine oxidase inhibitors, sympathomimetics, and tricyclic antidepressants.

Dilating the pupil has little or no effect on patients with open-angle glaucoma. Pupil dilation warnings only apply to patients with narrow-angle glaucoma who do not know they have narrow angles or who have narrow-angle glaucoma and have not had laser iridotomy. Thus, these drugs can unmask narrow-angle glaucoma in asymptomatic individuals who would have later spontaneously presented with the disease.

Dental alert: Recent population-based studies indicate that the risk of precipitating narrow-angle glaucoma by pharmacological pupil dilation is extremely low in the general population, but it is higher in the Asian population. Acute angle closure occurs when the pupil is in the mid-dilated, rather than fully dilated, position, and it is well known that the pupil is in the mid-dilated position in dimly lit settings. Therefore, being in a darkened room poses more risk in terms of precipitating acute glaucoma than that caused by pharmacological pupil dilation.

Therefore, keep the environment well lit when treating a patient with a history of glaucoma. Thoroughly assess the health history, and prior to treatment, ask specifically about glaucoma history. Use local anesthetics with no epinephrine or no more than 2 carpules of 1:200,000 epinephrine-containing local anesthetics when epinephrine is needed to minimize the risk of acute angle-closure glaucoma in the dental setting. However, one should encourage the patient to seek immediate medical attention if the symptoms of acute angle-closure glaucoma develop. Red painful eyes, blurry vision, nausea, and vomiting from acute angle-closure are cause for concern.

Diabetic Retinopathy

Diabetic retinopathy is a "microvascular complication" just as is kidney disease and nerve damage. Studies have shown that microvascular complications are related to high blood-sugar levels. Diabetic retinopathy is the leading cause of irreversible blindness in industrialized nations. If retinopathy is not found early and goes untreated it can lead to blindness. Tight blood sugar control can reduce the risk of retinopathy, nephropathy, or nerve damage (all microvascular complications). Treatment of diabetic retinopathy may involve laser procedures or surgery.

Macrovascular Disease

Macrovascular disease is associated with an increased incidence of CVA/stroke and myocardial infarction (MI) that is often silent because of underlying autonomic neuropathy. Macrovascular disease also affects the peripheral circulation causing peripheral vascular disease and narrowing of the blood vessels, and this can lead to amputation of the limbs.

Neuropathy

Poor diabetes control is associated with sensory and autonomic neuropathy, and the neuropathy has a classic glove-and-stocking type of presentation. Autonomic neuropathy causes gastroparesis, which is associated with a slowing down of the stomach and delayed gastric emptying time. The patient feels full after a few bites and experiences gastric reflux, halitosis, and vomiting. Because of small food intake there is a greater likelihood of hypoglycemia. Therefore, this patient will do better when given **shorter dental appointments** and treatment is provided in a semi-sitting position.

Skin or Mucus Membrane Infections

Yeast infections affect the oral cavity, and it is not uncommon for the uncontrolled diabetic to have oral candidiasis and/or esophageal candidiasis. Always ask the patient about dysphagia (difficulty swallowing) or odynophagia (painful swallowing) whenever you see oral candidiasis and/or elevated blood sugar values. Esophageal candidiasis is associated with dysphagia and odynophagia.

Urinary tract infection (UTI), abscess formation, otitis externa, unusual fungal infections, and genital yeast infection are also complications of hyperglycemia, and UTIs affect the female diabetic patient more commonly. Staphylococcal infections of the hair follicles cause chronic skin problems in the uncontrolled diabetic. It is not uncommon, therefore, to find frequent small pustules on the skin or specifically between the shoulder blades.

DIABETES MANAGEMENT

Type 1 Diabetes

The type 1 diabetic is treated with daily insulin by subcutaneous (SC) injections or via an insulin pump.

Type 2 Diabetes

The type 2 diabetic patient is treated with diet, exercise, oral anti-diabetic medications, insulin, or a combination of oral agents and insulin, and with bariatric gastric bypass surgery for weight control in the morbidly obese patient.

Medical Management

Insulin is used in the management of all type 1 diabetes and in some cases of uncontrolled type 2 diabetes. The patient is always on specific insulin preparations and doses, as dictated by the patient's physician. It is important to know the medication details from the patient along with dosage details and time(s) of intake. Tables 38.2 and 38.3 list the specifics for the most commonly used insulin preparations and oral agents.

Table 38.2. Time Course of Action of Insulin Preparation

Insulin Type	Onset	Peak	Duration
Regular Insulin:			
Humalin	30-60min	2–4h	6–8h
Humalin R U 500	30-60min	2–4h	24h
Novolin R	30–60min	2–4h	8h
Insulin Isophane			
Suspension (NPH):			
Novolin N	1.5h	4–12h	24h
Humulin N	1–2h	6–12h	18–24h
Insulin Isophane Suspension			
(NPH)/ Regular Insulin (R):			
Humulin 70/30	0.5h	2–12h	24h
Novolin 70/30	0.5h	2–12h	24h
Lente Insulin	1–2.5h	8–12h	18–24h
Ultralente	4–8h	16–18h	>36h
Insulin Anologs:			
1. **Lispro (Humalog)**	5–15min	1–2h	3.5–4.5h
2. **Insulin Aspart (Novolog)**	5–15min	1–2h	3–5h
3. **Glargine (Lantus)**	1.1h	None	≥24h
4. **Insulin Glulisine (Apidra)**	15–30min	1h	2–4h
5. **Insulin Determir (Levemir)**	1h	None	24h

DIABETES DENTAL ALERTS AND SUGGESTED MANAGEMENT GUIDELINES

The following are dental alerts and guidelines for diabetes:

1. Elevated sugar levels can predispose to the development of caries, periodontal disease, xerostomia, and parotid gland inflammation. Periodontal inflammation occurs because of poor blood sugar control. The patients have elevated C-reactive protein (CRP) levels, which are an indicator of inflammation. The inflamed periodontal tissues have very high counts of anaerobic bacteria. There is a definite improvement in the patient's blood sugar and HbA$_1$C levels with periodontal treatment. Excessive periodontal inflammation is associated with an increased risk of death from cardiovascular and renal disease. It is important to note that the 2010 Cochrane Review also suggests, "there is some evidence of improvement in metabolic control in people with diabetes, **after treating periodontal disease.**" HbA$_1$C was found to improve by 0.15–0.8%.

   Xerostomia predisposes to dental caries and oral candidiasis. Additionally, mucosal diseases such as lichen planus, lichenoid drug reactions from sulfonylurea use, candida infection due to xerostomia, altered taste, and parotid gland enlargement from uncontrolled diabetes are some of the other oral manifestations associated with diabetes.

2. Know the type and duration of the diabetes and determine the drugs in use for the patient's diabetes treatment.

Table 38.3. Oral Agents for the Management of Type 2 Diabetes

Category and Mech. of Action	Generic (Trade) Name	Side Effects, Special Facts
Sulphonylureas: Stimulate the pancreas to secrete more insulin	**First generation:** 1. Chlorpropamide (Diabinese) **Second generation:** 1. Glyburide (Glynase) 2. Glimepiride (Amaryl) 3. Glyburide (DiaBeta) 4. Glyburide (Glynase) 5. Glyburide (Micronase) 6. Glipizide (Glucotrol) 7. Glipizide (Glucotrol XL)	• All sulfonylureas may cause hypoglycemia and sun sensitivity. • Contraindicated during pregnancy and lactation. • Diabinese can cause a flushing reaction with alcohol use and may also cause low blood sodium problems. • Glucotrol XL cannot be chewed, crushed or divided. • Sulfonylureas (SU) can cause weight gain. • Dosing/day: 1-2
Meglitinides: Act by causing the pancreas to secrete more insulin.	8. Repaglinide (Prandin) 9. Nateglinide (Starlix)	• Prandin may be used with kidney disease. • Prandin is shorter and faster acting than sulfonylureas. • Prandin can cause hypoglycemia, but less than sulfonylureas. • Contraindicated with pregnancy/lactation. • Dosing/day: 3
Biguanides: Act by decreasing the liver glucose production	1. Glucophage (Metformin) 2. Metformin generic 3. Glucophage XR (Metformin long acting) 4. Metformin oral solution (Riomet)	• Rarely cause hypoglycemia. • Contraindicated with pregnancy/lactation. • Contraindicated with kidney disease, active liver disease, elderly, heart failure • Dosing/day: 2
Alpha-Glucosidase inhibitors: Act by working in the intestines to slow the digestion of some carbohydrates, and thus the after-meal blood glucose peaks are not so high.	1. Acarbose (Precose) 2. Miglitol (Glyset)	• These drugs block the action of enzymes in the digestive tract that break down carbohydrates. The sugars are absorbed more slowly into the blood, which helps prevent the rapid rise in blood sugar that usually occurs right after a meal. • They cause abdominal bloating, flatulence and diarrhea. • They are contraindicated with pregnancy/lactation. * Hypoglycemia may occur when used with Prandin, insulin, or sulfonylureas. Treat the hypoglycemic reaction with **pure glucose tablets/gel or milk** as Precose or Glyset **delay** absorption of other carbohydrates • Dosing/day: 3

(continued)

Table 38.3. Oral Agents for the Management of Type 2 Diabetes (*Continued*)

Category and Mech. of Action	Generic (Trade) Name	Side Effects, Special Facts
Thiazolidine-diones (TZDs or Glitazones): These drugs help the muscle cells respond to insulin and use glucose.	1. Rosiglitazone maleate (Avandia) 2. Pioglitazone HCL (Actos)	• TZDs require normal liver function. LFTs are done frequently. • Contraindicated during pregnancy, lactation and CHF. • Rarely cause hypoglycemia • Dosing/day: 1-2
Combination Drugs:	1. Glyburide + Metformin (Glucovance) 2. Glipizide + Metformin (Metaglip) 3. Rosiglitazone + Metformin (Avandamet) 4. Pioglitazone + Metformin (Actoplus Met) 5. Rosiglitazone + Glimepiride (Avandaryl)	
Newer Drugs: **1. Incretin Mimetics**	1. Exenatide (Byetta) 2. Liraglutide (Victoza)	• Injectable Incretin hormone analog, injected SC bid 1h prior to meals. • Used in combination with Sulfonylurea and/or Metformin. • **Pregnancy Category C** • Affects absorption of oral medications so take antibiotics or OCs **1 hour prior** to taking Byetta. • Dosing/day: 1-2 injections
2. Cannabinoid Receptor Antagonist	1. Rimonabant (Acomplia or Zimulti)	
3. Pramlintide (Symlin)		• Injectable • Gastroparesis • Dosing/day: 3 injections
4. Insulin		• Can precipitate hypoglycemia • Dosing/day: 1-4 injections
5. DPP-4 inhibitors: DPP-4 inhibitors release insulin in the presence of elevated blood sugar level. They decrease glucagon when needed thus minimizing hypoglycemia.	1. Sitaglyptin Phosphate (Januvia) 2. Saxagliptin (Onglyza) 3. Linagliptin) (Tradjenta)	• Stuffy nose, headaches • Dosing/day: 1

3. Assess the laboratory tests: FBS, PPBS, and HbA$_1$C to determine the level of disease control.

4. Avoid treating an uncontrolled diabetic. Elevated blood sugars can increase the risk of infection.

5. Determine the patient's meal and snack times and always treat the patient on a full stomach.

6. Ideally, morning appointments following a regular breakfast are best. It does not make sense, however, to schedule a morning appointment if the patient eats minimally in the morning or does not eat breakfast! Always check the patient's meal and snack times. Determine what and how much the patient consumes before you schedule the patient. The idea is always to treat the patient on a full stomach and with the patient having consumed complex carbohydrates instead of simple sugars, which can raise and drop the blood sugar levels rapidly.

7. Always plan breaks for snack times so the patient can eat. Snack times are usually around 10:00 AM/3:00 PM.

8. For outpatient routine dentistry, the type 1 patient **does not** need to cut back on the insulin dose. You need to check the blood sugar, particularly during longer major surgical procedures.

9. A well-controlled patient will have a FBS <120 mg/dL, a PPBS <160 mg/dL, and an HbA$_1$C <7%.

10. An HbA$_1$C level >8% indicates that the patient has been uncontrolled for the past one to two months.

11. Treat even a small infection aggressively with antibiotics, typically for five days. Failure to treat an infection can promote the occurrence of acute or chronic osteomyelitis, and this in turn can worsen the diabetes control.

12. Always provide aggressive pain management immediately.

13. Pain, infection, and inflammation cause epinephrine release. Epinephrine causes glycogen breakdown to glucose and this results in the precipitation of hyperglycemia.

14. Therefore, an insulin-dependent diabetic must follow "sick-day rules of insulin" during these temporary states of hyperglycemia to bring the diabetes under control and to have a better outcome with the pain, infection, or inflammation.

15. **Sick-day rules of insulin:** The patient needs to monitor the blood sugar levels in the presence of infection, inflammation, bleeding, trauma, or fever. If the levels are elevated, the patient contacts the physician and the physician orders short-term changes in insulin therapy to correct the temporary rise in the blood sugar values.

16. Delayed healing and increased incidences of opportunistic infections are common with uncontrolled diabetes.

17. Neutrophil action is decreased, and WBC migration to the site of the lesion is sluggish in patients with uncontrolled diabetes. These patients need antibiotics to promote the healing process.

18. Whenever needed, use stress management to reduce anxiety.

19. Maintain hygiene recall at three-to-four month intervals.

20. Use non-absorbable suture materials.

21. Patients on oral agents should take their normal dosage for all routine procedures done in a dental office. Exception to the rule will be patients on oral agents' glyburide, glipizide, glimepiride, repaglinide, and nateglinide, which **stimulate insulin release**. Consult with the patient's physician when you know that a patient

on one of these medications will undergo outpatient major dentistry that may prevent him/her from eating for several hours after the procedure. In such cases, the MD will hold a pre-procedure dose, even though the patient will eat prior to the procedure to avoid hypoglycemia post procedure. The MD will have the patient take the evening dose of the oral medication, only when meal consumption resumes.

22. Do not use NSAIDS or corticosteroids long term in diabetics because they promote hyperglycemia. Chronic NSAIDS and corticosteroid use raises the blood sugar levels by promoting the breakdown of glycogen to glucose. Ibuprofen for 2–3 days to control acute inflammation is acceptable, if the patient's underlying renal and liver statuses do not contraindicate NSAID use.

Suggested Modifications for Major Surgery in the Outpatient Setting

The following are insulin therapy modifications for use in the outpatient dental office setting:

1. Remember that the patient will be slow in resuming food intake post operatively.
2. The usual recommended protocol is for the patient to take **half** the dose of the intermediate or long-acting insulin (these are basal insulin preparations), and the **full dose** of the rapid or very rapid-acting insulin (these are bolus insulin preparations) prior to a full breakfast.
3. Following the procedure, when the patient is ready to resume meal consumption, the patient checks the sugar level prior to injecting insulin. The blood sugar level obtained at that time dictates the amount of insulin that is injected post operatively.
4. Once fully recovered, the patient resumes the routine insulin regimen.

Management Protocol for a Type I Diabetic Undergoing Inpatient Major Surgery Under General Anesthesia

Use the following protocol for a type 1 diabetic:

1. The patient is kept NPO (nil by mouth) overnight.
2. **Half** of the intermediate or long-acting insulin (Lantus/Levemir/NPH insulin, which are the basal insulin preparations) is given on the morning of the surgery and **all** rapid or very rapid insulin (the bolus insulin Humalog/NovoLog, most commonly) is **withheld**.
3. The basal insulin is continued with IV 5% dextrose in water.
4. The blood glucose is checked frequently intra-operatively and is maintained between 120–160 mg/dL. Blood glucose, when kept in this range intra-operatively, ensures better postoperative recovery and healing.
5. If the intra-operative blood glucose levels increase beyond 200 mg/dL, the patient is given a bolus dose of Humalog/NovoLog at a dose of 0.1 unit/kg body weight (BW). This may be followed by a continuous drip of 1–2 units of Humalog or NovoLog/h, if blood glucose remains >200mg/dL. The dosage per hour is calculated as follows: Total Daily Dose (TDD) ÷ 24 h = units given per hour.
6. The blood glucose is monitored every one to two hours during the postoperative period. Once meal consumption has been resumed, the patient resumes the routine insulin regimen as discussed previously.

Management During Major Surgery Under General Anesthesia for Patients on Insulin Pumps

Patients on insulin pumps use Humalog or NovoLog insulin only as the continuous basal insulin infused subcutaneously and take additional bolus before each meal via the pump. The patient tests his/her blood sugar prior to every meal and adds more insulin if needed.

NPO Surgical Procedures and the Insulin Pump

The patient is put on an insulin drip as previously described under inpatient protocol, and the pump is temporarily stopped.

Management Guidelines for a Type 2 Diabetic Undergoing Major Surgery Under General Anesthesia

Use the following guidelines for a type 2 diabetic:

1. If a type 2 patient is to undergo major surgery, the patient is kept NPO (nil by mouth) overnight.
2. The patient **does not take** the oral agent on the morning of the surgery.
3. During surgery, the patient's blood sugar levels are monitored and maintained with infusion of IV insulin.
4. Following surgery, when full meal intake is to be resumed, the patient monitors the blood sugar level **before** taking the oral agent. If the post-operation sugars are low, the patient can skip taking the oral agent. The patient resumes the routine oral agent intake on full recovery.

Blood Sugar Values and Suggested Dental Management Guidelines

The following are dental management guidelines for blood sugar values:

1. **The well-controlled patient will have an FBS <120 mg/dL, a PPBS <160 mg/dL, and an HbA$_1$C <7%.**
    -   Local anesthetics: Use 2% lidocaine (Xylocaine), 2% mepivacaine (Carbocaine) with 1:20,000 levonordefrin (NeoCobefrin), 0.5% bupivacaine (Marcaine), or 4% prilocaine HCL (Citanest Forte), maximum 2 carpules.
2. **The moderately uncontrolled patient will an have an FBS range of 120–180 mg/dL, a PPBS range of 160–250 mg/dL, and a HbA$_1$C range of 7–8%.**
    -   Local anesthetics: Decrease the amount of epinephrine in the local anesthetic. Use 4% prilocaine HCL (Citanest Forte) or 0.5% bupivacaine (Marcaine) local anesthetics with 1:200,000 epinephrine only, maximum 2 carpules.
    -   Antibiotics: If antibiotics are needed following major surgery a full dose of antibiotic can be used.
3. **The severely uncontrolled patient will have an FBS >180 mg/dL, a PPBS >250 mg/dL, and an HbA$_1$C >8%.**
    -   The patient receives dental treatment only if oral assessment indicates the presence of an acute dental infection. Infection worsens diabetes control, and

treatment of the acute dental infection will improve the blood sugar levels during the post-recovery period.

○ Defer routine dental treatment in this stage for *all* patients with poor sugar control until the diabetes is brought under better control.

○ Any dental emergency is treated using only 3% mepivacaine HCL (Carbocaine) or 4% prilocaine HCL (Citanest Plain). Give low-dose antibiotic coverage to promote healing for 3, 5, or 7 days.

Thyroid Gland Dysfunctions: Assessment, Analysis, and Associated Dental Management Guidelines

THE THYROID GLAND

Thyroid Hormones

Thyroid follicles secreting hormones include:

- **Thyroxine/Tetraiodothyronine (T_4):** T_4 accounts for 90% of thyroid gland secretions and is the "inactive" version of thyroid hormone.
- **Triiodothyronine (T_3):** T_3 is the "active" version of thyroid hormone. Low T_3 levels trigger TSH (Thyroid Stimulating Hormone) release from the pituitary, causing active conversion of T_4 to T_3. TSH levels drop when adequate T_3 levels are achieved.
- **Calcitonin:** The C cells of the follicles produce calcitonin (CT) in response to higher-than-normal concentrations of calcium ions in the extracellular fluids. Calcitonin stimulates osteoblasts, inhibits osteoclasts, and slows the intestinal absorption and renal conservation of calcium ions.

Role of Thyroid Hormones

- Thyroid hormones stimulate energy production and utilization by peripheral cells.
- The follicle cells manufacture thyroglobulin and store it as a colloid, filling the lumen of the follicle. The cells also actively transport iodine from the extracellular fluids into the follicular chamber, where they complex with the thyroglobulin molecules. Reabsorbed thyroglobulin is broken down into amino acids and thyroid hormones; the hormones diffuse into the circulation.
- Most of the thyroid hormones entering the bloodstream are attached to special thyroid-binding globulins. Unbound hormones affect peripheral tissues at once; the binding globulins gradually release their hormones over a week or more.
- The primary regulatory mechanism involves the production of TSH by the anterior pituitary.

Dentist's Guide to Medical Conditions, Medications, and Complications, Second Edition. Kanchan M. Ganda.
© 2013 John Wiley & Sons, Inc. Published 2013 by John Wiley & Sons, Inc.

- Thyroid hormone also increases the sensitivity of the cardiovascular system to sympathetic nervous system activity, and this effect helps maintain a normal heart rate.

HYPERTHYROIDISM

Etiology

Graves' disease is an autoimmune disorder associated with hyperthyroidism. The patient can present with hyperthyroidism due to a toxic nodular goiter, toxic adenoma, or exogenously, from excess thyroid hormone intake. Rarely, subacute thyroiditis (SAT) can cause temporary hyperthyroidism, which is associated with pain and tenderness over the thyroid area and with difficulty in swallowing.

Clinical Features

Hyperthyroidism can be associated with rapid heart rate, agitation, restlessness, anxiety, heat intolerance, fine tremors, polyphagia (excess appetite) with weight loss, excess perspiration involving the hands and feet, warm skin, menstrual irregularities, and frequent runs or diarrhea.

Graves' disease is associated with proptosis or protruding eyes/exophthalmus because of infiltration of adipocytes and involvement of the Mueller's muscles. This inflammation process can lead to double vision. The thyroid gland is firm and smooth in Graves' disease. Graves' disease patients can also have dermopathy that presents as pretibial myxedema or hypopigmentation of the skin.

Vital Signs and Cardiac Findings

The following are vital signs and cardiac findings for patients with hyperthyroidism:

- **Pulse:** The patient can have a rapid heart rate/tachycardia with irregular heartbeats and resting tachycardia, which is an increased pulse rate during sleep (the heart rate typically goes down during sleep in normal patients).
- **Blood pressure:** The systolic blood pressure (SBP) is elevated because the BMR is increased. The diastolic blood pressure (DBP) is decreased in the uncontrolled hyperthyroid patient. Thus, the pulse pressure (PP), which is the difference between the SBP and the DBP, is widened in uncontrolled hyperthyroidism and the PP is >40 mmHg (normal: 40 mmHg).
- **Cardiac findings:** Auscultation of the heart may often reveal a functional systolic murmur, which is a consequence of hyperdynamic circulation, secondary to the increased BMR and associated anemia. Arrhythmias can occur, and this is the reason why hyperthyroid patients often take digoxin (Lanoxin) and/or warfarin (Coumadin) long term.

Diagnosis

Blood tests will show high **T_4 and T_3, in addition to low TSH**. The high levels of T_4 and T_3 inhibit the release of the thyroid-releasing hormone (TRH) from the hypothalamus and this in turn inhibits the release of thyroid-stimulating hormone (TSH) from the pituitary. Thyroid function tests may also show a low TSH and high free T_4, possibly with elevated thyroid-stimulating immunoglobulin. If a patient has the classic history, exam, and lab values, no further testing is necessary. For patients with an uncertain diagnosis, imaging or fine-needle aspiration biopsy may be considered.

Treatment Options

Hyperthyroidism treatment options consist of the following:

1. **Antithyroid drugs:** Propylthiouracil (PTU) or methimazole (Tapazole). These drugs interfere with thyroid hormone production. Between the two drugs, PTU is considered second-line drug therapy, except in patients who are allergic or intolerant to methimazole, or in women who are in the first trimester of pregnancy.
2. **Radioactive iodine (I^{131}):** I^{131} causes gradual destruction of thyroid gland cells. It is important to note that I^{131} concentrates in the salivary glands causing xerostomia and caries, especially with higher doses, when it is used in the management of thyroid cancer.
3. **Surgery:** Thyroidectomy can be an option for patients of any age, and removal of part of the gland restores the euthyroid (normal thyroid) status.

Treatment Option Selection Protocol

The treatment option selected depends on the patient's age:

1. **Childbearing age:**
   a. **First option—antithyroid drugs:** Treatment with propylthiouracil (PTU) or methimazole (Tapazole) constitutes the first option.
   b. **Second option—surgery:** A part of the gland is removed and normal gland function is subsequently restored. Overtreatment with surgery can lead to hypothyroidism. Once the patient becomes hypothyroid, L-thyroxine is given as replacement therapy for life.
2. **Non-childbearing age:**

Radioactive I^{131}: This treatment is reserved for the non-childbearing age patient or patients who have had failures with antithyroid drug therapy. Radioactive I^{131} is given as a drink. In the initial two weeks following I^{131} treatment, the patient is isolated from pregnant patients and children to prevent radiation. One quarter of these patients can go on to develop hypothyroidism one year later. An important fact to remember is that I^{131} concentrates in the **salivary glands** and can cause xerostomia, caries, and salivary gland swelling.

Patients with subacute thyroiditis usually run a self-limited course without antithyroid medications.

Facts and Suggested Dental Guidelines

The following are dental facts and guidelines for hyperthyroidism:

1. Accelerated tooth development occurs in children with hyperthyroidism. Malocclusion can occur if eruptions of secondary teeth are precocious. However, teeth are usually normal but demineralization may occur.

2. **Local anesthetics:** Epinephrine in the local anesthetic and epinephrine cords must absolutely be avoided during the time the patient is on PTU/methimazole. Once the patient is off these drugs, the use of local anesthetics with epinephrine can resume; however, limit it to only two carpules.

3. PTU has anti–vitamin K activity and causes agranulocytosis and thrombocytopenia. Always check the CBC with platelet count and PT/INR when doing major dental work on such patients.

4. Calculate the absolute neutrophil count (ANC) in the patient with a decreased WBC count, and follow the ANC guidelines for antibiotic coverage. Antibiotics are needed to prevent infection and promote healing in the presence of agranulocytosis.

5. Sympathetic overactivity in the hyperthyroid patient is suppressed medically with the use of β-blockers. β-blockers decrease the associated tachycardia, agitation, and elevation of the blood pressure (BP).

6. β-blockers mask hypoglycemic symptoms, and sweating is the only symptom that occurs. Therefore, always suspect a hypoglycemic reaction if the patient starts to sweat in the chair and you know that the surroundings are not hot.

HYPOTHYROIDISM

Etiology

Autoimmune-associated Hashimoto's thyroiditis is the most common form of hypothyroidism. Hypothyroidism can also occur as a consequence to post-radioactive iodine treatment, post-hyperthyroid surgery, or after the acute phase of subacute thyroiditis.

Symptoms

Hypothyroidism commonly presents as a slowing in physical and mental activity, but the patient may be asymptomatic. When symptomatic, these patients are often lethargic, slow to react, have coarse dry skin and feel cold; they also complain of fatigue, suffer from constipation, and have puffiness around the face, gain weight, and experience cold intolerance. The classic symptoms and signs may not occur in many younger patients. Children with hypothyroidism may present with edema and thickening of the skin or a generalized reduction in mental acuity and physical activity. Cretinism occurs with congenital hypothyroidism.

Signs

The pulse is slow and the SBP is decreased because the BMR is decreased. The DBP is elevated because of severe vasoconstriction. The pulse pressure in an uncontrolled hypothyroid patient is <40 mmHg.

Diagnosis

Blood tests show low T_4 levels and high TSH levels. Screening is now done at birth to detect hypothyroidism by determining the T_4 and TSH levels.

Treatment

Levothyroxine (Synthroid/Levoxyl/Levothroid/Unithroid) is the treatment of choice. It takes five to six weeks for the drug to affect thyroid levels because the half-life of levothyroxine is 12 days. Levothyroxine is dosed to achieve normal TSH value.

DDIs with Levothyroxine/L-Thyroxine

The following are DDIs with levothyroxine:

- L-Thyroxine (Synthroid) decreases the effectiveness of digoxin (Lanoxin), so dose adjustments are needed in patients taking both these drugs.
- L-Thyroxine (Synthroid) enhances the catabolism of warfarin (Coumadin) in patients taking both these drugs.

Facts and Suggested Dental Guidelines

The patient with cretinism presents with maxillary prognathism and retardation of tooth development. Excessive caries plus macroglossia and swollen lips can occur due to myxedema, when the condition is advanced.

Hypothyroidism and Local Anesthetics

Use the following guidelines for local anesthetics:

1. **Uncontrolled hypothyroid patient:** Do not use epinephrine in the uncontrolled hypothyroid patient. The epinephrine will stay in the system longer because the BMR is decreased, plus the epinephrine can tax a sluggish heart.
2. **Controlled hypothyroid patient:** Use xylocaine with epinephrine, but limit it to two carpules.

Hypothyroidism and Sedatives, Hypnotics, and Narcotics

Use the following guidelines for sedatives, hypnotics, and narcotics:

1. The uncontrolled patient will have exaggerated response to narcotics and barbiturates.
2. Do not use diazepam (Valium), codeine, or other sedatives, hypnotics, or narcotics in the uncontrolled hypothyroid patient, because myxedema coma can occur.
3. The controlled hypothyroid patient can get diazepam (Valium), Tylenol #1–3, or other sedatives, hypnotics, or narcotics.

Adrenal Gland Disease States: Assessment, Analysis, and Associated Dental Management Guidelines

ADRENAL GLAND ANATOMY, PHYSIOLOGY, AND HORMONES

Adrenal Gland Anatomy

The adrenal glands consist of the outer adrenal cortex and the inner medulla, both of which produce hormones.

The Adrenal Cortex: The cortex contains three distinct zones: zona reticularis, zona fasciculata, and zona glomerulosa.

- The narrow **zona reticularis** surrounds the adrenal medulla and produces androgens of uncertain significance.
- The **zona fasciculata** produces glucocorticoids, cortisol (hydrocortisone), corticosterone, and cortisone. These hormones exert glucose-sparing and anti-inflammatory effects.
- The **zona glomerulosa** releases mineralocorticoids and aldosterone.

The Adrenal Medulla: The secretions of the adrenal medulla are controlled by the autonomic nervous system. The medulla secretes epinephrine (adrenaline) and norepinephrine (noradrenaline).

Adrenal Cortex Hormones

The adrenal cortex produces the following main hormones:

- **Glucocorticoids: mainly cortisol**
- **Mineralocorticoids: mainly aldosterone**
- **Androgens**

Glucocorticoids

Cortisol is released daily from the adrenal cortex and it helps the body regulate metabolism of protein, carbohydrates, and fat. Additionally, cortisol release helps fight

Dentist's Guide to Medical Conditions, Medications, and Complications, Second Edition. Kanchan M. Ganda.
© 2013 John Wiley & Sons, Inc. Published 2013 by John Wiley & Sons, Inc.

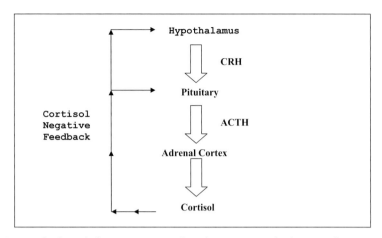

Figure 40.1. The hypothalamus-pituitary–adrenal cortex cortisol release cycle.

stress and suppress inflammation. Glucocorticoids also raise blood sugar levels by increasing gluconeogenesis, which is the synthesis of glucose from amino acid. This action ensures glucose supplies for the body when it is under stress.

Normal Mechanism of Cortisol Production

The hypothalamus releases the corticotropin hormone (CRH). CRH stimulates the pituitary to release the adrenocorticotropic hormone (ACTH). ACTH stimulates the adrenal cortex to release cortisol, which is also called "hydrocortisone." Cortisol, in turn, provides negative feedback to the pituitary and the hypothalamus when an adequate cortisol level is reached (see Figure 40.1).

Cushing's syndrome is associated with **excess** cortisol production, and Addison's disease is associated with a **deficiency** of cortisol and aldosterone.

Normal Release of Daily Cortisol and Corresponding Prednisone Equivalents

In a normal, healthy patient, **20 mg of cortisol** is released daily in the early morning between **2:00AM–8:00AM**, and this is equivalent to **5 mg prednisone**. The maximum output of endogenous cortisol released in response to severe stress by a **normal** gland is around **100–150 mg**; this is equivalent to about **25–40 mg prednisone**.

The anti-inflammatory potency of prednisone is **four times** that of hydrocortisone (Solu-Cortef). Thus, the **maximum** amount of steroid replacement given **during stressful** times should be about **25–40 mg prednisone PO or 100–150 mg hydrocortisone PO/IV**.

Mineralocorticoids

Aldosterone is the main hormone that helps maintain the plasma sodium and potassium balance. Aldosterone secretion is regulated by the renin-angiotensin system, ACTH, and the plasma sodium and potassium levels. When exposed to a decline in blood volume and/or low blood pressure, specialized kidney cells release the enzyme renin and the hormone erythropoietin into the circulation. Renin converts angiotensinogen, an inactive protein secreted by the liver, into angiotensin I. In the lungs, angiotensin I is converted to angiotensin II, and the zona glomerulosa then responds to the presence of angiotensin II in the circulation, stimulating aldosterone production by the adrenal cortex.

Erythropoietin that is also released by the kidney stimulates red blood cell production, elevating blood volume and improving oxygen delivery to peripheral tissues. Mineralocorticoids restrict sodium and water losses at the kidneys, sweat glands, digestive tract, and salivary glands and promote sodium or salt reabsorption by stimulating the kidneys to absorb more sodium from the blood.

When the blood volume becomes abnormally large, specialized cardiac muscle cells secrete the hormone atrial natriuretic factor (ANF). This hormone suppresses the secretion of ADH, aldosterone, and catecholamines, and it reduces thirst thereby encouraging water loss at the kidneys and lowering of the blood pressure. This response reduces blood volume and blood pressure. Aldosterone-secreting tumors are rare causes of hypertension that are resistant to conventional blood pressure treatment.

Androgens

The androgens released by the adrenal cortex help with protein anabolism and growth.

Adrenal Medulla Production

The adrenal medulla produces catecholamines, epinephrine (adrenaline), and norepinephrine (noradrenaline), which raise the blood sugar and fatty acid levels. The catecholamines increase the heart rate, myocardial contraction, myocardial excitability, blood pressure, and sympathetic tone, thus preparing the body for the "fight or flight" response. These hormones also promote vascular constriction of blood vessels supplying the skin, kidneys, gastrointestinal tract, and other areas of the body that are not needed for the response.

It is important to note that catecholamine-secreting tumors (pheochromocytoma) are rare causes of hypertension that are resistant to conventional blood pressure treatment. These patients are curable by surgery.

CUSHING'S SYNDROME

Etiology

Endogenous Causes

Pituitary, adrenal, or ectopic tumors in the lungs produce excess cortisol.

Exogenous Causes

Excessive steroids given for the management of, for example, asthma, rheumatoid arthritis, lupus, or chronic skin conditions can increase cortisol levels in the blood.

Symptoms and Signs

Patients with Cushing's syndrome may present with fatigue, weakness, ankle edema, central obesity from fat deposition, moon faces, "buffalo hump" around the neck, acne, purple striae that are most commonly located on the abdomen and thighs, alopecia, easy bruising, hirsutism, menstrual dysfunction or amenorrhea, hypertension, osteoporosis, peripheral muscle wasting/myopathy, and thinning of the limbs.

Treatment

Treatment options are surgery, radiation, or medication. In February 2012, the FDA approved mifepristone to control hyperglycemia in adult patients who are not good surgical candidates. Mifepristone is contraindicated during pregnancy because it promotes abortion.

Associated Dental Alerts

The following are dental alerts associated with Cushing's syndrome:

1. Patients with Cushing's syndrome have an increased risk for osteoporosis (because cortisol decreases bone formation), hypertension, heart failure, peptic ulcer, and diabetes (cortisol is antagonistic to insulin). When present, the status of any of these conditions must be assessed and dental management should be modified accordingly following the disease/condition-specific suggested dental guidelines discussed within this book.
2. The blood pressure should be routinely monitored during dentistry.
3. Aspirin and NSAIDS should be avoided because of the high incidence of peptic ulcer.
4. Patients with Cushing's syndrome also have an increased risk for periodontitis, oral candidiasis, and bleeding gums.
5. Excess steroids in the system lower the immune system activity, which increases the risk of infections and poor healing of wounds.
6. The practitioner should also provide adequate antibiotic coverage for five days following a major surgical procedure to promote healing.
7. The practitioner should assess and treat the oral cavity for oral and esophageal candidiasis when present.
8. Generalized osteoporosis can also affect the mandible and patients with dentures may need frequent re-adjustments.

ADDISON'S DISEASE

Addison's disease is associated with a lack of the adrenal hormones cortisol and aldosterone.

Etiology

Addison's disease occurs when the adrenal glands cannot produce enough cortisol or aldosterone. This disease affects both sexes and all age groups. About 80% of Addison's disease cases are idiopathic, autoimmune adrenocortical insufficiency resulting from autoimmune atrophy, fibrosis, and lymphocytic infiltration of the adrenal cortex. The adrenal medulla is usually spared. Tuberculosis accounts for nearly 10% of cases of Addison's disease. The disease causes pigmented mucous membrane patches and pigmentation around the mouth. Other causes include metastatic tumor and bilateral adrenal cortical hemorrhage.

Symptoms and Signs

Addison's disease patients experience tiredness, weakness, anorexia, weight loss, nausea, vomiting, lethargy, postural hypotension, and oral pigmentation. Blotchy melanin patches occur on the oral mucosa and skin. The melanocyte-stimulating hormone (**MSH**) is co-secreted **along with ACTH** causing the pigmentation. The pigmentation occurs on the buccal mucosa and spreads backward from the commissures.

Diagnosis

Blood tests show low levels of cortisol and aldosterone and high levels of ACTH and MSH.

Dental Alerts and Suggested Guidelines

The following are dental alerts and guidelines for Addison's disease:

1. Patients with Addison's disease have to be compensated with steroids to fight the stress associated with infection, inflammation, excessive bleeding, post-procedure starvation, pre- and postoperative pain (**very high risk factor**), and trauma associated with surgery, due to the lack of cortisol and aldosterone.
2. The dentist must consult with the patient's physician in these situations and provide adequate steroid coverage to compensate for the stress. Failure to provide coverage will precipitate acute adrenal insufficiency and collapse.
3. Patients taking steroids for more than two weeks may have adrenal insufficiency and consequently require additional steroid coverage for up to two years after treatment.
4. Oral infections must be aggressively treated in the Addison's disease patient to prevent hypoadrenal crisis or acute adrenal insufficiency.
5. Addison's patients benefit when given stress management with benzodiazepines or $O_2 + N_2O$, because stress reduction decreases cortisol demand.
6. It is best to treat this patient in the **first** appointment of the day because the cortisol secretion is at its highest in the morning between **2:00AM–8:00AM**. Cortisol secretion is **lowest** toward the **end** of the day.
7. Individuals working the night shift have a circadian rhythm reversal, and maximum cortisol release occurs during early evening, when they are awake.
8. If the patient is **currently** on steroids it is best for the patient to take the steroid for that day, **two hours prior** to dentistry.
9. Avoid barbiturates because they decrease cortisol levels.
10. Typically for minor procedures, no extra steroids are needed.
11. For major procedures, give **25–40 mg prednisone** PO, one hour prior to treatment on the day of surgery, and taper over two days. Alternatively, you can give **100–150 mg IV/IM hydrocortisone** one hour prior to the procedure if the patient has

to be NPO on the day of the surgery. This is followed by a taper to baseline within 48 hours using oral prednisone, once surgery has been completed.

CORTICOSTEROID FACTS AND SUGGESTED DENTAL GUIDELINES

The following are additional details and dental guidelines for corticosteroids:

1. During history-taking always evaluate for a history of corticosteroid therapy. Ask if the patient is currently on steroids or has been on corticosteroids for two weeks or longer within the past two years (**the rule of twos**). You must go back two years in the history because it can take **two weeks to two years** for the adrenal glands to return to **normal** function.

2. When exogenous steroids are taken by mouth or by injections, an inhibition of the endogenous cortisol release occurs because of negative feedback and associated inhibition of ATCH release.

3. Normal cortisol release occurs around **2:00AM–8:00AM** daily. Individuals working the night shift (as previously discussed) have a circadian rhythm reversal, and maximum cortisol release occurs in the late afternoon and early evening, when they are awake.

4. Exogenous corticosteroids will cause **minimal** endogenous corticosteroid suppression when the exogenous dose is given **prior to 9:00AM**.

5. Patients needing steroids prior to dentistry will benefit when treated as the **first** appointment in the morning.

6. Patients needing steroids will also benefit when given stress management with benzodiazepines or $O_2 + N_2O$, because stress reduction decreases cortisol demand.

7. In the dental setting, a patient with a history of steroid intake may need **extra** steroids in the presence of infection, fever, inflammation, bleeding, pain, or trauma due to surgery. Always consult with the patient's physician under such circumstances to determine the need for supplementation.

8. Corticosteroids decrease inflammation by inhibiting the migration of polymorphonuclear (PMN) leukocytes and by causing a reversal of increased capillary permeability.

9. The anti-inflammatory potency of prednisone is **four times** that of hydrocortisone (Solu-Cortef). This becomes important during a dental emergency when hydrocortisone (Solu-Cortef) is used instead of prednisone: **5 mg prednisone = 20 mg hydrocortisone**.

10. Prednisone, hydrocortisone, and dexamethasone are the most commonly used steroid preparations.

11. Dexamethasone is **40 times** stronger than hydrocortisone.

12. When extra steroids are needed for planned procedures, the intake or boost must begin **48 hours prior** to the surgery and, as previously discussed, the **maximum** amount of steroid replacement given **during stressful** times is about 25–40 mg **prednisone** PO or 100–150 mg **hydrocortisone** PO/IV.

13. For planned surgical procedures, the prednisone dose is increased gradually in a step-up pattern preoperatively and decreased gradually in a step-down pattern postoperatively, as shown in Figure 40.2.

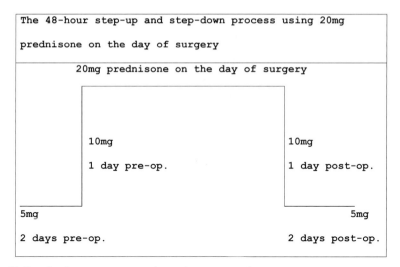

Figure 40.2.   Prednisone step-up and step-down protocol.

Alternate-Day Steroid Intake and Dentistry

Patients are often on alternate-day steroid intake, because this method of care is associated with a lesser degree of endogenous-steroid secretion inhibition. It is best to schedule surgery on the day of steroid intake. In most cases, depending on the magnitude of the procedure and the amount of steroid boost required, one can double the steroid dose on the day of treatment and taper the dose post operatively.

The step-up and step-down corticosteroid protocols using **10 mg/20 mg/40 mg** prednisone **on the day** of the surgical procedure in a patient on **0-5-0 mg** alternate-day steroid intake therapy are illustrated in Figure 40.3.

Suggested Steroid Dose Guidelines for Stress-Associated Dentistry

Mild Stress

This could be four or fewer extractions, or one quadrant flap surgery. Double the steroid dose if the patient is currently on steroids, or give 25 mg hydrocortisone PO/IV or

Surgery Day Dose	10mg/20mg/40mg Prednisone boost protocol with 0-5-0 alternate day Prednisone Therapy
10mg	Doubling of dose on the day of intake: 0 5 0 **10 5** 0 5 0 5 0 5 0 5 0 5 0 5 0 5 0 5 0 5
20mg	0 5 0 **10 20 10 5** 0 5 0 5 0 5 0 5 0 5 0 5 0 5 0
40mg	0 **10 20 40 20 10 5 0** 5 0 5 0 5 0 5 0 5 0 5 0 5

Figure 40.3.   Suggested step-up and step-down corticosteroid protocols.

Table 40.1. Suggested Steroid Dose Guidelines for Stress-Associated Dentistry

Stress Level	Suggestions

Mild stress: Stress equivalent to 1–4 extractions or 1 quadrant flap surgery	• If patient is currently on steroids: Depending on the procedure, double the steroid dose.
	• If patient is **not** currently on steroids: **Use 1 of 3 choices 1h before surgery:**
	  1. Give 6mg prednisone PO
	  2. 25mg hydrocortisone PO/IV
	  3. 5mg prednisone PO

Moderate stress: Stress equivalent to 5–16 extractions or 2 quadrants flap surgery	**Use 1 of 2 choices 1h before surgery:** 1. 15–20mg prednisone PO 2. 50–75mg hydrocortisone PO/IV
Severe stress: Stress equivalent to 17 or more extractions or 3 or more quadrants flap surgery	**Use 1 of 2 choices 1h before surgery:** 1. 25–40mg prednisone PO 2. 100–150mg hydrocortisone PO/IV

6.25 mg (round off to 6.0 mg) of prednisone PO, one hour prior to surgery if the patient is not currently on steroids but needs steroids. Giving 5 mg prednisone will also suffice.

Moderate Stress

This could be 5–16 extractions, or two quadrants flap surgery. Prescribe 50–75 mg hydrocortisone PO/IV or 12.5–18.75 mg (round off to 15–20 mg) of prednisone PO one hour prior to surgery.

Severe Stress

This could be 17 or more extractions, or three or more quadrants flap surgery. Prescribe 100–150 mg hydrocortisone PO/IV or 25–37.5 mg (round off to 25–40 mg) prednisone PO, one hour prior to surgery. **Note** that, when needed, it is better to err on the side of giving larger amounts of steroids than lesser amounts (Table 40.1).

Prednisone or Hydrocortisone Boost Protocol During Dental Emergency

Follow these steps:

1. During a dental emergency, the treatment cannot be delayed to implement the step-up protocol of steroid intake. Thus, the step-up protocol is completely skipped.
2. Dependent on the patient's needs and the major surgical procedure to be performed, approximately 25–40mg prednisone is given PO/IV/IM. The PO and IV dose are given one hour prior to surgery.
3. Alternately, the patient can be given PO/IV hydrocortisone (Cortef/Solu-Cortef) and as previously discussed the dose given is four times the prednisone dose required for the major dental procedure.

4. The postoperative steroid step-down is never skipped and is done with prednisone or hydrocortisone PO in the outpatient dental setting. Hydrocortisone IV is used for step-down in the inpatient dental setting.
5. Failure to give extra steroids when needed will result in very low cortisol levels, triggering a circulatory collapse from acute adrenal insufficiency.

Acute Adrenal Insufficiency Attack

In the presence of acute infection, inflammation, pain, trauma, or massive bleeding, acute adrenal insufficiency can occur if the patient is not given appropriate steroid supplementation when needed. Refer to Chapter 9 for discussion on clinical features and management of acute adrenal insufficiency.

Parathyroid Dysfunction Disease States: Assessment, Analysis, and Associated Dental Management Guidelines

PARATHYROID GLAND PHYSIOLOGY, FACTS, AND DYSFUNCTION OVERVIEW

Parathyroid dysfunction is frequently associated with disturbances in the bone. Presence of some form of bone pathology may prompt a dentist to evaluate tests to measure serum calcium, phosphorus, and alkaline phosphatase levels. These tests are primarily used to diagnose hyperparathyroidism, Paget's disease, metastatic bone disease, and disturbances in calcium absorption (Figure 41.1). Knowing the normal calcium metabolism and bone remodeling processes helps to better understand the changes in bone and blood tests that occur with associated disease states. The parathyroid glands, vitamin D, kidney, and gut are intricately involved in calcium metabolism and the remodeling of healthy bones.

Parathyroid Gland Physiology

There are two pairs of parathyroid glands embedded in the posterior surface of the thyroid gland, and there are several different populations of cells within the parathyroid glands.

The parathyroid glands are linked to the hypothalamus by **negative** homeostatic feedback mechanisms. Negative feedback mechanisms **decrease** the deviation from an ideal normal value and are important in maintaining homeostasis. The chief cells in the parathyroid glands secrete parathyroid hormone/parathormone/PTH, which activates vitamin D, affects bones and the kidney, and ultimately regulates the blood calcium level. If calcium ions decrease in the surrounding extracellular fluids, the parathyroid glands perceive the decrease and secrete more parathyroid hormone/PTH. The parathyroid hormone/PTH then stimulates calcium release from the bones by stimulating osteoclasts and inhibiting osteoblasts. PTH also increases intestinal absorption of calcium and reduces the urinary excretion of calcium ions through the kidneys. All of these mechanisms increase the calcium uptake into the bloodstream.

Dentist's Guide to Medical Conditions, Medications, and Complications, Second Edition. Kanchan M. Ganda.
© 2013 John Wiley & Sons, Inc. Published 2013 by John Wiley & Sons, Inc.

Disease State(s):	Parathyroid Hormone (PTH); Calcium and Phosphorus Patterns
Hyperparathyroidism:	↑ PTH, ↑ Calcium, ↓ Phosphorus
Hypoparathyroid or Renal Disease:	↓ PTH, ↓ Calcium, ↑ Phosphorus
Secondary Hyperparathyroidism:	↑ PTH, ↓ Calcium, ↑ Phosphorus

Figure 41.1. PTH, calcium, and phosphorus changes and associated disease states.

If blood calcium levels rise, the parathyroid glands reduce parathyroid hormone production. Thus, both responses are negative feedback responses and the effects are opposite of the stimulus.

Roles of the Gut, Parathyroid Glands, Vitamin D, and Kidney in Calcium Metabolism

- Calcium is an essential nutrient for mineralization of bone, increasing bone density, and decreasing the risk of fractures. Calcium increases bone density because it is a weak anti-resorptive agent that actually prevents bone breakdown and bone resorption, and also slightly modifies bone formation. Data show that patients given calcium have a greater decrease in alkaline phosphatase level, which confirms greater suppression of bone turnover, further showing that calcium works in terms of bone density.
- In terms of calcium supplementation and heart disease, high normal serum calcium is associated with increased carotid artery plaque thickness, an increased abdominal aortic calcification, an increased incidence of coronary heart disease and stroke, and an increased incidence of mortality. To prevent fractures, treatments with proven anti-resorptive agents are much better than calcium supplementation, but adequate calcium intake is important for normal bone health.
- Calcium balance is best determined by assessment of bone mass and a history of fracture rates.
- Elemental calcium is the calcium that is available for absorption, as with supplements containing calcium in addition to calcium from food sources. Most calcium is absorbed in the small intestine and the absorption in the gut occurs through active and passive mechanisms.
- **Active mechanism:** The active mechanism results in the trans-cellular movement of calcium, and this active transport is regulated primarily by $1,25(OH)_2D$, which is saturable. This regulated active transport of calcium is critically important when dietary calcium is very low. When there is no $1,25(OH)_2D$/calcitriol, active calcium absorption is essentially zero. As $1,25(OH)_2D$ levels increase in the gut, active calcium absorption increases. Patients with normal $1,25(OH)_2D$ levels can be in neutral calcium balance on very low calcium intakes because of the role of $1,25(OH)_2D$ in increasing gut calcium absorption.

- **Passive mechanism:** The passive, para-cellular calcium movement in the gut is not regulated by vitamin D, nor is it dependent on $1,25(OH)_2D$. Adequate calcium absorption can occur with passive absorption of calcium that is not dependent on vitamin D to maintain balance.
- Dietary vitamin D and vitamin D absorbed from sunlight are converted in the liver to 25(OH)D (25-hydroxycholecalciferol /Calcidiol/25-hydroxyvitamin D). 25(OH)D is the specific vitamin D metabolite that is measured in the serum to determine a patient's vitamin D status.
- PTH activates 1-alpha-hydroxylase in the kidney, which helps convert 25(OH)D to 1,25-dihydroxycholecalciferol (1,25-dihydroxyvitamin D_3/calcitriol). This hormone then circulates in the blood, regulating the concentration of calcium and phosphate in the bloodstream and promoting the healthy growth and remodeling of bone. It is important to note that excess vitamin D is associated with an excess of calcium and this can increase the incidence of renal stones in the patient.
- Kidney disease is associated with a decrease in the production of active vitamin D_3, causing hypocalcemia, secondary hyperparathyroidism, hyperphosphatemia, and renal osteodystrophy. Patients with renal osteodystrophy are prone to accelerated alveolar bone loss and it is not uncommon to discover **Brown** tumors in the jaws of such patients.
- **Secondary hyperparathyroidism** develops in chronic kidney disease because of hyperphosphatemia, hypocalcemia, decreased renal synthesis of 1,25-dihydroxycholecalciferol (1,25-dihydroxyvitamin D, or calcitriol), intrinsic alteration in the parathyroid gland, which gives rise to increased PTH secretion, as well as increased parathyroid growth and skeletal resistance to PTH.
- Calcium and calcitriol are primary feedback inhibitors for PTH; hyperphosphatemia is a stimulus to PTH synthesis and secretion. Phosphate retention begins in early chronic kidney disease. When the GFR falls, less phosphate is filtered and excreted, but serum levels do not initially rise because of increased PTH secretion, which increases renal excretion. As the GFR falls toward chronic kidney disease stages 4–5, hyperphosphatemia develops from the inability of the kidneys to excrete the excess dietary intake. Hyperphosphatemia suppresses the renal hydroxylation of inactive 25-hydroxyvitamin D to calcitriol, so serum calcitriol levels are low when the GFR is less than 30mL/min. Hypocalcemia develops primarily from decreased intestinal calcium absorption because of low plasma calcitriol levels. With the persistently elevated PTH levels, high-turnover bone disease or renal osteodystrophy occurs. Therefore, renal osteodystrophy is associated with hypocalcemia and high PTH levels.
- Therefore, bone disease and vascular calcification are common complications of chronic kidney disease (CKD). As previously discussed, CKD results in a fundamental disruption of the normal regulation of extracellular calcium, bone calcium, and vascular calcification. Abnormalities associated with serum phosphorus, PTH, vitamin D levels, and alkaline phosphatase occur as they relate to bone metabolism.
- According to the Institute of Medicine's recommendations on calcium intake for women ages 19–50, and for men ages 19–70, the recommended daily allowance of calcium from dietary and supplement intake should be 1,000mg, and for both men and women older than 70, it should be 1,200mg. No increased intake is recommended for pregnant or lactating patients.

The parathyroid hormone regulates the excretion of phosphate by the kidneys, and hyperparathyroidism is associated with low phosphorous levels. Phosphorous levels are increased in patients with hypoparathyroidism and renal disease.

Alkaline phosphatase (ALP) is a hydrolase enzyme that is responsible for the release of phosphate from proteins and other molecules. This enzyme is found in the liver, bones, bile duct, lining of the intestine, kidney, and placenta. Alkaline phosphatase is a product of osteoblasts and is therefore related to bone growth. This accounts for higher-than-normal ALP levels among growing children compared to adults. Likewise, during the third trimester of pregnancy, the ALP level is on the higher side, as it is normal for the placenta to produce additional ALP. This enzyme is needed for the synthesis of proteins in the cells, and it has a vital part in the calcification of bones and cartilage.

Biliary stasis, pregnancy, growing bones, Paget's disease, bone fractures, rheumatoid arthritis, osteoporosis, hyperparathyroidism, adrenal cortical hyperfunction, rickets, osteomalacia, osteosarcoma, metastatic bone disease, and renal and intestinal tumors can all cause increases in the alkaline phosphatase levels. Fatty liver, liver malignancy, hepatitis, cirrhosis, cholecystitis, cholangitis, and infection caused by Cytomegalovirus are other liver-related causes associated with elevated ALP. Phenytoin, ranitidine, erythromycin, carbamazepine, verapamil, and allopurinol are some of the drugs that can also elevate ALP levels.

Hyperparathyroidism

Hyperparathyroidism is associated with high calcium levels and high PTH. It usually manifests as a single adenoma but all four parathyroid glands may be affected. Autonomous production by the glands causes dysfunction of the negative feedback mechanism and consequent **elevation of calcium and PTH levels**. Oral findings encountered include bones of the jaw are less radio-dense, lamina dura may be absent, and radiolucent areas and central giant cell granulomas may occur.

Hypoparathyroidism

Hypoparathyroidism is associated with **low calcium and low PTH levels**. The condition is usually autoimmune. Hypoparathyroidism may be associated with oral candidiasis, hypoplasia of enamel, dentin, short roots, and delayed eruption of the teeth.

Osteomalacia

Osteomalacia is associated with vitamin D deficiency and it can be familial or acquired. Rickets and hypocalcification of dentin, enamel and alveolar bone are findings associated with vitamin D deficiency.

Vitamin D Excess

Excess vitamin D is associated with an excess of calcium. High vitamin D levels are associated with less bleeding on gingival probing.

Endogenous Causes

Endogenous causes of vitamin D excess include sarcoidosis, lymphoma, or TB. The immune cells make vitamin D in excess, which causes the calcium levels to be high.

Exogenous Causes of Vitamin D Excess

The exogenous cause is the presence of too much vitamin D in the milk.

Hypercalcemia from Tumors

Hypercalcemia can be caused by calcium-producing tumors from the lungs or breast.

BONE REMODELING PROCESS AND OSTEOPOROSIS

Bone Remodeling

Knowing the normal bone remodeling process and the associated blood tests demonstrating bone turnover rates helps to better understand the changes that occur with osteoporosis. The role of bone density tests and bone turnover markers in the diagnosis and management of osteoporosis is discussed at length in the following paragraphs.

Healthy bones are made up of living tissue—mainly collagen. Strong, healthy bones are maintained through a continuously balanced bone remodeling. Bone mass stays constant when bone resorption and bone formation are in balance. Bone turnover occurs exclusively on the surface of bone.

The bone remodeling process has two phases: breakdown/resorption and formation/deposition. Bone resorption, or bone breakdown, occurs first. Osteoclasts excavate small pits on the bone surface, releasing bone collagen and minerals in the circulatory system. Osteoclastic activity occurs over 7–10 days. The osteoclastic phase is then followed by bone formation/bone deposition, when osteoblasts deposit new tissue. Osteoblastic activity occurs over 2–3 months. The resting phase follows the bone remodeling phases, which are the combined osteoclastic and osteoblastic phases. The bone is mineralized in the resting phase, and the remodeling cycle begins again. The entire remodeling process takes 4–8 months (range: 3–24 months). **Bone-remodeling phase cycle: resorption phase + formation phase + resting phase.**

C-terminal telopeptide (CTx) and N-terminal telopeptide (NTx) markers: CTx and NTx are serum-based bone turnover biochemical markers of bone remodeling and particularly bone resorption. Together, these markers represent each end of the three strands of type 1 collagen, and each is used in tests that monitor bone turnover. Bone breakdown by-products appear in the urine and blood. CTx and NTx are **dynamic** measurements of the rate of bone breakdown. CTx and NTx tests measure these biochemical markers.

NTx test: NTx is a stable and specific breakdown product of bony collagen. NTx assay has been validated for the prediction of risk for osteoporosis and response to therapy. The serum NTx test is a very reproducible test demonstrating current osteoclastic activity. Increased serum NTx indicates increased bone turnover and increased risk for osteoporosis. Bisphosphonates decrease osteoclastic activity. Therefore, a decreased NTx value with bisphosphonate use indicates good response to bisphosphonate therapy. The NTx test is the more acceptable test compared with the CTx test.

N-telopeptide and creatinine are used to calculate the N-telo/creatinine ratio, which is the NTx test. After one year, menopausal women with baseline **NTx >38nM BCE** (Bone Collagen Equivalent)/mM creatinine have significant risk for decrease in bone mineral density (BMD), compared with women on hormone replacement therapy (HRT). The higher the baseline NTx, the greater the probability is for BMD decline. Indication that BP therapy is effective after three months is demonstrated **when the**

NTx value is ≤38nM BCE/mM CRT or the NTx value has decreased by ≥to 30% from baseline. Once therapy begins, NTx measurements can be repeated three months later and a reduction of 30% or more in NTx levels from baseline indicates good response. If treatment is stopped, NTx levels return slowly to the pre-Rx baseline.

Normal NTx range is 5–65 bone collagen equivalent (BCE) units/mMol creatinine. To check progress with treatment, the MD conducts follow-up tests every 6–12 months. Achieving a 30–mid-40s BCE units/mmol creatinine indicates a safe bone turnover. Values of <10 BCE units/mMol creatinine indicate significant osteoclastic suppression. Recovery from trauma following extractions or implant placements is less likely with over suppression.

In conclusion, the NTx test is a useful test that the physician can use to monitor the patient's response to antiresorptive therapy and/or poor adherence, but it is of **no** value to the dentist because the NTx test does not determine risk for anti-resorptive agent–induced osteonecrosis of the jaw (ARONJ).

Serum CTx test is a poorly reproducible test with a very wide normal range: 70–1,391pg/mL. CTx values can vary in a patient, depending on the time of day the blood is collected. Thus, the popularity of the CTx test has declined.

The DEXA/DXA scan is an x-ray/ultrasound bone scan that is measured at the hip, spine, or wrist, and the DEXA scan determines the amount of bone present in the patient at that given time.

Osteoporosis is diagnosed only with a DEXA scan/bone mineral density (BMD) test. The DEXA scan is reported as two scores: the T-score and the Z-score. The T-score measures bone density against the density of a healthy 20-year-old of the same gender, and this score should normally stay **above −1**. The Z-score measures bone density against the average bone density for the patient's age, gender, and race. **A normal DEXA score comprises** a T-score above −1 with an appropriate Z-score near 0. **Osteopenia/start of bone density loss is indicated** if the T-score is <−1 but >−2.5. **Osteoporosis diagnosis should be made** if the T-score is below −2.5.

CTx and NTx do not play a role in the diagnosis of osteoporosis. In both sexes, bone breakdown may increase with age due to a decrease in hormone levels. To assess complete bone status, DEXA scan and the NTx test should be considered, because, if present, increased levels of NTx will indicate faster bone break down compared to replacement, thus indicating a risk of osteoporosis. However, increased levels do not confirm a diagnosis of osteoporosis. BMD testing is spaced 12–24 months apart to identify significant bone loss. When spaced 60–90 days apart, the NTx test can identify increased bone breakdown.

Bisphosphonates (BPs) used for the treatment of osteoporosis are absorbed, stored, and excreted unchanged in skeletal bone. BPs disrupt the bone remodeling cycle by inhibiting osteoclastic activity, thereby decreasing bone resorption and consequently increasing bone mineral density (BMD). CTx and NTx levels decrease with BP therapy because of inhibition of osteoclastic activity. A reduction in CTx and NTx values indicates a slowing down of bone turnover and bone loss. Very low CTx and NTx values indicate over-aggressive treatment of osteoporosis with BPs. Be advised that very low CTx and NTx could mean that the bone turnover is quite low, making it less likely to recover from trauma associated with extractions or implant placements. An elevation of CTx and NTx values from depressed ranges with stoppage of BPs indicates recovery of osteoclastic activity and recovery of bone remodeling. Therefore, for optimal BP benefit, BPs should not overly suppress osteoclastic activity.

Osteoporosis

Facts

Risk factors for osteoporosis include thin body habitus, Caucasian or Asian decent, low calcium intake, and hyperthyroidism, which accelerates bone metabolism. Osteoporosis is most common in postmenopausal women but men can also develop osteoporosis. Osteoporosis is diagnosed by measurement of the bone density, mass, and volume of the lumbar spine, wrist, and hip by DXA/DEXA scan.

Treatment

Calcium and vitamin D supplementation, anti-resorptive agents (bisphosphonates), recombinant parathyroid hormone (rPTH), or denosumab are used in the treatment of osteoporosis.

ANTI-RESORPTIVE AGENTS

Classification

The three main categories of anti-resorptive agents currently in use are:

1. Bisphosphonates
2. Denosumab (Prolia)
3. Teriparatide (Fortea)

Bisphosphonates

Bisphosphonates (BPs) comprise a drug category that has been used for the longest in the management of osteoporosis and bone cancer therapy. The half-life of BPs is ten years. Bisphosphonates are subclassified into two distinct categories: nitrogen containing and non-nitrogen containing.
   Nitrogen containing amino-bisphosphonates include:

- Alendronate (Fosamax)
- Ibandronate (Boniva)
- Risedronate (Actonel)
- Pamidronate (Aredia)
- Zoledronic acid (Zometa 4mg IV; Reclast/Aclasta 5mg IV): Zoledronic acid has the highest incidence of bone necrosis in cancer patients.

   Non-Nitrogen containing bisphosphonates include:

- Clodronate (Bonefos)
- Etidronate (Didrocal)
- Tiludronate (Skelid)

   Bisphosphonates Mechanism of Action (MOA)

- BPs inhibit osteoclastic activity, which leads to a reduced in the activation of osteoblasts; consequently, this leads to reduced bone formation because of decreased osteoblastic activity.

- BPs inhibit Vascular Endothelial Growth Factor (VEGF). VEGF is a signal protein causing vascular growth; hence inhibition decreases vessel growth and angiogenesis.
- BPs activate the immune system. Tumor cells are directly killed by gamma delta T cells, which are activated by BPs
- BPs have anti-cancer activity; they induce tumor cell apoptosis, decrease the adhesion of cancer cells to bone, and decrease the invasive capacity of tumor cells.

Denosumab (Prolia)

Denosumab, a more recent non-bisphosphonate anti-resorptive agent, is a human monoclonal antibody that targets the receptor activator of the nuclear factor-kappa-B ligand (RANKL) protein, which acts as the primary signal to promote bone removal. By inhibiting the development and activity of osteoclasts, denosumab thus decreases bone resorption and increases bone density. Denosomab is used for the treatment of women with postmenopausal osteoporosis. Compared to alendronate, denosumab has shown to decrease the incidence of vertebral and hip fractures. It is a Pregnancy Category C drug. It is given as a single subcutaneous (SC) injection of 60mg every 6 months for osteoporosis, and as a single subcutaneous (SC) injection every month for cancer therapy. Higher prevalence of anti-resorptive agent–induced osteonecrosis of the jaw (ARONJ) has been demonstrated in patients taking denosumab, subcute (SC), once/month compared with zoledronic acid (Zometa), intravenous (IV), once/month.

Teriparatide (Fortea)

Teriparatide is the 1-34, N-terminal active fragment of parathyroid hormone (PTH). It is the first FDA-approved anabolic agent drug for osteoporosis that stimulates new bone formation leading to increased bone mineral density. Teriparatide is contraindicated in patients at risk for osteosarcoma or Paget's disease. Once-daily intramuscular (IM) injections of teriparatide lead to activation of osteoblasts more than osteoclasts. This, in turn, leads to new bone formation and increased bone mineral density. Teriparatide has shown some limited promise in the treatment of ARONJ. In a NIH supported study that compared teriparatide with placebo, teriparatide was shown to have improved clinical outcomes, with a reduction in periodontal probing depth and a gain in clinical attachment level, greater resolution of alveolar bone defects, and accelerated osseous wound healing in the oral cavity. It is postulated that teriparatide could potentially be therapeutic for localized bone defects in the jaw.

Anti-Resorptive Agent Uses

Anti-resorptive agents are used for the management of the following conditions:

- **Osteoporosis:** Bisphosphonates more commonly are given to decrease bone resorption in osteoporosis associated with menopause, prolonged immobility, or chronic corticosteroid use, which may be as little as 5mg prednisone × three months/longer. Typically, alendronate (Fosamax) 70mg, once/week oral, or once/year zolidronic acid (Reclast/Aclasta) intravenous (IV), are given for the management of osteoporosis.

- **Paget's disease:** Paget's disease of bone is a chronic bone condition that affects more men than women (3:2). Patients with Paget's disease experience rapid bone repair that causes symptoms ranging from softer bones to enlarged bone growth, typically in the pelvis, low back/spine, hips, thighs, skull, and arms. BP therapies have proven effective in reducing the frequency of pain, fractures, and arthritis that may be caused by Paget's disease.
- **Multiple myeloma (MM):** Multiple myeloma or plasma cell myeloma is a hematological cancer affecting the bone marrow in the spine, pelvic bones, ribs, shoulders, and hips. Plasma cells accumulate in the bone marrow, interfering with the normal bone marrow production. Infiltrating myeloma cells cause soft osteolytic bone lesions, resulting in bone loss. BPs are used as primary therapy along with chemotherapy drugs, corticosteroids and immune modulators/anti-VEGF drugs, thalidomide (Thalomid)/lenalidomide (Revlimid)/bortozomib (Velcade), in the management of MM.
- **Metastatic bone disease:** BPs are used as secondary therapy when metastasis occurs from primary tumor sites located in the lungs, breast, or prostate.

Anti-Resorptive Agent Side Effects

- **Esophagitis:** This side effect is BPs related and occurs most commonly with risedronate (Actonel). Patients on alendronate (Fosamax) are told to take the drug with water and remain upright for one hour. Because of this cumbersome requirement, many such patients now opt for zoledronic acid (Reclast) once/year.
- **Esophageal cancer:** Esophageal cancer is also BPs related and is associated more often with alendronate (Fosamax).
- **Atypical fractures:** Increasing numbers of atypical hip fractures have been reported among patients with history of bisphosphonate use for 5–7 years or longer.
- **ARONJ:** The 2008 terminology, bisphosphonate-associated osteonecrosis of the jaw (BONJ), was replaced in 2011 with new terminology: anti-resorptive agent–induced osteonecrosis of the jaw, or ARONJ. In addition to bisphosphonates, denosumab (Prolia), a non-bisphosphonate anti-resorptive drug approved for the treatment of postmenopausal osteoporosis, was reported to have been associated with osteonecrosis of the jaw (ONJ).

ANTI-RESORPTIVE AGENT–INDUCED OSTEONECROSIS OF THE JAW

The highest reliable estimate of anti-resorptive agent–induced osteonecrosis of the jaw (ARONJ) prevalence is approximately 0.10%. The prevalence rate for ARONJ is 1 in 30 for cancer and 1 in 2,000–3,000 for patients being treated for osteoporosis. The mandible-to-maxilla involvement ratio is 2:1. Of lesions, 33% are painless, and 60% of patients give a positive history of surgery. The risk of ARONJ in osteoporosis increases after the patient has been on bisphosphonates **for four or more** years. The **risk increases with monthly intravenous (IV)** bisphosphonates compared with once per year IV bisphosphonates or weekly oral BPs. The risk of ARONJ in cancer patients increases after being on bisphosphonates for **16–24 months**, but it could occur in less time, especially in multiple myeloma (MM) patients. Data show that the incidence of ARONJ increased in patients with MM when they were on once per month intravenous (IV) Zometa for three months. Because of these reasons, **all cancer patients** are now **reassessed after two years** of treatment in order to minimize the risk for ARONJ.

Risk Factors Associated with ARONJ

Risk factors include dento-alveolar surgery, including extractions, as bone turnover is higher in the alveolus than in the rest of the jaw; patients wearing dentures; presence of diabetes; elderly patients older than 65; obesity; patients on bisphosphonate for two or more years; periodontitis, periodontal pockets, or active-abscess associated, high bacterial load; significant family history of ARONJ due to of genetic predisposition; smoking; trauma from normal function or from dentures; and use of anti-vascular endothelial growth factor (VEGF) drugs such as thalidomide (Thalomid), lenalidomide (Revlimid), and bortozomib (Velcade). **It is important to note that chronic corticosteroid therapy has not been documented as a risk factor for ARONJ.**

Prevention Strategies

- The patient's physician and dentist must work collaboratively to eliminate all risk factors promoting ARONJ, and this can be done by targeting optimal oral health prior to the start of anti-resorptive therapy.
- Prior to osteoporosis or cancer therapy, the patient should have a complete oral assessment with panoramic radiograph and periapical films.
- The dentist should eliminate all foci of infection and complete all restorations, scaling and root planing (SCRP), root canal therapy, and extractions, when needed.
- Once the patient is cleared to start anti-resorptive therapy, daily excellent hygiene habits, optimal dental care, and routine dental follow-up visits should occur every 3–6 months.
- The MD should take caution not to over suppress bone turnover with the therapy.

Identification Criteria

- ARONJ-associated symptoms may include pain, swelling, cellulites, halitosis, and/or trismus.
- ARONJ-associated physical findings may include mandibular and/or maxillary bone exposure, pathologic fracture, oral-cutaneous fistula, and/or presence of infection.
- ARONJ is identified by the presence of exposed bone in the oral cavity for a period of **eight weeks**. If the lesion has been present for less than eight weeks, it should be considered suspicious. The sequestered bone, when cultured, can demonstrate Actinomycetes. Actinomycetes are a normal component of dental plaque-BIOFILM, colonizing dead bone as if it were tooth surface. It should be noted that there is no true Actinomycetes infection present. True Actinomycetes infection will show sulphur granules clinically and histologically. The patient will also experience significant pain, swelling, sinus tract formation, and pus.
- The patient has to have been exposed to bisphosphonates or denosumab.
- There has to be **no** history of exposure to radiation to the local site.

Radiographic, CT, and MRI Bone Findings Associated with Anti-Resorptive Agents

Radiographic Findings

It is important to note that radiographic changes related to BPs or denosumab are **non-specific** and **similar** to any other dental **inflammatory** changes. **Therefore, in the absence of clinical symptoms/necrotic sequestrate, we cannot predict ARONJ based on radiographs.** This view is also supported by the AAOMS position paper (See Figure 41.2 and 41.3).

- **Osteosclerosis:** The most common radiographic finding associated with ARONJ is osseous sclerosis. Varying degrees of osseous sclerosis commonly involve alveolar

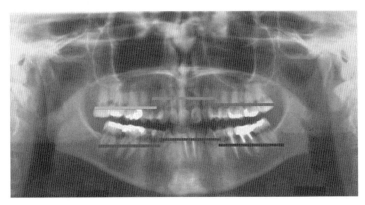

By dividing the maxilla and mandible into sextants, the clinical and radiographic findings can be accurately and reliably correlated with respect to the location of the lesion.

━━ Sextant 1 ━━ Sextant 2 ━━ Sextant 3 ━━ Sextant 4 ━━ Sextant 5 ━━ Sextant 6

Oral Diseases: Treister N, Sheehy N, Bae EH, Friedland B, Lerman M, Woo S. Dental panoramic radiographic evaluation in bisphosphonate-associated osteonecrosis of the jaws. 2008:15(1):88-92. DOI: 10.1111/j.1601-0825.2008.01494.x

Figure 41.2.   Panoramic radiographic evaluation in bisphosphonate-related osteonecrosis of the jaw.

Film A demonstrates: Persistent extraction sockets and surface irregularity

Film B demonstrates: Sclerosis and lysis

Film C demonstrates: Bone fragmentation

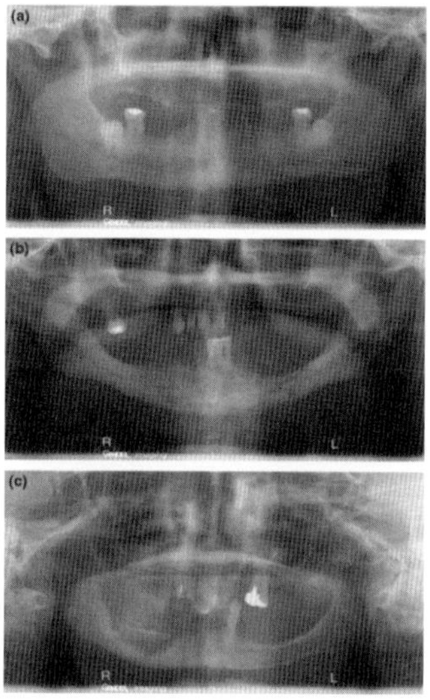

Oral Diseases: Treister N, Sheehy N, Bae EH, Friedland B, Lerman M, Woo S. Dental panoramic radiographic evaluation in bisphosphonate-associated osteonecrosis of the jaws. 2008:15(1): 88-92. DOI: 10.1111/j.1601-0825.2008.01494.x

Figure 41.3. ARONJ panoramic radiographic evaluation.

margin and the lamina dura. Sclerotic changes are often diffuse rather than localized to the area of clinical involvement. With sequential imaging, sclerotic changes are often progressive and can encroach on the mandibular canal causing the patient to experience excruciating pain. The sclerosis of the medullary cavity may be attenuated and reminiscent of osteopetrosis.

- **Thickened lamina dura:** This occurs especially around posterior teeth.
- ARONJ risk is higher if the patient has osteosclerosis and thickened lamina dura.
- **Widened periodontal ligament (PDL):** PDL widening may be a more sensitive indicator in predicting the risk of ARONJ.
- **Less-common findings**: Other less-commonly encountered findings include poorly healing or non-healing persistent extraction sockets, periapical lucencies, osteolysis, sequestra, oroantral fistula, soft tissue thickening, and periosteal new bone formation.

Computerized Tomography (CT) Findings

CT scans show increased medullary density, periosteal reaction, and bone sequestration. Cone beam computed tomography (CBCT) shows the extent of disease, especially if the patient has stage 0 ARONJ.

Magnetic Resonance Imaging (MRI)

With exposed bone, MRI shows a low signal in T-1 and T-2 images. Unexposed, diseased bone shows hypointensity in T-1 images and hyperintensity in T-2 images. Imaging is noninvasive and is likely to play a bigger role in confirming the diagnosis of ARONJ.

ARONJ Stages and Associated Treatments

ARONJ lesions are staged and treated as follows:
    Stage 0

- Stage 0 is further subclassified **Stage 0sa** (suspicious lesion, but the patient is asymptomatic) and **Stage 0ss** (Suspicious lesion and the patient is symptomatic).
- Patient gives a positive history of exposure to anti-resorptive therapy.
- There is presence of a suspicious lesion of less than eight weeks duration, but there is **no** exposed bone.
- Pain is typically absent.
- The patient may have non-specific symptoms, a deep periodontal pocket, or may show radiographic findings consistent with ARONJ, but there are **no** radiographic findings that indicate an odontogenic infection.

    Stage 0 Treatment

- Provide conservative local therapy, prescribe analgesics and antibiotics as needed, and advise routine dental care.
- Contact the MD to discuss the patient's status and the absolute need for bisphosphonate therapy.

    Stage 1

- Patient has exposed necrotic bone, is asymptomatic, does **not** have pain and there is **no** evidence of infection.

    Stage 1 Treatment

- Dispense non-alcoholic chlorhexidine 0.12% rinses, as they will help control Actinomycetes colonization in oral biofilms.
- Minocycline hydrochloride (Arestin) rinse may also be prescribed if periodontal pockets exist.
- Smooth out the sharp edges and, when possible, gently remove the dead bone non-surgically only.
- Use analgesics and antibiotics if needed
- Have the patient follow-up in 3–6 months.

    Stage 2

- The patient experiences exposed necrotic bone associated pain.
- The patient may or may not show symptoms for infection and there may or may not be any purulent sinus tract drainage.

- The provider must identify by culture if the infection is bacterial, viral, or fungal in nature.

Stage 2 Treatment

- As with stage 1, dispense non-alcoholic chlorhexidine 0.12% rinses and minocycline hydrochloride (Arestin) mouth rinse if periodontal pockets exist. Mouth rinse and antibiotics combined help to better control the pain.
- Prescribe analgesics.
- Prescribe standard dosing of single antibiotics such as, penicillin VK, amoxicillin, amoxicillin clavulanate, clindamycin, doxycycline, metronidazole or combination antibiotics such as, penicillin VK/amoxicillin + metronidazole, for 2–3 months, or longer, if culture indicates a bacterial infection. Antibiotic use prevents secondary soft tissue infection and progression to osteomyelitis, plus it enhances granulation tissue formation, which then promotes expulsion of dead bone. Antibiotic therapy may need to be continued until mucosal healing is observed.
- Use antifungals nystatin oral suspension 5–15mL, four times daily, 100,000units/mL, or 10mg clotrimazole (Mycelex) troches, five times daily if culture indicates localized fungal infection. Continue antifungal therapy until soft tissue healing occurs. Use fluconazole 200mg on day 1, followed by 100mg once daily, until mucosal healing is observed if systemic antifungals are needed.
- Prescribe acyclovir 400mg twice daily or valacyclovir 500mg–2g twice daily until mucosal healing occurs, when culture indicates a viral infection.
- Always remove dead bone non-surgically when possible and gently/atraumatically debride the area to promote granulation tissue formation.
- Fabricate a soft acrylic stent, if needed.
- Minimize soft tissue trauma with removable appliances.
- Follow-up must be more frequent: every two to six months.

Stage 3

- Lesion is as described in stage 2, but now the disease process could extend beyond the alveolar bone.
- There can be associated pathological fracture.
- There can be radiographic evidence of dissolution or degeneration of bone tissue through disease, extending to extra-oral areas or beyond, involving the sinus floor or the inferior mandibular border, with extra-oral fistula formation.

Stage 3 Treatment

- Treatment is the same as in stage 2.
- Additionally, the provider must be minimally invasive with dentistry. Do root canals instead of extractions, because root canal therapy is preferred over extractions.
- Provide surgical correction, debridement, or repair with minimal bone manipulation that promotes healing and creation of intact mucosa. Be advised that soft tissue injury with subsequent bacterial invasion and infection is the primary problem that can progress to bony necrosis.
- A **two to four week drug holiday** may be considered only to **promote soft tissue healing. A drug holiday lasting months is not advised because it has no direct impact on bones.** Furthermore, no study has confirmed that drug holidays are

effective in prevention of ARONJ without increasing the skeletally related risks of low bone mass, such as fractures.

- Post-operative antibiotics should be prescribed following all oral surgery procedures.

Dental Alerts Associated with Anti-Resorptive Therapy

- The provider must have good judgment and an understanding of the patient's health history and physical findings in order to appropriately plan for dentistry. Therefore, a thorough history and physical examination is very important during the initial visit. It is more important to know the patient's total bisphosphonate dose/year than to know if the bisphosphonate is given intravenously or orally. Be aware that cancer patients get 12 times the osteoporosis dose in the form of intravenous (IV) Zometa once/month, or IV Aredia once/month.
- The patient must be informed about the importance of having regular dental visits to further minimize the low risk of ARONJ ($\sim$0.10%), associated with anti-resorptive therapy for osteoporosis.
- The dentist must discuss, document, and gain written approval from the patient for all treatment options discussed openly and consented by the patient.
- The dentist must be conservative when planning surgical procedures to minimize tissue trauma and work **quadrant-by-quadrant, or per sextant,** to localize tissue trauma and observe tissue healing in a smaller area.
- The dentist must implement proper infection control, use non-alcoholic mouth rinse prior to all visits, and use oral antibiotics when needed. Once proper healing is observed, the dentist can proceed and provide treatment in multiple sextants if needed.
- The dentist should treat any active periodontal or dental disease immediately, irrespective of multiple-quadrant involvement, even if the risk of ARONJ exists. The risk of complications associated with untreated disease far outweighs the risk of developing ARONJ. Antiseptic mouthwash should be continued in order to decrease inflammation and to promote healing.
- Currently, there are no diagnostic tests that can predict the risk for ARONJ and there is no evidence showing that discontinuing therapy eliminates the risk for ARONJ. In fact, discontinuing therapy may increase the risk for fractures in patients with very low bone mass.
- Patients on anti-resorptive therapy with active chronic periodontal diseases should get nonsurgical hygiene therapy, and the patient should be reevaluated at an interval of three months or less. If surgical periodontal therapy is needed, it should be as atraumatic as possible, minimizing dento-alveolar manipulation.
- No published data exist on the risk of ARONJ following implant treatment after periodontal procedures, such as guided tissue regeneration or bone grafting. The success rates for implants placed in patients on bisphosphonate therapy appear to be no different than the success rates for implants placed in patients without a history of bisphosphonate therapy. Thus, anti-resorptive therapy is not a contraindication for dental implant placement.
- Invasive surgical procedures do have a small risk of developing ARONJ, but invasive procedures can occur if the benefits far outweigh the risks. After any surgical procedure involving bone or bone exposure, the surgeon should advise the patient

to rinse gently with a non-alcoholic chlorhexidine rinse twice daily, for four to eight weeks and prescribe antibiotic prophylaxis starting one day prior to the surgical procedure, continuing for three, five, or seven days following the surgical procedure to effectively prevent ARONJ.

- Once the patient has been on anti-resorptive therapy for two or more years, oral and maxillofacial surgery is not strictly contraindicated but procedures that minimize periosteal and/or intrabony exposures are preferred.
- As an alternate to extraction, the oral surgeon can advise endodontic treatment followed by removal of the clinical crown, thus allowing the roots to exfoliate. Then, fixed and removable partial dentures can be used.
- Endodontic therapy is a better option than surgical manipulation of a viable tooth in patients at greater risk for ARONJ. Manipulation beyond the apex should be limited.
- All routine restorative procedures can continue and prosthodontic appliances should be fitted promptly to avoid ulceration and possible bone exposure.
- Orthodontic movement of the teeth may be compromised by anti-resorptive therapy because of alteration in bone physiology caused by anti-resorptive therapy. Thus, the duration of orthodontic treatment may be longer in such cases.

42

Growth Hormone Dysfunction and Endocrine Tissues of the Reproductive System

GROWTH HORMONE DYSFUNCTION

Hypothalamus-Pituitary Growth Hormone (GH/Somatotrophin) Axis

The hypothalamus releases growth hormone-releasing hormone **(GHRH)**, which then stimulates the pituitary gland to produce GH. Secretion of GH by the pituitary into the bloodstream stimulates the liver to produce another hormone called insulin-like growth factor I (IGF-I). **IGF-I** is what actually causes tissue growth in the body. High levels of IGF-I, in turn, signal the pituitary to reduce GH production.

Somatostatin is another hormone made by the hypothalamus and it inhibits GH production and release. Normally, GHRH, somatostatin, GH, and IGF-I levels in the body are tightly regulated by one another and by sleep, exercise, stress, food intake, and blood sugar levels. If the pituitary continues to make GH independent of the normal regulatory mechanisms, the level of IGF-I continues to rise, leading to bone overgrowth and organ enlargement. High levels of IGF-I also cause changes in glucose and lipid metabolism, which can lead to diabetes, high blood pressure, and heart disease.

Growth hormone (GH) secreted by the anterior pituitary gland stimulates protein synthesis and cell division in cartilage and bone tissue. **Gigantism** results when excessive amounts of growth hormone are produced during childhood. **Pituitary dwarfism** occurs when too little growth hormone is produced and **acromegaly** occurs when too much GH is produced during adulthood.

GH-stimulated cell growth and protein synthesis occur via the release of somatomedins by the liver. This stimulation occurs almost immediately, when glucose and amino acid concentrations in the blood are elevated. A second effect appears hours later, as glucose and amino acid levels are declining. Under these conditions GH causes the breakdown of glycogen and lipid reserves, and directs peripheral tissues to begin using lipids instead of glucose as an energy source. As a result, blood glucose concentrations rise. These effects appear through an interaction between growth hormone and somatomedins.

Dentist's Guide to Medical Conditions, Medications, and Complications, Second Edition. Kanchan M. Ganda.
© 2013 John Wiley & Sons, Inc. Published 2013 by John Wiley & Sons, Inc.

Acromegaly Facts

The following summarizes acromegaly seen in dentistry:

- Acromegaly is associated with excess growth hormone (GH) from benign or non-cancerous pituitary tumors/adenomas. It is most often diagnosed in middle-aged adults, although symptoms can appear at any age. If not treated, acromegaly can result in serious illness and premature death. The hands and feet are big, with rapid increase in ring size or glove and shoe size; the patient often complains of excessive sweating, and there is an increased incidence of skin tags, moles, sebaceous cysts, colonic polyps, type 2 diabetes, hypertension, risk of cardiovascular disease, arthritis, and colon cancer.
- Accelerated tooth eruption occurs in children.
- Enlarged jaw with prognathism is common, the teeth are spaced and tipped outward, the facial features are coarse, there is excess deposition of cementum on the roots of teeth and macroglossia is often seen. The patient has larger than normal maxillary sinuses, and this is the cause of a booming voice in these patients.

Acromegaly Treatment

Acromegaly is treatable in most patients, but because of its slow onset, it often is not diagnosed early or correctly. Treatment options are surgery, radiation, or somatostatin therapy (an inhibitor of GH), and GH receptor blockade.

There are three options in the medical management of acromegaly:

- Somatostatin analogs (SSAs), such as octreotide or long-acting lanreotide, are the first line of therapy for management of acromegaly. SSAs shut off GH production and are effective in lowering GH and IGF-I levels in 50–70% of patients. SSAs also reduce tumor size to some extent in up to 50% of patients. SSAs are safe and effective for long-term treatment and in treating patients with acromegaly caused by non-pituitary tumors. Long-acting SSAs are given by intramuscular injection **once a month**. Temporary side effects occurring in about half the patients on SSAs include loose stools, nausea, and gas. Occasionally, elevated blood sugar levels can occur, but more commonly, SSAs reduce the need for insulin and improve blood glucose control in some people with acromegaly who already have diabetes.
- GH receptor antagonists (GHRAs) are the second line of therapy. GHRAs interfere with the action of GH. They normalize IGF-I levels in more than 90% of patients. They do not, however, lower GH levels. Given once a day through injection, GHRAs are usually well tolerated by patients. The long-term effects of these drugs on tumor growth are still being established. Side effects can include headaches, fatigue, and abnormal liver function.
- Dopamine agonists (bromocriptine mesylate, cabergoline) constitute the third line of therapy. These drugs are not as effective as the other medications in lowering GH or IGF-I levels, and they normalize IGF-I levels in only a minority of patients. Dopamine agonists are sometimes effective in patients who have mild degrees of excess GH and who have both acromegaly and hyperprolactinemia. Dopamine agonists can be used in combination with SSAs. Side effects can include nausea, headache, and lightheadedness.

Gigantism

Growth plates fuse after puberty, so the excessive GH production in adults does not result in increased height. However, increased growth of the long bones and increased height occurs when prolonged GH exposure occurs before the growth plates fuse. Gigantism should always be considered as a possibility if a child's growth rate suddenly and markedly increases beyond what would be predicted by previous growth and based on how tall the child's parents are. Treatment is along the lines of management of acromegaly.

ENDOCRINE TISSUES OF THE REPRODUCTIVE SYSTEM

The Gonads

The ovary is responsible for the synthesis of estrogen and progesterone. Estrogen is required for the formation of the ovum during oogenesis and prepares the uterus for implanting a fertilized egg. Progesterone works with estrogen to regulate the menstrual cycle and prepares the breasts for lactation during pregnancy. The testes produce the hormone testosterone, which is required for sperm formation during spermatogenesis and secondary sexual characteristics.

Interstitial cells of the male testes manufacture steroid androgens, particularly testosterone. Testosterone promotes the production of functional sperm, maintains the secretory glands of the male reproductive tract, and determines secondary sexual characteristics.

Follicle cells in the ovaries produce steroid estrogens while ova are developing. After ovulation, the cells reorganize into a corpus luteum that produces progesterone. If pregnancy occurs, the placenta then gradually develops endocrine functions of its own.

Seizure Disorders

Classic Seizures: Assessment, Analysis, and Associated Dental Management Guidelines

SEIZURE CLASSIFICATION, OVERVIEW, AND TREATMENT OPTIONS

Seizure Classification

Conditions associated with seizures are:

1. Vasovagal syncopal reaction
2. Orthostatic hypotension
3. Hyperventilation syndrome
4. Hypoglycemic reaction
5. Grand mal epilepsy
6. Petit mal epilepsy

The first four causes have been discussed in Chapter 9. Causes 5 and 6 are major seizure disorders and are discussed in this chapter.

General Introduction

Seizures are caused because of abnormal electrical discharges in the brain and they can occur as grand mal seizures, petit mal seizures, or temporal lobe seizures. Occurrence of repeat seizures leads to a diagnosis of epilepsy.

A seizure is **generalized** if the abnormal electrical discharges cross over the midline in the brain. When the seizures involve only a few muscles in the face, arms, or legs, it is a **focal** seizure. A grand mal seizure or a tonic-clonic seizure is characterized by loss of consciousness with the patient falling down, loss of bowel or bladder control, and rhythmic-to-arrhythmic convulsions.

Dentist's Guide to Medical Conditions, Medications, and Complications, Second Edition. Kanchan M. Ganda.
© 2013 John Wiley & Sons, Inc. Published 2013 by John Wiley & Sons, Inc.

Seizure Etiology

The following are etiological factors associated with seizures:

- **Familial:** Seizures can be familial affecting several members in the family.
- **Unknown etiology:** Often the etiology is unknown and there is no associated family history.
- **Metabolic disturbances:** Seizures can occur from chemical imbalance due to liver or kidney disease or very low levels of sodium, calcium, or magnesium.
- **Trauma:** Head injuries can cause seizures.
- **Space-occupying lesions:** Tumors or arterial-venous malformations in the brain can trigger seizures.
- **Cerebrovascular accidents (CVA) or strokes:** CVAs can cause seizures in older patients.
- **Drug addiction:** Withdrawal from recreational drugs can be associated with seizures.
- **Cerebral infection:** Meningitis or encephalitis can trigger a seizure.
- **Other causes:** Seizures can also be triggered by stress, lack of sleep, flickering lights, alcohol, or touch.

Seizure Diagnosis

Seizure diagnosis is established as follows:

1. **History and physical (H&P) examination:** A thorough H&P can reveal the etiology and presenting symptoms and signs of the seizure.
2. **Electroencephalography (EEG):** EEG measures the electrical activity in the brain and can show areas of increased activity.
3. **Magnetic resonance imaging (MRI):** MRI can detect brain pathology.

Seizure Treatment

Management of seizures consists of the following:

1. Treatment of the underlying cause, if known.
2. **Surgery** is an option when a tumor or vascular malformation is the cause of the seizure. Surgery is also an option when the patient does not respond to medications and has such frequent seizures that it significantly compromises the patient's life style.
3. Antiseizure medications.

SEIZURE MEDICATIONS: OVERVIEW

Grand Mal Seizure Medications

The most common medications used for grand mal epilepsy are phenytoin sodium (Dilantin), carbamazepine (Tegretol), phenobarbital (Barbita/Luminal), primidone (Mysoline), gabapentin (Neurontin), clonazepam (Klonopin), oxcarbazepine (Trileptal), and the benzodiazepines lorazepam (Ativan) or diazepam (Valium).

Petit Mal Seizure Medications

The following are the petit mal medications:

1. **Older medications:** valproic acid (Depakene), divalproex (Depakote), and ethosux-imide (Zarontin)
2. **Newer medications:** lamotrigine (Lamictal), topiramate (Topamax), and zonisamide (Zonegran).

SEIZURE MEDICATIONS: DETAILED DISCUSSION

To better manage a patient with a history of seizures, it is important to understand the medications used to treat the disorder. Significant facts relevant to dentistry have been highlighted with each drug.

Phenytoin Sodium (Dilantin)

Dilantin Facts

Phenytoin (Dilantin) is used in the management of grand mal epilepsy, and chronic use is associated with **gingival hyperplasia.** Dilantin **inhibits** the absorption of **folic acid** from the gut and predisposes the patient to develop folic acid deficiency/megaloblastic anemia. Evaluate the CBC and follow the suggested AAA guidelines for anemia if anemia is detected on the CBC. Chronic **alcohol** use or abuse decreases the serum levels of Dilantin and predisposes the patient to have more **frequent seizures.**

Dilantin and DDIs

The following are DDIs associated with Dilantin:

- Avoid the use of salicylates or diazepam (Valium) because these drugs can increase the serum levels of Dilantin.
- Avoid using doxycycline (Vibramycin) because the efficacy of doxycycline is impaired in the presence of Dilantin.

Carbamazepine (Tegretol)

Carbamazepine (Tegretol) is used for the management of grand mal seizures **and** trigeminal neuralgia.

Tegretol and DDIs

The following are DDIs associated with Tegretol:

- Avoid using doxycycline (Vibramycin) because carbamazepine (Tegretol) decreases the half-life of doxycycline.
- Macrolides and propoxyphene (Darvon) use should be restricted because they raise Tegretol levels.

Phenobarbital (Barbita/Luminal)

Phenobarbital Facts

Phenobarbital is the oldest and most widely used medication in the world. It is used for the management of generalized and partial seizures. Due to its sedative and hypnotic effects, phenobarbital is less preferred than benzodiazepines.

Phenobarbital (Barbita/Luminal) and DDIs

The following are DDIs associated with phenobarbital:

- Do not prescribe doxycycline with phenobarbital because phenobarbital induces the CYP450 enzymes in the liver, enhancing the utilization of doxycycline.
- Phenobarbital increases the effectiveness of sedatives, hypnotics, narcotics, and acetaminophen. It is suggested that you avoid using sedatives, hypnotics, and narcotics with phenobarbital and use only regular-strength Tylenol.

Primidone (Mysolin)

Primidone Facts

Primidone is used for the management of grand mal, complex, and focal seizures. Primidone is the first-line drug (along with propranolol) for the management of benign tremors. It is a GABA receptor agonist that also causes sedation because of its active metabolites, phenobarbital and phenylethylmalonamide. Primidone is associated with folic acid deficiency and poor calcium absorption. Evaluate the CBC for anemia and the dental radiographs for bone density in patients on primidone. Follow the AAA suggested guidelines for anemia if the CBC shows anemia. Primidone induces the enzymes in the liver and accelerates the metabolism of several medications.

Primidone (Mysolin) and DDIs

The following are DDIs associated with primidone:

- Primidone hastens the metabolism of doxycycline, dexamethasone, and other steroids due to liver enzyme induction and consequently decreases their effect.
- Avoid fentanyl use as primidone causes increase in fentanyl levels.

Gabapentin (Neurontin)

Neurontin is used for seizure disorders, non-specific neuralgia, trigeminal neuralgia, leg cramps, and postherpetic neuralgia. Alcohol increases the risk of side effects with Neurontin.

Gabapentin (Neurontin) and DDIs

The following are DDIs associated with gabapentin:

- Antacids decrease Neurontin absorption, and an interval of **at least two hours** must be maintained to avoid this DDI.

- Neurontin increases the effects of antihistamines, sedatives, centrally acting pain medications, benzodiazepines, and muscle relaxants, causing profound drowsiness. Avoid dispensing these medications in conjunction with gabapentin during dentistry.

Clonazepam (Klonopin)

Clonazepam is a benzodiazepine and is used for the treatment of petit mal seizures, restless leg syndrome, panic disorders, and neuralgia. Klonopin causes increased salivation.

Clonazepam (Klonopin) and DDIs

Avoid clarithromycin and metronidazole because they increase Klonopin levels via inhibition of the CYP3A4 enzyme.

Oxcarbazepine (Trileptal)

Trileptal is used in the management of partial seizures in adults and children. Trileptal works by decreasing impulses in the nerves that cause seizures and it is associated with significant xerostomia.

Valproic Acid (Depakene)

Valproic acid is used in the treatment of petit mal epilepsy. Valproic acid increases the effect of pain medications and anesthetics. Depakene causes hypofibrinogenemia, thrombocytopenia, inhibition of platelet aggregation, leukopenia, eosinophilia, and macrocytic, folic acid–associated anemia.

Always monitor the CBC, platelet count, and coagulation tests **prior** to major dental surgery in patients on Depakene. Always check the **LFTs** and avoid using other hepatotoxic drugs with valproic acid.

Valproic Acid (Depakene) and DDIs

Avoid aspirin, NSAIDS, barbiturates, and diazepam.

Ethosuximide (Zarontin)

Ethosuximide is an antiseizure medication used in the management of petit mal epilepsy. Zarontin can cause pancytopenia, so always assess CBC prior to major dental surgery.

Divalproex (Depakote)

The liver- and pancreas-associated side effects are similar to valproic acid. Depakote causes excessive sunburns because of increased photosensitivity.

Lamotrigene (Lamictal)

Lamictal is used for the treatment of partial seizures, generalized seizures in adults and children over 16 years of age, and for the treatment of bipolar disorder. Lamictal has relatively few side effects.

Topiramate (Topamax)

Topamax is used for the treatment of partial seizures and tonic-clonic seizures in children and adults. Topamax causes taste changes, feeling of pins and needles in the head and limbs, osteoporosis, gingivitis, xerostomia, and hyperthermia in children.

Zonisamide (Zonegran)

Zonegran is used for the treatment of partial seizures.

SEIZURE MEDICATIONS AND SUGGESTED DENTAL ALERTS

1. Always check for a history of alcohol use during history-taking, because alcohol decreases the potency of seizure medications.
2. All antiseizure drugs can increase the effectiveness of centrally acting pain medications and muscle relaxants, causing excess drowsiness.
3. Avoid centrally acting pain medications, sedatives, hypnotics, narcotics, and sedating antihistamines with antiseizure medications as they enhance sedation.
4. Use regular-strength acetaminophen (Tylenol) only.
5. Phenytoin (Dilantin), carbamazepine (Tegretol), primidone (Mysolin), and phenobarbital are the most potent hepatic enzyme inducers at therapeutic doses, and, as previously discussed, use doxycycline, clarithromycin, steroids, and metronidazole with extreme caution if you plan on using any one of them. It is best to avoid these medications.
6. Most of the seizure medications cause xerostomia. Always provide long-term xerostomia management, when needed.
7. Dilantin and primidone cause folic acid deficiency and macrocytic anemia. Obtain the **CBC** prior to dental treatment. Follow the AAA suggested guidelines for anemia, if CBC indicates changes associated with folic acid deficiency.
8. Phenytoin (Dilantin) additionally causes gingival hyperplasia. It is best to schedule hygiene recall every three to four months to control the hyperplasia. If the hyperplasia continues, alert the patient's physician who may switch to another medication.
9. Primidone (Mysoline) and topiramate (Topamax) cause osteoporosis. Always check the bone density on the dental radiographs. Presence of bone loss may cause frequent denture adjustments if the patient has removable appliances.
10. Topiramate (Topamax) additionally causes taste changes and parasthesias in the head and limbs. Always confirm the presence of these symptoms prior to injecting the local anesthetic.
11. Valproic acid enhances the effects of pain medications and anesthetics so use decreased doses or decreased amounts of the drugs.
12. Check the CBC, calculate the ANC, and determine the PT/INR, if the patient is on valproic acid for reasons previously discussed. The patient may need antibiotics to prevent and/or treat an infection.

13. Check the CBC for pancytopenia if the patient is on ethosuximide. The patient may need antibiotics to prevent and/or treat an infection.
14. Antiseizure medications, particularly phenobarbital and primidone (Mysolin), depress the CNS and the patient could be sleepy in the chair.
15. Limit the use of local anesthetics with epinephrine to two carpules in patients with well-controlled seizure activity, or in patients with a history of very infrequent seizures. Epinephrine should be avoided in patients with frequently recurring seizures.

GRAND MAL SEIZURE

Refer to Chapter 9 for discussion on clinical features and management of a grand mal seizure.

PETIT MAL SEIZURE

A petit mal seizure is also called an **absence seizure**, and although it is a type of seizure that occurs most often in children, adults can also be affected. An abnormal electrical discharge in the brain causes the seizure.

A petit mal seizure is brief with a sudden lapse of conscious activity, but the patient never falls to the ground. Each seizure lasts a few seconds or minutes, and hundreds of seizure attacks may occur each day.

There may be occasional jerking of the facial muscles or hands, or lip-smacking during the seizure phase. The patient usually resumes normal activities following the seizure and experiences no confusion, but has no recall of the seizure or the lost activity.

Petit mal seizures often occur when the child is inactive or alone; hence the diagnosis can often be delayed or missed if no adult supervision exists during the attacks. An observant mother will often state that the child has a "blank look" or is "staring at the TV without blinking."

Some children can outgrow the seizures and go on to discontinue the medications in adulthood. However, others may progress to develop grand mal seizures in adult life.

Etiology

The etiology is the same as with grand mal epilepsy.

Diagnosis

The process to diagnosis is the same as with grand mal epilepsy.

Treatment

Older Medications

Though older, valproic acid (Depakene) and ethosuximide (Zarontin) have been excellent standard drugs for the management of petit mal epilepsy.

Newer Medications

Lamotrigine (Lamictal), topiramate (Topamax) and zonisamide (Zonegran) are the newer medications available for petit mal epilepsy treatment.

Gastrointestinal Conditions and Diseases

XI

Gastrointestinal Disease States and Associated Oral Cavity Lesions: Assessment, Analysis, and Associated Dental Management Guidelines

ANGULAR CHEILITIS

Angular cheilitis is associated with cracking at the corners of the mouth, pain, and bleeding in severe cases.

Predisposing Factors

Nutritional anemias, and very particularly iron-deficiency anemia, ill-fitting dentures, improper bite, HIV/AIDS, cold weather, and constant lip-smacking are common etiological factors.

Superinfection with candidiasis is very common at the corners of the mouth. Some patients may have associated esophageal candidiasis and may complain of dysphagia and/or odynophagia.

Treatment

Prescribe topical antifungal therapy, pain medications in severe cases, and lip balm for those suffering due to the cold weather. Additionally, always treat the underlying cause of angular cheilitis.

APHTHOUS ULCERS

Etiology

Aphthous ulceration is often brought on by stress, local trauma, prolonged fever, or Crohn's disease (Table 44.1). Of Crohn's disease patients, 4–15% have aphthous ulcers. Aphthous ulceration is a rare finding with celiac disease. Aphthous ulcers can also occur in patients suffering from immunological conditions such as Sjögren's syndrome, systemic lupus erythematosus (SLE), and scleroderma.

Dentist's Guide to Medical Conditions, Medications, and Complications, Second Edition. Kanchan M. Ganda.
© 2013 John Wiley & Sons, Inc. Published 2013 by John Wiley & Sons, Inc.

Table 44.1. Treatment Options for Aphthous Ulcerations

Disease	Generic (Trade) Name	Treatment Instructions
Mild Disease	**1. Topical 0.15 Benzydamine** (Difflam or Tantum) oral rinse	Apply to the ulcers four times/day for two weeks or until the ulcers heal.
Mild Disease	**2. Protective Bioadhesives: Topical Carellose** (Orabase: pectin plus gelatin)	Apply to the ulcers four times/day for two weeks or until the ulcers heal.
Mild Disease	**3. Topical Corticosteroids, in adhesive base or as a spray/cream/pellet:** **a. 1% Triamcinalone dental paste** (Adrortyl or Kenolog in Orabase) **b. Hydrocortisone, 2.5mg pellets** (Corlan) **c. 0.12% or 0.2% Chlorhexidine gluconate aqueous mouth wash** (Peridex) or 1% Chlorhexidine gluconate gel	With any of the preparations for mild disease: Apply to the ulcers four times/day for two weeks or until the ulcers heal.
Severe Disease	**1. Systemic Corticosteroids:** Tablets/capsules	30–60mg prednisone daily for one week, followed by a one-week dose taper.
Severe Disease	**2. Thalidomide** (Thalomid)	50–200mg daily for four to eight weeks.

Treatment

The severity of the ulceration determines the type of treatment provided. Some of the treatment options available are listed in Table 44.1. For a complete list, refer to Chapter 48.

PEUTZ-JEGHER'S SYNDROME

Etiology

Peutz-Jegher's syndrome is associated with mucocutaneous hyperpigmentation and gastrointestinal hamatomatous polyps. The polyps can appear throughout the GI tract.

Clinical Manifestations

The macules appear in infancy and childhood and fade over time. The macules over buccal mucosa, however, do not fade over time. Occasional macules are seen on the palms, soles, digits, eyes, and mouth; 95% of the lesions occur on the lips and 83% occur on the buccal mucosa.

Complications

Complications associated with Peutz-Jegher's syndrome are intestinal obstruction, abdominal pain, and gastrointestinal (GI) bleeding.

ESOPHAGEAL CANCER

Esophageal cancer can be squamous cell cancer or an adenocarcinoma. However, both have poor prognosis. Squamous cell cancer is not associated with Barrett's esophagus. The cancer is usually located in the middle to proximal esophagus, and it may coexist with oropharyngeal cancer.

Risk Factors

Risk factors for esophageal cancer are smoking and alcohol use. The additional risk factors for adenocarcinoma of the esophagus are GERD, Barrett's esophagus, and being a Caucasian 40-year-old male patient.

GASTROESOPHAGEAL REFLUX DISEASE

Etiology

Gastroesophageal reflux disease (GERD) occurs when the lower esophageal sphincter (LES) does not close properly and stomach contents leak back into the esophagus causing heartburn, or the contents go into the back of the mouth, causing a water brash.

A hiatal hernia may contribute to GERD. Hiatal hernia can occur at any age and is not uncommon in people over ages 40–50. Obesity and pregnancy are often aggravating factors for GERD. Heartburn that occurs more than twice per week may be considered GERD.

Clinical Features

Patients with GERD experience substernal heartburn associated with burning, belching, water brush (from acid and water), and regurgitation. Heartburn may indicate severe disease. The symptoms occur after a meal and are aggravated by any change in position. The symptoms are also aggravated by certain foods: fatty foods, spicy foods, and tomato-based foods.

Extra-Esophageal Manifestation of GERD

GERD-associated extra-esophageal manifestations can be dental erosions, chronic cough and constant clearing of the throat, atypical chest pain, epigastric pain, and nausea.

Complications

Complications associated with GERD are esophagitis associated with linear ulcers seen on endoscopy, strictures caused by partially healed ulcers, and Barrett's esophagus that is diagnosed by barium swallow.

Treatment

Medical Management

GERD treatment includes the following medical management:

1. **Proton pump inhibitors (PPIs):** PPIs are acid suppressants and they are the most effective drugs prescribed to treat GERD. Esomeprazole (Nexium), lansoprazole

(Prevacid), omeprazole (Prilosec), and pantoprazole (Protonix) are the most commonly prescribed PPIs. **Side effects:** PPIs can interfere with the absorption of calcium because of the hypochlorhydria, and they also reduce bone resorption through inhibition of osteoclastic vacuolar-proton pumps. There is an increased risk of fractures associated with long-term PPI therapy and high doses of PPIs. Short-term PPIs use can prevent these serious adverse side effects.

2. **H$_2$ blockers:** H$_2$ blockers provide short-term relief and should not be used for more than a few weeks. Cimetidine (Tagamet), famotidine (Pepcid), and ranitidine (Zantac) are the commonly used H$_2$ blockers.

Surgical Management

1. **Surgery:** The goal with surgery is to tighten the stomach by fundoplication where the top part of the stomach is wrapped around the esophagus. Surgical management is not always efficient.
2. **Implant:** The FDA recently approved an implant for patients who want to avoid surgery. Enteryx is a solution that becomes spongy and reinforces the lower esophageal splinter (LES), thus preventing the stomach acid from flowing into the esophagus. Enteryx is injected during endoscopy. The implant has been approved for people who have GERD that has responded to PPIs. The long-term effect of the implant therapy is unknown.

Adjunct Treatment

Adjunct treatment guidelines for GERD are:

1. The patient should sleep with the head elevated with blocks. Trying to elevate the head with multiple pillows is not effective.
2. There should be no food consumption for **three hours** prior to sleeping.
3. The patient should stop smoking and avoid alcohol, caffeine, and mint-containing foods.
4. The patient should also avoid aspirin and NSAIDS to avoid further aggravation of symptoms.

PEPTIC ULCER DISEASE

Etiology

Heliobacter pylorus (H. pylori) is most often implicated as the leading cause of peptic ulcer. H. pylori can reside in the mucosal lining and causes no problem in some patients. When implicated however, it is found to erode the mucosa and cause ulceration.

The next leading cause is chronic NSAIDS use. Peptic ulcers can also be due to ischemia consequent to smoking. Stress and diet are no longer thought to be causative factors.

Classification

Peptic ulcers named according to their location in the GI tract are:

- **Gastric ulcer:** A peptic ulcer found in the stomach
- **Duodenal ulcer:** A peptic ulcer found in the duodenum

Symptoms

The following are symptoms associated with peptic ulcers:

- Pain: The most common type is a burning pain caused by the stomach acid coming into contact with the ulcer. The pain varies in location and can also be gnawing or hunger-like. The pain can last for a few minutes or a few hours. It is often relieved with food.
- Nausea and vomiting with or without blood.
- Black, tarry stools or dark blood in the stools.
- Indigestion, anorexia, early satiety, and bloating.

Diagnosis

Peptic ulcer diagnosis is made using the following tools:

1. **Barium studies:** Barium studies detect the location of the ulcer(s) and identify the ulcer status.
2. **Endoscopy:** Endoscopy visually detects the location of the ulcer(s) and identifies the ulcer status.
3. **Blood test:** The blood test is done to detect the presence of H. pylori antibodies. This test has a disadvantage because it cannot differentiate between past exposure and current infection with the bacteria. The test may be positive for several months after the bacterium has been eradicated.
4. **Breath test:** During the breath test a radioactive carbon atom as a part of urea is consumed as a clear liquid, and 30 minutes later the patient is asked to exhale in a small plastic bag. H. pylori, when present, break down the urea consumed and the radioactive carbon atom is then detected in the form of CO_2 in the exhaled air. The advantage of the breath test is its ability to detect bacteria eradication with treatment.
5. **Stool antigen test:** This test helps identify the presence of H. pylori in the stool. It also helps detect eradication with treatment.

Treatment

The treatment goal is to promote healing by eradicating H. pylori and decreasing the acid production that aggravates the ulcer. Successful treatment takes only a few weeks; the treatment options are as follows:

1. **Antibiotics:** H. pylorus is eradicated with antibiotic treatment, and antibiotic treatment reduces the recurrence rate down to 10–20%. Antibiotic treatment options include:
   a. **Combination antibiotics:** Combination antibiotics work best; the ones commonly prescribed for **two weeks** are amoxicillin (Amoxil), clarithromycin (Biaxin), and metronidazole (Flagyl).
   b. **Commercial preparations:** Commercial preparations containing two of the antibiotics along with a cytoprotective or acid suppressant are available under the names Helidac and Prevpac.

2. **Proton pump inhibitors (PPIs):** The PPIs shut down the tiny pumps in the acid-secreting cells in the stomach and promote healing. The PPIs are also found to inhibit H. pylori activity.
3. **Acid blockers:** H_2 blockers reduce the amount of acid released in the GI tract and promote healing.
4. **Cytoprotective medications:** Sucralfate (Carafate), misoprostol (Cytotec), or bismuth subsalicylate (Pepto-Bismol), are often prescribed. These medications protect the tissue lining of the stomach and duodenum, plus they appear to inhibit H. pylori activity.

Complications

Complications associated with peptic ulcer include bleeding, perforation, or obstruction. Note that bleeding ulcers do not perforate and perforated ulcers do not bleed.

ESOPHAGITIS, GERD, AND PEPTIC ULCER SUGGESTED DENTAL ALERTS

The following are dental alerts for esophagitis, GERD, and peptic ulcer:

1. Always check for a history of chronic intake of aspirin, NSAIDS, and corticosteroids because any one of these drugs taken long term can trigger peptic ulcer disease.
2. Therefore, aspirin, NSAIDS, or steroids should not be prescribed in patients with a history of peptic ulcers, because these drugs cause GI mucosal irritation.
3. Check if the patient is on antacids such as Mylanta, Maalox, or Gelusil. Always be aware that these agents contain aluminum hydroxide, which inhibits the absorption of all tetracyclines.
4. H_2 blockers such as cimetidine (Tagamet), famotidine (Pepcid), or ranitidine (Zantac) prolong the absorption of diazepam (Valium) or lorazepam (Ativan), and these stress-management drugs should be avoided in patients taking these H_2 blockers, or the benzodiazepines should be spaced at least two hours apart from the H_2 blocker.
5. Omeprazole (Prilosec) decreases the acid production in the stomach. Avoid the use of ampicillin in these patients because ampicillin needs the presence of acid in the stomach for absorption.
6. Sucralfate (Carafate) coats the stomach, promotes healing, and often causes constipation, so avoid the use of codeine with sucralfate (Carafate), or advise stool softener use if narcotics are needed.
7. Carafate can also decrease the bioavailability of certain drugs by binding with them. Dental used drugs that are affected are H_2 blockers and tetracyclines.
8. Always check the dental radiographs for bone density in patients on PPIs because PPIs affect calcium absorption.

PANCREATIC DISEASE: ACUTE PANCREATITIS

Gallstones and alcohol consumption are responsible for a majority of the cases of acute pancreatitis. Other factors responsible could be bile stones, bile duct obstructing tumors, and drugs such as diuretics, protease inhibitors, trauma, infections, hypercalcemia, or genetic predisposition can also be associated with acute pancreatitis.

Clinical Features

Acute pancreatitis is associated with epigastric pain radiating to the back, nausea, and vomiting.

Laboratory Tests

The following are tests associated with acute pancreatitis:

1. **Amylase test:** Amylase level assessment has a low specificity and cannot be used alone.
2. **Lipase test:** Lipase level determination has a high specificity and is more sensitive compared to the amylase test.

Diagnosis

Diagnosis of acute pancreatitis is made by evaluation of the clinical picture and laboratory tests.

Treatment

Treatment options are as follows:

1. Bowel rest and parenteral nutrition are paramount, and the patient is not allowed to consume any food by mouth.
2. Aggressive IV hydration is implemented to compensate for the loss of fluids from the pancreas.
3. Aggressive pain control is implemented immediately.
4. Treatment of the underlying condition precipitating the acute pancreatitis is simultaneously addressed.

CELIAC SPRUE

Celiac sprue is also called **gluten-sensitive enteropathy** or **nontropical sprue**. It is a genetic disease that causes the patient to be sensitive to wheat, rye, and barley. Caucasians are most affected with celiac sprue.

Clinical Features

The clinical features for celiac sprue can vary. Symptoms may occur in the digestive system or in other parts of the body. Typically, the patient presents with crampy abdominal pain, chronic diarrhea, bloating, weight loss, and steatorrhea.

Celiac disease prevents the body from absorbing nutrients appropriately. The patient can experience glossitis, burning mouth, large bruises, and deep tissue bleeding. To compensate for nutritional loss, the patient needs to receive supplementation for iron, folic acid, B vitamins, fluids, and electrolytes along with calcium, potassium, and magnesium.

Diagnosis

Diagnosis is established as follows:

1. **Biopsy:** Biopsy of the small intestine is the gold standard test that shows blunting of the villi in the small intestinal mucosa.
2. **Blood tests:** Diagnosis can be established with the detection of antigliadin antibody, antiendomysial antibodies, and tissue transglutaminase.

Treatment

Treatment options are a gluten-free diet along with nutritional supplements such as, iron, vitamin D, calcium, folic acid, and vitamin B_{12}.

Suggested Dental Alerts

The following are dental alerts for celiac disease:

1. The status of the iron deficiency anemia, osteoporosis due to poor calcium absorption, easy bruising due to malabsorption of vitamin K, and peripheral neuropathy due to poor absorption of folic acid and vitamin B_{12} should be assessed prior to dentistry by evaluating the CBC, PT/INR, and dental radiographs for bone density.
2. Both men and women with low bone density may require vitamin D replacement.
3. Associated conditions, such as lactose intolerance or diabetes, may need to be treated. Evaluate the FBS, PPBS, and Hb_1AC if the patient has associated diabetes.
4. These patients have under-functioning immune systems and may not handle infections well. Use antibiotics to **promote** the healing process, following major surgical procedures.
5. The patient may need less or sometimes even more of a particular vitamin, mineral, or medication because of inadequate absorption.
6. The dentist must work with the patient's physician; the MD will help determine the appropriate doses for specific antibiotics that can work optimally for the patient's infection.

IRRITABLE BOWEL SYNDROME

Irritable bowel syndrome (IBS) is the most commonly diagnosed condition that is chronic, recurrent, and involves the small intestines. The diagnosis is made by exclusion. Women are more commonly affected compared with men. Symptoms include abdominal pain, disturbed bowel movements with constipation or diarrhea, abdominal bloating, and abnormal peristalsis. The symptoms are not explained by any structural or biochemical abnormalities.

Diagnosis

Diagnosis is established using the following criteria:

1. **The Manning criteria:** The Manning criteria of diagnosis contains the following: pain that is relieved with defecation; more frequent bowel movements, occurring

at the onset of pain and associated with lesser amount of stools; visible abdominal distention; passage of mucus; and a sensation of incomplete evacuation.

2. **The Rome III criteria:** The Rome III criteria are more widely used and consist of recurrent abdominal pain or discomfort, occurring at least three days/month in last three months. This pain or discomfort is associated with at least two or more of the following: improvement of pain with defecation, onset associated with change in the frequency of stools, or onset associated with a change in the form or appearance of the stools.

Medical Management

Treatment options for IBS are as follows:

1. **Dietary modifications:** IBS is treated with lactose-free, gas-reducing food items that are high in fiber.
2. **Antispasmodic drugs:** Hyoscyamine (Levsin), an anticholinergic drug, may be prescribed.
3. **Antidiarrheal agents:** Diphenoxylate (Lomotil) or loperamide (Immodium) could be prescribed to control the diarrhea.
4. **Promotility: Tegaserod (Zelnorm)** is used for the short-term treatment of constipation only in women.
5. **Psychosocial therapy:** Behavior modification therapy could alleviate or lessen symptoms.
6. **Antidepressants:** Antidepressants are often prescribed as adjunct therapy.

CLOSTRIDIUM DIFFICILE INFECTION

Facts

Pseudomembranous colitis is antibiotic-associated colitis following antibiotic use. Any antibiotic, when used in high doses or for a prolonged period, can cause c. difficile colitis. Clindamycin has often been implicated as the antibiotic most responsible for c. difficile colitis, but recent literature has shown otherwise. Colonic bacterial flora is altered during c. difficile colitis.

Symptoms and Signs

C. difficile colitis is associated with fever and an elevated WBC count detected on the CBC. The patient has three or more unformed stools over 24 hours for two successive days and shows positive stool test results or has the presence of pseudomembranes in the stools.

Diagnosis

The initial test done to detect clostridium difficile colitis (CDI) is the enzyme immunoassay (EIA) test. The EIA accesses for toxins A and B and it is 79–97% sensitive. The cell culture toxin assay, considered the gold standard test, is done when the EIA is positive. The assay is observed for 24–48 hours.

Treatment

Treatment measures are as follows:

1. **Prevention:** Prevention is the best course of action and special attention should be placed on the dose, duration, and frequency of antibiotic prescriptions. The patient should be encouraged to use probiotics or acidophilus-containing yogurt with antibiotic intake, to maintain the intestinal flora. Bleach-based disinfectants are very effective in destroying c. difficile spores in the environment.
2. **Medical management:** Treatment provided is based on the extent of the disease, which can be mild, moderate, or severe. Mild or moderate CDI is associated with WBC <15,000 cells/mm^3 and serum creatinine <1.5 times the level, **prior** to the CDI. Severe CDI is associated with WBC ≥15,000 cells/mm^3 or serum creatinine >1.5 times the level, **prior** to the CDI.

Metronidazole, 500 mg TID for 10–14 days, is the first-line therapy for an **initial or first recurrence** of mild or moderate CDI. A second recurrence is treated with oral vancomycin. Oral vancomycin therapy is extremely effective in treating mild, moderate, or severe disease, but oral vancomycin is quite expensive, compared with metronidazole.

There is **no difference** in the effectiveness of metronidazole and oral vancomycin for a new or first recurrence mild/moderate CDI, but oral vancomycin is clearly **superior** for a second recurrence or severe CDI.

Patients respond within three days with oral vancomycin compared to four to six days with metronidazole, plus intestinal levels are higher with oral vancomycin because it is not absorbed by the colon.

Oral vancomycin, 125 mg qid for 10–14 days, is the first-line therapy for **initial** or recurrence of **severe** disease. **Second recurrence** is treated with oral vancomycin taper over four weeks, with or without pulse dosing, when 125 mg oral vancomycin is given every two to three days, for two to eight weeks.

INFLAMMATORY BOWEL DISEASE

Epidemiology

Crohn's disease and ulcerative colitis are the two most commonly occurring inflammatory bowel disease (IBD) states that affect the large bowel causing significant disease. There is an increased incidence of IBD in industrialized nations.

Peak onset of IBD occurs between the ages of 15–25, and a second peak occurs between the ages of 50–65. Males and females are equally affected.

CROHN'S DISEASE

Crohn's disease is an inflammatory bowel disease that can affect any area of the GI tract, from the mouth to the anus. However, it most commonly affects the lower part of the small intestine, the ileum.

All layers of the intestine may be involved, and normal healthy bowel can be found between sections of diseased bowel. White blood cells accumulate in the lining of the intestines, producing chronic inflammation, which leads to ulcerations and bowel injury.

Crohn's disease affects men and women equally and seems to run in some families. Crohn's disease is more often diagnosed in people between the ages of 20 and 30. People of Jewish heritage have an increased risk of developing Crohn's disease; African

Americans are at decreased risk for developing Crohn's disease. Some people with Crohn's disease also report that they experience a flare in disease when they are dealing with a stressful event or situation. Always provide **stress management** if dentistry is stressful for the patient.

Clinical Features

The most common symptoms experienced are abdominal pain, often in the lower right area, and diarrhea. Rectal bleeding, weight loss, arthritis, skin problems, and fever may also occur. Bleeding may be serious and persistent, leading to anemia. Always evaluate the CBC **prior** to dental treatment.

The swelling can cause pain and can make the patient have frequent bowel movements resulting in diarrhea. Crohn's can sometimes present with intestinal obstruction and appendicitis-like right-sided acute inflammation. Half of the cases present with ileocolitis, 30% of the cases present with ileitis, and 20% of the cases present with colitis. Extracolonic manifestations of Crohn's include uveitis, iritis, arthritis, rash, and hepatitis. Crohn's is characterized by rectal sparing, perianal disease, fistulization, and cobblestone appearance on endoscopy.

Diagnosis

Diagnosis is established as follows:

1. A thorough physical exam and a series of tests may be required to diagnose Crohn's disease.
2. Blood tests may be done to check for anemia, which could indicate bleeding in the intestines.
3. Blood tests may also show a high WBC count, which is a sign of inflammation.
4. An upper GI series will show the status of the small intestine.
5. Sigmoidoscopy can be done to examine the lining of the lower part of the large intestine, or a colonoscopy can be done to examine the lining of the entire large intestine.

Complications

The following are complications associated with Crohn's disease:

- Deficiencies of proteins, calories, and vitamins caused by inadequate dietary intake.
- Low protein levels, which can be associated with intestinal loss of protein due to malabsorption.
- Arthritis, skin problems, inflammation in the eyes or mouth, kidney stones, gallstones, or other diseases of the liver and biliary system.

Drug Therapy

The following are drugs used for Crohn's disease:

1. **Anti-inflammatory drugs:** Most patients are first treated with drugs containing mesalamine that helps control inflammation. Patients who have no relief from mesalamine or who cannot tolerate it are put on other mesalamine-containing

drugs, such as mesalamine (Asacol), olsalazine (Dipentum), or mesalamine (Pentasa).

2. **Corticosteroids:** Prednisone is usually prescribed in a large dose during the worst stage of the disease. Once symptoms resolve, the dose is decreased. Follow "the rule of twos" for major dentistry when the history is positive for steroid intake.

3. **Immune suppressants:** 6-mercaptopurine or azathioprine is usually prescribed. Always evaluate the CBC and determine the ANC counts prior to dental treatment.

4. **Infliximab (Remicade):** Infliximab (Remicade) is a tissue necrosis factor (TNF) drug that blocks the body's inflammation response. The FDA approved the drug for the treatment of moderate to severe Crohn's disease that does not respond to standard therapies and for the treatment of open, draining fistulas.

5. **Antibiotics:** Ampicillin, sulfonamide, cephalosporin, tetracycline, or metronidazole may be prescribed to treat intestinal infections. Before you prescribe an antibiotic for an oral infection, always determine if the antibiotic the patient is receiving is bactericidal or bacteriostatic in action.

6. **Antidiarrheal drugs:** Diarrhea and abdominal cramps often resolve when the inflammation subsides, but additional medication may also be necessary. Diphenoxylate (Lomotil) or loperamide (Immodium) could be used to control the diarrhea. Do not prescribe codeine because it will be additive in action promoting constipation.

7. **Fluid Replacements:** Patients dehydrated because of diarrhea need treatment with fluids and electrolytes.

ULCERATIVE COLITIS

Ulcerative colitis is also called **colitis**, **distal colitis**, **pancolitis**, or **ulcerative proctitis**. Ulcerative colitis causes inflammation and ulcers in the mucosal lining of the rectum and colon. Ulcers form where inflammation has killed the cells that usually line the colon.

Ulcerative colitis can occur at any age, but it usually starts between the ages of 15 and 30. It tends to run in families.

Symptoms

The most common symptoms experienced are pain in the abdomen (very particularly on the left side), bloody diarrhea, urgency, fever, nocturnal diarrhea, and frequent small-volume bowel movements.

Other symptoms may include anemia, severe tiredness, weight loss, loss of appetite, bleeding from the rectum, sores on the skin, and joint pain. Some patients have long periods of remission during which they are free of symptoms. In severe cases the colon may be removed. There is a higher incidence of colon cancer in these patients.

Diagnosis and Medical Management

- Recently published guidelines have suggested that treatment for UC be based on severity of symptoms. Most treatment algorithms are based on only the severity of disease. The guidelines describe mildly active disease, moderately active disease, severely active disease, and fulminant disease.

- **Mildly active disease** is characterized by fewer than four bowel movements per day with intermittent hematochezia (rectal bleeding), no sign of systemic toxicity, and a normal erythrocyte sedimentation rate (ESR).
- **Moderately active disease** is characterized by four or more bowel movements per day, hematochezia, and minimal systemic toxicity.
- **Severely active disease** is diagnosed when the patient has six or more bowel movements per day with bleeding, signs of toxicity (such as fever, tachycardia, and anemia), and an elevated ESR.
- **Fulminantly active disease** is diagnosed if there are more than ten bowel movements per day, continuous rectal bleeding, abdominal tenderness with distension, transfusion requirement, and possible colonic dilation.
- Patients who have mildly active disease are given mesalamine (Asacol), both orally and topically. Topical mesalamine in an enema preparation or a suppository is added to the regimen regardless of the extent of disease. Combination therapy with oral and topical mesalamine works better than oral or topical mesalamine alone. Oral corticosteroids and intravenous (IV) infliximab (Remicade) are often prescribed when the disease fails to respond to mesalamine.
- Patients who have severely active disease require hospital admission for IV corticosteroid therapy. Patients who fail to respond are usually prescribed IV cyclosporine (Sandimmune) or IV infliximab (Remicade). Patients responding to this therapy are then prescribed six months of oral cyclosporine, a tapering dosage of oral corticosteroids, and long-term thiopurine (azathioprine or 6-mercaptopurine). Such patients require regular assessment of cyclosporine levels and careful monitoring for toxicity.
- Patients whose disease fails to respond to IV corticosteroid therapy are started on infliximab. Patients who respond to corticosteroid therapy are then treated with infliximab, tapering doses of prednisone, and long-term thiopurine given along with infliximab.
- Recently, adalimumab, a drug FDA-approved for Crohn's disease, has been shown to be effective in UC. If approved for UC, adalimumab may be preferable to infliximab due to the convenience of subcutaneous administration
- A patient who has fulminant disease including toxic megacolon (transverse colon larger than 6cm) needs surgery.

Medications and Treatment Alerts

- Mesalamine is associated with interstitial nephritis. Monitor the creatinine level and avoid nephrotoxic drugs, including NSAIDS.
- Sulfasalazine is bacteriostatic and can cause hepatitis, pancreatitis, and skin rash. Monitor LFTs during dentistry.
- Long-term corticosteroids can cause osteoporosis, osteonecrosis, centripetal obesity, striae, cataracts, glucose intolerance, insomnia, anxiety, and hirsutism. Follow the rule-of-twos during major dentistry.
- Thiopurines are associated with leukopenia, pancreatitis, and allergy. Monitor the complete blood counts (CBC) prior to and during dentistry.
- Methotrexate (Trexall) use is associated with nausea. Monitor CBC during dentistry.
- Infliximab can be associated with tuberculosis and other opportunistic infections, hepatitis B, and lymphoma. Cyclosporine therapy warrants the monitoring of cyclosporine levels. Avoid nephrotoxic drugs during dentistry.

- Patients who require surgery usually get the ileal pouch-anal anastomosis. Patients with the ileal pouch have 4–7 soft bowel movements per day with nearly complete continence.

All alerts suggested for Crohn's disease apply to ulcerative colitis.

CROHN'S DISEASE AND ULCERATIVE COLITIS SUGGESTED DENTAL GUIDELINES

The following are dental guidelines for Crohn's disease and ulcerative colitis:

1. When needed, provide stress management for an anxious patient.
2. Always assess the CBC, serum creatinine, and LFTs in patients with Crohn's disease prior to dentistry.
3. Avoid codeine in patients already taking antidiarrheal medications because severe constipation may occur.
4. Determine what medications the patient is on for Crohn's disease or ulcerative colitis. With specific antibiotic intake, you need to determine if the antibiotic is cidal/static. Match the cidal/static status with an antibiotic you may need to give the patient for treatment of an oral infection. If the two antibiotics do not match with their status, keep a six-hour interval between the two. In such cases, you will have to opt for an antibiotic like, once/day azithromycin.
5. Check if the patient has been on steroids for two weeks or longer within the past two years, or if the patient is currently on steroids. You need to follow "the rule of twos" for major dentistry if the history is positive.
6. As with all chronic GI conditions, delay routine dentistry during the acute flare-up phase of the disease.

DIVERTICULITIS

Diverticulitis mainly affects the descending and pelvic colon, and symptoms include abdominal pain, constipation, and flatulence.

Suggested Dental Alerts

The following are dental alerts for diverticulitis:

1. Avoid codeine in these patients to prevent further worsening of the constipation.
2. Determine what medications the patient is taking for the management of diverticulosis or diverticulitis. With any specific antibiotic intake, you need to determine if the antibiotic is cidal/static. Match the cidal/static status with an antibiotic you may need to give the patient for treatment of an oral infection. If the two antibiotics do not match with their status, keep a six-hour interval between the two, as discussed under Crohn's disease.
3. Check if the patient has been on steroids for two weeks or longer within the past two years or if the patient is currently on steroids. You need to follow "the rule of twos" for major dentistry if the history is positive.
4. As with all chronic GI conditions, delay routine dentistry during the acute flare-up phase of the disease.

COLON CANCER

Facts

Colon cancer presents as colon polyps. There are two types of polyps:

- **Hyperplastic:** A hyperplastic polyp has no cancer risk.
- **Adenomatous:** An adenomatous polyp is premalignant.

Colon cancer is the second most common fatal cancer in the United States. A high-fiber and low-fat diet is protective against colon cancer. The right colon is most affected and the transverse colon is least affected with colon cancer.

All individuals older than age 50 should have a colonoscopy and flexible sigmoidoscopy to check the colon status for polyps, abnormal areas, or cancer.

Diagnosis

Biopsy specimens obtained from suspect areas are viewed under a microscope to check for signs of cancer.

Treatment

Treatment options depend on the following: the stage of the cancer, if the cancer has recurred, and the patient's general health.

ADDITIONAL ALERTS AND SUGGESTED DENTAL GUIDELINES

The following are additional alerts for GI diseases:

1. Bleeds in the upper GI tract cause black tarry stools, and the **Guiac test** will be positive showing the presence of blood in the stools in such patients.
2. Lower GI bleeds cause the presence of fresh blood in the stools.
3. No dental treatment should be done during an acute intestinal flare-up. Delay routine dental treatment by four to six weeks in the presence of an acute flare-up.
4. Do not prescribe codeine for **any** patient that has a history of **chronic constipation** or in the presence of diverticulitis, as previously discussed. Advise adjunct stool softener use if narcotics are absolutely needed.
5. Always obtain the CBC with platelet count and WBC differential if the patient is on immune-suppressant drugs, and always calculate the absolute neutrophil count (ANC) before proceeding with dentistry. Implement the ANC guidelines, when needed.

XII

Hepatology

Liver Function Tests, Hepatitis, and Cirrhosis: Assessment, Analysis, and Associated Dental Management Guidelines

LIVER FUNCTION TESTS

Liver function tests (LFTs) indicate how well the liver is functioning. LFTs should always be evaluated along with the patient's history and physical examination. LFTs are not very sensitive, nor are they very specific.

Albumin, bilirubin, and PT/INR are true indicators of the biosynthetic capacity of the liver or overall liver function. ALT (SGPT), AST (SGOT), gamma-glutamyltransferase (GGT), and alkaline phosphatase are markers of disease, and they all indicate the status of hepatocellular damage.

LIVER STATUS ASSESSMENT COMPONENTS

The components that typically assess the liver status are the total protein, serum albumin, serum globulin, prothrombin time/international normalized ratio (PT/INR), alanine aminotransferase (ALT/SGPT), aspartate aminotransferase (AST/SGOT), total bilirubin, conjugated plus unconjugated bilirubin, alkaline phosphatase, and gamma-glutamyltransferase (GGT).

When LFTs are requested, most laboratories provide information on all components listed above with the **exception** of the PT/INR. When needed, the PT/INR always has to be requested separately. The PT/INR and the partial thromboplastin time (PTT) are provided together when coagulation studies are requested for surgical preoperative assessment. For discussion purposes, PT/INR will be included in the next section because it assesses liver biosynthetic function.

DETAILED DISCUSSION

Total Protein

The total protein constitutes the amount of albumin and globulin in the blood. The total protein value helps with the diagnosis of kidney disease, liver disease, liquid (blood)

Dentist's Guide to Medical Conditions, Medications, and Complications, Second Edition. Kanchan M. Ganda.
© 2013 John Wiley & Sons, Inc. Published 2013 by John Wiley & Sons, Inc.

cancer, or malnutrition. The normal albumin to globulin ratio is 2:1; with cirrhosis, the ratio is reversed to 1:2. Normal total protein reference range is 6.5–8.2 g/dL.

Albumin

Albumin is a major protein and a true indicator of liver function. It is exclusively synthesized by the liver. The half-life of albumin is 20 days. Albumin, serum bilirubin, and prothrombin time are the three true indicators of liver function. Chronic liver disease causes a decrease in the amount of albumin produced. Therefore, in more advanced liver disease, the level of the serum albumin is reduced (less than 3.5mg/dL). Low albumin results in fluid leakage from the blood vessels into the tissues causing edema of the extremities. Albumin levels are always normal in acute liver disease and decreased in cirrhosis. Decreased levels, however, are not specific to liver disease, because protein-losing intestinal disease, colitis, acute or chronic infection, malnutrition, or chronic kidney disease can also cause a lowering of the albumin level. The normal albumin range is 3.5–5.0 g/dL.

Globulin

Globulins are made by the immune system and the liver cells. Globulins help fight infections. Globulin levels are increased in cirrhosis. Additionally, significant elevations of serum globulin in blood, associated with the presence of antinuclear antibodies or anti-smooth muscle antibodies, provide clues to the diagnosis of autoimmune hepatitis.

Low Albumin and Normal LFT Profile

Low albumin and normal LFTs are associated with proteinuria; acute inflammatory states caused by trauma, sepsis, and burns; and a chronic inflammatory state caused by active rheumatic disorders. **Note** that albumin values are lower in pregnancy.

Prothrombin Time/International Normalized Ratio

Prothrombin time or PT is a test that is used to assess blood clotting. Blood clotting factors are proteins made by the liver. When the liver is significantly injured, these proteins are not normally produced. The prothrombin time is also a useful test of liver function because there is a good correlation between abnormalities in coagulation measured by the prothrombin time and the degree of liver dysfunction. Thus, PT/INR, like albumin and serum bilirubin, is a true indicator of liver function.

- The liver produces Clotting Factors II, V, VII, IX, and X. An elevated PT/INR can result from a vitamin K deficiency in patients with chronic cholestasis (bile flow obstruction) or fat malabsorption from disease of the pancreas or small bowel and due to blood-thinning medications. Thus, a prolonged PT/INR is not specific to liver disease. The PT/INR does not become abnormal until more than 75–80% of liver synthetic capacity is lost. An abnormal PT/INR prolongation may be a sign of serious liver dysfunction. Bleeding will occur with INR >1.5.
- Factor VII has a short half-life of about six hours and it is sensitive to rapid changes in liver synthetic function. In fact, compared with other clotting factors, Factor VII has the shortest half-life. Thus, PT/INR is very useful for monitoring liver function in patients with acute liver failure. Normal PT/INR range is 0.9–1.2, average 1.

ALT and AST

Enzymes alanine aminotransferase (ALT)/SGPT and aspartate aminotransferase (AST)/SGOT are indicators of liver cell damage. The ALT and AST help the liver metabolize amino acids and thus make proteins. The ALT and AST show liver damage and are sensitive indicators of liver injury, especially acute liver injury. ALT is a more specific indicator of liver inflammation, as AST may be elevated in diseases of other organs. The ALT and AST are present in low levels in normal patients. ALT (SGPT) is predominately found in the liver and is present in the cytosol of the hepatocytes. The normal ALT range is 5–60 IU/L.

AST (SGOT) is found in the liver, cardiac muscle, skeletal muscle, kidney, brain, pancreas, lungs, RBCs, and WBCs, and in the cytosol and mitochondria of the hepatocytes. The normal AST range is 5–43 IU/L.

Mild or moderate elevations of ALT or AST are nonspecific and may be caused by a wide range of liver diseases. Mild elevations of ALT or AST in asymptomatic patients can be evaluated by initially considering alcohol abuse, hepatitis B, or hepatitis C. In acute viral hepatitis, the ALT and AST may be elevated to the high 100s or over 1,000IU/L. In chronic hepatitis or cirrhosis, the elevation of these enzymes may be minimal (less than two to three times normal) or moderate (100–300IU/L).

ALT, AST Levels of Elevation, and Hepatocellular Necrosis Etiology

The following are ALT and AST elevation levels:

- **Mild ALT and AST elevation (<250 IU/L):** Mild elevations can be due to drugs, bile stones, viral infection, alcohol, or exercise.
- **Moderate ALT and AST elevation (250–1,000 IU/L):** Moderate elevations can be due to EBV or HSV infection or NSAIDS.
- **Severe ALT and AST elevation (>1,000 IU/L):** Severe elevations can be drug- or toxin-induced, or due to an acute viral infection, choledocolithiasis, or primary graft failure.

Bilirubin

Bilirubin is formed primarily from the breakdown of "heme." It is taken up from blood processed through the liver, and then secreted into the bile by the liver. Normal individuals have only a small amount of bilirubin circulating in blood (less than 1.2mg/dL).

Conditions that cause increased formation of bilirubin, such as destruction of red blood cells or decreased removal from the blood stream, as with liver disease, may result in an increase in the level of serum bilirubin. Levels greater than 3mg/dL are usually noticeable as jaundice. The bilirubin may be elevated in many forms of liver or biliary tract disease, and thus it is also relatively nonspecific.

Thus, serum bilirubin is generally considered a true test of liver function, because it reflects the liver's ability to take up, process, and secrete bilirubin into the bile. Total bilirubin indicates the status of bile transportation, and bilirubin is the product of hemoglobin breakdown. Conjugated and unconjugated bilirubin are measured when LFTs are ordered.

Unconjugated Hyperbilirubinemia Etiology

Gilbert's syndrome is the most common cause of benign hyperbilirubinemia and it is associated with impaired uptake or impaired conjugation of bilirubin.

Conjugated Hyperbilirubinemia Etiology

Hepatocellular disease, intra- or extrahepatic bile duct obstruction, or sepsis are common causes of conjugated hyperbilirubinemia.

Alkaline Phosphatase

Alkaline phosphatase (AP) is found in the liver, bone, placenta, kidney, intestine, and WBCs. AP metabolizes phosphorus and thus is an energy source for the body. AP levels are higher in men than in women. The normal range of AP is 30–115 IU/L.

AP is a marker of chronic cholestasis disease due to bile duct obstruction caused by stricture/stones **or** infiltrative disease caused by sarcoidosis/TB/cancer. Nonpathologic elevations of AP may occur during the third trimester of pregnancy, during adolescence, or as a normal part of aging. With cholestasis, alkaline phosphatase is markedly elevated when compared with the aminotransferases or bilirubin levels. The total bilirubin will be increased with cholestasis disease.

Alkaline phosphatase (AP) and gamma-glutamyltranspeptidase (GGT) are elevated in a large number of disorders that affect the drainage of bile such as a gallstone or tumor blocking the common bile duct, or alcoholic liver disease or drug-induced hepatitis blocking the flow of bile in smaller bile channels within the liver. Alkaline phosphatase and GGT indicate obstruction to the biliary system, either within the liver or in the larger bile channels outside the liver. Thus, AP and GGT are often labeled "the cholestatic enzymes" because they spill from the liver into the bloodstream, with obstruction. The AP and gamma-glutamyltransferase (GGT) levels typically rise to several times the normal level after several days of bile duct obstruction or intrahepatic cholestasis. GGT helps differentiate if AP is coming from the liver or bone. With biliary obstruction, the GGT will be increased. With bone disease, the GGT is unaltered.

The highest AP levels, often greater than 1,000 U/L, or more than six times the normal value, are found in diffuse infiltrative diseases of the liver, such as infiltrating tumors and fungal infections. Both AP and GGT levels are elevated in about 90% of patients with cholestasis. An elevated AP value originating from the liver is usually accompanied by an elevated GGT value, an elevated 5'-nucleotidase value, and other LFT abnormalities. 5'-nucleotidase is a subset of alkaline phosphate.

Cholestasis Etiology

Etiological factors associated with cholestasis are:

1. **Obstructive causes:** partial bile-duct obstruction, primary biliary cirrhosis, primary sclerosing cholangitis, and drug-induced cholestasis
2. **Infiltrative causes:** sarcoidosis, TB, and primary or metastatic liver cancer

Isolated Elevation of AP in an Asymptomatic Patient with Normal GGT

Consider bone growth or injury, or primary biliary cirrhosis. AP levels rise in late pregnancy.

Gamma-Glutamyltransferase (GGT)

GGT is found in the hepatocytes and the biliary epithelial cells and brings oxygen to tissues. GGT is a sensitive indicator of hepatobiliary disease. It is **not** elevated in bone disease. GGT is most useful for confirming the hepatic origin of elevated alkaline phosphatase. Therefore, GGT is utilized as a supplementary test to ensure that the elevation of alkaline phosphatase is coming from the liver or the biliary tract. Unlike AP, GGT is not elevated in diseases of bone, placenta, or intestine.

Isolated Elevation of GGT Level Assessment

Isolated elevation of GGT level is induced by alcohol and there is usually no actual liver disease. The elevation of GGT alone, with no other LFT abnormalities, often results from enzyme induction by alcohol or seizure medications in the absence of liver disease. The GGT level is often elevated in persons who take three or more alcoholic drinks per day. A mildly elevated GGT level is a typical finding in patients taking anticonvulsants and by itself does not necessarily indicate liver disease. The normal GGT level is 5–80 IU/L.

Other Specific Tests Diagnosing Causes of Liver Disease

- Elevations in serum iron, the percent of iron saturated in blood, or the iron storage protein ferritin may indicate the presence of hemochromatosis, a liver disease associated with excess iron storage.
- Wilson's disease is associated with an accumulation of copper in the liver, a deficiency of serum ceruloplasmin, and excessive excretion of copper into the urine.
- Low levels of serum alpha-1-antitrypsin may indicate the presence of lung and/or liver disease in children or adults with alpha-1-antitrypsin deficiency.
- A positive anti-mitochondrial antibody indicates the underlying condition of primary biliary cirrhosis.

LFTs and Coagulation Studies: Medical Case Note/Medical Record Lattice Recording

LFTs, PT/INR, and PTT are often recorded in a standardized lattice pattern in medical records or medical case notes, and every practitioner should be able to read the tests when written as such. Figure 45.1 and 45.2 show the LFTs and coagulation studies lattice recordings.

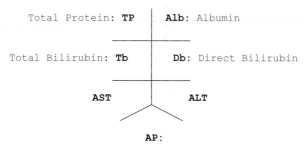

Figure 45.1. Liver function tests lattice recording.

Coagulation Tests

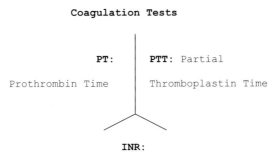

Figure 45.2.   Coagulation tests lattice recording.

ACUTE VIRAL HEPATITIS: HEPATITIS A AND E

Acute and Chronic Viral Hepatitis Introduction

Viral hepatitis can present as an acute or chronic disease state, and viral infections of importance in the dental setting are hepatitis A, B, C, D, and E. Hepatitis A and E are grouped as the acute types of hepatitis. Hepatitis B, C, and D are grouped as the chronic types of hepatitis.

Hepatitis A and E: General Overview

Hepatitis A and E are caused by the hepatitis A virus (HAV) and the hepatitis E virus (HEV), respectively. Hepatitis A is universal in occurrence and is associated with endemic outbreaks. Hepatitis A affects all age groups, and jaundice commonly co-occurs.

Hepatitis E occurrence in the United States is very rare; it is, however, prevalent in South Asia and North Africa. Hepatitis E is more prevalent among pregnant women and is a serious concern during the third trimester.

The incubation period is two to six weeks for hepatitis A and two to nine weeks for hepatitis E. There is no chronic state, nor is there any sexual transmission with either type of hepatitis.

Transmission

Transmission of both types is by contaminated food and water. Person-to-person transmission is more common with hepatitis A than with hepatitis E.

Symptoms and Signs

Nausea, vomiting, abdominal pain, loss of appetite, fatigue, dark urine, and jaundice occur with both types of hepatitis.

Infection Markers

The occurrence of jaundice heralds the start of recovery, especially with hepatitis A. Jaundice usually occurs in 70% of the cases infected with the hepatitis A virus. Infection with hepatitis A or E is indicated by the presence of anti-HAV IgM or anti-HEV IgM in the blood, respectively. The patient is infected and infectious to others during this phase. Presence of anti-HAV IgG or anti-HEV IgG indicates immunity to hepatitis A and E, respectively. The antibodies provide **lifelong immunity** following recovery from hepatitis A; lifelong protection with the hepatitis E antibody is questionable.

Acute Viral Hepatitis LFT Profiles

ALT levels often rise to several thousand units per liter in patients with acute viral hepatitis. The highest ALT levels, often more than 10,000 IU/L, are usually found in patients with acute toxic injury subsequent to acetaminophen overdose. AST and ALT levels usually fall rapidly after an acute insult. In typical viral or toxic liver injury, the serum ALT levels rise more than the AST value, reflecting the relative amounts of these enzymes in hepatocytes.

Vaccinations

Hepatitis A infection can be prevented with the hepatitis A vaccine, which is given in two doses, 6–18 months apart. The vaccine is recommended for children in day-care settings, cafeteria workers, and those traveling to areas with a high risk of transmission.

Of the adults vaccinated, 94–100% develop antibodies one month after the first injection, and 100% of the vaccinated adults develop protective antibodies after the second dose. Hepatitis A vaccine gives **lifelong immunity**. Immune globulin (IG) is given after the first dose to travelers who plan to travel in less than one month after the first dose of the vaccine. There is **no** vaccine for Hepatitis E.

CHRONIC HEPATITIS: HEPATITIS B, C, AND D

Hepatitis B, C, and D: General Overview

Hepatitis B is caused by the hepatitis B virus (HBV). HBV is a hepadnavirus that invades liver hepatocytes. The viral genome is a partially double-stranded circular DNA linked to a DNA polymerase. It is surrounded by a nucleocapsid and then by a lipid envelope. Embedded within the nucleocapsid are the hepatitis B core antigen (HBcAg) and the precore hepatitis B e-antigen (HBeAg), and on the envelope is the hepatitis B surface antigen (HBsAg).

Hepatitis C is caused by the hepatitis C virus (HCV). HCV is an enveloped virus, with a single-stranded RNA genome contained in a capsid. There are six genotypes of hepatitis C and genotypes 1 and 4 are associated with a lower rate of response to therapy. Most patients in the United States are infected with HCV genotype 1.

Hepatitis D is caused by the defective hepatitis D virus (HDV) that needs the presence of the hepatitis B virus to exist. Hepatitis D virus (HDV) is thus found associated with a first infection with HBV or with an HBV carrier state. HDV co-infection with HBV results in severe acute disease, fulminant hepatitis, and the risk of developing a chronic infection is 1–3%. HDV super-infection in the presence of chronic HBV infection results in the development of chronic HDV infection. There is high risk (70–80%) of progressing to chronic liver disease in such cases.

Transmission

Hepatitis B, C, and D are chronic or gradual in onset; the transmission is via contaminated blood.

Symptoms and Signs

Nausea, vomiting, diarrhea, constipation, fever, skin rash, anorexia, weight loss, joint pains, dark-colored urine, yellowing of the skin or eyes, and aversion to smoking are the common complaints.

Hepatitis B: Detailed Discussion

The incubation period for hepatitis B is two to six months. The hepatitis B virus is transmitted by exposure to contaminated blood and from intravenous (IV) drug use. Mother-to-child transmission can occur and there is a high rate of sexual transmission with the virus.

Jaundice occurs in 30% of the patients. For most adults, it is a form of infection that ultimately resolves; for most children it is a form of infection that persists as a chronic state of infection. HBV attacks the liver and it can cause lifelong infection, cirrhosis, liver cancer, and even death. Of adult patients, 1–3% are affected with chronic hepatitis. Hepatitis B can predispose to liver cancer in the absence of cirrhosis.

Hepatitis B: Serological Markers

Hepatitis B virus is associated with three distinct antigen markers: HBsAg, HBeAg, and HBcAg. Each antigen has a definite timeline of appearance during the infection cycle and each triggers the appearance of a corresponding antibody in the blood indicating recovery or otherwise. Anti-HBs, anti-HBe, and anti-HBc are the antibodies triggered by the antigens HBsAg, HBeAg, and HBcAg, respectively.

The Hepatitis B Antigen–Antibody Cycle Graph

Figure 45.3 depicts the sequential pattern of the rise and fall of the antigen–antibody markers associated with hepatitis B. Each of the markers is discussed in the following sections, and Figure 45.3 is used as a reference.

Serological Markers Facts

HBsAg (Surface Antigen)

The presence of HBsAg on hepatic serology indicates the presence of current infection. HBsAg is the first marker to appear in the blood, roughly around the seventh week from the start of an acute infection. In patients with a resolving infection, the HBsAg disappears completely from the blood by about the twentieth week from the start of infection.

A patient is said to be a simple "carrier" patient when the HBsAg **does not** disappear as expected and continues to be detected on serology, beyond the twenty-fourth week of infection. The carrier state occurs more commonly in children than adults.

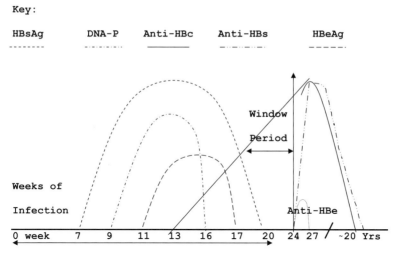

Figure 45.3. Classic hepatitis B antigen–antibody cycle.

Anti-HBs (Surface Antibody)

The presence of anti-HBs on hepatic serology indicates immunity. The presence of anti-HBs can be a result of hepatitis B immunization or it can appear in the blood **after** HBsAg from a natural infection that has completely cleared the system.

With a natural infection, anti-HBs appears around the twenty-fourth week from the start of the infection and persists for fifteen to twenty years, providing the patient with immunity during that time. It can be present, along with anti-HBc IgG, following recovery from a natural infection.

Anti-HBs is the only antibody formed with hepatitis B immunization. Anti-HBc IgM or anti-HBc IgG are not formed with vaccination.

HBcAg (Hepatitis B Core Antigen)

HBcAg resides inside the infected hepatocytes only and does **not** make its appearance in the blood. Hepatic serology does not record HBcAg, a marker of infection, and it is detected only on liver biopsy.

Anti-HBc IgM (IgM Core Antibody)

The presence of anti-HBc IgM indicates current infection **and** patient associated infectious status. Anti-HBc IgM develops **during the acute state** of hepatitis B and is generated due to a natural infection. Anti-HBc IgM is **not** associated with hepatitis B immunization.

Anti-HBc IgM is the only marker present during the "window period" of the typical hepatitis B infection cycle. The window period is the time interval during the cycle when the patient has shed the HBsAg but has not yet developed the anti-HBs. During the window period the patient is negative for HBsAg, DNA-P, HBeAg, and anti-HBs. Anti-HBc IgM typically appears in the blood around the thirteenth week from the start of infection and stays until about the twenty-fourth week, when anti-HBc IgG is formed.

Anti-HBc IgG (IgG Core Antibody)

Anti-HBc IgG is formed beyond the twenty-fourth week after the start of the hepatitis B infection. Once anti-HBc IgG appears in the blood, it can persist for fifteen to twenty years. Isolated presence of anti-HBc IgG on hepatic serology indicates that the patient was infected with the hepatitis B virus **more than** twenty-four weeks ago. When anti-HBc IgG is found along with anti-HBs on hepatic serology, it indicates definite recovery and immunity from a natural infection. The "interpretation" of an isolated presence of anti-HBc IgG on hepatic serology is essentially unclear. The presence could be interpreted as one of the following, a resolved infection with "undetectable" anti-HBs (most common); false-positive anti-HBc, thus susceptible to infection; "low level" chronic infection; or resolving acute infection.

HBeAg (Hepatitis B e-Antigen)

The presence of HBeAg on hepatic serology indicates active replication of the virus, and the patient is highly infectious at this time. During a typical cycle, HBeAg appears in the blood around the eleventh week from the start of infection and completely disappears from the blood around the seventeenth week from the start of infection. A carrier patient positive for HBsAg, who also continues to shed the HBeAg beyond the twenty-fourth week is called a **super infective carrier** patient.

During the acute state of hepatitis B, the patient will be positive for HBsAg, HBeAg, DNA-polymerase (DNA-P/viral DNA), anti-HBc IgM, and very high levels of ALT plus AST. Additionally, the patient will have symptoms associated with an acute infection.

Anti-HBe (Hepatitis B e-Antibody)

The presence of anti-HBe on hepatic serology indicates that the virus has ceased to replicate and there is an improvement in the patient's infectivity status compared to before. Anti-HBe usually appears around the twenty-fourth week and disappears by the twenty-seventh week from the start of the infection.

The Hepatitis B Carrier Patient

As stated in the previous sections, the simple carrier patient continues to shed HBsAg and the super infective carrier continues to shed HBsAg and HBeAg beyond the twenty-fourth week from the start of infection. Both these types of carrier patients do **not** develop anti-HBs, the marker of immunity, as long as HBsAg is detected on serology.

When the virus stops replicating and HBeAg is no longer detected on hepatic serology, the super infective status is lost but the patient will continue to be infective and infected, until the time HBsAg is detected on hepatic serology. The carrier patient's liver enzymes or LFTs will be normal or near normal. Past history assessment will in most cases indicate infection with the hepatitis B virus.

The carrier rate is inversely proportional to the age of the patient. The carrier rate is 80–85% among children, and pediatric patients are usually asymptomatic when infected. Adult patients are usually symptomatic and have a 10–20% carrier rate. Carrier patients can develop very severe hepatitis and about 25% of adult carriers go on to develop cirrhosis of the liver.

The Carrier Patient and Dentistry

Dental treatment is not contraindicated in the simple or super infective carrier patient. Always evaluate the LFTs prior to dentistry to determine if the carrier patient has underlying hepatitis or cirrhosis. Then follow the AAA suggested dental guidelines for either of the two disease states.

Hepatitis B Vaccine

Two single antigen hepatitis B vaccines are licensed in the United States for persons of any age. Children 1–10 years; adolescents 11–19 years and adults older than 20 years are all vaccinated at 0, 1, and 6 months. The second dose is given one month after the first dose and the third is given five months after the second dose. If the series is interrupted after the first dose, the second dose should be given immediately. The third dose should be given at least two months after the second. A delayed third dose should be given immediately.

When the vaccine is given according to the protocol of 0, 1, and 6 months, 30–50% protection occurs after the first dose. After the second dose 50–75% protection occurs, and after the third dose 90% protection occurs.

HIV patients may need several more shots beyond the routine three to gain immunity. Individuals who do not respond to the primary vaccine series may have to complete a second, three-dose series and be tested subsequent to the second set of vaccination.

Hepatitis B Post-Vaccination Testing

Testing for antibody response is **not** indicated after completion of the injections at 0, 1, and 6 months. Post-vaccination testing after completion of the routine series or interrupted series **may** be indicated in the following:

1. **Health-care workers (HCW):** HCW coming in close contact with blood or body fluids **may** be tested one to two months after the last vaccination dose.
2. **Chronic hemodialysis patients**: Chronic hemodialysis patients may be tested one to two months after the last vaccination dose.
3. **Sex partners of hepatitis B–infected persons**: Sex partners of hepatitis B–infected persons may be tested one to two months after the last vaccination dose.
4. **Infants born to hepatitis B–infected mothers**: Infants born to hepatitis B–infected mothers may be tested at nine to fifteen months of age.

Combined Hepatitis A and B Vaccine

Twintrix is the combined vaccine approved by the FDA for adults. Three doses of the combined vaccine are given over twenty-four weeks.

Hepatitis B Needle-Stick Exposure Rate

The transmission rate of hepatitis B by a single needle-stick is 30%, and this is why immunization against hepatitis B is required for dentists and others working in the dental setting.

HEPATITIS C (HCV)

Hepatitis C: Detailed Discussion

HCV infection is universal in occurrence. The incubation period for hepatitis C is 15–150 days. HCV is spread through the sharing of needles (accounting for 40% of infections), needle-sticks, sharps exposures on the job, transmission from an infected mother to her baby during birth, and through sexual transmission. The sexual transmission rate is quite low when compared with that for hepatitis B.

Globally, HCV infection is the leading cause of chronic hepatitis, liver cirrhosis, and hepatocellular carcinoma. Once the patient gets infected, chronic hepatitis develops within six months to ten years; progression toward cirrhosis occurs about 20 years from the start of the infection; and progression toward hepatocellular carcinoma (HCC) occurs about 30 years from the start of the infection.

About 15–35% of patients with HCV infection resolve spontaneously, with the HCV-RNA clearing the serum, followed by detection of HCV antibodies and about 65–85% of patients go on to develop chronic HCV infection. Of the patients with chronic HCV infection, 75% may progress to develop cirrhosis. Most patients with cirrhosis continue to stay stable, but about 25% of these patients may develop liver decompensation and liver cancer and die within five years. HCV-induced cirrhosis is the most common indication for liver transplantation in the United States. Thus, hepatitis C can be acute or chronic, and the chronic rate of hepatitis C is higher. Aggressive progression (70%) to chronic hepatitis occurs in the presence of co-infection with hepatitis B or HIV, at an older age, in male patients, and in the presence of alcohol use.

Within eight weeks from the start of the infection, anti-HCV antibody is formed. Anti-HCV antibody, unlike other antibodies, is **not** a protective antibody.

Hepatocellular Carcinoma (HCC) Risk Factors

Risk factors for HCC include Asian decent, male sex, advancing age, liver cirrhosis, heavy alcohol consumption, diabetes mellitus, and hemodialysis. Studies have shown that HCV therapy does decrease the incidence of HCC to some extent, but successful antiviral treatment in the presence of chronic hepatitis C may not always prevent the development of HCC.

Hepatitis C Needle-Stick Exposure Rate

Incidence of hepatitis C with a single needle-stick in health-care workers is less than 3%.

Hepatitis C Blood Tests

The five most common tests for hepatitis C are:

1. **Anti-HCV**
2. **HCV RIBA**
3. **HCV-RNA**
4. **Viral Load or Quantitative HCV**
5. **Viral Genotyping**

The provider must first order the qualitative test to make a diagnosis of HCV. This is followed by the HCV-RNA polymerase chain reaction assay. The qualitative test provides a positive or negative result, and the quantitative test determines the viral load.

HCV Antibody Tests

The anti-HCV test and the HCV RIBA test are the two tests that detect the antibody associated with hepatitis C. The anti-HCV testing is done by enzyme immunoassay (EIA). The RIBA test is the recombinant immunoblot assay. Both the anti-HCV tests (anti-HCV and RIBA) are reported as positive when they detect the presence of antibodies to hepatitis C. The tests indicate only exposure to the virus in the past. They are unable to indicate if the patient still has an active viral infection.

Anti-HCV Test

HCV antibodies usually appear around eight weeks into an infection and are always present in the later stages of the disease. It should be noted that because the hepatitis C virus (HCV) antibody remains active (even in a patient who has been treated and has achieved viral response, as well as in someone who clears the virus spontaneously), the HCV antibody is not sufficient for diagnosing chronic active hepatitis. A patient with a weakly positive anti-HCV antibody test should get the HCV RIBA test before final results are reported. The HCV RNA must be done if the hepatitis C antibody is positive. False negative results can occur in HIV or other immune-compromised patients. These patients also must be confirmed with the hepatitis C RNA test.

HCV RIBA Test

This test also confirms the presence of antibodies to the virus and, similar the anti-HCV test, the RIBA test cannot determine if the patient is currently infected. It indicates only that the patient has been exposed to the virus. A positive anti-HCV is reconfirmed with the RIBA test.

- **RIBA Positive:** Confirms exposure to HCV. Check the hepatitis C RNA by PCR in RIBA-positive patients.
- **RIBA Negative:** Indicates the positive anti-HCV was a false positive test.

HCV-RNA Test

The HCV-RNA test is a more reliable test and is positive one week after infection. The test is also used post treatment to see if the virus has been eliminated with therapy. This test detects the presence of the virus in the blood and indicates an active HCV infection. It is reported as HCV-RNA positive when the virus is detected.

● Positive HCV-RNA: Patient is chronically infected.
● Negative HCV-RNA: **Patient has cleared the infection.**

Viral Load or Quantitative HCV Test

This test measures the number of viral RNA particles in the blood. The Viral Load test is often used before and during treatment to help determine response to therapy by comparing the amount of virus present before and after treatment, and it is usually done after a period of three months. Successful treatment is associated with a decrease of 99% or more (2 logs) in the viral load within one to three months of starting treatment. Successful treatment usually leads to the viral load becoming undetected.

Viral Genotyping

This test is used to determine the virus genotype. Genotyping is often ordered before treatment has started to get a heads-up on the likelihood of treatment success and the length of time for which the treatment would be needed. There are six major types of HCV detected by genotyping. The most common genotype involved with infections in the United States is genotype 1, which is less likely to respond to treatment than genotypes 2 or 3. Genotype 1 usually requires **48 weeks** of therapy compared to **24 weeks** for genotype 2 or 3. Genotype 4 is also associated with a lower rate of response to therapy. Most patients in the United States are infected with HCV genotype 1.

HCV Tests Summary

● If the antibody test result is positive, the patient probably has been infected with hepatitis C or was exposed to hepatitis C.
● A positive RIBA confirms that the patient has been exposed to the virus.
● A negative RIBA indicates that the first test was probably a false positive and the patient has never been infected by HCV.
● A positive HCV-RNA means that the patient is **currently** infected by HCV.

Hepatitis C and Associated LFTs

The serum ALT level correlates only moderately well with liver inflammation in hepatitis C. Approximately one-third of the patients with chronic hepatitis C show constantly normal ALT levels. Liver cell death in hepatitis C occurs by a programmed cell death process, or apoptosis, and by necrosis. Liver cell death by apoptosis is associated with lesser amounts of AST and ALT because the liver cells wither away with time. This accounts for why one-third of patients infected with the hepatitis C virus have persistently normal serum ALT levels despite the presence of inflammation on liver biopsy. The liver histology is less severe in patients with normal ALT levels than in those with abnormal ALT levels. Chronic hepatitis C patients with persistently elevated ALT levels have a higher risk of HCC, and these patients should be treated as early as possible.

Hepatitis C Treatment

Mild Hepatitis C Treatment

Mild hepatitis C is treated with diet, exercise, abstinence from alcohol, and regular visits with the specialist to monitor the disease.

Current Traditional Chronic Hepatitis C Treatment

- Current therapy consists of interferon and ribavirin given in combination for 48 weeks. Interferon may be peginterferon alfa-2a (Pegasys) or peginterferon alfa-2b (PEG-Intron). Peginterferon alfa-2a (Pegasys) has been shown to be more effective. Peginterferon is given as an injection: alfa-2b once weekly or alfa-2a thrice weekly. Peginterferon causes potent side effects such as suicidal ideation, nausea, vomiting, fever, and chills.
- Ribavirin is taken daily by mouth. Side effects associated with ribavirin are anemia, rash, and neutropenia. Unlike interferon, ribavirin dose can be reduced to minimize the side effects. Erythropoietin is often added as supportive therapy.
- The patient is said to have a sustained virological response (SVR) when there is a loss of HCV-RNA by PCR for a minimum of six months after the end of chronic hepatitis C treatment. Studies have shown that once the patient has successfully established SVR, the risk of virological recurrence is very low (1–8%).
- Genotype 1 is associated with a lower treatment response rate, with less than 50% SVR rates occurring in these patients. SVR is associated with an improvement in occurrence of liver fibrosis, a reduction in liver failure/cirrhosis rates, and an overall reduction in liver-related morbidity and mortality rate.
- When IFN/PEG-IFN, alone or in combination with RBV, is used in the treatment of chronic hepatitis C patients with or without cirrhosis, there is a long durable response, improvement of fibrosis and cirrhosis, decreased risk of liver decompensation, decreased morbidity and mortality rates, increased survival, and better quality of life, especially in patients with SVR and biochemical responders compared with the non-responders or untreated controls.
- Ribavirin causes anemia, thrombocytopenia, neutropenia, rash, myalgia and chills. Therefore, it is important for the dental provider to review the CBC and the ANC count prior to dentistry.

New Triple Therapy for Hepatitis C

- Telaprevir (Incivek) and boceprevir (Victrelis) are the first oral medications specifically for HCV that recently received FDA approval. These oral agents have to be combined with the traditional therapy drugs interferon and ribavirin to prevent development of resistance.
- Dysgeusia (altered taste), anemia, and neutropenia are the major side effects of these new medications, which are given for a shorter duration of 28 weeks. Assess CBC and ANC count prior to dentistry.
- Both telaprevir and boceprevir are inhibitors of CYP3A4 inhibitors, thus affecting the concentration of medications that need the CYP3A4 enzyme to be metabolized.
- See Tables 45.1 and 45.2 for summaries of hepatitis vaccine protocols and LFT changes. See also Table 45.4.

Table 45.1. Hepatitis A, B, and C Summary with Vaccine Protocols, Post Needle-Stick Exposure Testing, and Prophylaxis

Indicators	Hepatitis A	Hepatitis B	Hepatitis C
Incubation: **Jaundice:**	2-6 weeks Affects all ages and jaundice is common	2-6 months Jaundice occurs in 30% of cases	2-24 weeks Jaundice occurrence is rare
Course:	It is an acute type of hepatitis	Acute for most adults, chronic for most kids	Can be acute or chronic, chronic rate is higher
Mode of **Transmission:** **Mother to Child** **Transmission:** **Sexual** **Transmission:**	– Contaminated food and water – No mother to child transmission – No sexual transmission	– Exposure by contact with contaminated blood and IV drug use – Mother to child transmission possible – High rate of sexual transmission	– Exposure by contact with contaminated blood and IV drug use – Mother to child transmission possible – Sexual transmission rate is low
Prevalence:	Universal with endemic outbreaks	Universal	Universal
Clinical **Features and** **Prognosis:**	**Pediatric patients:** Have a silent infection **Adult patients:** Are more symptomatic with flu-like symptoms	**Pediatric patients:** Are asymptomatic and have 90% carrier rate **Adult patients:** Are symptomatic, can get very severe hepatitis and have a 10-20% carrier rate	Hepatitis C usually has a silent acute onset (80%). Only 5-10% patients are symptomatic, having nausea and jaundice. The patient has a better chance of clearing the infection in the presence of symptoms. Hepatitis C has a high rate of progression to silent chronic hepatitis (55-85%). Aggressive progression to chronic hepatitis occurs in the presence of: Co-infection with hepatitis B or HIV, older age, male patient, and alcohol use (70%). Hep. C is associated with a slow evolution (~20-40 yr) to end-stage liver disease (1-5%).

Laboratory Tests and/or Hepatic Serology:

Anti-HAV IgM: Indicates acute infection

Anti-HAV IgG: Indicates recovery and life-long immunity

1. **Acute infection:**
   HBsAg: Positive
   Anti-HBs: Negative
   Anti-HBc IgM: Positive
   HBeAg: Positive
   Anti-HBe: Negative

2. **Recovery:**
   HBsAg: Negative
   Anti-HBs: Positive
   Anti-HBc IgM: Neg.
   Anti-HBc IgG: Positive
   HBeAg: Negative
   Anti-HBe: Positive

3. **Chronic Carrier with viral replication:** HBsAg: Positive
   Anti-HBs: Negative
   Anti-HBc IgM: Neg.
   Anti-HBc IgG: Positive
   HBeAg: Positive
   Anti-HBe: Negative

4. **Chronic Carrier without replication:**
   HBsAg: Positive
   Anti-HBs: Negative
   Anti-HBc IgM: Neg
   Anti-HBc IgG: Positive
   HBeAg: Negative
   Anti-HBe: Positive

5. **Vaccine:**
   HBsAg: Negative
   Anti-HBs: Positive
   Anti-HBc IgM: Negative
   Anti-HBc IgG: Negative
   HBeAg: Negative
   Anti-HBe: Negative

1. **Anti-HCV antibody test:** Positive antibody test indicates the patient probably has been infected with hepatitis C

2. **RIBA Test:**
   RIBA positive confirms exposure to the virus. Next check hepatitis C RNA by PCR
   RIBA Negative:
   Indicates the positive anti-HCV was a false positive test

3. **HCV RNA Test:** Positive HCV RNA indicates current chronic infection.
   Negative HCV RNA: Patient has cleared the infection

4. **Viral Load or Quantitative HCV test:** This test determines the number of viral RNA particles in the blood.

5. **Viral Genotyping Test:** This test determines the virus genotype

6. **LFTs:** In chronic hepatitis C the serum ALT level correlates only moderately well with liver inflammation.
   One-third of patients infected with Hepatitis C virus have persistently normal serum ALT levels

(continued)

Table 45.1. Hepatitis A, B, and C Summary with Vaccine Protocols, Post Needle-Stick Exposure Testing, and Prophylaxis (*Continued*)

Indicators	Hepatitis A	Hepatitis B	Hepatitis C
Complications:	Some severe infections need hospitalization. Full recovery following infection occurs in most cases, and no chronic state exists.	**Chronic Hepatitis:** 1-3% patients are affected with chronic hepatitis. Hepatitis B predisposes to liver cancer, in the absence of cirrhosis	Chronic Hep C is the number-one reason for liver transplant. 20% of the patients go on to develop cirrhosis. 2–3% patients with cirrhosis develop liver cancer.
Needle-stick exposure rate:	No exposure via needle-stick	6-30% chance of exposure with single needle-stick	<5% exposure rate with single needle-stick
Post needle-stick blood tests and follow-up:	None	**For Provider:** Check anti-HBs titer for immunity status. Hepatitis B vaccine and/or HBIG is given dependent on Provider's vaccination and antibody status. **Source:** Source is tested for HBsAg and HBeAg	**For Provider:** Check base-line anti-HCV status. **Source:** Source tested for anti-HCV and hep. C RNA. **If Source is positive:** Provider has follow-up serology tests at 6 and 12 weeks. With conversion, Provider is referred to MD for evaluation and treatment.
Vaccine:	Two doses of Hepatitis A vaccine given 6 months apart. Vaccine gives life-long immunity. First shot given 1 month prior to travel to endemic area. Immune Globulin (IG) also given with vaccine if travel will be in less than 1 month.	**Primary vaccine:** 3 shots. First 2 shots given at least 1 month apart. Third shot given 6 months from start or at least 2-4 months after second shot. No booster shots needed anymore.	No vaccine is available.

Table 45.2.   LFT Changes with Acute and Chronic Viral Hepatitis

LFT Markers	Acute Hepatitis	Chronic Hepatitis
Total Protein:	Normal	Normal
Albumin (A):	Normal	Normal
Globulin (G):	Normal	Normal
A:G ratio	Normal	Normal
ALT/SGPT:	>2,000 IU/L	Mild increase or normal
AST/SGOT:	>2,000 IU/L	Mild increase or normal
ALT:AST ratio	ALT>AST	ALT>AST
GGT:	Normal	Normal
Alk. Phos (AP):	Increased	Increased
PT/INR:	Normal	Normal
Total Bilirubin	Increased	Increased or normal
Direct-B	Increased	Increased or normal
Indirect-B	Increased	Increased or normal

ALCOHOLIC LIVER DISEASE

Alcoholic Liver Disease Facts

Alcoholic hepatitis leads to alcoholic cirrhosis, and 20% of chronic alcoholics develop advanced hepatitis or cirrhosis. Alcoholic fatty liver develops with transient alcohol use over days with binge drinking or chronic use. The patient is asymptomatic and the process is reversible with abstinence. With continued alcohol use, however, 20–30% of patients develop alcoholic hepatitis or cirrhosis.

Alcoholic Hepatitis

Alcoholic hepatitis develops after years of alcohol abuse. The patient develops fever; a tender, enlarged liver; and leukocytosis.

Alcoholic Liver Disease Laboratory Tests

Enzyme changes associated with alcoholic liver disease:

- Changes are often associated with minimal elevations of AST and ALT. AST is always greater than ALT and the AST-ALT ratio is >2:1.
- The serum AST level is almost never greater than 500 IU/L and the serum ALT value is almost never greater than 300 IU/L. The reasons for these limits on AST and ALT elevations are not well understood.
- The higher the AST-ALT ratio, the greater the likelihood that alcohol is contributing to the abnormal LFTs.
- The elevated AST-ALT ratio in alcoholic liver disease results in part from the depletion of vitamin B_6 (pyridoxine) in chronic alcoholics. ALT and AST both use pyridoxines as a coenzyme, and the synthesis of ALT is more strongly inhibited by pyridoxine deficiency compared to AST. Alcohol also causes mitochondrial injury, which releases the mitochondrial isoenzyme of AST.

Note that **ALT>AST** in nonalcoholic fatty liver disease.

Alcoholic Liver Disease LFT Pattern

AST:ALT >2:1 and AST is <500 IU/L and ALT is <300 IU/L.

CIRRHOSIS OF THE LIVER

Cirrhosis Symptoms and Signs

The symptoms and signs associated with cirrhosis are jaundice; flailing hands when the arms are raised out in front; muscle wasting, particularly in the temple area and the extremities; spider angiomas on the body and face; palmer erythema; caput medusa around the umbilicus and umbilical hernia; enlarged liver; testicular atrophy; chronic scarring; fibrosis of the liver; and portal hypertension and ascites. With ascites there is fluid buildup in the peritoneal cavity. The patient is treated with diuretics and a diet low in sodium. With **ascites, premedication** prior to dentistry is a must.

Cirrhosis Complications

The following are complications associated with cirrhosis:

- **Pressure changes:** Pressure changes include increased portal hypertension, decreased systemic BP, and esophageal varices that can be life threatening if they bleed.
- **Hepatic encephalopathy:** The liver is unable to clear the toxins that develop. Infection, GI bleeds, narcotics, excessive dietary protein, sedatives, constipation, uremia, and sedatives can trigger encephalopathy. A cirrhotic patient with normal mental status examination but a measurable deficit in learning capability, long-term memory, and intellectual performance is designated as having subclinical hepatic encephalopathy. Hepatic encephalopathy treatment consists of identifying and correcting the precipitating factor; prescribing lactulose and rifaximin; and liver transplant being a last resort.
- **Hepatorenal syndrome:** The liver is unable to clear toxins that affect the kidneys causing renal failure.
- **Hepatocellular carcinoma:** α-fetoprotein is measured for carcinoma of the liver.

Cirrhosis and Associated LFTs

The following are cirrhosis associated LFTs:

- Patients with cirrhosis often have normal or only slightly elevated serum AST and ALT levels. The levels do not rise beyond 300 IU/L with both, and AST level is greater than ALT.
- AST and ALT levels tend to be higher in cirrhotic patients with continuing inflammation or necrosis than in those without continuing liver injury.
- An increased AST-ALT ratio is often found in patients with cirrhosis.

Hepatic Function Derangement in Cirrhosis

Drug Metabolism and Cirrhosis

Cirrhosis is associated with decreased synthesis of plasma-binding proteins. Hypoalbuminemia impairs drug binding and metabolism and elevates serum drug levels.

Impaired drug metabolism, detoxification, and excretion by the liver can prolong drug half-lives. Thus, the absorption, distribution, metabolism, and excretion of anesthetics, muscle relaxants, analgesics, and sedatives can be affected. Drugs such as morphine, meperidine, benzodiazepines, and barbiturates should be used with caution because of their dependence on the liver for metabolism. When absolutely needed, the doses of these drugs should be decreased by 50%. However, fentanyl is the preferred narcotic, and no dose alteration is needed with fentanyl.

Cirrhosis and Vitamin K

Hepatic synthetic dysfunction (all of the coagulation factors, with the exception of von Willebrand factor and Factor VIII, are produced in the liver), malnutrition, and vitamin K malabsorption due to cholestasis contribute to this abnormality. Intravenous (IV) vitamin K supplementation and/or fresh-frozen plasma (FFP) can correct coagulopathy before surgery. Vitamin K by mouth is not recommended because oral absorption is impaired. Refer to Section V: Hemostasis and Associated Bleeding Disorders for a detailed discussion on coagulopathies associated with cirrhosis.

Cirrhosis Treatment

Treatment is as follows:

1. Cirrhosis patients are treated with a low-protein diet.
2. Lactulose and antibiotics are given to kill the ammonia-producing bacteria in the gut. When lactulose is broken down by bacteria in the gut, H^+ is produced and the hydrogen binds to ammonia, producing ammonium that cannot be absorbed by the gut. Thus, it gets excreted thereby decreasing the toxins in the blood.

SUGGESTED DENTAL GUIDELINES WITH HEPATITIS OR CIRRHOSIS

The following are dental guidelines for hepatitis or cirrhosis:

1. Always obtain the complete blood count (CBC) with platelets, hepatic serology, viral load, LFTs, and PT/INR.
2. Evaluate the laboratory results and determine the type of hepatitis or cirrhosis the patient has. The patient may have a history of one or more types of viral hepatitis.
3. Recovery is 100% with hepatitis A, and you do not need to obtain hepatic serology to confirm recovery if the patient is certain that it was hepatitis A.
4. Obtain the hepatic serology and viral load for each type of blood-transmitted hepatitis (B, C, or D) to determine current viral activity status for the virus infecting the patient.
5. Obtain the liver function tests (LFTs) in all patients with a history of any type of hepatitis or cirrhosis.
6. Look at the serum albumin level. The level will be normal with hepatitis, and it will be decreased with cirrhosis.
7. Elevated liver enzymes with a normal albumin level indicate active hepatitis.
8. Normal or mild elevation of liver enzymes with a normal albumin indicates chronic hepatitis.
9. Decreased albumin and AST>ALT is seen with cirrhosis.
10. In the presence of cirrhosis, always obtain the PT/INR prior to probing.

11. Prolongation of PT/INR depends on the **frequency and amount** of blood loss experienced by the cirrhotic patient and **not by the duration** of the disease.
12. Consult with the patient's MD if the PT/INR is prolonged or increased. The MD may give you the go-ahead to proceed with minor dentistry without transfusion therapy if the PT/INR is <2.
13. The patient will need blood plasma transfusion (fresh frozen plasma/FFP, whole blood, or vitamin K IV) for major and minor dentistry if the PT/INR is >2.
14. Cirrhosis can be associated with thrombocytopenia (decreased platelets) due to sequestration of the platelets by the spleen and/or decreased production by the liver.
15. Follow the platelet guidelines for dentistry (discussed in the hemopoietic section) and consult with the patient's MD for platelet replacement therapy, when required.
16. Calculate the absolute neutrophil count/ANC (discussed in the hemopoietic section) for all patients with hepatitis or cirrhosis. Follow the ANC guideline recommendations if the ANC is <1,500 cells/mm^3.
17. Follow the suggested anesthetic, analgesic, antibiotic (AAAs) guidelines listed in Table 45.3.
18. Premedicate a cirrhotic patient presenting with ascites to prevent bacterial growth in the ascetic fluid.
19. Minimize bleeding with dentistry and use the suction aggressively to prevent the swallowing of blood in the presence of cirrhosis. Swallowed blood is protein, which the cirrhotic patient's liver is unable to handle; this can lead to hepatic encephalopathy (see Table 45.4).
20. Limit treatment to one quadrant per visit in the cirrhotic patient to minimize local anesthetic use.

BILIARY DISEASE

Primary Biliary Cirrhosis

Primary biliary cirrhosis (PBC) is an autoimmune disease associated with destruction of intrahepatic bile ducts. Many patients are asymptomatic and eventually develop jaundice and cirrhosis. Middle-aged women are most affected with biliary cirrhosis. **Classic symptoms** experienced are intense itching, jaundice, and cirrhosis in the long term.

Primary Biliary Cirrhosis Blood Test

Antimitochondrial antibody (AMA) is a sensitive and specific test for PBC. It is 95% positive with this disease. Additionally, the AP is markedly increased.

Primary Sclerosing Cholangitis

Primary sclerosing cholangitis is also an autoimmune disease, but it is more common in men around age 40. It is often associated with ulcerative colitis.

Primary Sclerosing Cholangitis Pathology

Primary sclerosing cholangitis is associated with stricture of the intra- or extrahepatic bile ducts, and cirrhosis is a long-term complication.

Table 45.3. Anesthetics, Analgesics, Antibiotics (AAAs) Guidelines for Hepatitis and Cirrhosis

Medications	Prescriptions: Normal and Altered	Drug Alerts/Advice
LOCAL ANESTHETICS 1. **2% Lidocaine (Xylocaine)** with 1:100,000 epinephrine: 2. **4% Prilocaine HCL (Citanest Forte)** with 1:200,000 epi: 3. **4% Septocaine (Articaine)** with 1:100,000 and 1:200,000 epi: 4. **0.5% Bupivacaine (Marcaine)** with 1:200,000 epi: 5. **2% Mepivacaine (Carbocaine)** with 1:20,000 levonordefrin: 6. **3% Mepivacaine HCL** (Carbocaine) 7. **4% Prilocaine HCL** (Citanest Plain)	Any local anesthetic can be used. Use only 2 carpules per visit for hepatitis or cirrhosis	Amide LAs toxicity can occur with significant liver disease. Decreased liver enzymes and decreased hepatic blood flow are factors that alter the pharmacokinetics of LAs. Liver disease therefore increases the duration of the amides. Dental treatment with cirrhosis must be completed **over multiple visits one sextant at a time,** to minimize the total amount of local anesthetic used per visit
ANALGESICS: 1. **Acetaminophen** (Tylenol):	1. **Chronic inactive Hepatitis Dose:** 325-650mg q6-8h 2. **Chronic active hepatitis/cirrhosis Dose:** 325-650mg q8h	Avoid chronic use. Use low-dose therapy with liver disease. Maximum daily dose should be <2g/day with cirrhosis or chronic active hepatitis. Absolutely avoid with alcoholic liver disease.
2. Aspirin:	Avoid use as Aspirin promotes bleeding	Truly only contra-indicated with severe liver disease.
3. NSAIDS:	All NSAIDS are contraindicated with hepatitis and cirrhosis.	Avoid Aspirin and Ibuprofen with any liver disease. Patients with cirrhosis are at increased risk of kidney damage with NSAIDS.
4. COX-2 inhibitors:	Avoid COX-2 inhibitors with any hepatic impairment.	
5. Hydromorphone (Diludid):	**Normal Diludid Dose:** **Oral:** 2-4mg q4h **IV:** 0.2-1mg q4h	Recommended for use in liver failure
6. Fentanyl:	**Normal Oral Fentanyl Dose:** Start with one 200µg lozenge and use it over 15 minutes. Wait 15 minutes and use a second 200µg lozenge if the pain does not immediately subside. Do not use more than 2 lozenges at a given time	Recommended for use in liver failure

(continued)

Table 45.3. Anesthetics, Analgesics, Antibiotics (AAAs) Guidelines for Hepatitis and Cirrhosis
(*Continued*)

Medications	Prescriptions: Normal and Altered	Drug Alerts/Advice
7. Codeine:	**Dose for mild or chronic inactive Hepatitis:** Use the normal Codeine dose: 0-60mg: Dispense 1-2 Tylenol #3 q4-6h PRN. **Dose for moderate-severe or active Hepatitis:** Use 50% of the full dose of Codeine (15-30mg): Dispense 1-2 Tylenol #2 q6h PRN. **Dose for cirrhosis:** Use 25% of the full dose of Codeine (7.5-15mg): Dispense 1-2 Tylenol #1 q8h PRN.	Use caution with Hepatitis and Cirrhosis. Lower the dose and prolong the interval if an opioid has to be used in a patient with liver disease
8. Oxycodone + Acetaminophen (Percocet):	**Hepatitis dose:** One 2.5/325 tablet q6h PRN **Cirrhosis dose:** One 2.5/325 tablet q8h PRN	Limited, low-dose therapy for 2-3 days is usually well tolerated in hepatitis or cirrhosis
9. Hydrocodone + Acetaminophen (Vicodin):	**Dose schedule for Hepatitis:** Dispense 1 tab q6h PRN **Cirrhosis dose:** Dispense 1 tab q8h PRN	Limited, low-dose therapy for 2-3 days is usually well tolerated in hepatitis or cirrhosis. **Avoid chronic use**
10. Morphine: **11. Meperidine** (Demerol): **12. Propoxyphene** (Darvon): **13. Pentazocine** (Talwin): **14. Tramadol** (Ultram): **15.** Methadone	No doses specified as the drugs listed are contraindicated with any type of liver disease. Avoid Tramadol in severe liver disease Methadone is contraindicated in severe liver disease/cirrhosis.	Avoid with any form of liver disease.
ANTIBIOTICS:		
1. Penicillin VK:	**Rx:** 250mg/500mg/tab **Normal Dose:** 250/500mg q6h/qid x 5 days	Safe to use and no dose alteration needed with Hepatitis or Cirrhosis
2. Amoxicillin:	**Rx:** 250/500 875mg/capsules **Normal Dose:** 250/500mg q8h or 500-875mg PO q12h x 5 days	Safe to use and no dose alteration needed with Hepatitis or compensated Cirrhosis. Best to avoid use with decompensated cirrhosis. Can be used with 50% dose adjustment in a patient with **both** kidney and liver disease.
3. Ampicillin:	**Rx:** 250mg or 500mg/capsules **Normal Dose:** 250-500mg q6h for 5 days	Use caution in the presence of any liver disease, **best to avoid**
4. Dicloxacillin:	**Normal Dose:** 250-500mg qid x 5 days	Safe, use normal dose with Hepatitis or Cirrhosis

Table 45.3. Anesthetics, Analgesics, Antibiotics (AAAs) Guidelines for Hepatitis and Cirrhosis (*Continued*)

Medications	Prescriptions: Normal and Altered	Drug Alerts/Advice
Cephalosporins: **5. Cephalexin** (Keflex) **6. Cefadroxil** (Duricef)	**Cephalexin (Keflex):** **Rx:** 250mg or 500mg/capsule **Normal Dose:** 250-1000mg q6h/qid x 5 days, maximum 4g/day **Cefadroxil (Duricef):** **Rx:** 250mg or 500mg/capsules **Normal Dose:** 1-2g/day in two divided doses x 5 days	Safe, use normal dose with Hepatitis or Cirrhosis. Decrease the dose by 50% in patients with **both** kidney and liver disease
7. Clarithromycin (Biaxin):	**Rx:** 250mg or 500mg/capsules **Normal Dose:** 250mg or 500mg bid x 5 days	No dose adjustment is needed with **mild** liver disease **as long as** the renal function is **normal.** Dose adjustment is needed with moderate-severe liver disease as long as the renal function is **normal.** **Avoid** with any form of liver disease **if** renal function is **not** normal
8. Azithromycin (Zithromax):	**5-day supply:** 250mg bid or 500mg hs on the first day, and then 250mg/day for the next 4 days. **3-day supply:** 500mg/day x 3 days.	No dose change in patients with mild or moderate hepatic impairment. Use with caution in end-stage liver disease/cirrhosis. Either reduce the total daily dose or avoid using azithromycin altogether.
9. Clindamycin (Cleocin):	**Rx:** 150mg or 300mg/tablet **Normal Dose:** 150-450mg q6-8h/qid PO x 5 days. Prescribe the lower dose of clindamycin (150mg tid or q8h) routinely to minimize adverse side effects	No dose adjustment required with hepatitis. Decrease the dose by 50% in patients with cirrhosis. Decrease the dose by 50% in a patient with **both** kidney and liver disease.
10. Tetracycline HCl:	No prescriptions given because Tetracycline is contraindicated	Contraindicated with liver disease, kidney disease, or both liver and kidney disease.
11. Doxycycline (Vibramycin):	**Doxycycline, 100mg/capsule Normal dose:** 200mg PO 2 hours prior to bed on day one; 100mg 2 hours prior to bed/day: days 2-10 **Doxycycline, 50mg/capsule Normal dose:** 100mg PO 2 hours prior to bed on day one; 50mg 2 hours prior to bed/day: days 2-10.	No Doxycycline dose change is needed with any form of liver disease. Use doxycycline without dose change in a patient with **both** kidney and liver disease.
12. Metronidazole (Flagyl):	**Rx:** 250/500mg/tab **Normal Dose:** 250mg q6h or 500mg q8h x 5 days **OR** **Rx:** 7.5mg/kg BW, maximum 1g **Normal Dose:** Take q6h x 7 days	No dose alteration is needed with **mild** liver disease. The dose should be decreased in **moderate and severe** liver disease. Use 250mg q12h. Can be used in the presence of **both** liver and kidney disease but with a **reduced** dose, 250mg q12h

Table 45.4.   LFT Changes with Alcoholic Hepatitis, Cirrhosis, and Cholestatic Disease

LFT Markers	Alcoholic Hepatitis	Cirrhosis	Cholestatic Disease
Total Protein:	Normal	Decreased	Normal or decreased with chronic disease
Albumin (A):	Normal	Decreased	Normal or decreased with chronic disease
Globulin (G):	Normal	Increased	Normal or increased with chronic disease
A:G ratio	Normal	Reversed	Normal or reversed with chronic disease
ALT/SGPT:	Mild increase: <300 IU/L	Normal/Mild increase: <300 IU/L	>2,000 IU/L
AST/SGOT:	Mild increase: <500 IU/L	Normal/Mild increase: <300 IU/L	>2,000 IU/L
ALT:AST ratio	AST>ALT (>2:1)	AST>ALT	ALT>AST
GGT:	Increased	Normal or increased with alcoholic cirrhosis	Severely increased
Alk. Phos (AP):	Normal	Increased	Severely increased
PT/INR:	Normal	Normal/ prolonged	Normal/prolonged with chronic disease
Total Bilirubin	Normal	Increased	Increased
Direct-B	Normal	Decreased or normal	Severely increased
Indirect-B	Normal	Increased or normal	Increased

Primary Sclerosing Cholangitis Diagnosis

Primary sclerosing cholangitis is diagnosed with endoscopic retrograde cholangiopan-creotography (ERCP). There is no cure, and transplant is the only option for this disease state.

XIII

Postexposure Prevention and Prophylaxis

Needle-Stick Exposure Protocol and CDC Recommendations for Dental Health-Care Providers Infected with the Hepatitis B Virus

NEEDLE-STICK EXPOSURE OVERVIEW

Needle-stick exposure in the dental setting can predispose to hepatitis B, hepatitis C, or HIV infection. Every effort should be made to minimize risk and prevent such accidents from happening.

Exposure Risks with Percutaneous and Mucocutaneous Exposures

The risk of exposure with percutaneous injury is 0.3%, and with mucocutaneous exposure the risk is 0.09%. The risk increases with deep exposures and/or large volume exposure.

Risk-Reduction Steps

The two steps that can decrease the risk of infection are (1) development of an accident prevention protocol and (2) development of a percutaneous and mucocutaneous exposure protocol to implement once exposure occurs.

ACCIDENT PREVENTION PROTOCOL

An ideal accident prevention protocol should have the following steps implemented at all times during patient care:

1. Plan ahead and collect all instruments needed prior to the start of treatment. This is of particular importance in a dental-school setting where the student has to collect the instruments needed, and this increases the chances of injury when the provider is rushed.
2. Do not have two hands in the mouth at any time. Use the hand mirror to assist with the local anesthetic injection.

Dentist's Guide to Medical Conditions, Medications, and Complications, Second Edition. Kanchan M. Ganda.
© 2013 John Wiley & Sons, Inc. Published 2013 by John Wiley & Sons, Inc.

3. Do not recap the needles with two hands. Remove the needle from the syringe using the disengaging guard. Cover the burr after use with an inverted clean plastic cup to prevent injury.
4. Lay instruments in appropriate slots in the instruments box after use or in a single layer on the dental tray. Do not pile the instruments one over the other after use.
5. Never reach for instruments without looking.
6. Do not be distracted by others. Focus on the procedure being done.

All these steps should be periodically reviewed and reinforced, particularly in a large multi-provider office or student setting.

PERCUTANEOUS AND MUCOCUTANEOUS EXPOSURE PROTOCOL

In the event of an injury, every health-care setting must have a written percutaneous/needle-stick and mucocutaneous exposure protocol that must be implemented immediately. It is necessary to test and treat the exposed person within **one hour** of the exposure.

The dental office must designate in advance a neighboring physician's office or hospital emergency room as the site responsible for providing immediate and follow-up care for both the provider/health-care worker (HCW) and the source patient.

Every member of the dental setting should be familiar with the protocol, which should be visibly posted in the clinical care areas with all the appropriate telephone numbers listed.

The needle-stick exposure protocol should be periodically discussed among all members to ensure awareness. In the event of an accident, non-injured members can actively help, and this, in turn, decreases the anxiety experienced by the injured/exposed HCW.

EXPOSURE PROTOCOL

Postexposure Steps

Once exposure occurs, implement the following steps:

1. Stop dental treatment immediately, de-glove, and wash the injured area with soap and tepid water. If the oral mucosa or eyes have gotten contaminated, rinse the mouth or splash tepid water into the eyes accordingly. Do **not** be overly aggressive with the washing and do **not** use scalding hot water.
2. Inform your patient about the accident once you have completed the washing. Also inform the patient about your percutaneous and mucocutaneous protocol. The patient **needs to consent** for the blood tests that will be completed at the location implementing your protocol.

Postexposure Tests: Protocol for the Source and the Provider/Healthcare Worker (HCW)

Postexposure Tests for the Source

The source patient's status for HIV, hepatitis B, and hepatitis C are determined by conducting the following tests: rapid HIV test, HBsAg and HBeAg, anti-HCV, and hepatitis C RNA.

The rapid HIV test results are obtained within twenty minutes. If the source is positive for hepatitis C, the provider has to be tested at baseline and have follow-up serology tests at six and twelve weeks. If conversion occurs the provider/HCW is referred to an infectious disease specialist for hepatitis C infection evaluation and treatment.

Known HIV/AIDS-Positive Source

If the source patient is a **known** HIV-infected patient, the **HIV PCR or viral load of the source patient** is determined immediately. The viral load is also determined if the source tests positive with the rapid HIV test. In this case, it is clear that the source was unaware of the HIV status prior to the rapid HIV test. The designated physician will, in this case, inform the CDC about detection of a new HIV case, because it is mandatory for the MD to report all HIV sero-conversions.

Tests for the Provider/HCW

The provider must be tested for **baseline** HCV and HIV infections using the anti-HCV and the rapid HIV tests, respectively. Additionally, the anti-HBs titer test is done to determine the provider's immunity status with the hepatitis B vaccine. The hepatitis B vaccine and/or HBIG (hepatitis B immune globulin) are given dependent upon the provider's vaccination and antibody status.

The provider must be reevaluated at six weeks, twelve weeks, and six months. If the provider sero-converts for HIV or HCV, the testing is continued for an additional six months, for a total of twelve months from the time of exposure.

Postexposure Medications

When the source patient is a **known or newly discovered** HIV/AIDS patient, or the HIV/AIDS status of the source is unknown, the HCW must be protected immediately with postexposure medications. Postexposure prophylaxis (PEP) with three antiretroviral drugs must be given within 72 hours of a high-risk HIV exposure (such as percutaneous needle stick) involving an HIV-infected source. Postexposure prophylaxis is **not** recommended if the patient presents **72 hours after** an exposure **or** following a **negligible risk exposure**. Ideally, the treatment should begin as soon as possible after exposure (within hours) and continue for 28 days. With the **unknown** source, once the HIV/AIDS status of the source is confirmed to be negative with testing, the medications can be stopped immediately. The recommended drugs that should be started preferably within **one hour** of the exposure are:

1. **Two-drug regimen:** consists of efavirenz **plus** lamivudine, or emtricitabine **plus** zidovudine or tenofovir.
2. **Three-drug regimen:** consists of lopinavir/ritonavir **plus** lamivudine, or emtricitabine **plus** zidovudine.

An infectious disease expert should be consulted if treatment has been delayed by more than 24–36 hours, or if the provider is pregnant or breast-feeding.

THE CDC OCCUPATIONAL POSTEXPOSURE PROPHYLAXIS GUIDELINES

The CDC postexposure prophylaxis (PEP) guidelines to help the MD select the two- or three-drug regimen for the **exposed provider** are:

1. **If the source is HIV-positive, asymptomatic, and with a viral load <1,500 c/mL:** Two drugs are given for solid needle puncture or a superficial injury or if only a few drops splashed on the mucocutaneous areas. Three or more drugs are given for puncture with a large-bore, hollow needle, when deep injury occurs, or if there was visible presence of blood on the needle or instrument. Two or three drugs are given if there has been a major splash affecting the mucocutaneous areas.

2. **If the HIV-positive source is symptomatic, has AIDS, has acute retroviral syndrome, or has a known high viral load:** Three or more drugs are used immediately for all major or minor percutaneous or mucocutaneous exposures. Immediate consultation with an infectious disease expert is required if the source has demonstrated resistance to HIV medications. In some cases of known multidrug resistance to medications in the source, the physician will have to contact the CDC for further guidance or help in obtaining experimental/newer drugs that may prove to be beneficial.

3. **If the source is unknown:** The option is not to use medication for a low-risk/no-risk source, or to use two to three drugs dependent on the extent of exposure.

PEP Therapy Side Effects

The main side effects experienced are nausea, malaise, and fatigue.

PEP Guidelines for Toxicity Monitoring and Transmission Protection

The provider's CBC and LFTs are done at baseline and at two weeks. If protease inhibitors (PIs) are used, the provider's fasting blood sugar (FBS) is also done at baseline on the day of exposure and at the start of treatment. The provider's urine analysis is done at baseline if IDV/indinavir is used. The provider is asked to report any fever, rash, vomiting, body pain, hematuria (blood in the urine), dysuria (painful urination), or symptoms of hyperglycemia. The provider is also reminded to use protection during sex to prevent pregnancy, in the first 6–12 weeks after exposure, and not to donate blood or body tissues during the prophylaxis period.

This physician-generated protocol has been outlined to empower any provider accidentally injured during patient care. Realizing that the drug intake should be started immediately alleviates anxiety, as does knowing you have the CDC PEP protocol on hand to share with the MD. It is beneficial for the physician as well because it is not very often an MD treats percutaneous or mucocutaneous exposures.

CDC RECOMMENDATIONS FOR DENTAL PROVIDERS INFECTED WITH THE HEPATITIS B VIRUS

Introduction

The CDC recently published recommendations for hepatitis B infected providers that states that health-care providers do **not** have to notify patients of their hepatitis B virus status. The guidelines also state that hepatitis B virus DNA serum levels, in addition to hepatitis B e-antigen status, should be used to monitor the provider's infectivity, and that HBV DNA levels serve as a better prognostic gauge of infectivity. Also, a hepatitis B virus (HBV) DNA level of 1,000 international units (IU)/mL or 5,000 genome equivalents (GE)/mL, is the guideline threshold value recommended by the CDC as "safe" for practice. CDC recommendations, best practices, and HBV infection management protocols are all discussed in detail in the following sections.

New CDC Recommendations for the Management of Infected HCWs and Students

The CDC Recommendations

- Promotes patient safety and provides risk management and practice guidance to HBV-infected HCWs and students performing exposure-prone procedures (EPPs).
- Specifies injury prevention and blood exposure during EPPs.
- States that patient needs no prior notification of the HBV status of an infected HCW or student.
- Use HBV DNA serum levels rather than HBeAg status to monitor infectivity.
- HBV DNA titer is considered "safe" for practice at values that are <1,000 IU/mL.
- HBV infection alone does not disqualify an infected HCW or student from practice as long as infection control measures are optimal. This is of particular importance for the chronically infected provider/student.
- New data show that the risk for HBV and other blood-borne virus transmission from infected providers is extremely low; the infection-control practices have improved; nationally there have been decreasing trends in the incidence of acute HBV infection among HCWs and the general population; HBV vaccination rate is up following the adoption of universal infant vaccination along with catchup vaccinations for children and adolescents; improved HBV therapies are now available; and there is now strict implementation of standard precautions and Occupational Safety and Health Administration (OSHA) blood-borne pathogens standards.
- Standard precautions and double gloving for EPPs has further decreased the already low risk of transmission of HBV, HCV, and HIV from an infected HCW or student to the patient.

Current HBV Therapies

- HBV is currently treated with two types of interferon (α and peglated interferon) and five nucleoside or nucleotide analogs (lamuvidine, telbivudine, abacavir, entecavir, and tenofovir).
- Entecavir and tenofovir have potent antiviral activity and very low rates of drug resistance.
- Treatment with these drugs decreases HBV DNA to undetectable or almost undetectable viral loads in weeks or months of starting therapy.
- These newer medications effectively suppress viral replication and therefore can be very effective for decreasing viral load in infected HCWs with viral loads >1,000 IU/mL.

Dental Procedures and HBV infection

- Exposure-prone procedures (EPPs) are those where access to operate during surgery is difficult and exposure-prone fields tend to be very closed and un-visualized operating areas.
- Oral surgery procedures done by an oral surgeon are Category 1 procedures, and these procedures have an increased risk of infection transmission from doctor to patient.
- All other procedures in the dental setting are classified as Category 2 procedures and are not risk prone for the transmission of infection.
- EPPs performed specifically in the oral surgery setting have an increased risk of transfer of infection from provider to patient. Dependent on the infected provider's HBV DNA, certain procedures may then be restricted.
- Society for Health-Care Epidemiology of America (SHEA) states that infected HCWs or students may have to temporarily stop surgery, or, if they are to do invasive procedures, they should keep their viral loads below 2,000 IU/mL.
- Infected HCWs or students performing EPPs need to be monitored by a panel of experts to ensure balanced recommendations. Strict standard precautions and implementation of double-gloving will help prevent the transmission of infection.
- Exposure can be decreased by promoting single-use only instruments, not recapping needles, using puncture-resistant needles, and having a sharps disposal container.
- OSHA mandates that the HBV vaccine be made available by institutions or offices for all HCWs and students who are potentially at risk for infection.
- All HCWs should be vaccinated, especially those born to mothers from endemic parts of the world such as China and India. These individuals are vaccinated only after confirming that they have no infection, but if infection is found then these individuals are treated.
- Infected HCWs doing EPPs should be supervised by the hospital or clinic to ensure safe practices. Each infected person will need individual considerations.
- Some infected persons may be HBeAg negative in the presence of a very high viral load from viral replication, as the person may have pre-core mutants of the virus. Therefore, HBV DNA is better to detect infectivity. Also, HBV DNA monitors infectivity better.
- Real-time PCR testing is more sensitive than conventional testing and viral load <200 IU/mL is the threshold for this test. It should be noted that the newer, more sensitive assays detect viral loads as low as 20–30 IU/mL.
- If viral load continues to fluctuate, then one needs to consider failure in therapy.
- It is the ethical and professional responsibility of a provider to know the HBV status and implement appropriate steps for clinical care and prevention of infection transmission.
- If there is no exposure, then no routine mandatory disclosure of the HCWs status is required.
- Infected HCWs and students who are not conducting EPPs need to be monitored by their respective physicians, and not by the expert panel.
- Infected HCWs or students conducting EPPs must be monitored by an expert panel to oversee clinical progress and viral status; the practices of this person in the clinical setting; provide counseling and oversight; and report any breaches. The panel will

reinforce standard precautions—that is, double-gloving, changing gloves frequently, using blunt surgical needles, and so on.

Expert Panel Membership

The Expert Panel should include:

- One or two professionals from the infected HCWs area of practice
- The chief of Infectious Disease (ID) at the hospital
- A liver specialist or gastroenterologist
- The infected HCWs physician
- An ethics-qualified person
- Human resource professionals
- School administrators
- Legal counsel

The institution should have a needle-stick and percutaneous exposure protocol in place, and if exposure does occur, then the patient should be informed. The protocol should immediately be implemented for the patient and the patient should get postexposure vaccination or bepatitis B immune globulin and testing.

The infected HCW may or may not be identified to the panel, but if the panel gets to know the identity, then they have to respect confidentiality. **HBV infection should not prevent the study of dentistry because strict implementation of standard precautions protects patients and providers.**

Additionally, there should be no need to demonstrate persistently negligible viral loads at frequencies less than three months, with three months being the shortest interval for repeat testing. Furthermore, there is no need to notify patients, and there is no need to force any change of practice or enforce any exclusions from EPPs, which would hamper practice or student study.

HBV Vaccination and Screening

- The CDC recommends the three-dose series of vaccination followed by determination of anti-HBs titer >10m IU/mL to confirm immunity.
- Those with low titers should get re-vaccinated with the three doses.
- If the titers are still low, then the provider or student should get tested for HBsAg and anti-HBc, to determine infection status.
- Pre-vaccination testing is only recommended for those individuals born to mothers from endemic countries, if the individual is from an endemic country, if the person performs EPPs, or if the person is a sexually active gay man.
- Infected HCWs or students not conducting EPPs do not need monitoring, viral load testing, or any other restrictions; however, they must be monitored by their respective physicians. Additionally, they do not need to achieve low or undetectable viral loads.

HCWs Conducting Category 1 EPP

- Providers or students conducting EPPs should be monitored by the panel for procedures they can do. The panel should also provide oversight and maintain confidentiality.

- These HCWs can get tested every six months if the viral load is low or undetectable, but more frequent testing is required with high viral loads.
- CDC recommends HBV level <1,000 IU/mL or <5,000 GE/mL (genome equivalents/mL) as threshold for detection versus un-detection of infection.
- More sophisticated assays showing viral loads around 10–30 IU/mL can also be used.

XIV

Infectious Diseases

Human Immunodeficiency Virus, Herpes Simplex and Zoster, Lyme Disease, MRSA Infection, and Sexually Transmitted Diseases

HUMAN IMMUNODEFICIENCY VIRUS

Human Immunodeficiency Virus (HIV) Specifics

HIV is an infection caused by the human immunodeficiency virus that was formerly called the human T-lymphotropic virus-III (HTLV-III). HIV-1 and HIV-2 are the two species of HIV that infect humans. HIV-1 is the more aggressive of the two and it accounts for the majority of the infections worldwide. HIV-2 is less aggressive and is limited to western Africa.

The reverse transcriptase enzyme in the virus helps with the transfer of viral RNA into the DNA of the host cell. The virus attacks the CD_4 T cells causing them to become infected. The infected cells are destroyed in one of three ways: direct viral killing, death by apoptosis, and death through the cytotoxic effects mediated by CD_8 lymphocytes.

The T_4 lymphocytes are like the "pilots" of immunity that also govern the quality and quantity of the B lymphocytes. Defective cell-mediated and lymphokine-mediated humoral immunity consequently occurs. Impaired immunity accounts for the increased incidence of opportunistic infections when the patient becomes symptomatic.

In addition to the CD_4 cells, the virus affects the monocytes, macrophages, neural cells, or glial cells and crosses the blood-brain barrier. The virus has been isolated from almost all bodily fluids as free viral particles or embedded in previously specified cell. Isolation is most pronounced from the blood and the seminal fluid.

Gradual decline in immunity over time ultimately leads to the patient developing the acquired immunodeficiency syndrome (AIDS). The patient is said to have AIDS when the CD_4 count is <200 cells/mm^3. With the implementation of HIV/AIDS treatment, the CD_4 count can improve and rise >200 cells/mm^3. However, the patient will retain the diagnosis of AIDS even if the CD_4 improves. It is important to remember that throughout the asymptomatic phase the CD_4 count is on a steady decline.

Dentist's Guide to Medical Conditions, Medications, and Complications, Second Edition. Kanchan M. Ganda.
© 2013 John Wiley & Sons, Inc. Published 2013 by John Wiley & Sons, Inc.

Modes of HIV Transmission

HIV transmission can occur via the following:

1. Blood or Clotting Factors transfusion.
2. Intravenous drug use (IVDU).
3. Exchange of body fluids: unprotected sex can transmit the virus. Worldwide, the transmission rate by heterosexual sex is increasing at a greater rate.
4. Vertical transmission from mother to child: Transmission mostly occurs during birth, but there are data showing that some transmission may be intrauterine. Intrauterine transmission can be prevented by treating the mother with antiretroviral therapy. Vertical transmission is now prevented with implementing elective caesarian section prior to the rupture of membranes in the HIV-positive mother.
5. The virus can also be transmitted through breast-feeding, and this can be overcome by avoiding breast-feeding or treating the mother with antiretroviral therapy.

Epidemiology of HIV

Epidemiology of HIV in the Developed Nations

Initially in the developed world, men having sex with men (MSM) was the leading cause of HIV transmission. With increased awareness of risk practices and prevention strategies, those numbers declined in the 1990s, but the numbers are now increasing again. Current transmission types are as follows, MSM > heterosexual contact > injection drug use (showing small improvement).

Recently, there has been an increased rate of transmission of the virus in the heterosexual population because of unprotected sex and among people of color because of IV drug use (IVDU). However, injection drug use numbers have shown some improvement. Vertical transmission from mother to child is now rare in the developed world because of initiation of treatment during pregnancy and the implementation of elective caesarian section around the thirty-eighth week of pregnancy.

Epidemiology of HIV in the Developing Nations

About 33 million adults and children total are living with HIV, and 2.5 million children <15 years old are living with HIV. There are 2.6 million new infections in adults and children, and the incidence of infection in children <15 years old is 370,000. There are about 1.8 million AIDS-related deaths each year in adults and children, and last year the deaths among children <15 years old were 260,000, which is less than the number of new infections. Most people with HIV are in sub-Saharan Africa (22.5 million people) with the Middle East and northern Africa comprising a distant second (4.1 million people). In the developing nations, the highest rate of transmission has been encountered among the heterosexual population because of unprotected sex and IVDU. Mother-to-child vertical transmission is another leading cause for the increased numbers of infected cases.

There is a dire need to provide antiretroviral therapy (ART) in the developing nations along with improved prevention strategies to decrease the numbers. Prevention can be achieved by educating the population about HIV infection and the modes by which the virus is transmitted.

HIV Natural History

The following sections detail the ways in which the viral infection can progress, once exposure occurs.

Acute Retroviral Infection

An acute retroviral infection progresses in one of two ways:

1. Some patients on sero-conversion experience infectious mononucleosis-type symptoms, approximately two to four weeks post exposure. The mononucleosis-type illness simulates an actual mononucleosis attack, which lasts for 10–14 days. The patient usually recovers from the acute attack and progresses through an asymptomatic phase for years before becoming symptomatic again. However, once symptoms occur again, they are persistent and need to be addressed and treated.
2. The majority of patients are asymptomatic.

The Asymptomatic Patient

This patient has CD_4 >250 cells/mm^3 and a viral load up to 50–100 K/mL. The patient can stay asymptomatic for ten years, or even longer, while the CD_4 count gradually declines over time. No treatment is recommended in the presence of established disease if the patient is asymptomatic.

The Symptomatic Patient

This patient presents with AIDS-defining conditions (ADC): weight loss, oral candidiasis, opportunistic infections, tumors, and so on. The opportunistic infections that occur must be diagnosed and treated appropriately.

The Early Symptomatic Stage

The CD_4 count is >200 cells/mm^3 and the usual range at this stage is 250–300 cells/mm^3. MTB, candida infections, cryptococcus infection, histoplasmosis, and recurrent bacterial infections occur.

The Late Symptomatic Stage

Pneumocystis carinii pneumonia (PCP), now called **Pneumocystis jiroveci**, and chronic cryptosporidia diarrhea occur when the CD_4 count is <200 cells/mm^3. Toxoplasmosis, cytomegalovirus (CMV), and mycobacterium avium complex (MAC) infections can occur when the CD_4 is <100 cells/mm^3.

AIDS-Defining Conditions (ADC) in the Symptomatic Stage

The following are ADC conditions that can occur in the symptomatic stage:

- Recurrent bacterial infections.
- Candida infection affecting the esophagus, trachea, and bronchi.

- Disseminated coccidiomycosis, histoplasmosis.
- Extrapulmonary cryptococcosis.
- Chronic cryptosporidiosis.
- Cytomegalovirus (CMV).
- More advanced cases present with persistent mucocutaneous herpes simplex infection (HSV), HIV encephalopathy, Kaposi's sarcoma, primary lymphoma of the brain, non-Hodgkin's B-cell lymphoma, MAC, extrapulmonary TB (dissem TB), Pneumocystis jiroveci pneumonia, progressive multifocal leukoencephalopathy, recurrent salmonella infection, and toxoplasmosis of the brain.
- Cytomegalovirus (CMV) can affect the eyes, the brain, and the adrenal glands.
- Papilloma virus that causes warty cauliflower type of lesions on the gums.
- Mycobacterium avium complex (MAC) and mycobacterium kansasii (MK) occur only in the immune-compromised patients and not in healthy, immune-competent patients.
- Kaposi's sarcoma begins as a pink, pinhead-sized lesion that gradually enlarges and changes in color from pink to purple to black. Kaposi's sarcoma is usually multifocal and involves the trunk, the upper extremities, and the head and neck region.

HIV and AIDS Criteria Summary

HIV

The patient is said to have HIV when there is evidence that confirms presence of HIV. There is ongoing viral replication and progressive immune system decline.

AIDS

The patient is said to have AIDS when there is HIV infection and ADCs or the patient has CD_4 <200 cells/mm^3. There is ongoing viral replication and progressive immune system decline.

General Overview of HIV/AIDS in the United States

HIV is now one of the top-ten causes of death in the United States. However, people are now living longer with HIV due to effective antiretroviral therapy, and the death rate is decreasing. Numbers of new infections remain low but stable. Transmission-risk groups vary every year, but greater numbers of males than females are infected overall. The numbers of HIV cases among blacks and Hispanics have increased; the numbers among whites have declined. The numbers among Asians has stayed low throughout. Overall, the numbers by race show African Americans outnumbering Caucasians, Hispanics, Asians, and Native Americans.

Transmission by intravenous drug use (IVDU) has increased, and unprotected heterosexual contacts recorded the steepest rise. The numbers had decreased for men having sex with men (MSM) and MSM IV drug users, but these numbers are now increasing again.

HIV/AIDS TESTS

HIV tests detect the presence of the human immunodeficiency (HIV) antibodies, antigens, or RNA in the serum or saliva. There are three sets of tests associated with HIV/AIDS:

1. Diagnostic tests
2. Quantitative tests
3. Organ assessment tests with medication intake

DIAGNOSTIC TESTS

The average window period (the time from infection until antibodies develop) with the antibody tests is about 22 days. Occasionally, a patient may have a delay in forming antibodies and do so in about three to six months. There are two sets of diagnostic tests that help with the diagnosis of infection:

1. Non-rapid diagnostic tests
2. Rapid diagnostic tests

The Non-Rapid Diagnostic Tests

It takes about seven to ten days to obtain the results. The two non-rapid diagnostic tests are:

1. The Enzyme Linked Immunosorbent Assay (ELISA) test
2. The Western Blot test

The ELISA Test

The ELISA test is said to be reactive when it detects antibodies to HIV-1. Once positive, the blood is tested again to reconfirm that the ELISA test is indeed positive. Results from the ELISA test are reported as a number; the test is 99% sensitive.

The Western Blot Test

The Western Blot test is a more specific test that is 99.5% sensitive. The Western Blot test determines the size of the antigens binding to the antibodies in the test kit. Blood showing a positive ELISA is subjected to the Western Blot test. Thus, the Western Blot test is confirmatory testing for HIV infection. A positive Western Blot test confirms that the patient is infected with HIV.

Opt-Out Testing

It is estimated that one-third of those infected with HIV do not know their status. HIV testing requires written informed consent and the CDC recommends "opt-out" testing on the grounds that early treatment is effective. Therefore, early identification is especially encouraged. Furthermore, people with suppressed viral loads are at a lower risk of transmitting to someone, so this recommendation is not only good for the patient, it is also an excellent public health measure.

In opt-out testing it is assumed that every primary-care patient will get tested, unless they specifically request not to be tested, but no written consent is required. For any patient being seen for a general physical, the physician will test for HIV, unless there is an objection by a patient. This testing is not based on a person's risk factors. Consequently, this eliminates the necessity for informed consent. This measure will identify HIV-positive individuals in populations that may not otherwise undergo testing.

The First FDA-Approved OTC HIV Test Kit

The OraQuick in-home HIV test, manufactured by OraSure Technologies, is the first over-the-counter (OTC), self-administered FDA-approved HIV test kit to detect the presence of antibodies to HIV-1 and HIV-2. The patient collects an intraoral sample by swabbing the upper and lower gums and then places the sample into a developer vial. The patient obtains test results within 20–40 minutes. A positive test does not mean that an individual is definitely infected with HIV. A positive result indicates only that additional testing in a medical setting is necessary to confirm the result. A negative test result does not mean that an individual has definitely not been infected with HIV, especially when exposure may have occurred within the past three months. The OraQuick in-home HIV test has 92% test sensitivity and 99.98% test specificity. A version of this test for use by trained technicians in clinical settings was approved in 2004.

The Rapid Diagnostic Tests

These tests provide results immediately or within 20 minutes. The two rapid diagnostic tests are:

1. The OraQuick Rapid HIV-Antibody test
2. The Reveal Rapid HIV-Antibody test

The OraQuick Rapid HIV-1 Antibody Test

This test detects antibodies and is approved for use with a finger-stick or anticoagulated whole blood or serum or oral fluid specimens. Results are obtained within 20 minutes from the testing. The test is 99.6% sensitive and 100% specific. The specificity of the OraQuick assay is **higher** than the Reveal Rapid assay.

The Reveal Rapid HIV-1 Antibody Test

This test requires the use of a serum or plasma specimen that is added to the test cartridge. The result is read immediately after the solution is absorbed. If a serum sample is used, the Reveal Rapid assay is 99.8% sensitive and 99.1% specific. If a plasma sample is used, the test is 98.6% specific.

QUANTITATIVE TESTS

There are two tests:

1. The CD_4 count
2. The viral load

The Role of Quantitative Virology and Antiretroviral Therapy

CD_4 counts and HIV/RNA assays are of greatest clinical significance for efficient monitoring of the HIV infection. The CD_4 count provides an estimate of the patient's immune system status. CD_4 counts also are used to determine a patient's response to therapy. The CD_4 count should be repeated every three to six months, and the normal CD_4 count fluctuates between 900–1,200 cells/mm^3.

Correlation of CD_4 Count and Lymphocyte Percentage Reported on Laboratory Tests

Lymphocyte percentage reported on laboratory tests can be correlated to the appropriate CD_4 count to get a better understanding of the patient's immunity status.

Lymphocyte Percentage to CD_4 Count Conversion

- 29% lymphocytes = CD_4 count >500 cells/mm^3
- 14–28% lymphocytes = CD_4 200–500 cells/mm^3
- <14% lymphocytes = CD_4 count <200 cells/mm^3

HIV RNA or Viral Load

HIV RNA/viral load assays permit the detection of minute quantities of HIV RNA in the blood and tissues of the patient, in all stages of the disease. It is a strong predictor of disease progression. A threefold change with successive tests is said to be significant. If HIV RNA levels are repeatedly <10,000 copies/mL, therapy may be deferred. HIV RNA levels <50 copies/mL indicate an "undetectable viral load."

Serial HIV RNA assays must be repeated every three to four months. Longevity is increased if viral loads are kept constantly at negligible levels.

ORGAN ASSESSMENT TESTS WITH MEDICATION INTAKE

The following tests are required when the patient is on HIV/AIDS medications to detect adverse side effects with the medications:

1. **The CBC:** The CBC must be repeated every three to six months, or sooner, if indicated. HIV medications cause folic acid deficiency associated macrocytic anemia.
2. **Liver function tests (LFTs):** LFTs are done to monitor the liver enzymes that may be affected with the HIV/AIDS medications.
3. **Renal function tests:** Urinalysis and serum creatinine are monitored while the patient is on the HIV/AIDS medications.
4. **Fasting blood sugar (FBS):** The FBS is monitored for patients on Highly Active Antiretroviral Therapy (HAART), because HAART can raise the blood sugar levels. The FBS must be repeated every three to four months.
5. **Lipid profile:** The lipid profile is monitored for patients on HAART because the lipid levels can be affected with HAART. The lipid profile must be repeated every three to four months.

Table 47.1 provides a summary of HIV/AIDS medications.

Table 47.1. HIV/AIDS Medications

Drug Class	Drug Name	Side Effects
Nucleoside reverse transcriptase inhibitors (NRTIs): Tenofovir + Emtricitabine are primary therapy NRTIs. Abacavir + Lamivudine are alternate therapy NRTIs.	Tenofovir (Viread)	Causes renal insufficiency
	Emtricitabine (Emtriva)	Causes hyperpigmentation
	Abacavir (Ziagen)	Needs HLA*B5701 screening prior to administration to avoid hypersensitivity
	Lamivudine (Epivir)	Minimal toxicity, severe acute exacerbation of hepatitis may occur with HBV-coinfection upon discontinuation
	Stavudine (Zerit)	Causes peripheral neuropathy
	Didanosine (Videx)	Causes peripheral neuropathy, lactic acidosis
	Zalcitabine (Hivid)	Causes peripheral neuropathy and stomatitis
	Zidovudine (Retrovir)	Drug discontinued
Nonnucleoside reverse transcriptase inhibitors (NNRTIs): Efavirenz is primary therapy NNRTI Nevirapine or Rilpivirine are alternate therapy NNRTIs	Efavirenz (Sustiva)	Rash, hyperlipidemia
	Delavirdine (Rescriptor)	Rash
	Nevirapine (Viramune, Viramune XR)	Rash, hepatitis
	Rilpivirine (Edurant)	Rash
	Etravirine (Intelence)	Rash
Protease inhibitors (PIs): Primary therapy PIs are Ritonavir "boosted" Atazanavir or Ritonavir "boosted" Darunavir. Alternate therapy PI: Ritonavir "boosted" Lopinavir	Atazanavir (Reyataz): always combined with Ritonavir as "booster" drug	Prolonged PR interval, hyperglycemia, skin rash, hyperlipidemia
	Darunavir (Prezista): always combined with Ritonavir as "booster" drug	Hyperlipidemia, hyperglycemia
	Lopinavir/ritonavir (Kaletra): always combined with Ritonavir as "booster" drug	Hyperlipidemia, hyperglycemia
	Indinavir (Crixivan)	Hyperlipidemia, hyperglycemia
	Fosamprenavir (Lexiva)	Hyperlipidemia, hyperglycemia
	Nelfinavir (Viracept)	Hyperlipidemia, hyperglycemia
	Ritonavir (Norvir)	Hyperlipidemia, hyperglycemia, and oral parasthesias
	Saquinavir (Invirase)	Hyperlipidemia, hyperglycemia, and QT interval prolongation
	Tipranavir (Aptivus)	Hyperlipidemia, hyperglycemia, hepatotoxicity, and rash
Integrase inhibitor (II): II, Raltegravir is part of primary therapy	Raltegravir (Isentress)	CK elevations, myopathy, or rhabdomyolysis
Chemokine receptor antagonist (CCR5 antagonist)	Maraviroc (Selzentry)	CYP3A4 inducer and inhibitor effect Constipation, dizziness, infection
Fusion inhibitor (FI)	Enfuvirtide (Fuzeon), subcutaneous injection	Injection-site reactions

Table 47.1. HIV/AIDS Medications (*Continued*)

Drug Class	Drug Name	Side Effects
Combination Drugs	Epzicom − Abacavir + lamivudine Trizivir − Abacavir + lamivudine + zidovudine Truvada − Tenofovir + emtricitabine Atripla − Tenofovir + emtricitabine + efavirenz Complera − Tenofovir + emtricitabine + rilpivirine Combivir − Zidovudine + lamivudine	

Highly Active Antiretroviral Therapy (HAART)

HAART has been able to suppress the virus such that HIV is now considered a chronic disease. Once started, HAART has to be continued for life, so the question is when to start the treatment. The physician and the patient have to weigh the short- and long-term risks or toxicities associated with HAART. The biggest benefit has been a 50% reduction in mortality. The drawbacks have been lipodystrophy and metabolic abnormalities, thus increasing the risks for cardiovascular disease.

Not all HIV-associated disease states are reduced with HAART. Suppression of HIV does not mean that there is an associated decline in the replication of hepatitis C virus. In fact, it some cases it may worsen the hepatitis C co-infection. Incidence of Kaposi's sarcoma is decreasing, but the incidence of immunoblastic lymphoma, Hodgkin's lymphoma, invasive cervical cancer, and Burkitt's lymphoma are not.

HAART-Associated Lipodystrophy Syndrome and Metabolic Abnormalities

The resultant lipodystrophy syndrome is associated with abnormal fat accumulation causing central, intra-abdominal obesity and fat buildup around the back of the neck, which is known as a "buffalo hump." Subcutaneous fat atrophy between the skin and the muscles occurs, mostly affecting the face, arms, and legs. HAART is also associated with lipid metabolism changes demonstrating a low HDL and high triglycerides. Glucose metabolism changes showing insulin resistance and glucose intolerance is another side effect of HAART.

Cumulative Side Effects of HIV/AIDS Medications

The side effects associated with HIV/AIDS medications must be assessed and appropriately treated, when possible, by the dentist prior to the start of dentistry. The side effects that can occur are heart disease, liver disease (demonstrating elevated ALT levels and hepatic necrosis), xerostomia, change in prevalence and incidence of oral lesions,

Stevens-Johnson syndrome, lactic acidosis, pancreatitis, nephrotoxicity, marrow suppression, gastrointestinal intolerance, peripheral neuropathy, rash, CNS toxicity, insulin resistance, hyperlipidemia, fat atrophy, and fat accumulation.

PROPHYLAXIS AND TREATMENT OF OPPORTUNISTIC INFECTIONS

PCP occurs within one year in 60% of patients with HIV with CD_4 <200 cells/mm^3. Thus, prophylaxis against PCP is a must as a preventative therapy.

Primary and Secondary Opportunistic Infections Prophylaxis

Primary Prophylaxis

Primary prophylaxis is provided when there is no evidence of the disease against which the prophylaxis is being given. PCP prophylaxis is an example of primary prophylaxis. PCP prophylaxis is inexpensive and effective. Trimethoprim-sulfamethoxazole (Bactrim) is the recommended regimen for PCP prophylaxis. Bactrim also protects the patient from toxoplasmosis, salmonellosis, or any staphylococcal infection. Bactrim does not protect the patient against shigella, pneumococcal or pneumococcal strep, klepsiella, or pseudomonas.

All adults and adolescents are given prophylaxis when any one of these states occurs, regardless of whether they are taking HAART:

- The patient has CD_4 <200 cells/mm^3.
- There is a history of oral candidiasis.
- The CD_4 cells account for <14% of the lymphocyte count.
- There is a history of AIDS but without CD_4 <200/mm^3.

Secondary Prophylaxis

Secondary prophylaxis is provided **after** the disease against which the prophylaxis is being given has occurred. The patient gets treated for the disease **first**, and the prophylaxis is given after recovery to prevent any future attacks with the disease. Prophylaxis against CMV is secondary prophylaxis. It is expensive and its effectiveness is questionable.

HIV/AIDS TREATMENT

- Antiretroviral therapy (ART) guidelines are constantly updated on an ongoing basis by The US Department of Health and Human Services, in conjunction with the panels on International AIDS Society (IAS) and the World Health Organization (WHO).
- With the advent of highly active antiretroviral therapy (HAART), HIV-1 infection is now managed as a chronic disease, especially in patients who are being treated and who continue to maintain significant viral suppression. HAART therapy has nearly halved the mortality rate in patients with AIDS. Treatment should be based on at least two consistent determinations of CD_4 and viral load because they fluctuate.

- Current guidelines state that treatment must begin when a patient has a history of an AIDS-defining illness (symptomatic disease) or when the patient is asymptomatic but has a CD_4 count <350 cells/mm^3. Treatment must definitely begin with CD_4 <200 cells/mm^3. Treatment is also strongly recommended for asymptomatic patients with CD_4 counts from 350–500 cells/mm^3 and moderately recommended or optional for patients with CD_4 counts above 500 cells/mm^3, when associated with viral load >100,000 copies, or in the presence of CD_4 decline >100 cells/year.
- Pregnant women with HIV infection should get therapy regardless of CD_4 count, in order to prevent transmission of infection from mother to child. HAART therapy is started at the end of the first trimester.
- Antiretroviral therapy preserves renal function and prolongs survival regardless of CD_4 count in patients with HIV-associated nephropathy, so HAART therapy is started regardless of CD_4 count in patients with underlying kidney disease. Treatment is also started in the presence of cardiovascular risk factors or in the presence of active hepatitis B or C infection.
- The International Antiviral Society–USA panel (IAS-USA) for antiretroviral therapy (ART) issued recommendations at the XIX International AIDS Conference, and these provide the direction in which HIV/AIDS care will proceed in the future.

2012 Recommendations of the IAS-USA for ART

- New data show that antiretroviral therapy (ART) has dramatically reduced the numbers of opportunistic diseases and deaths in people infected with HIV; ART therapy results in viral suppression, thus decreasing human immunodeficiency virus (HIV) transmission, and when used consistently by HIV-uninfected persons ART may provide protection against HIV infection. Studies have shown that ART therapy was 96% effective in reducing HIV transmission from infected individuals to their non-infected partners. Thus, offering ART therapy to at-risk individuals or to their partners, especially in the absence of a vaccine, can benefit the population at large.
- All adults who are HIV-positive should get ART therapy as soon as possible, regardless of the CD_4 cell count, and the earlier the better. There is no CD_4 cell count threshold at which starting therapy is contraindicated.
- The aim of therapy is to trigger maximum, lifelong, and continuous suppression of HIV replication and to ultimately improve health.
- Initial therapy for HLA-B*5701-negative patients with baseline plasma HIV-1 RNA <100,000copies/mL consists of a combination of two nucleoside reverse transcriptase inhibitors (NRTIs) and a nonnucleoside reverse transcriptase inhibitor (NNRTI), a ritonavir-boosted protease inhibitor (PI/r), an integrase strand transfer inhibitor (InSTI), or, very occasionally, a chemokine receptor 5 (CCR5) antagonist. Regimens in fixed-dose combinations (FDCs) are used once daily, thus improving medication adherence. **Initial Therapy Drugs:** two nucleoside reverse transcriptase inhibitors (NRTIs), tenofovir/emtricitabine or abacavir/lamivudine + nonnucleoside reverse transcriptase inhibitor (NNRTI) efavirenz + ritonavir-boosted protease inhibitor (PI), atazanavir/darunavir, **or** integrase strand transfer inhibitor (InSTI), raltegravir (see Table 47.1).
- Alternatives in each class are selected if these drugs cannot be used.

- CD_4 cell count and HIV-1 RNA level should be monitored throughout therapy. Suppression of plasma HIV-1 RNA to less than 50 copies/mL by 24 weeks needs to occur with effective therapy, regardless of prior treatment.

- Current third-generation HIV-1 RNA assays show a lower limit of quantification of 40 or 20 copies/mL and can report qualitative RNA detection below these cutoffs. In addition, many patients receiving stable suppressive treatment show residual viremia of 1–10 copies/mL by research-based assays.

- Plasma HIV-1 RNA levels should be monitored at least every three months after beginning or modifying treatment, to confirm suppression of viremia <50 copies/mL.

- Once viral load is suppressed for one year and CD_4 cell count is stable at 350 cells/mm^3 or greater, HIV-1 RNA and CD_4 cell count can be monitored at intervals of up to six months in patients who are good about adhering to therapy.

- ART has a role in postexposure prophylaxis.

- **Preexposure prophylaxis (PrEP):** The FDA recently approved tenofovir disoproxil fumarate/emtricitabine (Truvada) for use as preexposure prophylaxis for HIV-seronegative gay men, in order to protect them from contracting the infection through sexual activity. Patients prescribed tenofovir disoproxil fumarate/emtricitabine for preexposure prophylaxis (PrEP) are required to take the drug daily, in addition to practicing safe sex and getting tested regularly for HIV.

- **When to initiate ART:** ART is recommended regardless of CD_4 cell count; the need increases as the CD_4 cell count decreases.

- **Acute HIV infection:** ART therapy is recommended for those with symptomatic, acute HIV infection, as well as individuals who were recently diagnosed. Patients with acute HIV infection have very high HIV-1 RNA levels in plasma and genital secretions, and this increases the risk of transmission by sexual encounter. Thus, offering persons with acute HIV infection early treatment is a high priority in preventing the spread of the infection.

- **Hepatitis B co-infection:** Liver-related morbidity and mortality is increased in persons with combined HIV and hepatitis B virus (HBV) infections, so treating both infections with the same medications can prove beneficial. The optimal ART regimen for people co-infected with HIV and HBV should include tenofovir and emtricitabine (or lamivudine) as the NRTI drugs.

- **Hepatitis C virus:** Liver-related morbidity and mortality is also increased in individuals with both HCV and HIV infections. Studies have shown that in patients with CD_4 cell counts >500 cells/mm^3 it is best to delay ART therapy until after completion of HCV treatment. Peginterferon alfa and ribavirin have been routinely used in people co-infected with HIV and HCV.

- **Older age and HIV-associated nephropathy:** Age 60 years and older is an indication to start ART regardless of CD_4 cell count. ART therapy improves survival and kidney function in patients with HIV-associated nephropathy. Hence therapy should begin as soon as the diagnosis is made in such patients.

- **Opportunistic infections:** Early initiation of ART is recommended after starting active treatment of opportunistic infections. ART therapy should begin even in the presence of opportunistic infections like cryptococcal disease and tuberculosis. ART should be started within the first two weeks of diagnosis in patients with opportunistic infections. ART is recommended in all HIV-infected persons with tuberculosis (TB) and should be started within two weeks of TB treatment when the CD_4

Table 47.2.   2004 Department of Health and Human Services (DHHS) Guidelines for the Indications for ART in Adult Patients

Clinical Status	CD$_4$ Count	Viral Load	Suggestion
Symptomatic Patient with or without AIDS	Any count	Any viral load	Start treatment (Rx)
Asymptomatic AIDS	<200 cells/μL	Any viral load	Start treatment
Asymptomatic Patient	CD$_4$: 200–350 cells/ μL	Any viral load	Rx may be suggested
Asymptomatic	CD$_4$: >350 cells/μL	>100,000 c/mL	Rx may/may not be considered
Asymptomatic	CD$_4$: >350 cells/μL	<100,000 c/mL	Defer Rx and observe

cell count is less than 50 cells/mm^3 and within 8–12 weeks for those with greater CD$_4$ cell counts.

- **Pregnancy:** All pregnant women should get ART to prevent HIV transmission to the infant and for the mother's health. Women who get pregnant while taking ART must continue the same therapy as before and the therapy should not be discontinued post partum.

Treatment Endpoints

HIV-RNA virology endpoints for therapy consist of the patient achieving:

- One log10 decline in HIV-1 RNA by weeks 2–8.
- Having fewer than 50 HIV-1 RNA copies/mL by weeks 16–24.

Tables 47.2 and 47.3 show a summary of the 2004 DHHS and IAS-USA guidelines for HIV/AIDS treatment initiation.

PREGNANCY AND HIV/AIDS

HAART can begin at the end of the first trimester. Efavirenz and a combination of D4T are avoided during pregnancy. Drug adherence is an issue because it has to be taken every day for the rest of the patient's life.

Table 47.3.   2004 International AIDS Society (IAS) USA Guidelines for the Indication for ART in Adult Patients

Clinical Status	CD$_4$ Count	Viral Load
Symptomatic Patient with/without AIDS	Treat	–
CD$_4$: **<200 cells/μL**	Treat	–
CD$_4$: **200–350 cells/ μL**	Consider Treatment	Especially if the Viral Load is >50,000–100,000c/mL and the CD$_4$ is closer to 200 cells or the CD$_4$ has declined by more than 100 cells/year
CD$_4$: **350–500 cells/ μL**	Monitor	Consider Treatment if the Viral Load is >100,000 c/ mL or the CD4 has declined by more than 100 cells/ year
CD$_4$: **>500 cells/μL**	Monitor	–

Table 47.4. List of Appropriate Drugs for the Management of Opportunistic Infections in the HIV/AIDS Pregnant Patient

Medication	Drug Category	Suggestion
Acyclovir	Category B	Safe: Follow Standard prescription guidelines
Amphotericin B	Category B	Safe: Follow Standard prescription guidelines
Azithromycin	Category B	Safe: Follow Standard prescription guidelines
Clindamycin	Category B	Safe: Follow Standard prescription guidelines
Metronidazole	Category B	Safe: Follow Standard prescription guidelines
Valacyclovir	Category B	Safe: Follow Standard prescription guidelines
Famciclovir	Category B	Limited data on the drug, **reserve** for **severe** herpes only
Clarithromycin	Category C	Contraindicated
Doxycycline	Category D	Contraindicated
Fluconazole	Category C	Avoid; use amphotericin B instead
Ganciclovir	Category C	Avoid
Itraconazole	Category C	Avoid

The treatment goal is to obtain maximum and durable suppression of the viral load, restoration and preservation of immunological function, improvement of quality of life, and reduction of HIV-related morbidity and mortality.

A C-section is done beyond 36 weeks if the pregnant patient has not received HIV treatment to prevent vertical transmission from mother to child. A C-section is done at 38 weeks if the patient has received HIV treatment.

Tables 47.4 and 47.5 present drugs for managing opportunistic infections in pregnant patients and also provide a summary of opportunistic infections treatment options.

Table 47.5. Summary of Opportunistic Infections (OIs) and Standard Treatments Options

Opportunistic Infection	Standard Preferred Treatment
Pneumocystis Jiroveci (Formerly PCP):	Trimethoprim-Sulphamethoxazole (TMP-SMX)
Toxoplasmosis:	Trimethoprim-Sulphamethoxazole (TMP-SMX)
Mycobacterium avium complex (MAC):	Azithromycin 1,200mg/wk and Clarithromycin 500mg bid
Oral Candida:	**Prescribe any one of the following:** 1. Clotrimazole troches 10mg PO 5 x/d 2. Nystatin suspension 5mL qid 3. Nystatin pastilles 4-5 x/d 4. Fluconazole 100mg qd PO 5. Itraconazole oral suspension 200mg qd
Esophageal Candida:	**Prescribe any one of the following:** 1. Fluconazole 100mg qd, (maximum 400mg qd), PO x 14-21 d 2. Itraconazole oral suspension 200mg qd PO
Cryptococcus:	Amphotericin B + Flucytosine
Cytomegalovirus (CMV):	Ganciclovir + Valganciclovir
Herpes Simplex:	Acyclovir 400mg 4-5x/d PO, continue until vesicles heal Provide maintenance with Acyclovir in relapse cases.

Highly Active Antiretroviral Therapy (HAART)

HAART therapy has categories of antiretroviral drugs:

1. Nucleoside reverse transcriptase inhibitors (NRTIs)
2. Nonnucleoside reverse transcriptase inhibitors (NNRTIs)
3. Protease inhibitors (PIs)
4. Integrase inhibitors (IIs)
5. Fusion inhibitors (FIs)
6. Chemokine receptor antagonists (CRAs)

Nucleoside Reverse Transcriptase Inhibitors (NRTIs)

The nucleoside/nucleotide reverse transcriptase inhibitors (NRTIs) are a main part of the current standard of care. NRTIs show activity against HIV-1 and HIV-2.
   The are seven NRTIs currently available:

- Abacavir (ABC, Ziagen)
- Didanosine (ddI, Videx)
- Emtricitabine (FTC, Emtriva)
- Lamivudine (3TC, Epivir)
- Stavudine (d4T, Zerit)
- Tenofovir (TDF, Viread)
- Zidovudine (ZDV, Retrovir)

Tenofovir and emtricitabine are available in once-daily, fixed-dosed combinations (FDCs). Tenofovir has been associated with renal damage that increases with prolonged use and when used in combination with PI/r. Emtricitabine is similar to lamivudine in mechanism of action, potency, toxicity, and patterns of resistance.

Abacavir and lamivudine FDCs are also available for once-daily use. HLA-B*5701 screening must be done prior to abacavir use in order to reduce the risk of potentially life-threatening hypersensitivity reaction to the drug. Patients unable to use abacavir or tenofovir are given zidovudine and lamivudine FDCs.

Dental alert: Renal function, along with bone density, must be monitored prior to and during dentistry, as tenofovir causes a decrease in bone mineral dentistry in the spine and hip, in addition to causing renal damage. Studies have shown that patients with HIV infection are at increased risk of osteoporosis-associated fragility fractures when compared with uninfected individuals, and the bone-loss effect is even more pronounced with tenofovir-containing therapies.

Nonnucleoside Reverse Transcriptase Inhibitors (NNRTIs)

NNRTIs show activity against HIV-1 and are part of the preferred initial regimens. Efavirenz has the most significant inhibition of viral infectivity among the NNRTIs. All NNRTIs exhibit the same mechanism of action. The currently available NNRTIs are **first-generation NNRTIs**, which include delavirdine (Rescriptor), efavirenz (Sustiva), and nevirapine (Viramune), and **second-generation NNRTIs**, which include etravirine (Intelence) and rilpivirine (Edurant).

Efivarenz is used once daily and is available in FDCs with tenofovir and emtricitabine. Nevirapine and rilpivirine are used as alternates when needed.

Protease Inhibitors

HIV protease inhibitors (PIs) are an integral part of treatment of HIV infection.
There are eight approved PIs:

- Atazanavir (Reyataz)
- Darunavir (Prezista)
- Fosamprenavir (Lexiva)
- Indinavir (Crixivan)
- Lopinavir/ritonavir (Kaletra)
- Nelfinavir (Viracept)
- Saquinavir (Invirase)
- Tipranavir (Aptivus)

Protease inhibitors are used in combination with two NRTIs as part of the initial ART therapy. PIs require coadministration with ritonavir that augments or "boosts" the levels of the PI through inhibition of the CYP34A enzyme.

Ritonavir-boosted atazanavir is used in initial therapy once daily. Alternately, ritonavir-boosted darunavir is used once daily in initial regimens and should be taken with a meal to improve bioavailability. Darunavir contains sulfa and may trigger an allergic reaction in those with sulfa allergy.

Lopinavir as FDCs with ritonavir is used as an alternate PI. Fosamprenavir or saquinavir boosted with ritonavir are also other alternate PIs that can be used.

PI side effects: All PIs are associated with mild-to-moderate nausea, diarrhea, and dyslipidemia. All PIs may be associated with cardiac conduction defects, particularly PR interval prolongation.

Integrase Strand Transfer Inhibitor (InSTI)

InSTIs are the newest class of potent antiretroviral drugs that are used with the two NRTIs in initial ART therapy. Raltegravir (Isentress) was the first InSTI approved by the FDA and elvitegravir is currently in phase III studies.

InSTI, raltegravir is used twice daily. Raltegravir combined with tenofovir/emtricitabine results in long-lasting viral suppression, fewer side effects, and smaller elevations in lipid levels.

Mechanism of action: HIV integrase is responsible for the transport and attachment of proviral DNA to host-cell chromosomes, thus allowing the transcription of viral proteins and subsequent assembly of virus particles. Raltegravir and elvitegravir competitively inhibit the strand transfer reaction by binding metallic ions in the active site.

Fusion Inhibitors

Fusion inhibitors (FIs) were the first class of antiretroviral medications to target the HIV replication cycle extracellularly. **Mechanism of action:** Fusion inhibitors (FIs) act extracellularly to prevent the fusion of HIV to the CD_4 or other target cell. The use of fusion inhibitors has been limited because of costs and route of administration (subcutaneous).

Chemokine Receptor Antagonists

Maraviroc (Selzentry) is the first FDA-approved medication in the class of antiretroviral drugs termed chemokine receptor 5 (CCR5) antagonists. **Mechanism of action:** The method by which HIV binds to CD_4 cells and ultimately fuses with the host cell is a complex multistep process, and maraviroc selectively and reversibly binds to the CCR5 co-receptor, thus inhibiting the fusion of the cellular membranes.

ART: Fixed-Dose Combinations (FDC)

- NNRTI: efavirenz/tenofovir/emtricitabine FDC (Atripla)
- Protease inhibitor: atazanavir + ritonavir + tenofovir/emtricitabine FDC (Truvada)
- Darunavir + ritonavir + tenofovir/emtricitabine FDC (Truvada)
- Integrase inhibitor: raltegravir + tenofovir/emtricitabine FDC (Truvada)
- Efavirenz + (Abacavir/Zidovudine)/lamivudine FDC (Epzicom, Combivir)
- Nevirapine + zidovudine/lamivudine FDC (Combivir)
- Atazanavir + ritonavir + (Abacavir or Zidovudine)/lamivudine FDC (Epzicom, Combivir)
- Fosamprenavir + ritonavir + (Abacavir or Zidovudine)/lamivudine (Epzicom, Combivir) or tenofovir/emtricitabine (Truvada) FDC
- Lopinavir/ritonavir + (Abacavir or Zidovudine)/lamivudine (Epzicom, Combivir) or tenofovir/emtricitabine (Truvada) FDC

HIV/AIDS DENTAL ASPECTS AND SUGGESTED DENTAL GUIDELINES

Always obtain the following laboratory tests from the patient's MD after obtaining a signed consent form from the patient:

- **The CBC with platelet count:** Megaloblastic anemia, neutropenia, and peripheral neuropathy (due to folic acid deficiency) are frequent side effects of anti-HIV medications. The use of opioids and block anesthesia are contraindicated when the hemoglobin is <10 g/dL.
- The CD_4 count.
- The viral load.
- The PT/INR if the liver is affected with cirrhosis.
- The LFTs.
- Serum creatinine.
- The FBS, PPBS, and HbA_1C.

Dental Guidelines

1. Use a nonalcoholic mouth rinse **prior** to every appointment to de-germ the oral cavity. Also have the patient use the mouth rinse once daily as home care. Follow this pretreatment mouth rinse protocol for all your patients.
2. When making a decision about which antibiotic to prescribe always **first** determine **which other** antibiotic the HIV patient is taking for another infection or as part of opportunistic infection (OI) prophylaxis. Determine if the antibiotic already in use is a cidal or a static antibiotic. To treat a dental infection in one such patient

you need to match the cidal or static criteria for the antibiotics to work. A cidal OI antibiotic works best with a cidal oral infection management antibiotic, and a static OI antibiotic works best with a static oral infection management antibiotic.

3. Prior to treatment, assess the current CD_4 count plus the WBC and ANC counts. If the CD_4 count is $\leq$200 cells/mm^3 and the WBC count is normal (3,500–11,000 cells/mm^3), proceed with the dental management as you would in a normal patient.

4. In patients with a decreased WBC count ($\leq$3,500 cells/mm^3) calculate the absolute neutrophil count (ANC).

ANC = total WBC $\times$ [neutrophils% + bands%]. The average ANC is 1,500–7,200/μL. Follow the ANC guidelines as discussed in Chapter 11 and summarized in Table 11.2.

Drugs Contraindicated with HIV/AIDS Medications

The following drugs are contraindicated in conjunction with HIV medications:

1. Protease inhibitors should not be combined with the following drugs due to DDIs associated with **the CYP3A4 enzyme:** Demerol, Darvon, clarithromycin, tetracycline, doxycycline, metronidazole, diazepam, lorazepam (diazepam and lorazepam may be used with caution as a small, single dose prior to a procedure, if approved by the patient's MD), and azole antifungals: clotrimazole, fluconazole, ketoconazole.

2. **Antihistamines: Avoid** asternizole and terfenadine.

3. **Psychotropics: Avoid** midazolam (Versed; may be used with caution as a small, single dose prior to a procedure if approved by the patient's MD), triazolam (Halcion), and alprazolam (Xanax).

4. **Antifungals: Avoid** itraconazole, ketoconazole, and voriconazole.

5. **Anticonvulsants: Avoid** phenobarbital.

6. **Antibiotics: Avoid** clarithromycin (Table 47.6).

7. **H_2 blockers: Avoid with H_2 blockers.** Keep a two-hour interval between the HIV medications and the H_2 blocker.

HERPES SIMPLEX AND HERPES ZOSTER INFECTIONS

Herpes Simplex

The herpes simplex viruses (HSV) comprise two distinct types of DNA viruses: HSV-1 and HSV-2. HSV-1 causes oral lesions in approximately 80% of cases and genital lesions in 20% of cases. In adolescents, as much as 30–40% of genital herpes is caused by HSV-1 because of increased orogenital contact. HSV-2 causes genital lesions in 80% of cases and oral lesions in 20% of cases. Antiviral drugs inhibit virus replication and suppress clinical manifestations, but they are not a cure for the disease.

For HSV infection to occur, intimate contact is required between a susceptible person without antibodies against the virus and an individual who is actively shedding the virus or has body fluids containing the virus. Contact must involve mucous membranes or open or abraded skin. The initial rash is typically "herpetic" in appearance: small vesicles grouped on an erythematous base. Treatment of herpes simplex is discussed in Chapters 8 and 48.

Table 47.6. Suggested Anesthetic, Analgesic, and Antibiotic Guidelines for Patients on HIV/AIDS Medications

Drug Category	Drug: Generic (Trade)	Suggested Guideline
Anesthetics	2% Lidocaine **(Xylocaine)**	Safe: Use maximum 2 carpules
	4% Prilocaine HCL **(Citanest Forte)**	Avoid with anemia
	0.5% Bupivacaine **(Marcaine)**	Safe: Use maximum 2 carpules
	4% Septocaine **(Articaine)**	Avoid with anemia
	3% Mepivacaine HCL **(Carbocaine)** **OR**	Safe: Use maximum 2 carpules
	2% Mepivacaine HCL (Carbocaine) **with Levonordefrin (NeoCobefrin)**	
	4% Prilocaine HCL **(Citanest Plain)**	Avoid with anemia
Analgesics	Codeine + Acetaminophen: **Tylenol #1–4**	Safe: Use Standard dose
	Oxycodone + Acetaminophen **(Percocet)**	Safe: Use Standard dose
	Hydrocodone + Acetaminophen **(Vicodin)**	Safe: Use Standard dose
	Meperidine **(Demerol)**	Avoid
	Propoxyphene **(Darvon)**	Avoid
Antibiotics	Penicillin **(Pen. VK)**	Safe: Use Standard dose
	Amoxicillin **(Amoxil)**	Safe: Use Standard dose
	Amoxicillin + Clavulanic acid **(Augmentin)**	Safe: Use Standard dose
	Cephalexin **(Keflex)**	Safe: Use Standard dose
	Cefadroxil **(Duricef)**	Safe: Use Standard dose
	Azithromycin **(Zithromax)**	Safe: Use Standard dose
	Clarithromycin **(Biaxin)**	Avoid
	Clindamycin **(Cleocin)**	Safe: Use Standard dose
	Tetracycline HCL	Avoid
	Doxycycline **(Vibramycin)**	Avoid with Protease Inhibitors; safe with other HIV drugs
	Metronidazole **(Flagyl)**	Avoid with Protease Inhibitors; safe with other HIV drugs
Antivirals	Acyclovir **(Zovirax)**	Safe: Use Standard dose
	Valacyclovir **(Valtrex)**	Safe: Use Standard dose
Antifungals	Clotrimazole **(Mycelex)**	Avoid with Protease Inhibitors, use Nystatin instead. Safe with other HIV drugs
	Mycostatin **(Nystatin)**	Safe: Use Standard dose
	Fluconazole **(Diflucan)**	May be used with caution with Protease inhibitors, safe with other drugs
	Ketoconazole **(Nizoral)**	Avoid
Benzo-diazepines	Diazepam **(Valium)**	Restrict. Use lowest dose if required after MD consult
	Lorazepam **(Ativan)**	Restrict. Use lowest dose if required after MD consult

Herpes Zoster

Varicella-zoster virus (VZV), which is the agent causing chicken pox, lies dormant in the spinal dorsal root ganglia, following primary varicella infection, until reactivation results in herpes zoster/shingles. "Shingles" is a syndrome characterized by a painful, unilateral vesicular rash usually restricted to a dermatomal distribution. After years of latency, the virus travels along the nerve to the skin, resulting in a dermatomal distribution. Lesions are often preceded by pain and hyperesthesia of the skin. Zoster is more common in patients who are older or immune suppressed, including organ transplant recipients and patients with human immunodeficiency virus (HIV).

Herpes zoster usually has a benign course, but complications can occur that range from mild to life threatening. Common complications of herpes zoster infections include acute pain, post-herpetic neuralgia, persistent neuropathy, hemorrhage, ulceration, necrosis, necrosis of bone, and, occasionally, secondary bacterial infection.

The classic lesions of herpes zoster consist of umbilicated vesicles on an erythematous base. The vesicles occur in small clusters referred to as herpetiform groupings. With time, the vesicles become confluent, crusted, and often heal with scarring. Pain and weakness can persist for months.

The dermatomal distribution of zoster typically stops abruptly at the midline. Dermatomes on the trunk have a horizontal distribution, whereas those on the arms and legs have an arc-like or roughly linear distribution. Within the dermatome, the clusters of vesicles and crusts often have a patchy distribution in clustered herpetiform groupings. The hypersensitivity of the overlying skin to light touch and presence of spontaneous pain are helpful diagnostic features.

Herpes zoster oticus involves the inner, middle, and external ear. Herpes zoster oticus presents as excruciating otalgia with an associated cutaneous vesicular eruption involving the external ear canal and pinna. When associated facial paralysis is present, the disease is called Ramsay Hunt syndrome.

Herpes zoster may involve the ophthalmic (V1) division of the trigeminal nerve, leading to involvement of the forehead and eye, and may extend to the tip of the nose. This involvement is associated with complications such as conjunctivitis, keratitis, corneal ulceration, iridocyclitis, glaucoma, and blindness. Early consultation with an ophthalmologist is recommended. Treatment with antiviral medication usually leads to a good visual outcome for patients with trigeminal herpes, although they can develop late VZV dendriform keratitis, which can recur even with treatment.

VZV diagnosis: The Tzanck smear is a classic test for the diagnosis of VZV. The base of an ulcerated lesion is typically scraped and then stained. The Tzanck smear shows multinucleated, giant cells. The Tzanck test cannot differentiate between VZV and herpes simplex. Polymerase Chain Reaction (PCR) has high sensitivity and specificity that approaches 100%. PCR is inexpensive and has replaced direct fluorescent assay (DFA) as the assay of choice in many large laboratories. Viral cultures have high false-negative rates and take two weeks for a result. Bacterial cultures can help exclude secondary bacterial infection, but do not confirm a diagnosis of zoster.

VZV treatment: Treatment for zoster usually involves a one-week course of an antiviral medication, such as acyclovir (Zovirax), valacyclovir (Valtrex), or famciclovir (Famvir). Standard adult doses are 1g of valacyclovir every eight hours (three times daily) or 500mg of famciclovir every eight hours (three times daily) for seven days. The dosing for acyclovir is 800mg five times daily. All three drugs have comparative efficacy and safety profiles. If initiated within 72 hours of the rash onset, antiviral medication can suppress viral replication, reduce the length of acute pain, and speed up the cutaneous healing. Herpes zoster treatment is also discussed in Chapters 8 and 48.

Postherpetic neuralgia (PHN): Postherpetic neuralgia (PHN) is a more common complication in patients older than 50 years. Short-acting opioids in combination with acetaminophen or a NSAID are part of the protocol for managing PHN. Gabapentin (Neurontin), followed by a tricyclic antidepressant (nortriptyline or desipramine), can be added if conventional analgesics are not effective in treating the herpes zoster pain. PHN can also be treated with lidocaine as a transdermal patch. The patient can use a maximum of three patches simultaneously for 12 hours on and 12 hours off. Studies have shown that patients treated with the lidocaine patch have reduced intensity of pain and improved quality of life.

Zoster vaccine: A zoster vaccine, Zostavax, is now available in the United States. Studies have shown it to be safe and effective in reducing the occurrence of herpes zoster and the consequent development of postherpetic neuralgia in older patients. It is recommended for people older than 60 years of age. Vaccination is the single most important tool for the prevention of complications related to herpes zoster.

LYME DISEASE

Overview

Lyme disease (LD) was first described in 1975 among residents of Lyme, Connecticut, when they presented with an outbreak of juvenile arthritis that was preceded by a rash. Spirochete Borrelia burgdorferi, the bacterium that causes LD, infects the deer ticks. These infected ticks feed and mate on deer during part of their life cycle. The animals that most often carry these spirochetes are white-footed field mice, deer, raccoons, skunks, foxes, chipmunks, squirrels, and horses. An infected tick transmits the spirochete to humans and animals it bites. Once a tick latches onto human skin it generally climbs upward until it reaches a creased area, often the back of the knee, groin, navel, armpit, ears, or nape of the neck. It then begins inserting its mouthparts into the skin to reach the blood supply. The tick has to be attached to its host for about **36–48 hours** before it can transmit the spirochetes. Therefore, it is best to remove any ticks before they become engorged with blood. If the tick is not removed, the spirochetes can become blood borne and infect various parts of the body.

LD is an inflammatory disease with clinical manifestations that most often involve the skin, joints, nervous system, and heart. Spirochete Borrelia burgdorferi concentrates in collagen-rich connective tissues. Initially, the patient presents with flu-like symptoms and a skin rash. The infection then progressively spreads to the joints, nervous system, and other organ systems in the later disseminated stages. If diagnosed and treated early with antibiotics, the disease can be cured. Generally, LD in its later stages can also be treated effectively, but because the rate of disease progression and the response to therapy varies from patient to patient, some individuals may have symptoms that last for months or even years after treatment has been completed. In rare instances, LD causes permanent damage.

In the United States, LD is prevalent in the coastal northeast, mid-Atlantic states, Wisconsin, Minnesota, and northern California; but is most prevalent in the highly endemic northeast areas associated with a high tick infection rate. Outside the United States, LD has been detected in large areas of Asia, Europe, and South America.

Prevention and Precautions

When outdoors in tick-infested areas, it is best to wear enclosed shoes and light-colored clothing; use insect repellant containing DEET (Diethyl-meta-toluamide) on skin and clothes, or permethrin on clothes, but not skin; avoid sitting directly on the ground or on stone walls; keep long hair tied back and do a final, full-body tick-check at the end of the day. Upon returning home, clothes can be spun in the dryer for 20 minutes to kill any unseen ticks. A shower and shampoo may help to remove crawling ticks but will not remove attached ticks. Inspect carefully after a shower. Baby deer ticks are the size of poppy seeds; adult deer ticks are the size of apple seeds.

Presenting Features

Erythema migrans (EM), arthritis, and cardiac and neurological manifestations are the classic presenting features of LD. The diagnosis and treatment of LD can often be difficult or challenging because of its diverse manifestations. The clinician should be highly suspicious of LD if a patient gives a history of having had a tick bite about a month ago and is now presenting with a red rash surrounding the tick bite, flu-like symptoms, or joint pains. As previously discussed, the duration of tick attachment and feeding is a key factor in transmission. The early symptoms of LD can be mild and easily overlooked. People who are aware of the risk of LD in their communities and who do not ignore the sometimes subtle early symptoms are most likely to seek medical attention and treatment early enough to be assured of a full recovery.

Erythema migrans (EM) rash: Early cutaneous infection with B. burgdorferi is called erythema migrans, and this is the most common clinical manifestation of LD. Initially, during the early or acute phase of LD, the patient has a localized rash with associated lymph glandular swelling, generalized body ache, and headache. The expanding erythema migrans (EM) rash occurs in 70–80% of cases. An EM rash generally radiates from the site of the tick bite and appears as a solid, red, expanding rash or blotch, or a central spot surrounded by clear skin that is ringed by an expanding red rash (which looks like a bull's-eye, or a doughnut). The rash appears an average of 3–30 days after disease transmission; has an average diameter of 5–6 inches, but is occasionally larger; persists for about 3–5 weeks; may or may not be warm to the touch; and is usually not painful or itchy. EM rashes appearing on brown-skinned or sun-tanned patients may be more difficult to identify because of decreased contrast. A dark, bruise-like appearance is more common on dark-skinned patients.

Ticks prefer to target body creases such as the armpit, groin, back of the knee, and nape of the neck; rashes are therefore commonly found affecting these areas. Multiple rash areas may occur after the initial rash at sites away from the bite area.

Arthritis: After several weeks of being infected with LD, about 60% of untreated patients develop recurrent attacks of painful and swollen joints that last a few days to a few months. The arthritis can be fleeting, with one or more joints affected at any given time; the knee is most commonly affected. About 10–20% of untreated patients go on to develop lasting arthritis. The knuckle joints of the hands are only very rarely affected.

Cardiac symptoms: Palpitations, dizziness, atrioventricular heart block and/or myopericarditis are common cardiac manifestations associated with LD.

Neurological symptoms: Progressively toward the later stages, the patient develops neurological symptoms in addition to migrating pains in joints/tendons, severe fatigue, and cardiac abnormalities. Headache, stiff achy neck, facial palsy similar to Bell's palsy, tingling or numbness in extremities, and CNS involvement (leading to disorientation, confusion, dizziness, inability to concentrate, changes in vision, and mental "fog") occurs and may appear weeks, months, or even years after a tick bite.

Stages

Presenting features can be divided into the following stages:

- **Early localized stage:** This stage occurs within 3–30 days after a tick bite and is characterized by the presence of erythema migrans (EM), flu-like symptoms, joint pains, and enlarged lymph nodes.
- **Early disseminated stage:** This stage occurs days or weeks after the tick bite. When the disease is untreated and the infection disseminates causing additional EM lesions, progressive neurological manifestations and progressive arthritis, shooting pains resulting in sleep disruption, palpitations, and dizziness.
- **Late disseminated stage:** This stage occurs months or years following a tick bite when the patient develops intermittent bouts of arthritis with severe joint pain and swelling; chronic neurological symptoms; and short-term memory loss.
- **Post-treatment LD syndrome (PTLDS):** The exact etiology of PTLDS is unknown but it is thought to be an autoimmune response consequence. Months or years after treatment with antibiotics, approximately 10–20% of patients develop muscle and joint pains, cognitive defects, sleep disturbance, or fatigue.

Diagnosis

The EM rash is specific for LD, and once the rash has been identified, treatment should begin immediately. The LD bacterium is difficult to isolate or culture from body tissues or fluids. In the absence of an EM rash, diagnosis of early LD is made on the basis of suspicion, if the individual is living in or has been to the endemic area, by assessing presenting symptoms and evidence of a tick bite but not by blood tests.

Clinical findings, as evident during the early stages of the disease, are adequate for the diagnosis of erythema migrans. However, clinical findings alone are not enough to make a diagnosis of extracutaneous manifestations or late stages of LD.

Blood tests can often give incorrect results if performed in the first month after initial infection. These tests are considered more reliable and accurate when performed **at least a month after initial infection** when the body's immune system has had a chance to produce antibodies. Also, antibody production can be negatively impacted by antibiotics that are given early in the infection, thereby preventing antibodies from reaching detectable levels.

Therefore, history-taking and physical examination are most reliable for disease detection in the early stages. The ELISA and Western Blot tests are more reliable for disease detection weeks, months, or years after exposure. The **ELISA** test measures the levels of antibodies against the LD bacteria that are present in the body. The **Western**

Blot test identifies antibodies directed against a panel of proteins found on the Lyme bacteria. This test is done when the ELISA test is either positive or uncertain. The **Polymerase Chain Reaction (PCR)** test can detect the spirochete DNA. PCR testing has limitations and is not useful for the diagnosis of LD.

Treatment

- Individuals who may or may not have received antibiotic prophylaxis following removal of attached ticks should be monitored closely for symptoms and signs of LD for up to 30 days. Close attention should be paid to the development of erythema migrans at the bite site. Medical care must be immediately implemented once the rash develops or if the patient develops flu-like illness within one month after removing an attached tick.
- Early treatment implemented prior to four weeks after initial infection almost always results in a full cure. The cure rate decreases the longer the treatment is delayed.
- Doxycycline, amoxicillin, and cefuroxime (Ceftin), in order of preference, are the three oral antibiotics most recommended for treatment of early localized or early disseminated LD with no associated neurologic manifestations or advanced atrioventricular heart block (manifestations of advanced or disseminated disease). Each of these antimicrobials has been shown to be very effective for the treatment of erythema migrans and associated symptoms. Studies support that the 14-day therapy with doxycycline is effective; however, the efficacy of 14-day regimens with the other first-line agents is unknown.
- **A single dose of doxycycline may be given to adult patients (200mg dose) and to children ≥8 years of age (4mg/kg, up to a maximum dose of 200mg) when all of the following circumstances exist:**
  - The attached tick can be reliably identified as an adult or nymphal I. scapularis tick that is estimated to have been attached for ≥36 hours, on the basis of the degree of engorgement of the tick with blood or of certainty about the time of exposure to the tick.
  - Prophylaxis can be started within 72 hours of the time that the tick was removed.
  - The local rate of infection of these ticks with B. burgdorferi is ≥20%.
  - Doxycycline treatment is not contraindicated.
- **Recommended treatment of adult patients with early localized or early disseminated LD associated with erythema migrans:**
  - **Doxycycline:** 100mg twice per day, for 14 days (range of therapy, 10–21 days).
  - **Amoxicillin:** 500mg three times per day, for 14 days (range of therapy 14–21 days).
  - **Cefuroxime axetil:** 500mg twice per day, for 14 days (range of therapy 14–21 days).
- Doxycycline is relatively contraindicated during pregnancy or lactation and in children <8 years of age.
- **Antibiotics used for children include:**
  - **Amoxicillin:** 50mg/kg per day in three divided doses, maximum of 500mg per dose.
  - **Cefuroxime axetil:** 30mg/kg per day in two divided doses, maximum of 500mg per dose.

- – **If the patient is ≥8 years of age:** Doxycycline 4mg/kg per day in two divided doses, maximum of 100mg per dose.
- Macrolides are not that effective and are reserved for patients who are intolerant of, or should not take, amoxicillin, doxycycline, and cefuroxime axetil. Patients treated with macrolides should be closely observed to ensure resolution of the clinical manifestations.
- **Recommended adult dosage regimens for macrolide antibiotics are as follows:**
  - – **Azithromycin,** 500mg orally per day for 7–10 days.
  - – **Clarithromycin,** 500mg orally twice per day for 14–21 days, if the patient is not pregnant.
  - – **Erythromycin,** 500mg orally four times per day for 14–21 days.
- **Recommended dosages of macrolides for children are as follows:**
  - – **Azithromycin,** 10mg/kg per day, maximum of 500mg per day.
  - – **Clarithromycin,** 7.5mg/kg twice per day, maximum of 500mg per dose.
  - – **Erythromycin,** 12.5mg/kg four times per day, maximum of 500mg per dose.
- Regardless of the clinical manifestation of LD, complete response to treatment may be delayed beyond the treatment duration.
- Relapse may occur with any of these regimens; patients with objective signs of relapse may need a second course of treatment.
- **Preferred parenteral regimens for adults with early onset acute neurological disease or atrioventricular heart block and/or myopericarditis associated with early LD:**
  - – **Ceftriaxone (Rocephine):** 2g intravenously once per day for 14 days. An oral regimen may then be substituted to complete a course of therapy or to treat ambulatory patients. A temporary pacemaker may be required for patients with advanced heart block.
  - – **Other good parenteral alternatives for advanced LD:** Parenteral therapy with cefotaxime: 2g intravenously (IV) every eight hours, or penicillin G in the presence of normal renal function: 18–24 million U per day in divided doses every four hours.
  - – Alternate oral therapy for advanced LD: Patients intolerant to β-lactam antibiotics can get doxycycline: 200–400mg per day in two divided doses orally for 10–28 days.
- Oral antibiotic treatment is recommended for patients presenting with seventh cranial nerve palsy to prevent any further disease advancement.
- Doxycycline is not used in the management of pregnant patients with LD. However, all other management guidelines are the same, as previously outlined.
- Late-stage LD can usually be treated effectively, but individual variations in the rate of disease progression and response to treatment are deciding factors. In some of these patients, the disease may persist for many months or even years. These patients will experience slow improvement and resolution of their persisting symptoms following oral or IV treatment that eliminated the infection. Dependent on the presenting symptoms, in some cases several courses of either oral or IV antibiotic treatment may be indicated for no more than four to six weeks to avoid adverse side effects.
- There is currently no scientific evidence to support that long-term antibiotic courses are more effective than the recommended course of four to six weeks.

- Symptomatic therapy consists of NSAIDS, intra-articular injections of corticosteroids, or disease-modifying antirheumatic drugs (DMARDS) such as hydroxychloroquine, and consultation with a rheumatologist.
- If persistent synovitis is associated with significant pain, or if it limits function, then arthroscopic synovectomy can reduce the period of joint inflammation.

Dental Alerts

- Defer routine dentistry during the acute phase of LD. However, the patient should get palliative dental care to alleviate acute dental distress, including incision and drainage (I&D) of an abscess and/or pain medications.
- Do a thorough medical history and physical examination prior to the start of dentistry.
- Determine if the patient is currently on an antibiotic and for how long. Match cidal with cidal or static with static if an antibiotic is needed. Also, establish if the patient is on NSAIDS, DMARDS, or corticosteroids. You may have to follow the rule of twos if the patient has been on oral steroids. Intra-articular steroids do not call for you to follow the rule of twos.
- Prior to dentistry obtain the basic laboratory tests such as CBC, serum creatinine, and LFTs. Obtain the patient's current cardiac and/or neurological assessment from the patient's physician in patients with advanced disease.
- Avoid electrical appliances in patients with cardiac pacemakers.
- Avoid the 4% local anesthetics in patients presenting with neurological symptoms/dysfunction or cardiac arrhythmias.

METHICILLIN-RESISTANT STAPHYLOCOCCUS AUREUS (MRSA)

Introduction

The CDC's definition is "Methicillin-resistant Staphylococcus Aureus (MRSA) is a type of staph bacteria that is resistant to certain antibiotics called beta-lactams. These antibiotics include methicillin and other more common antibiotics such as oxacillin, penicillin, and amoxicillin. In the community, most MRSA infections are skin infections. More severe or potentially life-threatening MRSA infections occur most frequently among patients in healthcare settings. While 25–30% of people are colonized in the nose with staph, less than 2% are colonized with MRSA."

MRSA infections involving the skin can present as cellulites, abscess, draining fistula, pustules, furuncles, carbuncles, impetigo, or necrotizing fasciitis. Severe forms of MRSA infection can present as osteomyelitis, bacteremia, endocarditis, wound infections, pneumonia, gastroenteritis, and occasionally toxic shock syndrome. Skin infections, if not treated appropriately, can also progress and become severe. S. aureus thrives on human skin and mucous membranes, growing rapidly under anaerobic or aerobic conditions, and the bacteria can be carried by its host for a long period of time without causing clinical consequences. Populations found to be at high risk for MRSA include patients on dialysis, individuals in daycare settings, prisons, elder housing, or long-term care facilities. The elderly and athletes are also at high risk.

Prevention is the key to stop the spread of MRSA infection. Standard Precautions as detailed in the 2007 "Guideline for Isolation Precautions: Preventing Transmission of Infectious Agents in Healthcare Settings" should control the spread of MRSA in most instances and should be used for all patient care. Optimal infection control measures can interrupt transmission and arrest the survival and growth of the bacteria in a susceptible host.

Studies have shown that aerosolization can deposit bacteria on dental surfaces and on exposed skin surfaces of individuals involved with patient care. The bacteria can very easily be transmitted by soiled hands from exposure to infected blood, by body fluids that may or may not contain blood, by saliva, by aspiration of infected aerosolized particles during patient care or from infected droplets from a coughing or sneezing patient, by skin contact with recently contaminated surfaces, by instruments or devices, and by exposure to the bacteria through injured skin, mucous membranes, or needle-stick injuries. Saliva often contains blood and is therefore considered potentially infectious.

Classification

- **Community acquired (CA-MRSA):** Most CA-MRSA cases begin as skin or soft tissue infections (SSTI) in previously healthy members of a community.
- **Hospital acquired or health-care associated (HA-MRSA):** Most HA-MRSA cases start out as skin infections at areas that have come in contact with medical devices or areas at open surgical sites or wounds.

Terminology

- **Colonization:** Colonization is when MRSA organisms are found growing at a tissue site without causing any damage at the site. The most common body site for MRSA colonization in humans is the anterior nares, but colonization has also been found in the oral cavity, in biofilms, on dentures, in open wounds, in the respiratory tract from aspiration of infected saliva, on the extremities, in the umbilicus, and in the axilla. Colonized patients are asymptomatic carriers of the infection and can transmit the bacteria to others.
- **Decolonization:** Decolonization refers to the elimination of the MRSA carrier state through the use of infection control measures and/or antibiotics. Decolonization decreases the risk of transmission to populations previously specified.
- **MRSA infection:** MRSA infection occurs when the bacteria enter the host and multiply in the tissues causing tissue injury, and the patient becomes symptomatic for the infection. Infected patients can also transmit MRSA.
- **MRSA diagnosis:** Per the CDC, general screening of patients for MRSA is not recommended but high-risk patients who are being admitted to the hospital should be screened for MRSA, and if found positive, the provider and the hospital should follow infection-control guidelines during the patient's hospital stay. **MRSA diagnosis can be made by culture or PCR.**

    Culture: Culture is commonly used to diagnose MRSA and is less costly. It can take 48–72 hours to identify MRSA-colonized patients. Clinical infection can be identified by cultures of blood, sputum, urine, percutaneous aspiration or surgically obtained specimens. Swabs can be obtained from the following infected areas: nares, rectum, or skin. Two successive negative nasal swabs when obtained within 24–48 hour intervals indicate successful decolonization.

Polymerase chain reaction (PCR): In 2008, the FDA approved a rapid PCR-based blood test (StaphSR assay) that detects the presence of MRSA genetic material in a blood sample in about **two** hours. Additionally, there are new screening tests that provide reports in about five hours. Even though PCR provides rapid results, the test is more expensive.

Clinical Presentation

Most MRSA infections present as skin infections that may appear red, swollen, painful, and are warm to the touch, filled with pus or other drainage, and/or may resemble a "spider bite." Common lesions seen are:

- **Abscess:** Pus-filled mass below skin structures.
- **Cellulitis:** Inflammation of skin that causes the infected area to be warm, red, swollen, and tender.
- **Folliculitis:** Infection of the hair follicle that appears as a group of red bumps and may develop into pus-filled blisters.
- **Furuncles:** Most frequently appear on the neck as red nodules up to 1cm in size that are tender, pinkish-red, swollen, and firm, and will feel like a water-filled balloon or cyst upon inspection.
- **Impetigo:** Bullous lesions that develop from red bumps, which rupture and ooze fluid or puss into honey-colored crust; most commonly appear around children's nose and mouth.
- Recurrent **intraoral aphthous ulcers** presenting as painful, red spots or bumps that develop into open ulcers can also occur. These ulcers are usually less than 1cm in size and have a white- or yellow-colored center.

Treatment

- CA-MRSA infections presenting as simple boils and abscesses are treated in the outpatient setting with incision and drainage (I&D) and **no antibiotics**. Optimal wound hygiene and personal hygiene are emphasized in the care of all forms of MRSA infections.
- Antibiotic therapy for MRSA should be considered pending culture data for multiple abscesses that are severe, rapidly progressive, associated with cellulites, systemic symptoms and signs, occurring in the immune suppressed, affecting the very young or elderly, or when the lesion has not responded to I&D. Purulent cellulites is treated with five to ten days of antibiotic therapy with any of the following oral antibiotic options: clindamycin, trimethoprim-sulfamethoxazole (TMP-SMX/Bactrim), doxycycline, minocycline, or linezolid.
- For hospitalized patients with complicated SSTI in addition to I&D, broad-spectrum antibiotic therapy should be considered pending culture data. Options include: intravenous (IV) vancomycin, oral or IV linezolid 600mg twice daily, daptomycin 4mg/kg/dose IV once daily, telavancin 10mg/kg/dose IV once daily, or clindamycin 600mg IV or oral, three times a day. Depending on the patient's clinical response 7–14 days of therapy is recommended.
- Cultures from abscesses and other purulent SSTIs are recommended, particularly in patients with severe, symptomatic infections, and in those that have not responded well to initial treatment.

- Decolonization is recommended for recurrent SSTI only, with mupirocin 2% topical ointment twice daily for 5–10 days, or mupirocin 2% topical ointment twice daily for 5–10 days, along with a skin antiseptic, chlorhexidine solution baths for 5–14 days, or dilute bleach baths given for 15 minutes twice weekly for approximately three months. **Oral antibiotics are not recommended for decolonization.** Follow-up cultures are **not** routinely done following decolonization if there is **no active** infection.
- Serious CA-MRSA and HA-MRSA patients have to be hospitalized and treated with IV vancomycin, alone or in combination with other antibiotics. All isolated MRSA strains are tested for antibiotic sensitivity to select the most appropriate antibiotic therapy. For hospitalized patients with severe CA-MRSA or for HA-MRSA, the patient is treated with IV vancomycin or linezolid 600mg PO/IV twice daily or clindamycin 600mg PO/IV three times daily for 7–21 days.

In patients with normal renal function, IV vancomycin 15–20mg/kg/dose every 8–12 hours, and not to exceed 2g per dose, is recommended. A loading dose of 25–30mg/kg given over two hours may be considered for seriously ill patients. For most patients with SSTI who have normal renal function and are not obese, IV vancomycin doses of 1g every 12 hours is adequate.

Vancomycin failures are treated with high-dose daptomycin (10mg/kg/day) if the isolate is susceptible, in combination with gentamicin 1mg/kg IV every eight hours, rifampin 600mg PO/IV daily or 300–450mg PO/IV twice daily, linezolid 600mg PO/IV BID, or TMP-SMX 5mg/kg IV twice daily.

- Several reports now suggest that MRSA is becoming more and more resistant to clindamycin.

Prevention Steps in the Dental Setting

- All members in the dental setting must be educated about MRSA and how the infection can be transmitted. Particular emphasis must be placed on standard precautions during all patient encounters.
- Safe work practices are a must and this includes the covering of computer keyboards; not touching surfaces with contaminated gloves; proper hand hygiene; use of personal protective equipment (PPE); cough etiquette; and safe injection practices. PPE protects both the provider and the patient. When present, the clinician must cover all skin cuts immediately.
- Use of protective clothing over street clothes prevents them from contamination and possible cross-contamination to other patients.
- Correct hand-washing and hand-rubbing techniques must be clearly posted.
- Hands should be washed with soap and water when soiled; after touching contaminated surfaces; before and after touching patients; prior to wearing gloves; and immediately after removing gloves.
- It is best to use disposable single-use masks that should be changed between patients and when the mask becomes wet during patient care.
- Protective eyewear, face shield with side protectors, and goggles for patients are necessary to prevent transmission. Reusable goggles or shields must be thoroughly cleaned and properly stored after use.

- Every dental office must have written infection-control policies and procedures for occupational health and safety, disinfection, sterilization, safe handling of patient-care items, and the proper disposal of hazard waste material. A designate should be assigned for coordinating the infection control program.
- Every dental office should have an optimal and updated needle-stick/percutaneous injury protocol and one that must be implemented immediately following accidental exposure.
- Infection transmission is minimized when dental offices have more single-use items or instruments.
- Environmental surfaces, including dental chairs, trays, and equipment, should be regularly cleaned with detergent, and visible contaminants should be wiped off or scrubbed away. Surface barriers should be used whenever possible.
- Dental devices that can be removed from the waterline should be cleaned and heat sterilized.
- In between patient appointments, devices connected to the dental air/water system must be flushed for at least 20–30 seconds to remove any material that might have entered the air and waterlines.
- Bacterial burden in aerosolized particles can be decreased by using pre-procedural antiseptic oral rinses.
- Environmental contamination during dentistry can be decreased by using a rubber dam during procedures.

Routine Dental Care

- Neither the American Dental Association nor the CDC make a recommendation about avoiding dental treatment for patients with invasive MRSA disease. Standard or universal precautions should be applied when treating all patients who are colonized or infected with MRSA.
- Standard precautions and safe work practices are all that is needed when treating known MRSA carriers or patients known to have a MRSA infection. Any visible red lesion or pustule that may or may not be draining should be covered with sterile gauze prior to dentistry.
- Routine dental care should be deferred until you have contacted the physician to confirm clearance for dentistry, if the known symptomatic MRSA patient is receiving IV vancomycin decolonization therapy or has received IV vancomycin and is now on short-term or long-term trimethoprim-sulfamethoxazole (Bactrim) or any other oral antibiotic. You need to obtain physician clearance to proceed with routine dentistry and you need to get the time line when routine procedures can begin.
- MRSA does **not** contraindicate dental treatment, but you need to have a good understanding of the patient's level or extent of infection so you can optimally care for the patient.
- The physician will most probably not give you clearance if the patient is on IV vancomycin, but clearance may be given if the patient is on long-term oral antibiotics. Typically, you should wait for completion of short-term oral antibiotics before proceeding with routine dentistry if the patient still continues to have cellulites. You want the acute cellulites to clear prior to routine dentistry.
- Once clearance has been obtained, Standard Operating Procedures (SOP) for operatory preparation and operatory cleaning must be followed according to standard

infection control protocols, which include application of appropriate PPE and cleaning and disinfection of operatory.

- Additionally, for all patients that have not yet cleared the infection, including MRSA carrier patients, it is best to use the disposable blood pressure (BP) cuff sleeve and the disposable stethoscope diaphragm sleeve prior to monitoring the patient's blood pressure. This extent of barrier protection is needed in the clinical setting to prevent infection transmission.
- Furthermore, emphasis should be on using sterile, single-use disposable instruments as much as possible. All reusable instruments should be heat sterilized when possible or processed with standard recommended disinfectants.
- Have the patient use an antiseptic mouth rinse prior to treatment and provide treatment using a rubber dam.
- All blood-soaked gauze from infected patient care should be disposed in the hazard waste container, and all sharps should go into the sharps container.

Acute Dental Care

- Patients experiencing acute dental symptoms while on acute MRSA therapy should get palliative dental care to alleviate acute dental distress, including I&D of an abscess, and/or pain medications. Dental emergency-associated antibiotic, when needed, will need to be compatible with the MRSA-associated antibiotic that the patient is taking. Dental emergency should always be addressed at any stage of MRSA therapy.
- Always obtain medical clearance prior to initiation of care. Once clearance is obtained, Standard Operating Procedures (SOP) for operatory preparation and operatory cleaning must be followed according to standard infection control protocols, which include application of appropriate PPE and cleaning and disinfection of operatory.
- Additionally, you will need to use the disposable blood pressure (BP) cuff sleeve and the disposable stethoscope diaphragm sleeve, prior to monitoring the patient's blood pressure. This extent of barrier protection is needed in the clinical setting to prevent infection transmission.
- Furthermore, emphasis should be on using sterile, single-use disposable instruments as much as possible. All reusable instruments should be heat sterilized when possible or processed with standard recommended disinfectants.
- Have the patient use an antiseptic mouth rinse prior to treatment and provide treatment using a rubber dam.
- All blood-soaked gauze from infected patient care should be disposed of in the hazard waste container and all sharps should go in to the sharps container.

MRSA Prevention Protocol and Dental Alerts

- Clean hands with soap and water or use an alcohol-based hand rub, before and after caring for each patient.
- Carefully clean all operatories.
- When caring for patients with MRSA use contact precautions, which include:
  - Wearing gloves, gown, and eye protection while treating patients with MRSA.
  - If allowed in the operatory, visitors may be asked to wear gowns and gloves.

- Appropriate device handling of patient equipment and instruments/devices.
  - When leaving an operatory, dentists and visitors should remove their gloves and gowns and clean their hands.
- Patients with recurrent MRSA skin and soft-tissue infections should be educated on proper wound care and personal and environmental hygiene.
- MRSA may be more resistant to killing when commercially available agents such as sodium hypochlorite are not sufficiently concentrated.
- MRSA biofilms are more resistant to killing by the disinfecting agents typically used, and dental impressions can show evidence of contamination even after disinfection.
- It has been determined that soaking dentures in 2% chlorhexidine gluconate solution for ten minutes and microwave irradiation irradiation for three minutes at 650W completely disinfects dentures contaminated with MRSA for both the short and the long term. Despite being effective, the soaking of dentures in the disinfectant solution is discouraged because of the possible detrimental effects on the denture material. Soaking in sodium hypochlorite solution is only effective as a short-term disinfectant.
- Optimal oral and denture hygiene prevents the spread and recurrence of local and systemic infections associated with MRSA.

SEXUALLY TRANSMITTED DISEASES

Overview

Chlamydia, genital herpes, gonorrhea, and syphilis are discussed in the following sections. The occurrence of STDs in the past must always be confirmed during patient assessment. Always confirm what STDs were diagnosed in the patient. Is there a history of **completion** of treatment in a patient presenting with a positive history of STDs? STDs, when left untreated or incompletely treated, can lead to pelvic inflammatory disease (PID) in the female patient and consequent infertility. An astute dental provider could recognize STD lesions in the oral cavity and refer the patient for thorough evaluation and treatment.

Chlamydia

Facts

Chlamydia is caused by the bacterium, Chlamydia trachomatis. Chlamydia can infect both males and females. An untreated infection causes irreversible damage and infertility. It is considered to be a relatively silent disease because symptoms caused by the infection are usually mild or absent. Symptoms, when present, occur within one to three weeks of the start of the infection. The patient usually experiences a vaginal discharge or burning on urination. Chlamydia infection has gained much prominence and concern because it is now being considered an important etiological factor for periodontal and coronary artery diseases.

Treatment

Chlamydia infection is treated with a **single dose** of 500 mg azithromycin (Zithromax) or doxycycline (Vibramycin) 100 mg bid for seven days. To completely eradicate the infection, all sex partners of the patient must be tested and treated accordingly.

Genital Herpes

Facts

Genital herpes can be caused by HSV-1 and HSV-2. However, most genital herpes are caused by HSV-2. With the initial genital herpes outbreak, the patient experiences vesicles or blisters around the genitals or the rectum. The initial infection is painful and ulcerative and lasts for two to four weeks. Subsequent outbreaks are less severe and can reoccur with variable frequency. The virus is present in the secretion from the vesicles and can be transmitted by sexual contact.

Treatment

Genital herpes cannot be cured, but the outbreaks can be attenuated with antiviral medications. The patient is typically on chronic suppressive therapy to reduce symptoms and transmission of the disease.

Gonorrhea

Facts

Gonorrhea is caused by the bacterium Neisseria gonorrhoeae. The bacterium grows in warm, moist areas of the reproductive system, rectum, anus, mouth, throat, and eyes.

Men are usually more symptomatic than women and experience clear-to-purulent discharge, painful urination, or soreness of the genitals. Symptoms are usually minimal in women and often simulate a urinary tract infection.

Treatment

The patient with nonresistant bacteria is usually treated with ceftriaxone 125 mg IM in a single dose, **or** cefixime 400 mg is given orally in a single dose or 400 mg by suspension (200 mg/5 mL).

Syphilis

Facts

Syphilis is caused by the bacterium Treponema pallidum. Syphilis infection can manifest in three ways: primary, secondary, or tertiary. An observant dental provider could occasionally encounter a primary syphilis chancre sore in the oral cavity. Immediate treatment at this point will prevent progression to the secondary and tertiary stages.

Primary Stage

The primary stage of syphilis is usually characterized by the appearance of a single chancre, or sore, on the genitalia within 2–12 weeks of infection. The chancre is painless and can heal in 3–6 weeks without treatment. When left untreated, the infection will progress to the secondary stage.

Secondary Stage

The secondary stage is characterized with the appearance of a non-itchy skin rash on the palms of the hands and soles of the feet. Additionally, the patient also presents with mucous-membrane lesions, fever, lymphadenopathy, sore throat, weight loss, and flu-like symptoms. When left untreated, the secondary stage manifests soon after the primary stage.

Tertiary Syphilis

Tertiary syphilis occurs many years after the disappearance of the symptoms and signs experienced in the secondary stage. The infection ultimately causes neurological, cardiac, and musculoskeletal damage leading to dementia, paralysis, and blindness.

Treatment

Syphilis should be treated immediately in the primary stage, to prevent progression to the secondary and tertiary stages. A single intramuscular injection of penicillin results in complete cure.

Oral Lesions and Dentistry

XV

48

Therapeutic Management of Oral Lesions in the Immune-Competent and the Immune-Compromised Patient in the Dental Setting

OVERVIEW

The common oral lesions seen in the immune-competent and the immune-compromised patient will be collectively discussed because many of the lesions in the two populations overlap. However, the severity and duration often differ.

Immunity can be compromised because of many factors including HIV/AIDS, chemotherapy, radiotherapy, leukemias, lymphomas, connective tissue disorders, and poorly controlled diabetes. Stress, chronic corticosteroid therapy, severe sun exposure, and broad-spectrum antibiotic use are often the cause of oral lesions in the immune-competent patient. Thus, presence of oral lesions by themselves is not diagnostic of HIV infection or other causes of decreased immunity.

With the presence of oral lesions, the clinician must assess the medical history and decide if appropriate laboratory tests need evaluation to confirm the presence or absence of all causes of decreased immunity, including HIV infection. However, once confirmed, the underlying cause or disease state should be addressed and appropriately managed **along** with the care of the oral lesions.

When treating an HIV patient, the dentist must refer a formerly asymptomatic, untreated, known HIV patient to the physician upon discovery of new oral lesions. The physician will evaluate the patient's current health status, including the CD_4 count and the viral load, to determine if antiretroviral treatment is necessary. The oral lesions can resolve with improvement of the patient's immunity following antiretroviral treatment. Recurrence of oral lesions following resolution in the HIV/AIDS patient can indicate failure of oral lesion therapy or worsening of the HIV infection. In spite of tremendous advances in antiretroviral therapy, oral lesions do occur and they must be appropriately managed.

The oral lesions have a tendency to recur more often with reduction of immunity, and in the HIV patient it can herald the start of the symptomatic phase. Oral herpes simplex or zoster, oral and/or esophageal candidiasis, angular chilities, xerostomia, and aphthous ulcers can affect the immune-competent or the immune-compromised patient.

Dentist's Guide to Medical Conditions, Medications, and Complications, Second Edition. Kanchan M. Ganda.
© 2013 John Wiley & Sons, Inc. Published 2013 by John Wiley & Sons, Inc.

Table 48.1. Prescriptions Management of Oral Lesions in the Immune-Competent and the Immune-Compromised Patient

Infection/Lesion; Medication(s); Drug Category	Prescription/Treatment Guidelines
HERPES SIMPLEX:	
Valacyclovir (Valtrex): Prganancy Category B	1. **Rx: Valtrex caplet,** 1g/caplet Disp: 4 caplets Sig: Take 2g q12h for 1 day only 2. **Therapy for first herpes infection:** Rx: Valtrex 1g bid x 10 days 3. **Therapy for recurrent herpes infection:** Rx: 500mg bid x 5 days
Acyclovir (Zovirax): Pregnancy Category B	1. **5-day Rx:** Zovirax capsules, 200mg/cap Disp: 25 capsules Sig: 1 capsule q4h while awake or take 5 capsules per day. Start when symptoms begin. 2. **5-day therapy with kidney disease:** GFR <10mL/minute or dialysis: 200mg q12h for 5 days
Acyclovir (Zovirax) capsules: Pregnancy Category B	1. **14-day Rx:** Zovirax capsules, 200mg/capsule Disp: 70 capsules Sig: 1 cap. 5 times/day x 2 weeks 2. **14-day Rx with kidney disease:** GFR <10mL/minute or dialysis: Dose 200mg q12h
Famciclovir (Famvir): Pregnancy Category B	**Recurrent cold sores in immune-competent patient:** 1,500mg as a single dose. **HIV-infected patients (cold sores or genital herpes):** 500mg 3 times/day x 7 days.
Acyclovir (Zovirax) ointment: Pregnancy Category B	**Rx: 5% Zovirax ointment for recurrent herpes:** Disp: 15g tube Sig: Apply to sores 5-6/day. Zovirax ointment is most effective when used with Zovirax capsules.
HERPES ZOSTER:	
Valacyclovir (Valtrex): Pregnancy Category B	1. **Rx: Valtex caplet,** 1g/caplet Disp: 21 caplets Sig: Take 1g tid for 7 days 2. **Kidney disease dose:** GFR <30mL/minute or s.creatinine >3mg/dL to predialysis: 1g q24h
Acyclovir (Zovirax): Pregnancy Category B	1. **Rx: Zovirax capsules,** 200mg/capsule Disp: 140 capsules Sig: 800mg 5 times/day x 7 days 2. **Kidney disease dose:** a. GFR 10-25mL/minute or s.creatinine >3mg/dL to predialysis: Rx: Dose 800mg q8h b. GFR <10mL/minute or dialysis: Rx: Dose 800mg q12h

Table 48.1. Prescriptions Management of Oral Lesions in the Immune-Competent and the Immune-Compromised Patient (*Continued*)

Infection/Lesion; Medication(s); Drug Category	Prescription/Treatment Guidelines
Famciclovir (Famvir):	1. **Famciclovir Herpes Zoster Rx:** 500mg every 8 hours x 7 days. 2. **Famciclovir dosing for Herpes Zoster with GFR [40–59mL/min/1.73m^2]:** 500mg q12h. 3. **Famciclovir dosing for Herpes Zoster with GFR [20–39mL/min/1.73m^2]:** 500mg q24h. 4. **Famciclovir dosing for Herpes Zoster with GFR [<20mL/min/1.73m^2]:** 250mg q24h. 5. **Famciclovir dosing for patients on dialysis:** 250mg after each dialysis.
HERPES CHRONIC SUPPRESSIVE THERAPY:	
Valacyclovir (Valtrex): Pregnancy Category B	**Rx: Valtrex caplet,** 500mg/caplet Disp: Dispensed for 6 months to 1 year according to the patient's immunity Sig: 500mg OD (once a day) or bid
Acyclovir (Zovirax): Pregnancy Category B	1. **Rx: Zovirax capsules,** 200mg/capsule Disp: Variable Sig: 200mg tid for up to 6 months or 400mg bid/tid, for up to 3 years 2. **Chronic suppressive Rx with kidney disease:** GFR <10mL/minute or dialysis: Dose 400mg q12h or 200mg q12h
HIV-GINGIVITIS:	
0.12% nonalcoholic Chlorhexidine Gluconate (Peridex):	– Oral hygiene and scaling with Betadine irrigation **Rx: Chlorhexidine (Peridex):** Disp: 3 x 16 oz bottles Sig: Rinse with 1/2 oz. for 30 seconds bid after oral hygiene
HIV-PERIODOTITIS:	
Treat with 0.12% nonalcoholic Chlorhexidine Gluconate (Peridex) AND Antibiotics: **First Choice:** Metronidazole **Second Choice:** Clindamycin, Cephalexin (Keflex) or Amoxicillin with Clavulanate potassium or Ciprofloxacin	– Oral hygiene and scaling with Betadine irrigation **Rx: Chlorhexidine (Peridex)** Disp: 3 x 16 oz bottles Sig: Rinse with 1/2 oz for 30 seconds bid after oral hygiene **Rx: Metronidazole (Flagyl):** 250mg/tablet Disp: 20 tablets x 5 days Sig: 1 tab qid **Clindamycin:** 150/300mg tid/qid x 5 days **Cephalexin (Keflex):** 250/500mg bid/tid x 5 days

(continued)

Table 48.1.   Prescriptions Management of Oral Lesions in the Immune-Competent and the Immune-Compromised Patient (*Continued*)

Infection/Lesion; Medication(s); Drug Category	Prescription/Treatment Guidelines
	Amoxicillin with Clavulanate potassium (Augmentin): 250/500mg tid x 5 days **Ciprofloxacin (Cipro):** 500mg bid x 5 days
ORAL CANDIDIASIS: PSEUDOMEMBRANOUS or HYPERTROPHIC or ERYTHEMATOUS	**As first choice:** Use Topicals **Refractory/severe cases:** Use systemic antifungals.
Clotrimazole (Mycelex) Troche: Pregnancy Category B/C Topical Azole antifungal	**Rx: Clotrimazole (Mycelex)** Troches, 10mg/Troche Disp: 70 troches Sig: Use 1 troche 5x/day, **swallow saliva**. No eating/drinking for 30 minutes after use. **Also dispense:** Chlorhexidine to all patients. In patients with removable appliances, re-infection can be avoided by dropping a clotrimazole (Mycelex) troche into water and soaking the appliance over night for 14 days. Clotrimazole is **not** an ideal drug to dispense in the presence of xerostomia.
Nystatin (Mycostatin) Prescriptions: Pregnancy Category B Topical Polyene antifungal	a. **Rx: Nystatin (Mycostatin)** Lozenge 200,000 units/Lozenge Disp: 70 Lozenges (14 day supply) Sig: Dissolve 1 Lozenge in the mouth 5 times daily. There should be **no** eating or drinking for 30 minutes after use. b. **Rx: Nystatin Oral Suspension 100,000 units/mL** Disp: 473mL (1 pint) bottle (14 day supply) Sig: Use 1 teaspoonful or 5mL, qid. Rinse and hold in the mouth as long as possible before swallowing. There should be **no** eating or drinking for 30 minutes after use. c. **Rx: Nystatin Oral Suspension 100,000 units/mL for dentures** Disp: 473mL (1 pint) bottle Sig: Add 5–10mL of 1:100,000 units Nystatin to half cup of water and soak the dentures overnight daily, for 14 days. Rinse the dentures before use. d. **Rx: Nystatin Pastille 200,000 units/pastille** Disp: 70 pastilles Sig: Dissolve 1 pastille in the mouth 4–5 times/day for 14 days. e. **Nystatin (Mycostatin) Cream:** The cream can be applied to dentures before insertion or can be used for angular chielitis. Rx: 100,000 units/g Disp: 15/30g tube Sig: Apply to the affected area 4–5 times/day. Do **not** eat or drink for 30 minutes after use. f. Re-infection can be avoided in patients with removable appliances by dropping a Nystatin lozenge/troche into a 1/4 cup of water and soaking the appliance overnight for 14 days. Also, Nystatin powder or Nystatin ointment can be applied to appliances prior to insertion.

Table 48.1. Prescriptions Management of Oral Lesions in the Immune-Competent and the Immune-Compromised Patient (*Continued*)

Infection/Lesion; Medication(s); Drug Category	Prescription/Treatment Guidelines
Amphotericin B: Topical Polyene antifungal; Pregnancy Category B	a. **Rx: 3% Topical Amphoteric B Cream** Disp: 20g tube Sig: Apply to the affected area 3–4 times/day for 2–4 weeks b. **Oral Amphotericin B:** Oral Amphotericin B is dispensed as a capsule or a suspension. The oral forms are poorly absorbed. (i) **Rx: Amphotericin B 500mg/capsule** Disp: 56 capsules Sig: Take 500mg capsule PO qid for 2 weeks. (ii) **Rx: Amphotericin B suspension: 500mg/mL** Disp: 56mL suspension Sig: Use 1mL of the suspension, swish and swallow qid for 2 weeks.
REFRACTORY ORAL/SYSTEMIC CANDIDIASIS:	
Fluconazole (Diflucan): Systemic Azole antifungal; Pregnancy Category C	**Rx: Fluconazole (Diflucan) 100mg/capsule** Disp: 15 capsules Sig: Day 1: Take 2 capsules. Days 2–14: Take 1 capsule daily.
ESOPHAGEAL CANDIDIASIS:	
Fluconazole (Diflucan): Systemic Azole antifungal; Pregnancy Category C	**Rx: Fluconazole (Diflucan)** 100mg/capsule Disp: Variable Sig: 100mg qd (maximum 400mg qd) for 14–21 days
Itraconazole (Sporanox): Triazole antifungal; Pregnancy Category C	**Rx: Itraconazole Oral Suspension** Sig: 200mg qd PO x 10–21 days
ANGULAR CHEILITIS:	
Clotrimazole (Mycelex) Cream: Pregnancy Category B/C	**Rx: Clotrimazole (Mycelex) Cream** Disp: 15g tube Sig: Rub on lesions 2–3 times daily
Nystatin (Mycolog) Ointment: Pregnancy Category B	**Rx: Mycolog cream (Nystatin)** Disp: 15g tube Sig: Rub on lesions 2–3 times daily
Clioquinol and Hydrocortisone (Corque Topical): Pregnancy Category C	**Rx: Clioquinol and Hydrocortisone (Corque Topical)** Disp: 15g tube Sig: Rub into affected area 2–3 times daily

(continued)

Table 48.1. Prescriptions Management of Oral Lesions in the Immune-Competent and the Immune-Compromised Patient (*Continued*)

Infection/Lesion; Medication(s); Drug Category	Prescription/Treatment Guidelines
RECURRENT APHTHOUS ULCERS:	
Tetracycline Capsules Pregnancy Category D	**Tetracycline Capsules:** Dissolve a 250mg Tetracycline capsule in 180mL water. Swish and spit qid for several days until ulcers heal. Do not eat or drink for 30 minutes.
Tetracycline suspension: Pregnancy Category D	**Tetracycline suspension:** Dispense 250mg Tetracycline/5ml. Swish and expectorate qid until ulcers heal. Do not eat or drink for 30 minutes. Avoid in children and pregnant women.
Triamcinolone 0.1% (Kenalog in Orabase): Topical steroid; use sparingly for pain relief.	**Triamcinolone 0.1% (Kenalog in Orabase):** Apply the paste to ulcers bid/qid until the ulcers heal. Disp: 5g tube Sig: Apply a thin film *without rubbing*, on affected areas up to 3 times daily
0.05% Flucinonide (Lidex) ointment mixed 50/50 with Orabsase:	**Rx: 0.05% Lidex ointment mixed 50/50 with Orabsase** Disp: 30g total Sig: Apply a thin layer on the lesions 4–6 times daily
Dexamethasone Elixir	**Rx: Dexamethasone Elixir,** 0.5mg/5mL Disp: 250mL Sig: Rinse with 1 teaspoon solution in the mouth for 1 minute 4–5 times daily and **expectorate**
Thalidomide (Thalomid): Pregnancy Category X	**Thalidomide (Thalomid),** 200mg OD/bid x 3–8 weeks is reserved for HIV/AIDS or refractory patients.
Xylocaine 2% Viscous:	**Rx: Xylocaine 2% Viscous** Disp: 100mL or 450mL Sig: Use 2tsp to rinse the oral cavity, as needed and **expectorate**.
Diphenhydramine (Benadryl) Syrup with Liquid Bismuth Subsalicylate (Kaopectate):	**Rx: Diphenhydramine (Benadryl) Syrup (5mg/mL) with Liquid Bismuth Subsalicylate (Kaopectate), mix 50/50** Disp: 8oz total Sig: Rinse with 2tsp, as needed for pain relief; **expectorate**
Diphenhydramine (Benadryl) Syrup with Magnesium Hydroxide antacid:	**Rx: Diphenhydramine (Benadryl) Syrup (5mg/mL) with Magnesium Hydroxide antacid, mixed 50–50** Disp: 8oz total Sig: Rinse with 2tsp, as needed for pain relief; **expectorate**
Topical 0.15 Benzydamine (Difflam or Tantum) oral rinse:	**Rx: Topical 0.15 Benzydamine (Difflam/Tantum) oral rinse:** Apply to the ulcers 4x/day for 2 weeks or until the ulcers heal. Treats mild disease.
Topical Carellose: (Orabase: Pectin plus Gelatin)	**Rx: Topical Carellose (Orabase: Pectin plus Gelatin):** Apply to the ulcers qid for 2 weeks or until the ulcers heal. A protective bio-adhesive preparation for mild disease.

Table 48.1.   Prescriptions Management of Oral Lesions in the Immune-Competent and the Immune-Compromised Patient (*Continued*)

Infection/Lesion; Medication(s); Drug Category	Prescription/Treatment Guidelines
Topical Corticosteroids: Spray/cream/pellet For mild disease	a. **Rx: 1% triamcinalone dental paste (Adrortyl or Kenolog in Orabase):** b. **Rx: Hydrocortisone, 2.5mg pellets (Corlan)** c. **Rx: 0.12% or 0.2% chlorhexidine gluconate aqueous mouthwash (Peridex) or 1% chlorhexidine gluconate gel.** Apply to the ulcers qid with any one of the **3** preparations for 2 weeks/ until the ulcers heal.
Rx: Systemic Corticosteroids: For severe disease.	**Rx: 30–60mg prednisone** PO daily for 1 week, followed by a 1 week dose taper.
XEROSTOMIA:	
	Xerostomia Treatment Options: Daily oral hygiene; 3–6 month recall; nonalcoholic Peridex mouth rinse; topical Fluorides; saliva substitutes; saliva stimulants. A calcium-containing remineralizing oral rinse such as Caphsol (Eusa Pharma) is also recommended as calcium has a remineralizing effect on dental enamel. Use fluoride therapy in the form of professionally applied concentrated sodium fluoride varnishes and daily use of 1.1% sodium fluoride prescription strength fluoride toothpaste (PreviDent 5000 Dry Mouth), all to prevent tooth decay.
Saliva Substitutes:	The combined use of Biotene and Oralbalance is very effective in the management of xerostomia.
Biotene Products	**Biotene** available as sugar-free gum, alcohol-free mouthwash, and toothpaste. **Biotene mouthwash:** Use one tablespoon PRN, swish, and expectorate. It works best when used with Biotene toothpaste. **Biotene toothpaste:** This toothpaste is non-irritating and it contains the protective enzyme systems needed for optimal oral health. The toothpaste should be used post meals and at bedtime.
Oralbalance	**Oralbalance** is available as a moisturizing gel.
Saliva Stimulants:	
1. **Pilocarpine HCL (Salagen)** Increases saliva secretion by systemic cholinergic stimulation 2. **Cevimeline (Evoxac)**	**Pilocarpine HCL (Salagen), Strength:** 5mg/tab **Disp:** Variable **Sig:** 1–2 tablets tid/qid per day taken 30 minutes **prior** to meals **Cevimeline (Evoxac)** **Strength:** 30mg/capsule **Disp:** Variable **Sig:** 30mg three times a day, taken with meals.
CHEMOTHERAPY/ RADIOTHERAPY ASSOCIATED SIDE EFFECTS:	Refer to Table 51.2 for chemotherapy or radiotherapy associated oral lesions or side-effects and suggested management guidelines

Oral viral leukoplakia (OVL) or hairy leukoplakia (HL), HIV-gingivitis, HIV-periodontitis, HIV necrotizing stomatitis, Kaposi's sarcoma, cytomegalovirus, or papilloma virus infections are found only in the HIV/AIDS patient. Oral lesions occur in 30–80% of the affected patient population and highly active antiretroviral therapy (HAART) has decreased the incidence, frequency, and severity of most, but not all, HIV-associated oral lesions.

The treatment guidelines for oral herpes, oral candidiasis, xerostomia, and aphthous ulcers in the HIV/AIDS and the non-HIV/AIDS patient are the same. The viral infections in the HIV/AIDS patient are generally treated for a longer duration when compared with the non-HIV/AIDS patient. The HIV/AIDS patient also often needs chronic suppressive therapy.

COMMON ORAL LESIONS

The following are common oral lesions that are encountered in dentistry:

1. **Viral infections:** Herpes simplex and herpes zoster are the viral infections encountered in the immune-competent or immune-compromised patient. Cytomegalovirus infection occurs in only the immune-compromised patient.
2. **Oral viral leukoplakia (OVL) or hairy leukoplakia (HL):** OVL or HL is specific for HIV/AIDS.
3. **Fungal infections:** Oral and/or esophageal candidiasis and angular cheilitis are seen in both populations.
4. **HIV-gingivitis (HIV-G):** HIV-G is specific for HIV/AIDS.
5. **HIV-periodontitis (HIV-P):** HIV-P is specific for HIV/AIDS.
6. **HIV necrotizing stomatitis:** This lesion is also specific for HIV/AIDS.
7. **Kaposi's sarcoma:** Kaposi's sarcoma is specific for HIV/AIDS.
8. **Oral warts:** Oral warts are caused by the papilloma virus and occur specifically in the HIV/AIDS patient.
9. **Aphthous ulcers:** These ulcers occur in both populations.
10. **Xerostomia:** This occurs in both populations.
11. **Petechiae and ecchymosis:** These occur in both populations.

DETAILED DISCUSSION OF COMMON VIRAL INFECTIONS

Herpes Simplex, Herpes Zoster, and Cytomegalovirus

Herpes Simplex (HSV)

HSV lesions may be solitary, multiple, or confluent, and they may be vesicular or keratinized. There is no erythematous halo associated with the vesicles, but the margins are round-to-slightly irregular.

The lesions may be in the periodontal region, dorsum of the tongue, hard palate, or attached gingiva. The lesions resolve in less than a week in the immune-competent patient, but HSV outbreaks in the HIV patients usually last longer. Refer to Chapters 8 and 47 for additional discussion on this topic.

Herpes Zoster

Herpes zoster consists of unilateral vesicular erosive eruptions of the skin and oral mucosa along the distribution of the trigeminal nerve. It is often preceded or accompanied by **pain.** Refer to Chapters 8 and 47 for additional discussion on this topic.

Cytomegalovirus (CMV)

CMV presents as oral ulcers from which cytomegalovirus can be isolated.

VIRAL INFECTION TREATMENTS

Drugs commonly prescribed for recurrent herpetic infections are:

- Valacyclovir HCL (Valtrex)
- Acyclovir (Zovirax)
- Famciclovir (Famvir)

All three drugs have comparative efficacy and safety profiles. If initiated within 72 hours of the rash onset, antiviral medication can suppress viral replication, reduce the length of acute pain, and speed up the cutaneous healing. Herpes infection treatments are also discussed in Chapters 8 and 47.

VALACYCLOVIR HCL (VALTREX)

Facts

Valtrex is a Category B prodrug that rapidly converts to acyclovir on ingestion. It acts on HSV-1, HSV-2, and the varicella zoster virus (VZV). Valacyclovir (Valtrex) is recommended for the treatment of herpes zoster, genital herpes, and herpes labialis (cold sore). A 50–75% dose reduction is recommended in patients with end-stage renal disease (ESRD). Patients on hemodialysis should get Valtrex after the dialysis. No dose adjustments are needed in patients with cirrhosis. Valacyclovir should not be prescribed with SSRIs as SSRIs inhibit the 2D6 enzyme needed to activate the drug.

Valtrex is a better choice than acyclovir (Zovirax) because of its shorter duration of treatment time. Valtrex strength per caplet is 500 mg or 1 g per caplet.

Prescriptions

1. **Valacyclovir (Valtrex) therapy for recurrent herpes simplex (cold sore lasting less than one week/shorter duration cold sores):**
   Rx: Valtrex caplet, 1 g/caplet.
   Disp: 4 caplets.
   Sig: Take 2 g q12h **for 1 day only.**
2. **Valacyclovir (Valtrex) therapy for first/initial/primary herpes infection (patient is highly symptomatic):**
   Rx: Valtrex 1 g bid × 10 days.
3. **Five-day duration valacyclovir (Valtrex) therapy for recurrent herpes infection (for cold sores lasting for 1–2 weeks/longer duration cold sores):**
   Rx: 500 mg bid × 5 days.

4. a. **Valacyclovir (Valtrex) therapy for herpes zoster:**
        Rx: Valtex caplet, 1 g/caplet.
        Disp: 21 caplets.
        Sig: Take 1 g tid for 7 days. Begin the drug with the start of symptoms or within 48 hours of the rash.
    b. **Valacyclovir (Valtrex) therapy for herpes zoster in the presence of kidney disease:**
        GFR <30 mL/min or s. creatinine >3 mg/dL to predialysis:
        Rx: 1 g q24h.
5. **Valacyclovir (Valtrex) chronic suppressive therapy: For chronic cold sores/zoster suppression:**
    The chronic suppressive therapy should be dispensed for any type of herpes recurrences.
    Rx: Valtrex caplet, 500 mg/caplet.
    Disp: Dispensed for six months to one year according to the patient's immunity.
    Sig: 500 mg OD (once a day) or bid.

ACYCLOVIR (ZOVIRAX) PRESCRIPTIONS

Acyclovir is a Pregnancy Category B drug and is safe to use during pregnancy:

1. **Acyclovir (Zovirax) ointment for recurrent herpes:**
    Rx: 5% Zovirax ointment.
    Disp: 15 g tube.
    Sig: Apply to lip sores 5–6 times daily.
    Zovirax ointment is most effective when used in conjunction with Zovirax capsules.
2. a. **Five-day duration, acute acyclovir (Zovirax) therapy:** The five-day therapy is usually given if the cold sores last for less than one week. This is less likely in an immune-compromised patient and more likely in an immune-competent patient.
        Rx: Zovirax capsules, 200 mg/capsule.
        Disp: 25 capsules.
        Sig: 1 capsule q4h while awake or total of 5 capsules/day. Start the intake as soon as the symptoms begin.
    b. **Five-day duration, acute acyclovir (Zovirax) therapy with kidney disease:** The five-day therapy is usually given if the cold sores last for less than one week. This is less likely in an immune-compromised patient and more likely in an immune-competent patient.
        GFR <10 mL/min or dialysis:
        Rx: 200 mg q12h × 5 days.
3. a. **Fourteen-day duration, acute acyclovir (Zovirax) therapy:**
        The 14-day therapy is usually given for primary herpes simplex infection or if the recurring cold sores last for 1–2 weeks. This is more likely to happen in an immune-compromised patient.
        Rx: Zovirax capsules, 200 mg/capsule.
        Disp: 70 capsules.
        Sig: Take 1 capsule 5 times/day × 2 weeks.
    b. **Fourteen-day duration, acute acyclovir (Zovirax) therapy with kidney disease:**
        GFR <10 mL/min or dialysis:
        Rx: Dose 200 mg q12h.

4. a. **Acyclovir (Zovirax) chronic suppressive therapy:**
        Rx: Zovirax capsules, 200 mg/capsule.
        Disp: Variable.
        Sig: 200 mg tid or 400 mg bid/tid for up to one year and then reevaluate.
    b. **Acyclovir (Zovirax) chronic suppressive therapy with kidney disease:**
        GFR <10 mL/min or dialysis:
        Rx: Dose 400 mg q12h or 200 mg q12h.
5. a. **Acyclovir (Zovirax) normal dose for herpes zoster therapy:**
    b. **Rx: Zovirax** capsules, 200 mg/capsule.
        Disp: 200 capsules.
        Sig: 800 mg (4 capsules) 5 times/day × 7 days.
    c. **Kidney disease and acyclovir (Zovirax) dose for herpes zoster therapy:**
        GFR 10–25 mL/min or s. creatinine >3 mg/dL to predialysis:
        Rx: Dose 800 mg q8h.
        GFR <10 mL/min or dialysis:
        Rx: Dose 800 mg q12h.

FAMCICLOVIR (FAMVIR)

Famciclovir Facts

Famciclovir is a Pregnancy Category **B** antiviral drug which is active against the herpes viruses, including herpes simplex 1 and 2 (cold sores and genital herpes) and varicella-zoster (shingles and chickenpox). Famciclovir is a prodrug that is converted to penciclovir, which is then active against the viruses. Famciclovir has a longer duration of action and it can be taken fewer times each day. A 50–75% dose reduction is recommended in patients with end-stage renal disease (ESRD). Patients on hemodialysis should get famciclovir after the dialysis. No dose adjustments are needed in patients with cirrhosis. Famciclovir should **not** be prescribed with SSRIs as SSRIs inhibit the 2D6 enzyme needed to activate the drug.

Famciclovir Dosing

Famciclovir can be taken with or without food. It is available in tablet form in strengths such as 125, 250, and 500mg. The recommended doses are:

1. **Recurrent cold sores in the immune-competent patient:** 1,500mg as a single dose.
2. **Recurrent genital herpes in the immune-competent patient:** 1,000mg every 12 hours for one day.
3. **Suppression of recurrent genital herpes in both populations:** 250mg twice daily.
4. **Herpes zoster/shingles in both populations:** 500mg every 8 hours for 7 days.
5. **HIV-infected patients (cold sores or genital herpes):** 500mg three times daily for 7 days.
6. a. **Famciclovir dosing in kidney disease with GFR [40–59mL/min/1.73m^2]:**
        Herpes zoster: 500mg q12h.
        For other regimens: No changes needed.
    b. **Famciclovir dosing in kidney disease with GFR [20–39mL/min/1.73m^2]:**
        Herpes zoster: 500mg q24h.
        Recurrent genital herpes (GH): 125mg q24h.
        GH suppression: 125mg q12h.

c. **Famciclovir dosing in kidney disease with GFR [<20mL/min/1.73m^2]:**
   Herpes zoster: 250mg q24h.
   Recurrent GH: 125mg q24h.
   GH suppression: 125mg q24h.
d. **Famciclovir dosing in patients on dialysis:**
   Recurrent genital herpes or suppression: 125mg after each dialysis.
   Herpes zoster or genital herpes in HIV patient: 250mg after each dialysis.

ORAL VIRAL LEUKOPLAKIA AND HAIRY LEUKOPLAKIA

Oral viral leukoplakia (OVL) and hairy leukoplakia (HL) are specific for HIV/AIDS and consist of vertically corrugated, slightly elevated white surface alterations of the lateral or ventral tongue margin that do not wipe off.

Hairy leukoplakia is caused by the Epstein-Barr virus. No definitive therapy has proven to be effective in the treatment of OVL. Several antiviral drugs including acyclovir have been investigated as potential treatments for OVL. Further studies are necessary in order to determine the treatment effectiveness of these agents.

Antifungal therapy should be implemented if candida is found to superinfect the OVL lesion. If the lesion is traumatized or not esthetic to look at, OVL may be treated with Zovirax at doses greater than 1 g/day until the lesion resolves. Usually, however, no treatment is necessary.

HIV-GINGIVITIS

HIV-gingivitis (HIV-G) is specific to HIV/AIDS. Combination antiretroviral therapy has reduced the incidence of severe gingivitis in people with HIV. HIV-G consists of an erythematous gingival band along the gingival margin and it extends into the adjacent attached and alveolar mucosa. HIV-G does not respond to calculus and plaque removal. It also does not respond to all measures used for oral hygiene.

HIV-G General Guidelines of Care

The general guidelines of care consist of the following:

1. The patient must be given intensive oral hygiene instructions. Scaling and root planing should be done with 10% povidone-iodine (Betadine) irrigation; 0.12% nonalcoholic chlorhexidine gluconate (Peridex) home rinses should be prescribed. Chlorhexidine (Peridex/PerioChip/PerioGard) is an antibiotic used to control plaque and gingivitis in the mouth or in periodontal pockets.
   Prescription is as follows:
   Rx: 0.12% nonalcoholic chlorhexidine gluconate (Peridex).
   Disp: 3 × 16 oz bottles.
   Sig: Rinse with 1/2 oz for 30 seconds bid after completion of oral hygiene.
2. There should be careful follow-up and maintenance and use Peridex short term as it stains the oral mucosa. Use any nonalcoholic mouth rinse in all medically complex patients to minimize alcohol related xerostomia.

HIV-PERIODONTITIS

HIV-periodontitis (HIV-P) is specific to HIV/AIDS. The HIV-P lesions are severely destructive. They are characterized by soft tissue ulceration and necrosis. There is rapid progressive loss of bone and periodontal attachment.

HIV-P is frequently associated with deep pain and spontaneous bleeding. The tissue loss, which is very rapid, may occur within a period of four weeks. Without treatment, HIV-periodontitis may progress to necrotizing stomatitis.

HIV-P Treatment

Treatment is as follows:

1. Initial debridement with 10% betadine irrigation should be done. In cases of severe necrosis, pain, and fever antibiotics and analgesics may become necessary.
2. 0.12% nonalcoholic chlorhexidine gluconate (Peridex) home rinses should be prescribed. Intensive oral hygiene instructions should be provided and the patient must be reevaluated in one week.
3. Follow-up should consist of scaling and root planing by quadrants, using 10% betadine irrigation, and the Peridex home rinses should be continued.
4. Oral hygiene instructions should be reinforced. There should be careful follow-up and maintenance.
5. The patient should be recalled every four weeks until stable. Thereafter, three-month recalls should be scheduled.

HIV-P Recommended Antibiotic Therapy

1. **First drug of choice:**
   Rx: Metronidazole (Flagyl) 250 mg/tablet
   Disp: 20 tabs for 5 days.
   Sig: 1 tab qid until gone.
   Metronidazole, a Category B drug, is safe during pregnancy.
2. **Alternate antibiotic choices:** Dispense any one of the following anaerobic complex organism effective antibiotics, if metronidazole is contraindicated due to DDIs with the patient's HIV medications or due to associated liver disease or alcoholism. All the antibiotics listed below, with the exception of Cipro (Category B/C), are Pregnancy Category B drugs and are safe for use during pregnancy.
   a. **Clindamycin:** 150/300 mg tid/qid × 5 days.
   b. **Cephalexin (Keflex):** 250/500mg bid/tid × 5 days.
   c. **Amoxicillin with Clavulanate potassium (Augmentin):** 250/500 mg tid × 5 days.
   d. **Ciproflaxim (Cipro):** 500 mg bid × 5 days, in refractory cases.

It is best to use the lower dose of the antibiotics to prevent candida-associated superinfection. All scaling and root planing should be completed during the five days of antibiotic intake.

Chlorhexidine as a chip can also be used as an adjunct to scaling and root planing procedures for reducing the depth of pockets around the teeth in patients with periodontitis. It is used as a nonalcoholic mouth rinse, which provides antimicrobial activity between dental visits. As previously mentioned, chlorhexidine may cause staining of the teeth, dentures, or appliances.

HIV NECROTIZING STOMATITIS

HIV necrotizing stomatitis is specific to HIV/AIDS. It is an acute localized, painful, necrotizing, ulcerated lesion of the oral mucosa. It results in exposure of the underlying bone. The lesion may extend into contiguous tissues. The margins are undermined and sharply defined.

The exact etiology cannot be identified even by biopsy. Without treatment, HIV-G may progress from a mild gingivitis to a destructive periodontitis, and this progression may take place within weeks.

HIV Necrotizing Stomatitis Treatment

Treatment of necrotizing stomatitis is essentially the same as that recommended for HIV-P. Initial debridement should be done with 10% betadine irrigation. Antibiotics are necessary in cases of severe necrosis, pain, and fever. Antibiotic suggestions are the same as with HIV-P; 0.12% nonalcoholic chlorhexidine gluconate (Peridex) home rinses should be prescribed. Intensive oral hygiene home instructions should be provided. The patient must be reevaluated one week later.

This should be followed by scaling and root planing by quadrant using 10% betadine irrigation. Continue Peridex home rinses after the scaling and root planing and reinforce oral hygiene instructions. Also reinforce careful follow-up and maintenance. Recall the patient every four weeks until stable and then schedule three-month recalls.

ORAL AND ESOPHAGEAL CANDIDIASIS

Oral candidiasis can occur in either the immune-competent or the immune-compromised patient. Long-term or high-dose antibiotic use, chronic corticosteroid therapy, xerostomia anemia, stress, and ill-fitting dentures are some of the causes for candidiasis in the immune-competent patient. The underlying cause must always be addressed and treated to completely eradicate the fungus, along with antifungal prescriptions for local or systemic use.

In either population oral candidiasis can present as pseudomembranous candidiasis or as hypertrophic or erythematous candidiasis. Oral candidiasis can extend down toward the esophagus causing the patient to experience dysphagia (difficulty swallowing) and/or odynophagia (painful swallowing).

All fungal infections must be treated for 14 days and significant esophageal candidiasis is treated for at least 21 days. In addition to the antifungal prescription, the dentist must also prescribe an antifungal soaking solution for all removable oral appliances that must be soaked daily for 14 days to completely eradicate the fungus.

The suggested guidelines for treatment of pseudomembranous candidiasis or hypertrophic or erythematous candidiasis are all the same: antifungals plus nonalcoholic chlorhexidine mouth rinse. Always start with topical antifungals and avoid the azole antifungals in HIV/AIDS patients taking protease inhibitors. **Nystatin is an ideal oral antifungal in the immune-compromised patient because it does not interact with the**

HIV medications, and the patient can use it comfortably even in the presence of xerostomia. Use systemic antifungals in refractory cases or in patients with systemic fungal infections.

Dispense nonalcoholic chlorhexidine or any other nonalcoholic mouth rinse for use after oral hygiene, for all types of candidiasis. **Rx:** nonalcoholic chlorhexidine (Peridex); **Disp:** 3 × 16 oz bottles; **Sig:** Rinse with 0.5oz for 30 seconds twice/day after oral hygiene.

ANTIFUNGAL DRUGS
Antifungal Drugs Classification

Refer to Chapter 7 for a complete discussion on antifungal classification and facts.

CLOTRIMAZOLE (MYCELEX) TROCHES
Clotrimazole (Mycelex) Troches Facts

Clotrimazole is more popular because it is very convenient to use, but it is costly. It looks more like a peppermint candy and less like a medication so the patient compliance rate is higher. The troches contain sucrose so the risk of caries exists if the drug is used for more than 3 three months. Do not prescribe Clotrimazole clotrimazole troches if the HIV patient is on protease inhibitors, or there is significant xerostomia, as.because the patient is unable to adequately suck on the troche due to lack of saliva

Clotrimazole Prescription

Rx: Clotrimazole (Mycelex) Troches, 10 mg/troche.
Disp: 70 troches (14-day supply).
Sig: Dissolve 1 troche in the mouth five times daily and *swallow the saliva*. There should be **no** eating or drinking for 30 minutes after use. In patients with removable appliances, re-infection can be avoided by dropping a clotrimazole (Mycelex) troche into water and soaking the appliance over night for 14 days. Also, clotrimazole ointment can be applied to appliances prior to insertion.

NYSTATIN (MYCOSTATIN)

Nystatin (Mycostatin) is available as a lozenge, pastille, cream, or oral suspension. The nystatin oral suspension contains alcohol and sucrose. In patients with removable appliances, the suspension should be dispensed, along with the oral antifungal lozenge, for 14 days.

Oral nystatin suspension is the preferred antifungal preparation over clotrimazole troches or nystatin lozenges for patients with xerostomia. Lack of saliva makes it difficult for the patient to suck on the troche or lozenge. Nystatin is **the** topical agent for an HIV patient on protease inhibitors.

Nystatin (Mycostatin) Prescriptions

1. **Nystatin (Mycostatin) lozenge/troche:**
   Rx: Nystatin (Mycostatin) lozenge/troche 200,000 units/lozenge.

Disp: 70 lozenges (14-day supply).
Sig: Dissolve 1 lozenge in the mouth 5 times daily.

There should be **no** eating or drinking for 30 min after use.

Re-infection can be avoided in patients with removable appliances by dropping a nystatin lozenge/troche into a $\frac{1}{4}$ cup of water and soaking the appliance over night for 14 days. Also, nystatin powder or nystatin ointment can be applied to appliances prior to insertion.

2. **Nystatin oral suspension:**
   Rx: Nystatin oral suspension 100,000 units/mL.
   Disp: 473 mL (1 pint) bottle (14-day supply).
   Sig: Use 1 tsp or 5 mL, qid.

   Rinse and hold in the mouth as long as possible before swallowing. There should be **no** eating or drinking for 30 min after use.

   Note that nystatin oral suspension also comes in a 60 mL bottle.

3. **Nystatin oral suspension for dentures:**
   Rx: Nystatin oral suspension 100,000 units/mL.
   Disp: 473 mL (1 pint) bottle.
   Sig: Add 5–10 mL of 1:100,000 units nystatin to half a cup of water and soak the dentures overnight daily, for 14 days. Rinse the dentures before use.

4. **Nystatin pastille:**
   Rx: Nystatin pastille 200,000 units/pastille.
   Disp: 70 pastilles.
   Sig: Dissolve 1 pastille in the mouth 4–5 times/day, for 14 days.

5. **Nystatin (Mycostatin) cream:**
   The cream can be applied to dentures before insertion or can be used for angular cheilitis.
   Rx: Nystatin (Mycostatin) cream 100,000 units/g.
   Disp: 15g or 30 g tube.
   Sig: Apply to the affected area 4–5 times/day.

   Do **not** eat or drink for 30 min after use.

AMPHOTERICIN B

Facts

Amphotericin B can be used in the pregnant patient because it is a Pregnancy Category B drug. It can also be used in HIV patients on protease inhibitors. It is minimally absorbed and relatively nontoxic.

Prescriptions

1. **Topical amphotericin B:**
   Rx: 3% topical amphotericin B cream.
   Disp: 20 g tube.
   Sig: Apply to the affected area 3–4 times/day, for 2–4 weeks.

2. **Oral amphotericin B:**
   Oral amphotericin B is dispensed as a capsule or a suspension. The oral forms are poorly absorbed.

2a. **Rx: amphotericin B 500 mg/capsule.**
    Disp: 56 capsules.
    Sig: Take 500 mg capsule PO qid for 2 weeks.
2b. **Rx: amphotericin B suspension: 500 mg/mL.**
    Disp: 56 mL suspension.
    Sig: Use 1 mL of the suspension, swish and swallow qid, for 2 weeks.

FLUCONAZOLE (DIFLUCAN)

Fluconazole (Diflucan) Facts

Fluconazole (Diflucan) is prescribed if the patient fails to respond to topical antifungal treatments, and it is also prescribed for esophageal candidiasis. Diflucan is the drug of choice for systemic antifungal treatment. Diflucan is a Pregnancy Category **C** drug. It should be avoided in the pregnant patient and amphotericin B should be prescribed instead.

Fluconazole (Diflucan) Prescriptions

1. **Treatment for refractory oral or systemic candidiasis:**
    Rx: Fluconazole (Diflucan) 100 mg/capsule.
    Disp: 15 capsules.
    Sig: Day 1: Take 2 capsules. **Days 2–14:** Take 1 capsule daily.
2. **Fluconazole (Diflucan) treatment for esophageal candidiasis:**
    Rx: Fluconazole (Diflucan) 100 mg/capsule.
    Disp: Variable.
    Sig: 100 mg qid (maximum 400 mg qid) for 14–21 days.

ANGULAR CHEILITIS

Angular Cheilitis Facts

Angular cheilitis can occur in the immune-competent or the immune-compromised patient. The common etiological factors are stress, flu, ill-fitting dentures, malnutrition, and anemia. The underlying cause must be simultaneously eradicated while treating the angular cheilitis with topical creams.

Candidiasis is a frequent superinfection associated with angular cheilitis, so the candidiasis must also be treated with appropriate antifungal therapy. Clotrimazole (Mycelex) or nystatin (Mycolog) creams are more commonly dispensed for angular cheilitis. Clioquinol-hydrocortisone (HC; Vioform-HC) cream is reserved for the refractory or very severe cases when the patient is experiencing profound cracking and pain.

Angular Cheilitis Prescriptions

1. **Clotrimazole (Mycelex) cream:**
    Rx: Clotrimazole (Mycelex) cream.
    Disp: 15 g tube.
    Sig: Rub into the affected area 2–3 times daily, for 2 weeks.

2. **Nystatin (Mycolog) cream:**
   Rx: Nystatin (Mycolog) cream.
   Disp: 15 g tube.
   Sig: Rub into the affected area 2–3 times daily, for 2 weeks.
3. **Clioquinol-hydrocortisone (HC; Vioform-HC) cream:**
   Rx: Clioquinol-Hydrocortisone (HC; Vioform-HC) cream.
   Disp: 15 g tube.
   Sig: Rub into affected area 2–3 times daily, until the patient is symptom free.

ORAL KAPOSI'S SARCOMA

Oral Kaposi's sarcoma (KS) is specific to HIV/AIDS, and the incidence of KS has significantly decreased with the advent of newer therapies. Kaposi's sarcoma in the oral cavity presents as a brown, red, blue, or purple macule, papule, or nodule. Kaposi's sarcoma has a predilection for the hard palate and the attached gingiva, but KS can appear on other mucosal sites as well. These lesions can also become secondarily infected with candida, as happens with oral viral leukoplakia. Nonalcoholic clorhexidine (Peridex) mouth rinse used twice a day can help prevent any secondary infections. Patients with AIDS-associated Kaposi's sarcoma usually die not because of the sarcoma but as a result of an associated systemic opportunistic infection. Many asymptomatic patients do not require treatment. Treatment modalities include surgery, radiation, and chemotherapy.

ORAL WARTS

Oral warts are specific in HIV/AIDS. They are papillary outgrowths of the oral mucosa and are caused by the papilloma virus, the same virus that causes genital warts. The diagnosis is confirmed by routine histopathologic analysis. Oral warts tend to be troublesome and frequently recur after removal. Treatment for oral warts usually consists of simple surgical excision. This form of treatment is used alone or in conjunction with cryotherapy.

RECURRENT APHTHOUS ULCERS

Aphthous ulcers frequently affect young adults and their occurrence can also be familial. The exact etiology is not known, but stress, localized trauma, food allergy, or infection (HSV or Helicobacter pylori) are frequently implicated as etiological factors. Patients with aphthous ulcers may have associated cell-mediated immunity problems along with systemic B and T cell–mediated immunity concerns.

Classification

Aphthous ulcers can be classified into three categories:

1. Minor aphthous ulcers
2. Major aphthous ulcers
3. Herpetiform aphthous ulcers

Minor Aphthous Ulcerations

Minor ulcers are benign aphthae. They tend to be small, shallow, single, or multiple lesions. They are highly recurrent, well-circumscribed, painful lesions, occur on non-keratinized tissue, and measure 0.2–0.5 cm in diameter. They are usually located on labial or buccal mucosa, the soft palate, or the floor of the mouth. Minor ulcers have no systemic symptoms and signs.

Major Aphthous Ulcerations Overview

The major aphthous ulcers measure more than 0.5 cm in diameter and are extremely painful and recurrent. They are larger and deeper ulcerations that tend to scar on healing and are serious aphthae. These ulcers are associated with systemic symptoms and signs such as uveitis, conjunctivitis, arthritis, genital ulcerations, fever, or adenopathy.

Etiological Factors

Major aphthae can be due to infections, autoimmune conditions, or hematological causes such as:

1. **Infections:** Human immunodeficiency virus (HIV) infection, herpes, CMV, bacteria, fungus (cryptosporidium, mucormycosis, histoplasma), and syphilis can be associated with major aphthae.
2. **Autoimmune conditions:** lupus erythematosus, Behçet's syndrome, Reiter's syndrome, bullous pemphigoid, Pemphigus vulgaris, and Crohn's disease patients often suffer from major aphthae.
   a. **Behçet's syndrome:** Behçet's syndrome is an autoimmune vasculitis that causes recurrent oral and genital ulcerations, uveitis, and retinitis.
   b. **Reiter's syndrome:** Reiter's syndrome is associated with oral ulcers, uveitis, conjunctivitis, and HLA B27-positive arthritis following nongonococcal urethritis or bacillary dysentery.
   c. **Crohn's disease:** These patients may present with associated oral ulcerations.
   d. **Lupus erythematosus, bullous pemphigoid, and pemphigus vulgaris:** Always determine the disease-associated symptoms to differentiate benign from recurrent aphthae.
3. **Hematological cause:** Patients with cyclic neutropenia can suffer from major aphthae. Cyclic neutropenia should be considered when the patient has oral ulcers with fever, which this happens during the neutropenic period. Cyclic neutropenia is a chronic type of neutropenia that is marked by regular, periodic episodic recurrences associated with malaise, fever, stomatitis, and various infections.

Herpetiform Ulcerations

The herpetiform ulcers are less than 0.2 cm in diameter and are painful lesions. They tend to be more numerous in number and are vesicular in nature.

Treatment Options and Prescriptions

Aphthous ulcers can be treated with any of the following medications:

- Antibiotics
- Anti-inflammatory medications

- Immune modulators
- Topical anesthetics
- Other agents

Antibiotic Therapy Prescriptions

Tetracycline and minocycline antibiotics are used because infectious agents are postulated to be one of the causes for aphthous ulcers.

1. **Tetracycline Capsules:**
   Rx: Dissolve a 250 mg tetracycline capsule in 180 mL water.
   Sig: Swish for a few minutes and **then expectorate**, qid for several days until the ulcers heal.
   Reduction of pain and reduction of duration of ulcerations may result. Do not eat or drink for 30 minutes afterward. Avoid use in children and pregnant women.
2. **Tetracycline Suspension:**
   Rx: Dispense 250 mg tetracycline/5 mL.
   Sig: Swish for a few minutes and **then expectorate**, qid until ulcers heal.
   Do not eat or drink for 30 minutes afterward. Avoid use in children and pregnant women.

Anti-inflammatory Agents Prescriptions

Local Anti-inflammatory Agents

Topical agents provide quick relief and can attenuate the duration of the ulcers. Triamcinolone 0.1% (Kenalog in Orabase) is a topical corticosteroid that should be used sparingly to gain temporary pain relief associated with oral ulcerations.

1. **Triamcinolone 0.1% (Kenalog in Orabase):**
   Rx: Triamcinolone 0.1% (Kenalog in Orabase):
   Disp: 5 g tube.
   Sig: Apply a thin film, *without rubbing*, on affected areas up to three times daily until the ulcers heal.
2. **Flucinonide (Lidex):**
   Rx: 0.05% Lidex ointment mixed 50/50 with Orabase.
   Disp: 30 g total.
   Sig: Apply a thin layer on the lesions 4–6 times daily.
3. **Dexamethasone (Decadrone) elixir:** Use dexamethasone (Decadron) elixir for severe ulcers as a rinse and expectorate. A secondary fungal infection could develop.
   Rx: Dexamethasone elixir, 0.5 mg/5mL.
   Disp: 250 mL.
   Sig: Rinse with 1tsp solution in the mouth for 1 min 4–5 times daily and **expectorate**.

Immune Modulators Prescriptions

1. **Rx:** Thalidomide (Thalomid) 200 mg OD/bid × 3–8 weeks.
   Thalidomide is a Pregnancy Category X drug and it is reserved for HIV-infected, non-pregnant patients only.

2. **Rx:** Oral prednisone, 5mg/tablet. Start at 30–40mg daily, with taper over one month, for severe disease resistant to topical agents.

Topical Anesthetics Prescription

Rx: Xylocaine 2% Viscous.
Disp: 100 mL or 450 mL.
Sig: Use 2tsp to rinse the oral cavity, as needed to relieve pain, and **expectorate**.

Prescription of Other Agents for Recurrent Aphthous Ulcerations

1. **Diphenhydramine (Benadryl) syrup (5 mg/mL) with liquid bismuth subsalicylate (Kaopectate):**
   Rx: Diphenhydramine (Benadryl) syrup (5 mg/mL) with liquid bismuth subsalicylate (Kaopectate), mix 50/50.
   Disp: 8oz total.
   Sig: Rinse with 2tsp, as needed, to relieve pain or burning, and **expectorate**.
   Expectoration will prevent constipation because Kaopectate is an anti-diarrhea preparation. You may have to suggest that the patient take Maalox if the patient swallows the mixture and constipation occurs.
2. **Diphenhydramine (Benadryl) syrup (5 mg/mL) with magnesium hydroxide antacid:**
   Rx: Diphenhydramine (Benadryl) syrup (5 mg/mL) with magnesium hydroxide antacid, mixed 50/50.
   Sig: Rinse with 2tsp, as needed, to relieve pain or burning, and **expectorate.**

XEROSTOMIA (DRY MOUTH)

Xerostomia is a condition associated with decreased saliva production and an alteration in the saliva composition such that the saliva gets thickened and viscous. A diagnosis of xerostomia is positive when the un-stimulated salivary flow is less than 0.1mL/min. Xerostomia causes a reduction of the protective proteolytic enzymes and antibodies in the saliva, thus increasing the incidence of oral infections, candidiasis, and caries.

Xerostomia is associated with impaired chewing, speech impairment, decreased taste sensation, halitosis, and an increased incidence of caries and oral infections.

Etiology

Xerostomia can be caused by:

1. **Medications:** Medications with anticholinergic effects: antipsychotics, antidepressants, antiretroviral drugs, sedatives, hypnotics, antihistamines, anticonvulsants, and muscle relaxants can cause xerostomia.
2. **Age:** Xerostomia is more common in the elderly.
3. **Sjögren's syndrome:** Sjögren's syndrome is an autoimmune condition that is associated with lymphocytic infiltration of the salivary glands. It is more common in women than in men. Primary Sjögren's syndrome is associated with xerostomia and keratoconjunctivitis. Secondary Sjögren's syndrome is associated with systemic

lupus erythematosus, scleroderma, and other connective tissue disorders. Presence of anti-Ro/SSA or anti-La/SSB on blood tests is very suggestive of Sjögren's syndrome.

4. **Diabetes:** Uncontrolled diabetes is often associated with xerostomia.
5. **Head and neck radiation therapy:** The amount of salivary gland destruction with treatment depends on the amount of radiation dose given during radiation therapy. The destruction is often permanent with higher doses, but with lower doses, the glands may bounce back in 6–12 months. Doses that are greater than 30 Gy can cause permanent damage of the salivary glands.

Manifestations

Xerostomia can be associated with dental caries, erythematous oral mucosa, oral and/or esophageal candidiasis, angular cheilitis, mucositis, and oral ulcerations.

Treatment Options

Xerostomia treatment options are discussed here and in Chapter 50. The reader is advised to view both discussions. Treatment options for xerostomia discussed here are as follows:

1. Daily, good oral hygiene.
2. Xerostomia sufferers should have frequent, comprehensive dental exams with x-ray evaluations to detect any new carious or any other oral disease lesions. These patients are also at high risk for periodontal disease and should get periodontal prophylaxis every three months.
3. **Rinses:** Nonalcoholic chlorhexidine or any other nonalcoholic mouth rinse to assist with the care of gingivitis and plaque formation. A calcium-containing remineralizing oral rinse such as caphsol (Eusa Pharma) is also recommended because calcium has a remineralizing effect on dental enamel.
4. **Saliva substitutes:** The use of saliva substitutes Biotene products, Salivart, or Xerolube is highly advocated.
5. **Saliva stimulants:** Pilocarpine and cevimeline (Evoxac) are saliva stimulants that are reserved for refractory cases.
6. **Topical fluorides:** These patients need fluoride therapy in the form of professionally applied concentrated sodium fluoride varnishes and daily use of 1.1% sodium fluoride prescription strength fluoride toothpaste (PreviDent 5000 Dry Mouth). Fluoride is used to prevent tooth decay. Patients with severe xerostomia should get 1.23% acidulated phosphate fluoride gel for four minutes four times per year.

Saliva Substitutes Detailed Discussion

Common saliva substitutes are as follows:

1. **Water:** Water intake should be frequent throughout the day.
2. **Milk:** Milk buffers oral acids and provides calcium and phosphate.
3. **Biotene and Oralbalance:** These products contain three enzyme systems and a protein similar to that found in natural saliva. These enzyme systems penetrate the plaque-forming bacterial cell walls and maintain a healthy oral flora. The combined

use of Biotene and Oralbalance has been found to be very effective in the management of xerostomia. Oralbalance is available as a moisturizing gel. Biotene is available as a sugar-free gum, alcohol-free mouthwash, and toothpaste.

a. **Biotene mouthwash:** Use 1tbsp PRN, swish, and **expectorate**. It works best when used with Biotene toothpaste.

b. **Biotene toothpaste:** The toothpaste is nonirritating and it contains the protective enzyme systems needed for optimal oral health. The toothpaste should be used post-meals and at bedtime.

Saliva Stimulants Detailed Discussion

Parasympathetic nervous system stimulation causes salivary secretion, and this can be achieved by the simple process of chewing or sucking on sugar-free candy. Nonselective muscarinic receptor agonists such as pilocarpine (Salagen) or cevimeline (Evoxac) can also promote salivary function.

Pilocarpine HCL (Salagen) Overview

Pilocarpine increases saliva secretion by systemic cholinergic stimulation. Pilocarpine's effectiveness relies on the presence of intact salivary gland tissue and nerve supply. In the case of the irradiated patient, it would be the intact tissue outside the area of radiation. Pilocarpine HCL should be reserved for radiation, drug-induced, or Sjögren's syndrome–associated xerostomia.

Increased frequency of cardiovascular and pulmonary side effects contraindicates the use of pilocarpine HCL (Salagen) in patients with moderate-to-severe asthma, COPD, and cardiac arrhythmias. It is also contraindicated in patients with a history of renal stones, gallstones, and narrow angle glaucoma.

Pilocarpine HCL Side Effects

Common side effects experienced are perspiration (earliest side effect), nausea, dizziness, lacrimation, headaches, tachycardia, tremors, dysphagia, and heartburn.

Pilocarpine HCL (Salagen) Prescription

Rx: Salagen, 5 mg/tablet.
Disp: Variable.
Sig: 1–2 tablets tid/qid per day **taken 30 min prior to meals**.

The patient should be treated for a minimum of 90 days for optimal effect. Pilocarpine effect begins in 15 minutes and lasts for two to three hours. The patient should drink 2 L of water daily when taking pilocarpine HCL. Please inform the patient that it can take a few weeks for pilocarpine to become optimally effective.

Cevimeline (Evoxac)

Cevimeline is a Pregnancy Category C drug that is used to treat the symptoms of dry mouth that are often experienced by patients with Sjogren's syndrome.

Contraindications: Cevimeline is contraindicated in the presence of uncontrolled asthma, cholelithiasis (gallstones), heart disease, nephrolithiasis (kidney stones), acute iritis and narrow-angle glaucoma, or pulmonary disease other than asthma.

Cevimeline alerts: Cevimeline should be administered with caution to patients taking beta-adrenergic antagonists, because of the possibility of conduction disturbances. Drugs with parasympathomimetic effects administered along with cevimeline can have additive effects. Cevimeline might interfere with desirable antimuscarinic effects of drugs used concomitantly.

Drugs that inhibit CYP2D6 and CYP33A4 also inhibit the metabolism of cevimeline. Cevimeline should be used with caution in patients known or suspected to be deficient in CYP2D6 activity based on previous experience, because they may be at a higher risk of adverse events.

Cevimeline dose: 30mg three times a day, with meals. If a dose is missed, the patient should take it as soon as possible. However, if it is almost time for the next dose, then the missed dose should be skipped and the patient should go back to the regular dosing schedule and **not** double the doses.

Cevimeline side effects: Cevimeline may cause drowsiness, dizziness, decreased alertness, difficulty breathing, tachycardia, itching, swelling of the gums or tongue and change in vision, especially at night.

XVI

The Female Patient: Pregnancy, Lactation, and Contraception

Pregnancy, Lactation, and Contraception: Assessment and Associated Dental Management Guidelines

PREGNANCY, LACTATION, AND CONTRACEPTION

Many providers in the past were hesitant about providing care during pregnancy out of fear for the safety of the fetus and the mother and uncertainty of the safety of local anesthetics, analgesics, and antibiotics. We now know that pregnancy does not contraindicate dentistry and dentistry can occur throughout pregnancy, give or take a few weeks. Dentistry is safe for the mother and safe for the fetus. Maintaining optimal oral health helps control oral disease, and this in turn reduces the transmission of pathogens from mother to child. Preventative services should be given during early pregnancy, and the provider must treat acute infections immediately.

A knowledgeable provider is a more confident provider. The goal of this section is to provide you with the knowledge of the current concepts associated with pregnancy, lactation, and contraception so you can proceed with confidence in the dental setting.

Pregnancy Overview

In order to know how and when to proceed with dentistry one needs to understand the symptoms, signs, and tests associated with pregnancy. The practitioner should be aware of the medications that can and cannot be used during pregnancy, as well as facts regarding radiation exposure during pregnancy.

Pregnancy and Trimesters

The 40 weeks of pregnancy are divided into three trimesters: **The first trimester** spans from 1–14 weeks, **the second trimester** spans from 14–28 weeks, and **the third trimester** spans from 28–40 weeks.

Some facts to remember: Development of organ systems occurs during the first trimester, and many organ systems are laid down by about eight weeks. By the third trimester, the placenta and the fetus together weigh about 13lb, on average. Therefore,

Dentist's Guide to Medical Conditions, Medications, and Complications, Second Edition. Kanchan M. Ganda.
© 2013 John Wiley & Sons, Inc. Published 2013 by John Wiley & Sons, Inc.

in the supine position, this mass can potentially exert pressure on the thin walled inferior vena cava (IVC), causing it to collapse, or the gravid uterus can actually obstruct the IVC, leading to supine hypotension. The aorta is not affected, as it is a thick-walled blood vessel. Supine hypotension can be avoided by giving the patient a left lateral semi-sitting position in the chair to begin with, so the gravid uterus no longer presses on the IVC.

Assessment during the initial dental visit: During the pregnant patient's first dental visit, determine the stage of her pregnancy. Determine if she is experiencing any pregnancy-associated symptoms that need to be accommodated. Assess if she is presenting with acute dental problems or if the patient is in for routine dental care. All emergency and routine care can continue during pregnancy. You must make provisions for and confirm her comfort in the dental chair throughout the duration of the dental appointment.

Pregnancy-Associated Symptoms and Signs

The early symptoms and signs of pregnancy are described in the following sections.

Amenorrhea

Conception occurs 14 days after the first day of the previous menstrual cycle. A patient having regular menstrual periods will know when her cycle is delayed and if she is pregnant. It is always important to ask your patient if she could be pregnant and when was the last menstrual period (LMP).

Nausea and Vomiting

"Morning sickness" can occur at any time of the day; it does not have to be in the morning only! It lasts for a few days or weeks and it is best **not** to schedule dentistry during this period of discomfort.

Urinary Frequency

Urinary frequency exists throughout pregnancy and the patient may need to excuse herself during dental treatment.

Fatigue

The patient more commonly complains of fatigue in the first and third trimester. It is better to schedule shorter appointments to prevent further exhaustion.

Pregnancy Tests

Tests confirming pregnancy are:

1. **Urine pregnancy test:** This test detects the monoclonal antibodies in the urine and the test is positive two weeks after conception, which is just around the time of the missed menstrual period.
2. **The serum pregnancy test:** This test detects β-HCG; the test becomes positive nine days after conception.

PREGNANCY-ASSOCIATED CHANGES

Pregnancy-associated changes experienced by the mother are generalized and knowing what areas are affected will help you better manage your patient. There are dietary, cardiovascular, gastrointestinal, and oral-cavity related changes.

Dietary Changes

The daily caloric, protein, and folic acid requirements increase, and lack of folic acid can lead to spina bifida in the fetus. The patient gains about 25–35 lb throughout the pregnancy.

Cardiovascular Changes

Several cardiovascular changes occur as the pregnancy advances.

Pulse

The pulse rate increases by 10–15 beats/min during pregnancy. Having knowledge of the baseline pulse rate **prior** to pregnancy always helps to calculate the actual change in pulse rate for the patient.

It is always advisable to **decrease** the amount of **epinephrine** in the local anesthetic, or to avoid epinephrine in a patient visibly affected with tachycardia.

Cardiac Output

The cardiac output increases by 40% in the first trimester. There is increased stroke volume from increased plasma volume. This is associated with increased vascularity in all areas of the body, including the gum tissue.

Cardiac output changes cause blood pressure changes in the mother. It is always important to monitor the blood pressure throughout the pregnancy. A diagnosis of hypertension is made when the current BP shows changes compared with the pre-pregnancy BP or the BP prior to 20 weeks of pregnancy.

An increase in the systolic BP by 30 mmHg and/or the diastolic BP by 15 mmHg indicates hypertension. Any BP reading >140/90 mmHg, if previous readings are unknown, also indicates hypertension.

It is important to remember that the blood pressure usually decreases in the second trimester because of vasodilatation. You need to stop all planned/routine dental treatment and refer the patient to the obstetrician immediately **if the second trimester BP shows no change, or if there is an increase** when compared to the first trimester BP readings. The obstetrician needs to evaluate and treat this patient for any pregnancy-associated hypertension before you can continue with dentistry.

Supine Hypotension

Supine hypotension as previously discussed usually occurs in the third trimester due to compression of the inferior vena cava by the gravid uterus. Supine hypotension must be prevented in the dental chair because it can cause the patient to pass out. When the patient passes out, the uterine blood flow gets affected and this causes the baby's heart rate to decrease.

The best preventive treatment for supine hypotension is to turn the patient, preferably to the left side, to displace the uterus away from the inferior vena cava. The patient can also be placed in a sitting position with the knees flexed.

Supine hypotension presentation and management: During supine hypotension, the patient feels faint and the vision goes gray, plus the patient experiences dizziness. The blood pressure drops because of decreased venous return and decreased blood flow to the uterus. Also, with the supine position and consequent compression of IVC, there is lack of venous return from the lower extremities, which results in decreased cardiac output, adding to the hypotension due to the supine position.

Treatment of supine hypotention consists of sitting the patient up, or you can fully recline the chair and roll the patient toward her left side (this is the all-important left lateral position) to push the weight of the gravid uterus off to the left and away from the IVC.

Gastrointestinal Changes

The gums can become hyperemic and bleed during pregnancy. It is advisable to stress good, daily oral hygiene and schedule hygiene appointments at shorter intervals. The gastric emptying is delayed and this accounts for the increased risk of aspiration. This increased risk of aspiration is especially of concern during general anesthesia, so spinal or epidural anesthesias are preferred. This also avoids any threat of sedating the baby. General anesthesia is best avoided in the dental setting.

Oral Cavity Changes

Pregnancy-related oral cavity changes seen are pregnancy gingivitis, pregnancy tumor, and periodontal disease. Periodontal disease affects about 15% of individuals in the childbearing age and up to 40% of pregnant women. There is a disproportionate burden among low-income women, and advanced age, smoking, and diabetes increase the risk for periodontal disease. Dental carious lesions may become exacerbated during pregnancy, but the incidence of caries is **not** increased by pregnancy.

Pregnancy Gingivitis

Pregnancy gingivitis is relatively common and occurs in 50–70% of patients. There is an increased incidence of inflammation, erythema, edema, and hypertrophy of the gums with pregnancy gingivitis.

Pregnancy-associated hormonal changes cause increased growth of gum capillaries resulting in hypertrophy of the gums. The shift in hormonal changes also causes a shift in the bacterial flora and increased bacterial growth at the gum-line. The gums swell, bleed easily, and become sensitive.

The process begins around the second month of pregnancy and peaks in the middle of the third trimester. However, pregnancy gingivitis usually disappears postpartum. The dentist may need to implement scaling and root planing to correct or improve the gingivitis and prevent plaque growth.

Pregnancy gingivitis was thought to cause premature birth and low birth weight. The hypothesis was that bacteria from the pregnancy gingivitis–associated plaque entered the bloodstream and stimulated the patient's immune system to produce prostaglandins. Prostaglandins in turn were thought to trigger uterine contraction leading to early labor, premature birth, and a smaller-sized baby. All these theoretical concerns that gram-negative bacteria associated with periodontitis increase the risk through bacteremia, causing an increase of preterm delivery and low birth weight, have now been put to rest. The study by Novak et al. (2008) examined periodontal treatment starting before 21 weeks pregnancy, and this study showed that even though periodontal care significantly reduced levels of bacteria associated with periodontitis, these periodontitis-associated bacteria were not associated with preterm birth. Thus, meticulous oral hygiene should continue in the pregnant patient, but periodontal care has no effect on birth weight or premature birth.

Pregnancy Tumor

The pregnancy tumor or "pyogenic granuloma" is a pedunculated outgrowth from the palatal surface of the gingiva and is usually found between the teeth or is associated with areas of local trauma or irritation. The tumor is usually anterior and maxillary in location. It is an inflammatory immune system response to an irritant, and in this case plaque acts as an irritant. Pregnancy tumors occur in about 10% of all pregnancies, but they disappear after birth. Pregnancy tumors can also be found on the face, hands, or arms.

The pregnancy tumor is painless and appears as a soft, gray tissue mass with a red border. Surgical excision after birth is the treatment of choice, but it can recur.

TERATOGENIC DRUGS AND FDA DRUG CATEGORIES

Teratogenic Drugs Facts

Teratogens are drugs or factors that can cause permanent alteration in the formation, functioning, or anchoring of the fetus. Organogenesis occurs during **weeks 3–10,** and structural malformations or morphological abnormalities due to teratogens can occur during these weeks. The CNS, limbs, heart, palate, and teeth are formed during this time. The brain and heart are vulnerable organs, and outcomes of insult include functional defects and morphological abnormalities. It is best to **avoid** dental drugs and routine dentistry during these weeks. The baby is completely formed at 35 weeks, and prior to this point the fetus is vulnerable to changes caused by adverse teratogenic drugs or factors.

Some of the **Category B opioid** pain medications that are safe during pregnancy **become Category C/D** toward the time of delivery and should not be used **closer to term**. These specific drugs are discussed in further detail in this chapter.

To have a better understanding of what medications should be used and what should be avoided in the pregnant patient, one has to have a good understanding of the FDA drug categories and specific drug facts. Drugs that are Category A or B are safe drugs to use during pregnancy.

FDA Drug Categories

The following are FDA drug categories:

Category A: Drugs in this category demonstrate no fetal risk and their safety has been documented by controlled studies.

Category B: Animal studies have shown no risk with the drugs in this category, but there are no well-documented human studies to demonstrate the safety of these drugs.

Category C: Animal studies have shown adverse effects; no controlled studies have been done in women, and there are no studies available in animals or women to demonstrate the safety of these drugs.

Category D: Drugs in this class have evidence of human risks, but the benefits may sometimes outweigh the risks when the drug is needed.

Category X: There is definite demonstration of risk, and the risks far outweigh the benefits. These drugs should not be given to pregnant mothers.

DRUGS CONTRAINDICATED DURING PREGNANCY

Drugs Absolutely Contraindicated During Pregnancy

- **Accutane:** Accutane is associated with severe congenital abnormalities.
- **Amiodarone:** Amiodarone is an anti-arrhythmia drug.
- **Angiotensin-converting enzyme (ACE) inhibitors.**
- **Ciprofloxacin (Cipro):** Cipro affects fetal kidneys and it should be completely avoided during pregnancy.
- **Live attenuated vaccines:** Includes varicella and MMR.
- **Methotrexate:** Methotrexate is associated with a high rate of miscarriage.
- **Oral hypoglycemic drugs:** These drugs can cause hypoglycemia in the fetus.
- **Prostaglandins:** These drugs promote miscarriage.
- **Radioactive iodine:** Radiation exposure occurs.
- **Sumatriptan succinate (Imitrex):** An anti-migraine drug, vasoconstrictor in action, that can cause growth restriction.
- **Tetracyclines:** These affect teeth and bone growth.
- **Warfarin (Coumadin):** Heparin is used instead, if blood thinning is required.

RADIATION AND PREGNANCY

The following are important facts to know about radiation:

- No single diagnostic x-ray procedure results in radiation exposure to a degree that would threaten the well-being of the developing pre-embryo, embryo, or fetus. Radiation exposure <5 RADS is considered safe. Risk of anomalies, growth restriction, or abortions is not increased with exposure >5 RADS. Even multiple x-ray exposures seldom result in this level.
- During routine maternal dental x-rays, the fetal exposure is <0.01 RADS and <.004 RADS for a skull film. This is because exposure to mother and fetus are not the same. Additionally, shielding is used and that minimizes exposure.

- Daily background radiation is 0.0004 RADS. Moderate amount of radiation exposure is not harmful in pregnancy. It is important to inform and educate your patient in order to minimize anxiety.
- Chest x-ray exposure radiation dose is 0.008 RADS.

Fetal Risks with Improper Radiation Exposure

The following are fetal risks with radiation exposure:

1. **Embryonic death resulting in miscarriage:** This occurs if there is too much radiation exposure in the first trimester and especially in the first week of pregnancy.
2. **Congenital abnormalities:** Congenital abnormalities occur mostly during weeks 3–10 of the pregnancy, when organogenesis occurs.
3. **Intrauterine growth:** Intrauterine growth restriction occurs after the first trimester.
4. **Leukemia:** There is a slightly increased risk of childhood leukemia with fetal radiation exposure.

GENERAL ANESTHESIA AND PREGNANCY

General anesthetic can affect the fetus if it crosses through the placental circulation. General anesthesia should not be given near the time of delivery because it will impair the infant's breathing. General anesthesia will also prolong the gastrointestinal transition time in the mother and thus increase the risk of aspiration.

Chronic N_2O exposure can be hazardous. This is more relevant to women working in your office rather than the pregnant patient. Women chronically exposed to N_2O have an increased rate of spontaneous abortions or give birth to infants with congenital abnormalities. Chronic N_2O exposure also accounts for the reduced rate of fertility among such women.

SUGGESTED GENERAL PRINCIPLES OF PREGNANT PATIENT CARE

Follow these guidelines:

1. Always have the patient sign a case note in the dental record giving consent to dentistry before you start the dental treatment.
2. Dental treatment can be conducted throughout pregnancy with the exception of the following periods:
   a. Organogenesis or fetal organ formation occurs in weeks 3–10, and the highest risk to the fetus occurs during these weeks. Consequently, all potentially harmful drugs should be avoided during the organogenesis weeks; this is also true for drugs used for dentistry.
   b. Avoid treatment during the weeks of morning sickness in the first trimester for obvious reasons.
3. The safest and most comfortable time for dentistry during pregnancy is the last 2–3 weeks of the first trimester, the entire second trimester, and the first half of the third trimester.
4. Give the patient a left lateral position during dental treatment in the latter half of the third trimester. Dentistry is not contraindicated in the latter half of the third

trimester, but it may be uncomfortable for the patient. The lateral position displaces the gravid uterus and prevents putting pressure on the inferior vena cava.

5. You should provide dental treatment only if the patient is comfortable going through it.
6. Do not use $O_2 + N_2O$, because N_2O has teratogenic effects.
7. Restrict the taking of excessive radiographs during pregnancy, and take only those that are needed. If absolutely needed, a full-mouth radiographic survey can be done as long as you protect the patient with a full body and thyroid lead shield. The full-mouth survey radiation dose is 1.6 mGy.
8. All essential dental treatment can continue during pregnancy. This includes routine extractions, periodontal treatment, restorations, continuation of orthodontic treatment, and placement of removable and fixed prosthodontics and crowns.
9. In general, during dentistry, use a minimum amount of epinephrine and minimum number of carpules of the local anesthetic.

SPECIFICS OF PREGNANT PATIENT CARE IN THE DENTAL SETTING

- The importance of oral health and overall health should be relayed by the practitioner to the mother. This tenet comes from the "Oral Health During Pregnancy and Early Childhood: Evidence-Based Guidelines for Health Professionals," a consensus formed following deliberations by the California Dental Association Foundation (CDA Foundation) and the American College of Obstetricians and Gynecologists District IX (ACOG District IX), following extensive review of medical and dental literatures.
- Treating the mother during pregnancy reduces the risk of bacterial transmission to her children.
- Prevention, diagnosis, routine dental care, and treatment of oral diseases can occur **anytime** during the pregnancy. **Deferring care during pregnancy can increase the bacterial count in the mother and this consequently increases the risk of caries in her children.**
- Preventive and restorative dental treatment during the perinatal period is safe and results in better health outcomes. Delaying necessary dental treatment can result in harm to the mother. **Rubber dam use is encouraged.**
- Dentistry during the first trimester does **not** increase the risk of spontaneous abortion.
- Studies demonstrate that scaling and root planing treatment during pregnancy is safe and improves the status of periodontal disease in the mother.
- Periodontal care during pregnancy does **not** affect the outcomes of preterm labor, the risk of preterm birth, or low birth weight infants.
- Periodontal care during pregnancy **should occur as early as possible,** and **acute oral disease should be addressed immediately at any time during the pregnancy.**
- Periodontal disease increases the risk of preeclampsia, but preeclampsia is **not** a contraindication to dentistry if dental care has been approved by the obstetrician.
- The second trimester is associated with decreased immunoglobulin (IgG) levels, and this is largely responsible for oral tissues becoming more susceptible to disease as bacteria multiply.

- Pregnancy is associated with a mild decrease in platelet count (gestational thrombocytopenia), a mild increase in the white blood cell (WBC) count, and decreased neutrophil function. This accounts for the increased incidence of plaque-induced gingivitis and pregnancy-associated periodontal disease.
- Scaling root planning (nonsurgical periodontal therapy), and vigorous oral hygiene instructions are highly recommended to eliminate plaque buildup. Dental caries must be aggressively treated to reduce the bacterial burden in the pregnant patient.
- Cariogenic bacteria can be transmitted from mother to child, and this should prompt caregivers to discourage kissing the baby on the mouth, sharing utensils, and so on. Streptococcus mutans and Lactobacillus are the two cariogenic bacteria found in dental plaque and they are the two main organisms used to assess susceptibility to caries.
- There is documentation that pregnancy increases the risk of dental erosion and periodontal disease. Advise mouth rinses and chewing xylitol-containing or sugar-free gum, to decrease oral bacterial count in the mother. Xylitol reduces S. mutans levels in the plaque and saliva, thus slowing the transfer of bacteria; xylitol is also antibacterial in action.
- **Chlorhexidine and xylitol:** Pregnancy category is undetermined and both have not been evaluated for pregnancy adversity or side effects.
- **Other dental drugs:** Amlexanox (Aphthasol) and sodium fluoride (Fluoridex) are safe to use.
- Mothers experiencing nausea should rinse with a teaspoon of baking soda (sodium bicarbonate) in a cup of water and expectorate.
- Pregnant women with gestational diabetes are at an increased risk for periodontal disease, which, in turn, worsens the control of diabetes. Gestational diabetes is also associated with newborns having increased birth-weight. Smoking and advanced age, along with diabetes, are risk factors for periodontal disease, and this gets compounded in the pregnant patient.
- The rate of congenital anomalies increases with diabetes that is **not** in control, particularly during the first trimester. Good diabetes control decreases the risk of preeclampsia and newborns larger for their gestational age.
- The second trimester is associated with a drop in blood pressure because of increases in plasma volume and cardiac output and associated decrease in peripheral vascular resistance.
- Because of the physiologic changes the body undergoes during pregnancy, delayed gastric emptying, and reduced HCL production in the stomach, drug metabolism could be affected. **First-pass drug metabolism is typically not affected, but second-pass metabolism associated with liver enzymes does get affected and may be increased or decreased.**
- Shorter appointments and explaining the care to the patient helps reduce anxiety.
- Studies document that essential dental treatment in pregnant women during weeks 13–21 (the second trimester) is **not** associated with an increased risk of serious medical adverse events or adverse pregnancy outcomes.
- **Teeth whitening** products associated with hydrogen peroxide release inorganic mercury from dental amalgams, so they should be **avoided** during pregnancy.
- Use the rubber dam and high-speed suction when removing or placing amalgam restorations to minimize mercury vapor inhalation. If both cannot be used, then the practitioner must delay restorations removal until after delivery. Note, however,

that FDA approval does exist, which demonstrates safety of amalgam material. No adverse effect has been demonstrated with this safe practice. Alternatively, composite resins, porcelain and gold restorations may be used.

- Preterm birth is when delivery occurs before the end of 37 weeks of gestation.
- Guidelines allow the use of dental radiographs for diagnosis and dental treatment planning. **Digital radiography has the advantage of reduced radiation, no chemical processing, and instant imaging.**
- Provide frequent position changes during treatment, particularly as the pregnancy advances.
- **Anesthetics:** Guidelines allow the use of local anesthesia to adequately manage oral diseases in the mother. Epinephrine is **not** contraindicated and Category B local anesthetics are considered safe.

Safe Local Anesthetics

The following are safe **Category B** local anesthetics that can be used during pregnancy:

1. 2% lidocaine (Xylocaine) with 1:100,000 epinephrine
2. 4% prilocaine HCL with 1:200,000 epinephrine (Citanest Forte)
3. 4% prilocaine HCL without epinephrine (Citanest Plain)

It is best to use local anesthetics with little or no epinephrine, particularly in the presence of an increased pulse rate during the pregnancy. With any of the anesthetics, use a maximum of two carpules.

Avoid epinephrine completely when treating a mild-to-moderate hypertensive pregnant patient. Use 4% prilocaine HCL without epinephrine (Citanest Plain) after obtaining clearance for dentistry from the patient's obstetrician.

Unsafe Local Anesthetics

The following are **Category C** local anesthetics that are contraindicated during pregnancy:

1. 0.5% bupivacaine (Marcaine)
2. 4% septocaine (Articaine) with 1:100,000 or 1:200,000 epinephrine
3. 2% mepivacaine (Carbocaine) with 1:20,000 levonordefrin (NeoCobefrin)
4. 3% mepivacaine HCL (Carbocaine)

Pregnancy and Anesthetics, Analgesics, Antibiotics, Antivirals, and Antifungals

- **Analgesics:** Acetaminophen (Category B) is **the** analgesic and antipyretic of choice during pregnancy.
- Avoid NSAIDS in the first and third trimesters, and prescribe for no more than two to three days if NSAIDS are absolutely necessary. If given in the first trimester, NSAIDS may be associated with abdominal-wall birth defect causing herniation of intestinal contents (gastroschisis).
- **Naproxen and ibuprofen (both Category B):** Even though ibuprofen and naproxen are classified as Category B, NSAIDS should generally be avoided in pregnancy. There is good evidence showing that ibuprofen and naproxen should **not** be used

in first and third trimesters. There is a risk of miscarriage with NSAIDS use in the first trimester, and premature ductus arteriosus closure can occur if used in the third trimester. If benefits far outweigh the risk, and if cleared for use by the obstetrician, ibuprofen or naproxen should not be dispensed for more than 48–72 hours.

- Aspirin (Category C) use during pregnancy should be for only medical reasons, not dental reasons, and should be short term if benefits far outweigh the risks. Avoid use during the first and third trimesters.
- **Celecoxib (Celebrex):** Pregnancy Category C/D with chronic use or high doses. **Avoid** during pregnancy.
- Occasional narcotic use is allowed in pregnancy when benefits far outweigh the risks. **There is no known safe level of narcotic use during pregnancy.** Risks to the fetus include miscarriage, stillbirth, or premature delivery, **especially with pro-longed and high-dose use.** At birth, the baby is also at increased risk for low birth weight, and may experience breathing difficulties and extreme drowsiness, which can then lead to feeding problems.
- Opioids should be avoided in pregnancy, unless absolutely needed, and it is important to remember that first trimester use may be associated with heart defects and spina bifida.
- **Narcotics with "no risk in controlled animal studies":** Narcotics that can be used short term for two to three days in the first or second trimester of pregnancy are oxycodone (Category B), morphine (Category C), meperidine (Category C), fentanyl (Category C), and hydromorphone (Category C).
- **Category C narcotics that become Category D with prolonged use or in high doses, and with "a small risk in controlled animal studies":** codeine (Tylenol with codeine), hydrocodone (Vicodin), propoxyphene (Darvocet), and tramadol (Ultram).
- **Codeine:** Codeine (Category C) is considered "less safe" during pregnancy, compared with Percocet. Post ingestion, codeine is converted to morphine. Some individuals are genetically predisposed to metabolize codeine much faster and more completely than others. These individuals are called ultra-rapid metabolizers. They are more likely to have higher-than-normal levels of morphine in their blood after taking codeine. Ultrarapid CYP2D6 metabolism occurs in 3% African Americans, 10% Caucasians, and 1% of Chinese and Hispanics.
- **Morphine and meperidine:** Both drugs are Category C and these analgesics become Category D in high doses or with prolonged use. Short-term use of these drugs is acceptable during the first or second trimesters of pregnancy, as these drugs are found to have "no risk in controlled animal studies."
- **Oxycodone:** Category B becomes Category D in high doses or with prolonged use. Oxycodone with acetaminophen (Percocet) is Category C. The drug is safe to use short term during the first or second trimester, as it has been found to have "no risk in controlled animal studies."
- **Hydrocodone:** Acetaminophen hydrocodone (Vicodin) has been assigned to Category C by the FDA and becomes Category D with prolonged use. Vicodin has been found to have "small risk in controlled animal studies," so its use is considered "less safe," per say, during pregnancy compared with Percocet.
- **Fentanyl and hydromorphone:** Both are Category C drugs and are excreted in breast milk. It is best to avoid these drugs during breast-feeding.

- **Propoxyphene (Darvon):** Category C, and D with prolonged use. Avoid during pregnancy.
- **Tramadol:** Category C, and D with prolonged use. Tramadol is found to have "small risk in controlled animal studies," so it is "less safe" than Percocet during pregnancy and should **not** be used.
- **Category D analgesics** aspirin, etodolac (Lodine), ketorolac (Toradol): These analgesics demonstrate strong evidence of risk to the human fetus. Aspirin is the only one medication by the physician with specific indications in pregnancy when benefits far outweigh the risks. Low-dose aspirin may be safer, but the risk of neonatal hemorrhage or perinatal death exists.
- **Safe antibiotics:** Penicillin V potassium (Veetids), amoxicillin (Amoxil), amoxicillin (Trimox), amoxicillin/clavulanic acid (Augmentin), ampicillin sodium/sulbactam sodium (Unasyn), azithromycin (Zithromax), cefaclor (Ceclor), cefazolin (Ancef), cephalexin (Keflex), clindamycin (Cleocin), and metronidazole (Flagyl). Metronidazole is safe only in second and third trimesters and is contraindicated in the first trimester. Metronidazole safety prior to 14 weeks has not been established.
- **Sulfa antibiotics**, even though considered safe when prescribed prior to third trimester, should be avoided because they cause hyperbilirubinemia and kernicterus.
- **Unsafe antibiotics:** Erythromycin estolate, clarithromycin (Biaxin), doxycycline, tetracycline HCL, minocycline, vancomycin nitrofurantoin, and fluoroquinolones are considered unsafe during pregnancy. Fluoroquinolones (Category C) should not be used during pregnancy and lactation because animal studies have shown cartilage malformation. Tetracyclines are associated with discoloration of teeth and they affect growing bones. Nitrofurantoin can cause hemolytic anemia in an infant with G6PD deficiency.
- **Antivirals:** Category B drugs showing **no risk** in controlled animal studies are **valacyclovir (Valtrex) and acyclovir (Zovirax).**
- **Antifungals:** As per the CDC, it is best to prescribe topical antifungals during pregnancy and it is best to avoid prescribing systemic antifungals in the first trimester. Category B drugs showing **no risk** in controlled animal studies are **nystatin (Mycostatin), amphotericin B lipid complex (Abelcet), and amphotericin B liposome (Ambisome)**.
- **Category C antifungals showing small risk in controlled animal studies that should be avoided during pregnancy:** clotrimazole (Mycelex, Lotrimin), fluconazole (Diflucan), itraconazole (Sporanox), and ketoconazole (Nizoral),

Trimester Dental Guidelines

Follow these guidelines:

1. **During the first trimester:** Evaluate the dentition and perform ongoing and maintenance dentistry.
2. **During the second trimester:** Perform any routine or major procedures necessary because this is the best time to treat the pregnant patient.
3. **During the third trimester:** Continue established maintenance programs and perform only major, required procedures.

Table 49.1.   Suggested Safe AAAs During Pregnancy

Safe Medications	Precautions/Remarks
LOCAL ANESTHETICS: 1. 2% Lidocaine (Xylocaine), 1:100,000 epinephrine 2. 4% Prilocaine HCL with 1:200,000 epinephrine (Citanest Forte) 3. 4% Prilocaine HCL without epinephrine (Citanest Plain)	It is best to use local anesthetics with less or no epinephrine in the presence of tachycardia. Use a maximum of 2 carpules. Avoid epinephrine in presence of mild to moderate hypertension. Use 4% prilocaine HCL without epinephrine (Citanest Plain) after obtaining a **clearance** for dentistry from the patient's obstretrician.
ANALGESICS: 1. Acetaminophen (Tylenol) 2. Codeine + Tylenol 3. Hydrocodone + Tylenol (Vicodin) 4. Oxycodone + Tylenol (Percocet) 5. Morphine and Meperidine 6. Fentanyl 7. Hydromorphone	**ALWAYS GET MD/OBSTRETRICIAN APPROVAL PRIOR TO PRESCRIBING ANALGESICS DURING PREGNANCY** **Acetaminophen** is **the** analgesic and antipyretic of choice during pregnancy. **Narcotics with "no risk in controlled animal studies":** Narcotics that can be used short term for 2–3 days in the first or second trimester of pregnancy are oxycodone, morphine, meperidine, fentanyl, and hydromorphone. **Oxycodone is the safest and ideal narcotic.** **Hydrocodone** is less safe during pregnancy compared with Percocet. **Codeine** rapidly crosses the placenta and is considered "less safe" during pregnancy, compared with Percocet. Avoid aspirin and NSAIDS, especially in first and third trimester, and prescribe Pregnancy Category B ibuprofen or naproxen, with MD approval, for no more than 2–3 days if NSAIDS are absolutely needed at other times during the pregnancy.
ANTIBIOTICS: Use Standard dose of: 1. All Penicillins 2. All Cephalosporins 3. Erythromycin (not used now) 4. Azithromycin (Zithromax) 5. Clindamycin (Cleocin)	Use Pen. VK to treat acute oral infections (symptomatic for less than three days). *Use clindamycin with penicillin or if the infection has been symptomatic for more than three days.

Suggested Guidelines for Anesthetics, Analgesics, Antibiotics Use During Pregnancy

Refer to Table 49.1 for a list of AAAs and guidelines for their safe use during pregnancy.

LACTATION/BREAST-FEEDING

American Association of Pediatricians (AAP) recommendations for breast-feeding:

- Infants should be breast-fed exclusively for first six months.

- Breast-feeding should continue until one year of age, with supplementation of solid foods after six months.
- **Benefits of breast-feeding include:**
  - Colostrum, which is the first flow, helps the digestive system so the baby has less gas, fewer feeding issues, and less constipation, which are typically associated with formula use.
  - Breast milk contains antibodies that help the baby's immune system, thereby lowering the risk of asthma, obesity, and allergies.
  - The incidence of sudden infant death (SIDS) is less.
  - Cheap and convenient.
- **Contraindications for breast-feeding include:**
  - Mother taking antineoplastic, thyrotoxic, and immunosuppressive drugs.
  - Mother receiving radioactive isotopes.
  - Mother undergoing chemotherapy or radiation therapy.

Outlined in the following sections are the anesthetics, analgesics, and antibiotics that are safe for use in the lactating patient, after breast-feeding has occurred.

Safe Local Anesthetics During Lactation

The following local anesthetics are safe for use during lactation (Table 49.2):

1. 2% lidocaine with 1:100,000 epinephrine (Xylocaine)
2. 0.5% bupivacaine with 1:200,000 epinephrine (Marcaine)
3. 4% septocaine with 1:100,000 or 1:200,000 epinephrine (Articaine)
4. 4% prilocaine HCL with 1:200,000 epinephrine or without epinephrine (Citanest Forte/Citanest Plain)
5. 2% mepivacaine (Carbocaine) with 1:20,000 levonordefrin
6. 3% mepivacaine (Carbocaine)

In a hypertensive lactating patient with stage I hypertension, use a local anesthetic with 1:200,000 epinephrine, and avoid epinephrine in the local anesthetic in the stage II hypertension patient.

Safe Analgesics During Lactation

The following analgesics are safe when used short-term during lactation. The mother should "pump and dump" the breast milk when taking narcotics to avoid sedating the baby.

1. Acetaminophen (Tylenol)
2. Codeine + Tylenol (Tylenol #1–3)
3. Hydrocodone + Tylenol (Vicodin)
4. Oxycodone + Tylenol (Percocet)

Opioids pass through the breast milk; therefore, accordingly use lower doses and prescribe opioids only when absolutely needed. Avoid prescribing opioid analgesics such as codeine, hydrocodone, and oxycodone that are converted to active metabolites by CYP2D6 or need CYP2D6 for clearance in mothers who happen to be very rapid CYP2D6

Table 49.2. Suggested Anesthetics, Analgesics, and Antibiotics Guidelines During Lactation

Safe Medications	Precautions/Remarks
LOCAL ANESTHETICS:	
1. 2% Lidocaine, 1:100,000 epinephrine (Xylocaine)	Inject the local anesthetic **after** the baby has been fed.
2. 0.5% Bupivacaine with 1:200,000 epinephrine (Marcaine)	For stage I hypertensive lactating patient: Use a local anesthetic with 1:200,000 epinephrine.
3. 4% Septocaine with 1:100,000 and 1,200,000 epinephrine (Articaine)	Avoid epinephrine in the stage II hypertension patient. Defer routine dental treatment in a stage III hypertensive lactating patient.
4. 4% Prilocaine HCL with 1:200,000 epinephrine or without epinephrine (Citanest Forte/Citanest Plain)	
5. 3% Mepivacaine (Carbocaine)	
6. 2% Mepivacaine (Carbocaine) with 1:20,000 Levonordefrin (NeoCobefrin)	
ANALGESICS:	
1. Acetaminophen (Tylenol)	The patient should take the pain medication **after** breast-feeding and keep a **2-hour** interval with the next feed.
2. Codeine + Tylenol (Tylenol #1–3)	
3. Hydrocodone + Tylenol (Vicodin)	
4. Oxycodone + Tylenol (Percocet)	Opioids pass through the breast milk. Use lower doses and prescribe opioids only when absolutely needed.
ANTIBIOTIC:	
1. All Penicillins	The patient should take the antibiotic **after** breast-feeding and keep a **2-hour** interval with the next feed.
2. All Cephalosporins	
3. All Macrolides	
4. Clindamycin	Minimize antibiotic use because of the risk of altering the baby's intestinal flora and promoting the growth of resistant pathogens.

metabolizers. Risk of opioid overdose exists in the babies of mothers who happen to be very rapid CYP2D6 metabolizers.

Some individuals are genetically predisposed to metabolize codeine much faster and more completely than others. These individuals are called ultra-rapid metabolizers. They are more likely to have higher-than-normal levels of morphine in their blood after taking codeine. Ultra-rapid CYP2D6 metabolism occurs in 3% African Americans, 10% Caucasians, and in 1% of Chinese and Hispanics.

Mothers who are ultra-rapid metabolizers may have higher-than-usual levels of morphine in their breast milk. Excess morphine in a nursing baby will cause increased sleepiness, difficulty breast-feeding, breathing difficulties, or limpness. Be aware that codeine can cause drowsiness in lactating newborns. Chronic use of morphine or meperidine can cause drowsiness in the breast-feeding infant.

The patient should pump and discard breast milk while taking the opioid and should switch to acetaminophen or NSAIDS as soon as possible. It is best to use the lowest dose of the shortest-acting NSAIDS and advise the patient to consume the medication, post feeding.

The following analgesics are safest to use during lactation: acetaminophen (Tylenol), ibuprofen (Motrin), and tramadol (Ultram); **note** that small amounts of tramadol cross into breast milk.

Safe Antibiotics During Lactation

The following antibiotics are safe for use during lactation (Table 49.2):

1. All penicillins
2. All cephalosporins
3. All macrolides
4. Clindamycin

Unsafe Antibiotics During Lactation

The following antibiotics are unsafe for use during lactation: tetracycline HCL and doxycycline (Vibramycin).

ORAL AND SYSTEMIC CONTRACEPTIVES

Hormonal Contraception

Some oral contraceptive pills contain estrogen and progestin, and are called combination oral contraceptive pills (COCPs). The COCPs contain progesterone and estrogen, which are more commonly in the form of ethinylestradiol and less commonly as estradiol valerate/mestranol. Most patients take the combination pills.

Some contraceptive pills contain only progestin. The progesterone-only pill contains progesterone in the form of desogestrel/gestodene/drospirenone. The higher progestin strength in some preparations may increase the risk for blood clots when compared with other birth control pills with lower progestin strength. Progestin can also raise potassium levels in the blood, and this could cause heart and health problems.

COCP method of action: Estrogen interferes with ovulation and progesterone thickens the cervical mucosa, blocking sperm passage and thinning the uterine mucosa, thus preventing embryo implantation.

Commonly Available Contraceptives

NuvaRing

NuvaRing is a once-a-month contraceptive that contains estrogen and progestin. It works similar to the hormones in oral contraceptive pills (OCPs). With NuvaRing, the hormone release is activated once the ring comes into contact with the vagina. The hormones are absorbed and distributed into the bloodstream. The ring is kept in place for three weeks and then removed. Menstruation occurs during the fourth week, after which a new ring is inserted by the patient. When used appropriately, NuvaRing is found to be 99% effective in preventing pregnancy.

Levonorgestrel-Releasing Intrauterine System (Mirena)

Mirena is a soft, flexible intra-uterine device (IUD) that releases small amounts of hormone locally into the uterus. It protects against pregnancy for up to five years.

Silicone-Free Insert: Essure

Essure is a permanent, hormone-free transcervical sterilization procedure, whereby the gynecologist inserts small, soft silicone-free inserts into the fallopian tubes. These inserts mold to the shape of the fallopian tubes and stay in place to prevent pregnancy. During the first three months after insertion when the body is creating a natural barrier to stop the sperm from reaching the ovary, the patient needs to use barrier protection to prevent pregnancy.

Birth Control Implant (Implanon and Nexplanon)

Birth control implants are safe, effective, and convenient methods of contraception, and their effectiveness lasts for three years. A very thin progestin-releasing implant is inserted into the patient's arm by the gynecologist. The implant prevents pregnancy by inhibiting ovulation and thickening the cervical mucus.

Birth Control Patch (Ortho Evra)

Ortho Evra is an ethinyl estradiol and norelgestromin combination, transdermal patch that is safe, effective, and conveniently sticks to the skin. The patch prevents pregnancy by releasing estrogen and progestin. A new patch is placed on the skin once a week for three weeks in a row, followed by a patch-free week.

Birth Control Shot (Depo-Provera)

Medroxyprogesterone is given as an intramuscular (IM) or subcutaneous (SC) injection. Each shot in the arm delivers progestin that prevents pregnancy by inhibiting ovulation. It is safe, convenient, and effective for three months.

Long-Acting Contraception Alerts

- The effectiveness of long-acting reversible contraception is superior to that of contraceptive pills, patch, or ring, and it is not altered in adolescents and young women.
- Dental alert: Long-acting contraception injections can cause bone thinning that reverses once the injections are stopped.

Antibiotic Use with Oral Contraceptives

It was long thought that because oral antibiotics interfered with estrogen metabolism and estrogen levels, dentists were required to advise patients on oral contraceptives to use barrier protection until the end of the next cycle. **It has now been documented sufficiently well that the commonly prescribed antibiotics in the dental setting do not interfere with estrogen metabolism, and the dentist no longer needs to advise additional barrier contraception measures when prescribing oral antibiotics in the presence of COCPs.**

Estrogen Metabolism

- Once estrogen is absorbed from the small intestine, it undergoes first-bypass metabolism in the liver getting conjugated with glucuronic acid. This conjugate is then excreted into the bile; thus, estrogen re-enters the small intestine and then the large intestine as a conjugate. Hydrolytic enzymes contained in the intestinal bacteria cleave the glucuronic-estrogen conjugates, enabling estrogen to be reabsorbed in the large intestine and enter the entero-hepatic circulation. It is important to note that progesterone does **not** have an enterohepatic recycling like estrogen.

- Oral antibiotics up until now were postulated to interfere with estrogen metabolism by decreasing or destroying the intestinal flora. This concept has now been negated by recent evidence based studies, which have demonstrated that only CYP450 enzyme inducer drugs accelerate estrogen metabolism and impact the efficacy of estrogen-containing combined oral contraceptives (COCPs).

- **Antibiotics in dentistry:** Penicillins, cephalosporins, clindamycin, macrolides, tetracyclines, and quinolones **do not** induce the CYP450 enzyme, and consequently do not affect estrogen level and no barrier protection is needed for short- or long-term use of routine antibiotics prescribed in the dental setting.

- **"Low-Dose" COCPs:** The hormone doses/strengths of the low-dose (<35μg of estrogen) COCPs are now much lower than they used to be. Patients can show greater hormone level reductions, thus putting them at risk of unintended pregnancy, when pushed a little lower by co-administration of drugs that accelerate estrogen metabolism. The provider must suggest alternative contraception or barrier protection when prescribing the estrogen metabolism accelerator drugs in conjunction with COCPs. The same warnings should apply for both intravenous (IV) and oral contraceptives, as the warnings have not been specifically differentiated between the two.

- **Estrogen metabolism accelerator drugs:** As strong competitors in the cytochrome P450 chain, rifampin, anti-epileptics, atypical antipsychotics, azole antifungals and St. John's wort have significant impact on the metabolism of COCPs, because they accelerate the metabolism of the estrogen component of the pill. Note that azole antifungals are the only "interfering" drugs on this list that can potentially be prescribed in the dental setting. Therefore, when prescribed, the patient should be advised to use an alternative method of contraception or be advised to switch to a higher-dose COCP (if using low-dose contraceptives), for the duration of intake of the estrogen-accelerator drug. It is best for the dental provider to **dispense nystatin** instead of the azoles when an antifungal is needed.

- **Diarrhea/vomiting and contraceptive pills:** Vomiting and significant, persistent diarrhea can affect pill potency by interfering with the absorption of both progesterone-only contraceptive pills **and** COCPs. Be aware that antibiotics, including those used in dentistry, can cause vomiting and/or diarrhea. Vomiting that occurs within two hours of taking the pill can also affect pill potency. When faced with any one of these situations always advise your patient to use extra barrier protection **for one week minimum** post vomiting/diarrhea or until the end of the next cycle for complete safety and to avoid accidental pregnancy.

- Always check during history-taking if the patient uses birth control or oral contraceptive pills and details of the type of contraception. **Let the patient know that it is firmly established now that oral antibiotics can only decrease the potency** of combined oral contraceptive pills (COCPs) or progesterone-only contraceptive pills when antibiotics cause severe, persistent diarrhea or vomiting, essentially "washing out" the pills. It is only then that the patient will have to use extra barrier protection to prevent pregnancy, until one-week post vomiting and/or diarrhea, or, if conservative, until the end of the next cycle.

- Always enter a case note in the record stating that the patient has been so informed.

Rheumatology: Diseases of the Joints, Bones, and Muscles

XVII

Classic Rheumatic Diseases: Assessment and Associated Dental Management Guidelines

RHEUMATOLOGY OVERVIEW, FACTS, AND DISEASE CLASSIFICATION

Rheumatic diseases are chronic conditions that cause significant morbidity and affect the patient's quality of life. The patient is often on immunosuppressants to control the underlying inflammation and to improve the long-term outcome of the disease.

It is important to remember that immunosuppressants **decrease** inflammation but **increase** the incidence of infections. This increased incidence of infections, coupled with the poor oral hygiene and increased dental decay found in this population, stresses the importance of regular dental intervention for these patients.

Arthritis affecting the hands can also make it difficult for the patient to keep up with the routines of daily oral care. Extractions are often needed when the decay is extensive because the patient has neglected going to the dentist. Thus, the patient must incorporate regular dental visits as an important part of the multidisciplinary care to stay dentally healthy.

Classification of Rheumatic Diseases

Rheumatic diseases are classified as follows:

1. **Classic rheumatic diseases that commonly affect the joints:** Systemic lupus erythematosus (SLE), scleroderma, Sjögren's syndrome, Reiter's syndrome, Behçet's syndrome, temporal or giant cell arteritis, rheumatoid arthritis (RA), osteoarthritis, ankylosing spondilitis, diffuse idiopathic skeletal hyperostosis (DISH), Forestier disease, and gout.
2. **Diseases affecting the bones:** Paget's disease.
3. **Diseases affecting the muscles:** Malignant hyperthermia, polymyositis, Parkinson's disease, myasthenia gravis, and multiple sclerosis.

Dentist's Guide to Medical Conditions, Medications, and Complications, Second Edition. Kanchan M. Ganda.
© 2013 John Wiley & Sons, Inc. Published 2013 by John Wiley & Sons, Inc.

SYSTEMIC LUPUS ERYTHEMATOSUS

Overview

Systemic lupus erythematosus (SLE) is a chronic autoimmune condition associated with a hyperactive immune system that attacks normal tissue. The exact cause for this adverse action is unknown. Systemic lupus is a multisystem disease that can affect the skin, joints, blood, lungs, kidney, heart, brain, and the nervous system. SLE typically affects women in the child-bearing age, and it is postulated that estrogen plays a role with this disease state. Antibody production is important for the diagnosis of SLE.

Eleven Criteria Associated with SLE

To make a diagnosis of SLE at least four of the following eleven criteria must be present:

1. **Anemia:** Lupus-associated CBC will show leukopenia, lymphopenia, and thrombocytopenia.
2. **Arthritis:** SLE-associated arthritis affects the major and minor joints.
3. **Discoid rash:** Discoid lupus or cutaneous lupus affects the skin causing a discoid rash. The discoid lupus patient, similar to the SLE patient, experiences increased photosensitivity.
4. **Increased photosensitivity:** The least amount of sun exposure causes blistering and sunburn with lupus.
5. **Neurological disorder:** SLE can be associated with seizures and/or psychosis.
6. **Oral ulcers:** Lupus-associated ulcers are nonspecific, shallow, and painless. Nasal ulcerations often coexist.
7. **Renal disease:** Lupus-associated renal disease is demonstrated by an elevated serum creatinine and BUN levels.
8. **Serositis:** SLE causes inflammation of the pericardial and pleural linings.
9. **The malar or the butterfly rash:** This lupus-associated rash occurs on the face, spanning over the nose and the cheeks, but not occurring below the nasolabial fold.
10. **Positive ANA test:** The antinuclear antibody (ANA) test is a screening test for lupus. Active lupus is associated with high levels of antinuclear antibodies. The majority of patients with SLE have a positive ANA test at some point during their disease. However, the ANA test is not specific for lupus. It can be positive in healthy people and in patients suffering from other connective tissue disorders.
11. **Other blood tests:** Other blood tests that can assist with the diagnosis of lupus are the LE test, the anti-ds DNA test, the anti-Sm test, the anti-Ro test, and the anti-La test.

The LE (lupus erythematosus) cell test is positive in only 50% of patients with SLE. In some cases the patient may be tested for specific ANA subtypes. Anti–double-stranded DNA (anti-ds DNA) is usually found only in SLE patients. Anti-Sm antibodies are also usually found only with SLE. When the ANA is negative and there is a strong suspicion for lupus, the anti-Ro and anti-La antibodies, when detected, can identify a rare form of lupus called **Ro lupus**.

Symptoms and Signs

No two patients with lupus will have similar symptoms. Symptoms will vary according to the organ systems affected. Additionally, these patients can have alopecia and may present with oral candidiasis due to the underlying xerostomia commonly affecting the majority of these patients. Overwhelming infection and kidney failure are two of the common causes of death in people with lupus.

Treatment

The treatment is aimed at decreasing inflammation with high dose NSAIDS, corticosteroids, and cytotoxic drugs.

Drug Precautions

Patients with lupus are **often** allergic to multiple drugs. Always go through the allergy history very carefully. Drug history may show that the patient has responded adversely to sulpha antimicrobials and penicillin in the past. All drugs causing even a minimal form of allergy should be avoided.

SCLERODERMA

Scleroderma is an autoimmune condition associated with excessive fibrosis or scar tissue formation involving organs and the skin of the face and distal extremities. Scleroderma causes thickness and firmness of the affected areas. Vascular reactivity causing Raynaud's phenomenon is quite significant with scleroderma. Auto-antibodies are useful in the diagnosis of the disease.

Forms of Scleroderma

There are two forms of the disease: diffuse scleroderma and limited scleroderma.

Diffuse Scleroderma

Diffuse scleroderma is the more severe form of scleroderma, which begins with thickening of the skin of the trunk and extremities. This rapidly progresses to fibrosis and involvement of vital organs. Heart, lungs, esophagus, and the kidneys can be affected. Renal insufficiency occurs in >10% of patients. Antiscleroderma-70 antibodies are present in 40% of the patients.

Limited Scleroderma/Limited Form (CREST)

This is the more benign form of scleroderma and it affects mainly the skin of the face and the digits. This form progresses slowly. CREST represents the clinical pattern associated with this form and it stands for calcinosis, Raynaud's phenomenon, esophageal involvement, sclerodactyly, and telangiactasias. There is less cardiac and pulmonary involvement with this form of scleroderma. Anticentromeric antibodies are exhibited by 80% of the patients.

Clinical Features

The scleroderma patient can present with the following features:

1. **Microstomia:** Microstomia is a classic oral manifestation of scleroderma.
2. **Retracted skin of the face and hands:** The skin on the face is retracted, the lips are pursed, and the skin is tightly bound around the digits. This can cause a "mouse face" appearance in the late stages.
3. **Swollen hands:** Swollen hands are caused by diffuse edema.
4. **Raynaud's phenomenon:** Raynaud's phenomenon causes the patient to experience white, painful fingers and toes due to vasoconstriction.
5. **Arthritis:** Scleroderma-associated arthritis affects the major and the minor joints.
6. **Dysphagia or regurgitation:** Smooth muscle dysfunction involving the lower two-thirds of the esophagus occurs, causing dysphagia or regurgitation. The patient can swallow but cannot get the food down.
7. **Pulmonary fibrosis:** Pulmonary fibrosis is progressive and is associated with significant breathing difficulty as the condition worsens.
8. **Myocardial fibrosis:** Myocardial fibrosis causes arrhythmia and spells poor prognosis.
9. **Kidney disease:** Renal involvement also indicates poor disease prognosis.

Diagnosis

The diagnosis of scleroderma is based on the presence of the clinical features of the disease and specific blood tests. Most scleroderma patients are antinuclear antibody (ANA)–positive.

The CREST or the limited form is exclusively positive for the anticentromere antibody. The Anti-Scl 70 antibody (anti–topo-isomerase I antibody) is positive in most cases of the diffuse form of scleroderma.

Treatment

Treatment is directed toward the organs affected. Special emphasis is placed on the monitoring and control of the blood pressure (BP) to slow the progression of associated kidney disease.

SJÖGREN'S SYNDROME

Introduction

Sjögren's syndrome is a chronic autoimmune condition associated with hypofunction of the lacrimal glands, causing dry eyes or keratoconjunctivitis sicca and hypofunction of the salivary glands, which causes xerostomia.

The "old" Sjögren's syndrome (SS) classification that is now considered obsolete was based on the presence or absence of other autoimmune conditions with SS. It was classified as "Primary," when the autoimmune condition was present alone and "Secondary" when the condition was present with other autoimmune conditions such as systemic lupus erythematosus (SLE), rheumatoid arthritis (RA), or scleroderma.

The "new" American-European classification system for the diagnosis of primary Sjögren's syndrome is based on the fulfillment of objective criteria. It requires the patient to have four of the six criteria, and either criterion number 5 or criterion number 6 must be met. In the Sjögren's syndrome patient that has no sicca symptoms, the diagnosis of SS can be made if the patient has met three of the four objective criteria (criteria numbers 3–6).

Criteria

The six diagnostic criteria are as follows:

1. **Ocular symptoms:** The patient has a history of having had dry eyes for more than three months, having a foreign-body sensation in the eyes, and having used tear substitutes more than three times daily.
2. **Oral symptoms:** The patient complains of having a history of feeling dry in the mouth, having recurrently swollen salivary glands, and frequently drinks water or other liquids to help with swallowing.
3. **Ocular signs:** Schirmer's test shows <5mm tearing in five minutes, and ocular staining shows a score ≥3, thus confirming the diagnosis of xerophthalmia or keratoconjunctivitis sicca.
4. **Oral signs:** Oral signs demonstrate abnormal salivary scintigraphy findings, abnormal parotid sialography findings, and abnormal sialometry findings, showing unstimulated salivary flow <1.5mL in 15 minutes.
5. **Positive blood test:** The blood test shows a positive serum anti-SSA/Ro and/or anti-SSB/La or a positive rheumatoid factor and antinuclear antibody titer ≥1:320.
6. **Positive minor salivary gland biopsy:** The labial minor salivary gland biopsy shows focal lymphocytic sialadenitis with a focus score ≥1 focus/4mm^2.

Sjögren's syndrome patients need coordinated care provided by experts in the fields of oral health, rheumatology, and ophthalmology to achieve the optimal evaluation and management of this condition. Treatment is largely based on symptoms, and the patient should be monitored for the potential development of lymphoma.

Most Sjögren's syndrome patients present with sicca symptoms: xerophthalmia (dry eyes), xerostomia (dry mouth), and parotid gland enlargement. Additionally, the patient may also have arthralgia, arthritis, Raynaud's phenomenon, myalgia, pulmonary disease, gastrointestinal disease, leucopenia, anemia, lymphadenopathy, neuropathy, vasculitis, renal tubular acidosis, and lymphoma. Almost 50% of patients with SS have cutaneous findings such as dry skin (xeroderma), palpable and nonpalpable purpura, and/or urticaria.

Complications

General complications associated with SS are:

- **Other autoimmune conditions:** There can be an emergence of systemic lupus erythematosus (SLE) and rheumatoid arthritis (RA).
- **Lacrimal gland occlusion:** Occlusion of the lacrimal puncta is corrected surgically by electrocautery and other techniques for permanent punctal occlusion.

- **Parotid gland infection:** Typically staphylococcal, streptococcal, or pneumococcal infection can occur. The patient can present with unilateral worsening of symptoms, along with tenderness, warmth, and erythema. An elevated amylase level may occur from parotid gland involvement.
- **Parotid tumors:** The provider should always be on the lookout for any new unusually hard or unilateral parotid enlargement.
- **Pregnancy outcome:** Pregnant patients with a positive SS-related blood test are at risk for fetal loss, complete heart block in the fetus, and neonatal lupus syndrome in the newborn.
- **Lymphomas:** The patient can present with pseudo-lymphomas, showing pleomorphic cells, and non-Hodgkin B-cell lymphomas.

Xerostomia-Associated Oral Side Effects and Dental Alerts

Side effects and dental alerts include:

- Inability to eat crackers because they stick to the roof the mouth.
- The tongue often sticks to the roof of the mouth.
- Drinking water at night, resulting in nocturia.
- Difficulty speaking for long periods of time or of hoarseness.
- Higher incidence of dental caries and periodontal disease, which warrants more frequent visits to the dentist and hygienist.
- Altered sense of taste.
- Difficulty wearing dentures due to xerostomia, and the patient needing frequent dentire adjustments.
- Development of oral candidiasis with painful angular cheilitis.
- Lack of saliva may lead to impaired clearance of acid, and this may result in gastroesophageal reflux and esophagitis.
- Patients with Sjögren's syndrome are at increased risk for delayed gastric emptying, upper abdominal discomfort, nausea, and vomiting. Always have the patient seated in a semi-sitting position in the chair.
- Cranial neuropathies, particularly trigeminal neuropathy, or facial nerve palsy can develop along with CNS involvement in general. Avoid using the 4% local anesthetics in SS patients.
- A progressively elevated erythrocyte sedimentation rate (ESR) indicates active/ progressive inflammation, and this warrants consultation with the patient's physician. Routine dentistry must be temporarily deferred.
- CBC may show anemia, leucopenia, and/or eosinophilia. Pernicious anemia may be associated with the atrophic gastritis. An abnormal WBC, count, especially with an abnormal differential count, should trigger concerns for a lympho-reticular malignancy. In addition, although a low platelet or WBC count can occur in persons with primary Sjögren's syndrome, the finding should also prompt the provider to consider coexisting SLE. Half of the SS patients present with mild, normochromic, normocytic anemia, and leukopenia occurs in almost half of the SS patients. Implement appropriate anemia or ANC-associated guidelines, when required.
- Renal stones, progressive weakness, and paralysis secondary to hypokalemia from underlying renal tubular acidosis and osteomalacia are not uncommon with SS. Severe hypokalemia can lead to periodic paralysis. Renal tubular acidosis can also be

associated with a low bicarbonate level. Always obtain serum creatinine and electrolytes prior to dentistry, and implement appropriate deviations in AAAs in the presence of decreased renal function.

- High total protein level or a low albumin level should prompt the clinician to perform serum protein electrophoresis
- The patient can have high alkaline phosphatase level due to associated primary biliary cirrhosis that commonly affects SS patients.
- Chronic active hepatitis or hepatitis C can also occur with SS, causing an elevated transaminase levels. Mild (less than twofold) increases in transaminase levels are not uncommon with SS, so always obtain LFTs prior to dentistry.

Prognosis

Per say, the prognosis for Sjögren's syndrome is good if the patient does not develop a lympho-proliferative disorder. Declining exocrine gland function from infiltration with lymphocytes does increase the morbidity associated with Sjögren's syndrome. The SS-associated mortality rate increases when disorders such as RA, SLE, primary biliary cirrhosis, and/or lymphoma occur, which cause a decline in function.

Treatment

No curative agents for Sjögren's syndrome exist. The treatment of the disorder is essentially symptomatic. In secondary Sjögren's syndrome, treatment is based on the accompanying disease and its clinical features. Sjögren's syndrome and associated SLE improve more than primary Sjögren's syndrome. In Sjögren's syndrome associated with polymyositis, monthly cyclophosphamide pulse therapy has been successful. Long-term anticoagulation may be needed in patients with vascular thrombosis related to antiphospholipid antibody syndrome. Among the biologic therapies, etanercept has failed to demonstrate benefit in Sjögren's syndrome, whereas rituximab appears promising in the treatment of vasculitis and intravenous immunoglobulin (IVIG)–dependent ataxic neuropathy.

Dry Mouth Therapy

Dry mouth therapy consists of:

- Frequent sips of water.
- Sugar-free lemon drops to stimulate salivary secretion.
- Patients should avoid medications with anticholinergic and antihistamine effects.
- Humidifier use can possibly help.
- Regular dental check ups and fluoride treatments.
- Use toothpaste without mouth irritation: Recommend Biotene toothpaste, Biotene mouth rinse, Dental Care toothpaste, and Oral Balance gel.
- Assess for oral candidiasis and angular cheilitis. Treat infection with topical antifungal such as nystatin troches, but oral fluconazole may occasionally be needed. Denture wearers should disinfect their dentures.
- Treat all sinus-related issues immediately because these issues, when untreated, can promote mouth breathing and worsening of xerostomia.

- The patient should use isotonic sodium chloride solution nasal sprays and avoid antihistamine use.

Topical and Systemic Therapies

Topical and systemic therapies are also discussed in Chapter 48. The reader is advised to review those contents and the contents discussed here.

Topical Therapies

Artificial saliva preparations contain methylcellulose, sorbitol, and salts to moisten and lubricate the mouth. Topical therapy for Sjögren's syndrome should be prioritized, but pilocarpine or cevimeline should be opted for treatment of xerostomia when local therapy is not successful.

Common OTC artificial saliva preparations:

1. **Oasis:** Contains glycerin and hydrogenated castor oil, is ethanol and sugar free, and has a mild mint flavor.
   Rx: 1–2 sprays PRN; not to exceed 60 sprays/day.
2. **Aquoral:** Oxidized glycerol preparation that delivers 400 citrus-flavored sprays.
   Rx: 2 sprays oral (PO), tid/qid PRN.
3. **Caphosol:** Caphosol is packaged in two 15mL ampoules that when mixed together provide one 30mL dose.
   The patient should swish and spit contents and should not use more than 10 doses/day.
4. **SalivaSure:** Lozenge contains xylitol.
   Rx: Dissolve lozenge in mouth PRN; dose should not to exceed 16 lozenges/day.
5. **XyliMelts:** XyliMelts as xylitol in time-release discs is dispensed in 500mg strength.
   Rx: During the day, use can be as needed. At night, the patient applies two discs before bed, one on each side of the mouth in the lower or upper part of the cheek. The patient swallows as the disc slowly dissolves.

Systemic Therapies

1. **Pilocarpine (Salagen):** Pilocarpine, a saliva stimulant, is a cholinergic parasympathetic drug that enhances exocrine glands secretion.
   Radiation-induced xerostomia dose: 5mg oral (PO) tid; dose may be titrated up to 10mg oral tid, but should not exceed 30mg/day.
   Xerostomia associated with Sjögren's syndrome dose: 5mg oral qid.
   Pilocarpine dose for all indications, in the presence of moderate hepatic insufficiency: Start with 5mg PO bid, then adjust dose according to patient tolerance and treatment benefit. Pilocarpine is not recommended for severe liver insufficiency.
2. **Cevimeline (Evoxac):** Cevimeline is also a saliva stimulant, indicated for xerostomia in Sjögren's syndrome.
   Rx: 30mg PO tid.
3. **Rituximab** is an up-and-coming drug that has shown significant improvement of saliva flow rate and lacrimal gland function in studies with patients with primary Sjögren's syndrome.

Other Therapies

1. **Artificial Tears:** Nu-Tears, Murine Tears, Refresh, and Tears Naturale are preparations that contain the equivalent of 0.9% sodium chloride and are used to maintain ocular tonicity. They replace the aqueous layer of tears that is lost in patients with Sjögren's syndrome. Preparations that have hydroxymethylcellulose or dextran are more viscous and therefore can last longer before reapplication is needed.
2. **Cyclosporine ophthalmic (Restasis):** Cyclosporine ophthalmic is used to relieve dry eyes caused by suppressed tear production secondary to ocular inflammation. It is thought to act as a partial immune modulator, but the exact mechanism of action is not known.
3. **Cyclophosphamide (Cytoxan):** Cyclophosphamide is an alkylating agent with potent immunosuppressant properties. It is used in patients with Sjögren's syndrome who develop a major organ manifestation such as interstitial lung disease. The CBC should be monitored when the patient is on cyclophosphamide.
4. **Hydroxychloroquine (Plaquenil):** Hydroxychloroquine is an antimalarial drug that is used to treat Sjögren's syndrome–associated arthritis that unresponsive to NSAIDS. The mechanism of action in inflammatory arthritis is unknown.
5. **Prednisone:** Prednisone decreases inflammation by reversing increased capillary permeability and suppressing polymorphonuclear cell activity. Prednisone stabilizes lysosomal membranes and also suppresses lymphocytes and antibody production and activity.
6. **Methylprednisolone (A-Methapred, Solu-Medrol, Depo-Medrol):** Methylprednisolone is available in intravenous (IV)/intramuscular (IM) or oral (PO) form. Like prednisone, methylprednisolone also decreases inflammation by reversing increased capillary permeability and suppressing polymorphonuclear (PMN) leukocyte activity.

REITER'S SYNDROME

Reiter's syndrome or reactive arthritis is an autoimmune condition that affects white males, most commonly, ages 20–40. It occurs in response to a genitourinary or gastrointestinal infection. It is an HLA-B27–linked inflammatory arthritis that damages the cartilage of the joints, which triggers subacute or chronic inflammatory disease. The inflammatory response triggers a triad of symptoms: arthritis, uveitis, and urethritis.

Characteristic Features

The characteristic features associated with Reiter's syndrome are conjunctivitis, nonspecific urethritis, arthritis affecting mostly the joints of the lower extremities (feet and heels), and painless, shallow oral and genital ulcers.

Treatment

Treatment consists of providing adequate antibiotics to treat the precipitating infection, NSAIDS, and corticosteroids.

BEHÇET'S SYNDROME

Behçet's syndrome, or Behçet's disease, is associated with inflammation of the blood vessels. Behçet's syndrome affects patients who are 20–30 years old. The disease is chronic and recurrent with asymptomatic periods in between, but the flare-ups are unpredictable. It is prevalent in North Africa, Turkey, the Middle East, Korea, and Japan.

Clinical Features

Behçet's syndrome is characterized as follows:

1. Features include painful, deep oral ulcers involving the mucous membrane of lips, gingiva, cheeks, and tongue; painful genital ulcers; and anterior or posterior uveitis that can lead to blindness.
2. **Pathergy:** This is a hyperirritable reaction to needle puncture such that blistering occurs at the puncture site.
3. **Arthritis:** Pain and swelling of the joints is quite significant.
4. Thrombophlebitis.
5. Meningitis.
6. Thrombosis.
7. Neurological symptoms can occasionally occur but are rare.

Behçet's Syndrome Treatment

Treatment is symptomatic and focuses on pain relief and prevention of serious problems.

TEMPORAL OR GIANT CELL ARTERITIS

Temporal or giant cell arteritis is a vasculitis that affects medium and large blood vessels, particularly in the head. It is called **temporal arteritis** because the temporal artery is frequently affected. The alternate name, giant cell arteritis reflects the cells seen on biopsy of the affected blood vessel.

It is not a permanent disease because it completely disappears in 1–2 years. The disease affects the elderly, and women are more affected than men. It is rare before age 50 and is most common around age 70.

Classic Features

The patient typically complains of temporal headache that is associated with a tender, thickened, and nodular temporal artery. However, temporal arteritis can also affect other vessels such as the opthalmic, facial, or lingual arteries. Ophthalmic and posterior ciliary arteries, when involved, can lead to blindness.

Facial artery involvement is rare, but when it occurs it is associated with painful jaw swelling or claudication. Lingual artery involvement is rare and when affected it causes color change, paresthesias, and necrosis of the tongue. Oral pain may be prominent at the level of the gums.

Diagnostic Test

Temporal or giant cell arteritis characteristically shows immediate elevation of the ESR with values rising at the rate of 100mm/h. Definitive diagnosis is established only with tissue biopsy of the affected vessel.

Treatment

Treatment consists of high-dose corticosteroids, which rapidly correct the symptoms and prevent blindness. Steroids should be given immediately even before the return of biopsy results if the suspicion is high. The corticosteroids are continued if the biopsy results are positive and discontinued with negative results. Once started, the steroids are gradually decreased over months.

RHEUMATOID ARTHRITIS

Rheumatoid arthritis (RA) affects more women than men and occurs around age 30 or older.

Clinical Features

The patient experiences symmetrical inflammation of the distal joints: digits, wrists, feet, and knees. The pain in the joints is worst upon waking up. The knuckles and the proximal interphalangeal joints of the hands and feet are affected. The cervical spine is involved in severe cases, but involvement of the spine is rare. Lumbar spine is always spared. The patient complains of prolonged morning stiffness, malaise, and sometimes a low-grade fever.

Cervical Spine Involvement

RA-associated cervical spine changes are prominent at the uncovertebral joints and bursae. Uncovertebral joints are small synovial joints formed secondarily between the lateral lips (uncinate processes) of the superior surfaces of the bodies of the lower cervical vertebrae, and the inferior surface of the superior vertebral body. The synovial bursae surrounding the dens are often affected, causing lysis and disruption of the transverse ligament of atlas and atlantoaxial subluxation. This can lead to impingement of the spinal cord. Cervical spine involvement is associated with the **Lehrmitte's sign** in which the patient experiences flashes of pain in all four extremities.

Cervical Spine Involvement Diagnosis

RA-associated cervical spine involvement is diagnosed with review of the cervical spine films taken with the neck in forward flexion. Diagnosis is confirmed by identifying an increased distance between the dens and the anterior arch of atlas.

Cervical Spine Involvement Treatment

Treatment consists of prompt surgical stabilization and consists of wiring of the C-1 and C-2 posterior arches.

Cricoaritenoid Arthritis

This is a frequent manifestation of RA. The patient experiences pain, dysphagia, fullness or tension in the throat, hoarseness, and stridor.

Rheumatoid Arthritis Blood Tests

CBC often shows thrombocytopenia and anemia in patients with RA.

Rheumatoid Arthritis Treatment

Treatment is symptomatic and focuses on pain relief: NSAIDS, corticosteroids, DMARDs, and chemotherapeutic drugs. Please also refer to the "Antirheumatic Medications" section in this chapter for detailed discussion of RA drug therapy.

Tocilizumab (Actemra) is a newly approved drug used to treat adult patients with moderately-to-severely active RA, who have had an inadequate response to tumor necrosis factor (TNF)-alfa inhibitors, as well as patients who have not responded well to methotrexate and other oral DMARDS.

Tocilizumab (Actemra) adverse effects: Tocilizumab use could be associated with upper airway infection, hypertension, hepatotoxicity as evidenced by an increased ALT, neutropenia, thrombocytopenia, demyelinating disorders, lipid abnormalities potentially precipitating cardiac disease, neurotoxicity, and gastrointestinal perforation. The provider must always assess the CBC with ANC counts prior to dentistry if the patient is on tocilizumab. Tuberculosis (TB), invasive bacterial, viral, and fungal opportunistic infections can occur with tocilizumab (Actemra). The drug is interrupted temporarily if a serious infection develops.

OSTEOARTHRITIS

Facts

Osteoarthritis is differentiated from RA in that osteoarthritis is associated with pain on rotation, negligible morning stiffness, and bony enlargements, especially affecting the hands. The pain of osteoarthritis is most pronounced at the end of the day. Joint involvement is unilateral and the major joints or distal interphalyngeal joints of the hands are affected. The patient does not experience any systemic symptoms, and there are no associated changes seen on the CBC. Treatment is symptomatic with NSAIDS or steroids.

ANKYLOSING SPONDILITIS

Young men are more affected than women, and the majority of these patients are HLA-B28 positive. Ankylosing spondilitis is associated with inflammation of vertebral attachment or outermost fibers of intervertebral discs. This results in ossification and spinal fusion.

Clinical Features

The patient experiences lack of motion and brittle cervical spine due to lack of muscle pulling. The patient finds it difficult to turn and complains of a stiff back and prolonged morning stiffness lasting for more than 30 minutes.

Diagnosis

Classic "bamboo spine" is seen on radiographs.

General Anesthesia

These patients present significant risk during general anesthesia because minor forces can fracture the neck precipitating quadric-paresis.

DIFFUSE IDIOPATHIC SKELETAL HYPEROSTOSIS OR FORESTIER DISEASE

Facts

Diffuse idiopathic skeletal hyperostosis (DISH) is characterized by the fusion of four vertebrae that are welded together by heavily ossified anterior longitudinal ligaments. This condition is limited to the dorsal spine area, and the cervical spine is often involved. Massive flame-shaped anterior osteophytes (bone spurs) can produce dysphagia. Compression of the cord is rare.

GOUT

Facts

Gout is an inherited disorder associated with an abnormality in the body's ability to process uric acid. Thus, there is an overload of uric acid in the body, recurring attacks of joint inflammation, and gouty arthritis.

Chronic gout is associated with kidney stones, decreased renal function, and progressive renal failure. Gouty arthritis is precipitated by deposits of uric acid crystals in the synovial fluid and the synovial lining. Intense joint inflammation occurs as white blood cells engulf the uric acid crystals and release lysosomal enzymes associated with inflammation, which causes pain, heat, and redness of the joint tissues.

Gout is more common in males. However, the numbers increase in females after menopause. Diseases often associated with gout are hypertension, obesity, leukemia, and lymphomas.

Symptoms and Signs

Gout attacks are very sudden in onset. The pain escalates rapidly as the joint gets inflamed. It is characteristic for only a single joint to be affected. The big toe, knees, ankle, small joints of the hands, and so on can be affected.

Clinical Features

During an attack, the joint swells and the skin over the joint becomes red, hot, and extremely painful. Chronic deposition of uric acid crystals causes tophi (tiny nodules/outgrowths), and these can be found at the outer rim of the pinna upon examination of the head and neck.

Diagnosis

Diagnosis of gout is established as follows:

1. **Medical history** will show the classic disease presentation, joint involvement history of sudden onset, and single joint involvement history.
2. **Blood tests** will show increased uric acid levels.
3. **Arthrocentesis**, finding uric acid crystals in the fluid aspirate from the joint, confirms the diagnosis.

Treatment

Treatment is as follows:

1. **Weight reduction:** Weight loss along with decreased alcohol consumption helps control the disease state.
2. **Dietary changes:** Diet should be low in animal protein and purine-containing food items.
3. **Water consumption:** The water intake should be increased to dilute the urine and decrease the formation of renal stones. Literature shows that dehydration increases the incidence of gout attacks.
4. **Medications:** Gout **therapy** is divided into three stages.

Medications: Acute and Maintenance Drugs

Acute Gout Medications

Treatment is provided with medications that treat acute gout and maintenance drugs that keep the patient symptom free between attacks. The following are classic acute gout medications:

1. **NSAIDS:** NSAIDS are given until symptoms abate. NSAIDS are contraindicated in the presence of kidney disease. Use maximal dosing of NSAIDS and continue for 24 hours after symptoms have improved, then taper over two to four days. Aspirin is not used for treatment at this time because of the effects of aspirin on uric acid transport.
2. **Corticosteroids:** Steroids are given short term to decrease the inflammation and are a useful alternative to NSAIDS in patients with associated kidney disease. Steroids can be taken by mouth, as intramuscular (IM) injection, or intra-articular injection. Generally, when given by mouth, the patient gets 40–60mg prednisone daily until symptoms resolve. Then the dose is tapered every three days.
3. **Colchicine:** As stated previously, during an acute gout attack, intense joint inflammation occurs as white blood cells engulf the uric acid crystals and release lysosomal enzymes associated with inflammation, causing pain, heat, and redness of the joint tissues. Colchicine helps suppress inflammation associated with the acute attack by decreasing WBC motility and phagocytosis in the joint. It also inhibits lactic acid production, and this, in turn, slows down the deposition of urate crystals in the joints. Colchicine is very effective in the management of an acute attack and it is given every few hours until the symptoms resolve. A double dose of colchicine is

followed by a third dose one hour later. Ideally, a patient can often prevent an attack if the patient begins colchicine when experiencing a "twinge."

Prophylaxis Therapy Immediately Following an Acute Attack

Once the patient is symptom free from an acute attack, the patient is then switched to the following prophylaxis regimen:

1. **Ibuprofen:** 400mg PO/oral tid.
2. **Colchicine:** BID, to every three days.
3. **Steroids:** Prednisone 5–7.5mg daily.

Maintenance Drugs

Urate-lowering therapy cannot be initiated until the patient is **symptom-free for two weeks**, and the treatment is typically life-long. Uricosuric drugs have generally fallen out of favor and cannot be used in patients with GFR <30mL/mm^3.

The following are drugs used to prevent gout:

1. **Allopurinol (Zyloprim):** Allopurinol is a maintenance drug that causes decreased uric acid production. Allopurinol is a first-line treatment drug and is dosed at 100–800mg daily. Decreased GFR increases the half-life of the drug, thus increasing the risk of toxicity.

    Allopurinol side effects: Agranulocytosis, rash, cytopenias, diarroea, drug fever, nausea, and vomiting can occur. The risk for rash increases when combined with ampicillin. Monitor CBC and ANC during dentistry.

2. **Probenecid (Benemid) and sulfinpyrazone (Anturane):** These are maintenance drugs and are uricosuric drugs that increase the clearance of uric acid and thus prevent gout.

    Probenecid: Dosed initially at 250mg PO/oral bid, and can be titrated up to 3g total daily. Probenacid requires adequate fluid intake and is associated with numerous DDIs. This is why it is now a second-line drug.

    Probenacid side effects: Rash, agranulocytosis, nephrolithiasis, or GI intolerance. Monitor CBC and ANC during dentistry.

3. **Newer therapies:** Febuxastat, pegloticase, URAT 1, and GLUT 9 inhibitors are emerging options in the treatment of gout.

ANTIRHEUMATIC MEDICATIONS

Rheumatic disease management drugs are not used solely for the classic rheumatic diseases; they are also used for diseases affecting the bones and muscles. They can be classified into three basic classes of drugs:

1. **Biologic response modifiers** (BRMs)
2. **NSAIDS**
3. **Older Drugs:** corticosteroids (see Chapter 40)

BIOLOGIC RESPONSE MODIFIERS

The biologic response modifiers (BRMs) stimulate or restore the ability of the immune system to fight arthritis, rheumatic diseases, and infections. BRMs interfere with inflammatory activity by binding to and inactivating TNF-alpha, thus ultimately decreasing joint damage.

Classification

BRMs can be classified into:

1. Tumor necrosing factor (TNF) blockers
2. The biologic disease-modifying antirheumatic drugs (DMARDS)

Common TNF Blockers

TNF blockers are often the first-line drugs. The common drugs in this category are:

1. D2E7/Adalimumab (Humira)
2. Etanercept (Enbrel)
3. Infliximab (Remicade)

Side Effects

The side effects associated with TNF blockers are leukopenia and risk of serious infection such as MTB and lymphoma. In the presence of these drugs, always monitor the CBC and the ANC count during dentistry.

DMARDS

DMARDS are often prescribed early on in the treatment of rheumatic diseases in addition to NSAIDS.

Common DMARDS

The common DMARDs prescribed are azathioprine (Imuran), chlorambucil (Leukeran), cyclophosphamide (Cytoxan), hydroxychloroquine (Plaquenil), injectable gold (Myochrysine), leflunomide (Arava), methotrexate (Rheumatrex, Trexall), minocycline (Minocin), mycophenolate (CellCept), penicillamine (Cuprimine, Depen), ridaura/oral gold (Auranofin), gold injections (they cause metallic taste and stomatitis), cyclosporine (Sandimmune), and sulfasalazine (Azulfidine).

Methotrexate Facts

Methotrexate (MTX) blocks purine synthesis and inhibits the activity of the immune system, thus reducing inflammation. As a cytotoxic drug it may slow the rapid growth of cells in the synovial membrane that lines the joints. MTX is currently the most frequently used disease-modifying antirheumatic drug (DMARD) in the treatment of rheumatoid arthritis (RA) and other forms of chronic inflammatory arthritis. MTX can be used as a monotherapy, in combination with glucocorticoids, or with other synthetic DMARDS, and biologic agents to enhance their efficacy. MTX is as effective as anti-TNF agents. It is one of the safest DMARDS and is associated with lower mortality, especially from cardiovascular causes. MTX is discussed here in reference to **RA** because it **is the most common form of chronic arthritis**. However, the information is applicable to the management of all forms of chronic inflammatory arthritis disease states.

Universally, MTX is regarded as the first medical treatment option for all forms of chronic inflammatory arthritis. The combination of MTX with biologic agents is considered the most effective therapy currently for RA. MTX was shown to improve signs and symptoms of RA, disease activity, and function to a similar degree as the TNF blockers in monotherapy.

The safety profile of MTX indicates that it is among the safest of all drugs used for the treatment of chronic inflammatory arthritis. An increased risk of leukemia, non-Hodgkin's lymphoma and lung cancer is found in patients with RA, but the overall standardized mortality ratio of cancer is no higher than expected. However, RA patients with kidney or lung cancer have a higher mortality than expected.

RA is a systemic, debilitating inflammatory arthritis but with the use of MTX, the overall survival of RA patients has definitely improved because of its beneficial effects on cardiovascular mortality. MTX suppresses inflammation and has an atheroprotective effect. Recent studies have shown MTX to facilitate cholesterol outflow from foam cells of the arterial wall involved in the atherosclerosis process.

Following MTX monotherapy in patients with persistently active, but not progressively rapid disease, DMARD combination therapy may be used in combination with MTX. These drugs include leflunomide, cyclosporine A, sulfasalazine, and hydroxychloroquine (HCQ). Early use of biologics is considered in patients at risk for rapid disease progression.

Inhibition of radiographic progression is found to be greater with biologics, probably because TNF inhibitors, in addition to their anti-inflammatory effects, directly reduce osteoclast activity. The efficacy of biologics is significantly augmented when combined with MTX. All clinical trials have shown a good performance of MTX in comparison with biologics.

MTX Mechanism of Action

MTX decreases cell proliferation, increases T-cell apoptosis, increases endogenous adenosine release, and influences cytokine production in addition to other humoral responses and bone formation. Adenosine release suppresses the inflammatory functions of neutrophils, macrophage/monocytes, dendritic cells, and lymphocytes in the pathogenesis of joint inflammation.

MTX Pharmacology

Studies have shown that patients getting subcutaneous (SC) MTX have a better clinical outcome when compared to those treated with oral MTX. Thus, patients with an inadequate response or patients intolerant to oral MTX can benefit from SC MTX.

MTX Side Effects

Frequent side effects include mild liver transaminase elevation, minor gastrointestinal side effects, stomatitis, anemia, leucopenia, and thrombocytopenia, which are reversible after dose reduction or discontinuation of treatment.

Serious side effects include pancytopenia, hepatotoxicity and interstitial pneumonitis. In such cases, MTX is usually withdrawn.

Prevention of side effects: Supplementation with folic acid (FA) effectively reduces MTX associated hepatic adverse effects. FA exerts a beneficial effect on homocysteine metabolism and may prevent the formation of the less effective metabolite 7-hydroxy-MTX. Patients on MTX should not drink alcohol.

Multinational Evidence-Based Recommendations for the use of MTX in RA

- The therapeutic goal in RA treatment is remission or low disease activity.
- Today, MTX is considered the main drug for the treatment of RA–not just as monotherapy, but also in combination with other DMARDS or biologics. Supplementation with at least 5mg folic acid weekly is strongly recommended when prescribing MTX.
- The standard of care is for DMARDS to be started within the first three months of disease onset, with MTX being the most common DMARD of choice. It should be started very early in the treatment of RA and the overall effectiveness of MTX is higher than other DMARDS after five years of therapy.
- Before starting MTX, patients are assessed for risk factors for MTX toxicity, including alcohol intake, complete blood count, serum transaminases, albumin and creatinine levels, and chest x-ray, serology for HIV, hepatitis B or C, fasting blood sugar (FBS), serum lipid profile, and pregnancy test.
- Oral MTX is started at 10–15mg/week, with gradual increase every 2–4 weeks by 5mg up to the dose of 20–30mg/week, depending on response and tolerance. Parenteral administration is considered in cases of inadequate clinical response or poor tolerance
- At doses between 7.5 and 25mg weekly, MTX relieves pain, reduces the number of tender and swollen joints, and improves function. Treatment withdrawals due to adverse events are infrequent at the doses used.
- In regard to radiographic outcome, MTX inhibits radiological progression more than other DMARDs. MTX has similar results in efficacy and radiological progression compared with biological monotherapy.
- When starting MTX or increasing the dose, alanine aminotransferase (ALT) with or without aspartate aminotransferase (AST), creatinine, and complete blood count should be checked every 1–1.5 months, until a stable dose is attained, and then every 1–3 months. Clinical assessment for adverse effects and risk factors are performed at each visit.
- MTX is discontinued if there is a confirmed increase in ALT/AST larger than three-times the upper limit of normal (ULN), but it can be reintroduced at a lower dose after normalization. If the ALT/AST levels are persistently elevated up to three times the ULN, then the MTX dose is adjusted. Diagnostic procedures are considered if elevated ALT/AST more than three-times the ULN persists after discontinuation.
- In patients undergoing elective orthopedic surgery, MTX can be safely continued in the perioperative period.

- Both men and women are advised not to use MTX for at least three months before planned pregnancy, and women should not use MTX during pregnancy or breast-feeding.
- DMARD combination therapy may be used from the beginning or after a patient has failed initial MTX monotherapy. The most frequently used combinations include: MTX plus leflunomide, MTX plus cyclosporine A, MTX plus sulfasalazine, MTX plus HCQ, and triple therapy with MTX plus sulfasalazine plus HCQ. Less common and presently outdated combinations include MTX plus azathioprine and MTX plus gold.
- Azathioprine, antimalarials, cyclosporine A, cyclophosphamide, D-penicillamine, leflunomide, gold salts, and sulfasalazine are not more effective than MTX. Some are less effective and are more toxic.
- In patients at risk for rapid radiographic progression, the early use of biologics in combination with MTX is considered. In the case of poor response to a single DMARD or to a DMARD combination, a biologic is invariably added to MTX.
- The most frequent biologic treatment is TNF inhibition with etanercept, adalimumab, infliximab or the newer inhibitors, certolizumab pegol and golimumab.
- Most studies have shown that all biologics (with the exception of anakinra) have comparable efficacy. The combinations of MTX plus abatacept, MTX plus rituximab, and MTX plus tocilizumab are very effective in both producing clinical improvement and inhibiting radiographic progression. The efficacy of biological therapy is far better using MTX combination than monotherapy.
- In patients in whom treatment with TNF antagonists has failed, a combination of rituximab or abatacept or tocilizumab or golimumab plus MTX is more effective than MTX alone.

NSAIDS

Classification

NSAIDS interfere with the inflammatory process. They are classified into the following:

1. Acetylated salicylates: aspirin
2. Nonacetylated salicylates
3. Traditional NSAIDS
4. COX-2 selective inhibitors: celecoxib (Celebrex) and etoricoxib (Baxtra)

Acetylated Salicylate: Aspirin

Aspirin permanently affects platelets, and patients are often on large doses of aspirin. Consult with the MD when major surgery is planned; it may take 7–10 days to reverse the effects of high doses of aspirin if the go-ahead is given to stop the aspirin.

Nonacetyl Salicylates

Common nonacetyl salicylates are the following:

1. Choline salicylate (Arthropan)
2. Magnesium salicylate (Magan/Mobidin)
3. Nonprescription magnesium salicylate (Arthritab or Bayer Select or Doan's Pills)

Nonacetylated Salicylates Facts

These drugs are not used as much now. Choline and magnesium salicylate **do not** affect platelets and **do not** affect the bleeding time (BT). Nonacetylated salicylates **do not** need to be stopped prior to any kind of dental surgery.

Traditional NSAIDS

The traditional NSAIDS include diclofenac potassium (Cataflam), diclofenac/ miso-prostol (Arthrotec—the first NSAID protective against ulcers), diclofenac sodium (Voltaren), diflunisal (Dolobid), etodolac (Lodine), fenoprofen (Nalfon), flurbipro-fen (Ansaid), ibuprofen (Motrin, Advil), indomethacin (Indocin), ketoprofen (Orudis, Oruvail), meclofenamate sodium (Meclomen), mefanamic acid (Ponstel), meloxicam (Mobic), nabumetone (Relafen), naproxen (Naprosyn, Aleve), oxaprozin (Daypro), piroxicam (Feldene), sulindac (Clinoril), and tolmetin sodium (Tolectin).

NSAIDS Facts

NSAIDS affect platelet adhesiveness, resulting in prolonged bleeding. Ibuprofen has a reversible inhibitory effect that lasts only hours. All NSAIDS, with the exception of aspirin and nonacetylated salicylates, should be stopped for at least 24 hours prior to major surgery, but only after consulting with the patient's MD.

Cyclo-oxygenase (COX)-2 Inhibitors

The only COX-2 inhibitor prescribed today is celecoxib (Celebrex). Valdecoxib (Baxtra) and rofecoxib (Vioxx) were withdrawn because of life-threatening side effects.

COX-2 Inhibitor Facts

COX-2 inhibitors are associated with some extent of increased cardiovascular complica-tions and potentially life-threatening gastrointestinal bleeding. Baxtra was withdrawn because it had increased cardiovascular events. Vioxx was associated with deaths from sudden cardiac arrhythmias. Thus, valdecoxib (Baxtra) and rofecoxib (Vioxx) were with-drawn because the risks with both the drugs far outweighed the benefits.

Celecoxib (Celebrex) also was temporarily withdrawn, but because the benefits out-weighed the risks, Celebrex was reintroduced with specific warning labels about its side effects posted prominently.

COX-2 inhibitors act by inhibition of prostaglandin synthesis via inhibition of cyclo-oxygenase-2 (COX-2). COX-2 inhibitors do not affect COX-1.

COX-2 inhibitors are metabolized in the liver by the CYP450 enzyme and are excreted through the kidneys. The COX-2 inhibitors are primarily used to treat pain associated with osteoarthritis and rheumatoid arthritis. These drugs do not cause GI ulcers, nor do they affect platelet aggregation, so they do not need to be stopped prior to major surgery. Reduction of the total daily dose by 50% is recommended in patients with hepatitis, and COX-2 inhibitors are contraindicated in patients with cirrhosis or any form of kidney disease. Celecoxib should not be prescribed to patients with a history of allergy to sulfa antimicrobials.

COX-2 Inhibitors and DDIs

Do not prescribe the following drugs to patients on COX-2 inhibitors:

- Fluconazole (Diflucan)
- Tetracycline HCL
- Doxycycline (Vibramycin)
- Clarithromycin (Biaxin)

SUGGESTED DENTAL GUIDELINES FOR RHEUMATIC DISEASES

In general, these guidelines are applicable for diseases of the joints, bones, or muscles:

1. Always determine the type of rheumatic disease affecting your patient and the extent of the disease.
2. Determine what organ systems are affected because this will help guide you in the request of laboratory tests to determine the patient's current medical and vital organ status.
3. At the minimum, request the CBC, serum creatinine, and LFTs. Review the CBC and determine if the patient has leucopenia, anemia, thrombocytopenia, or increased monocyte count.
4. Incorporate the leucopenia, anemia, and thrombocytopenia suggested anesthetics, analgesics, and antibiotics (AAA) guidelines if corresponding changes are seen on the CBC.
5. Increased monocyte count is associated with flare-ups, and routine dental treatment must be deferred for four to six weeks until the acute state resolves.
6. Always calculate the absolute neutrophil count (ANC) count and follow the ANC guidelines when the immunity is affected (not uncommon with these diseases).
7. Follow the kidney and liver AAA suggested guidelines if the serum creatinine and LFTs are affected.
8. Discuss with the patient to determine if the spine is affected and what the patient's mobility status is as far as the TMJ, cervical, and lumbar spine areas are concerned. Provide TMD care if the TMJ is affected.
9. Patients with limited cervical spine mobility should be asked to move their neck themselves when a change in position is needed. Do not rotate the neck yourself because this could negatively affect the patient and cause nerve pains in the upper extremities.
10. A patient with lumbar spine involvement may not be able to stay in the chair for too long and may need help getting out of the chair. Have the patient bring in a lumbar pillow if the patient uses one.
11. A patient with moderate-to-severe arthritis-associated hand deformities may need to use an electric toothbrush or have a bulky, taped wrapping around the toothbrush handle for a better grip. The toothbrush can also be taped in place after inserting it through small cuts made into the top and bottom of a tennis ball.
12. Know and analyze each medication the patient is on for the management of underlying rheumatic disease.
13. Always confirm if the patient is currently on corticosteroids or has been on steroids for two weeks or longer, in the past two years. If the response is positive, you

will have to follow "the rule of twos" for major surgery after consulting with the patient's physician.

14. Patients on bisphosphonates or any other anti-resorptive therapy must be educated about maintaining a healthy dental status and have more frequent hygiene recalls to prevent any adverse side effects from the drug. All infections must be aggressively treated with antibiotics and pain medications in these patients.

15. Patients experiencing xerostomia should be treated with saliva substitutes. Optimal oral hygiene should be maintained, and any oral candidiasis that develops should be immediately treated as outlined in this chapter under Sjögren's syndrome and in Chapter 48.

16. As previously discussed, there are several antirheumatic medications, and the specifics of each should be noted and implemented appropriately during patient care. Of particular importance are the TNF blockers, which usually need to be stopped two weeks prior to dentistry if the WBC count is low. This temporary cessation will help increase the WBC count and promote healing.

DISEASES OF THE BONES: PAGET'S DISEASE

Paget's is a bone disease that is more common in people over 40, and men are more frequently affected than women. The exact etiology is not known, but it does seem to run in families. The bones affected are the skull, extremities, pelvis, and spine. The disease could be limited to one or two bones, or it could be widespread, affecting several bones.

Pathophysiology

Paget's disease is associated with a disruption of bone remodeling. In the initial stages of the disease, bone breakdown is more rapid than bone remodeling. With time, however, bone remodeling is rapid but the new bone formed is soft and weak. This leads to bone pain, bone deformity, and bone fractures.

Symptoms and Signs

Symptoms and signs associated with Paget's depend on the extensiveness of the disease. Some patients can be asymptomatic, whereas others are quite bothered by their symptoms.

Common Symptoms

The following are common symptoms experienced:

1. **Bone pains:** The pains may be constant and deep and are more aggravating at night.
2. **Joint pains:** Joint pains are due to the loss of cartilage and the progressive osteoarthritis that follows.
3. **Nerve pains:** Enlargement of the bones causes compression of the nerves in close proximity to the spine. This causes severe radiating pains, tingling, numbness, and weakness along the distribution of the nerves affected.
4. **Neurological symptoms:** Headaches, vision problems, facial weakness, and hearing loss are the neurological symptoms experienced.

5. **Other symptoms:** Fractures, increased head size, loss of teeth, and bowlegs are some of the symptoms that are classically associated with the disease as it progresses with time.

Diagnosis

Paget's disease diagnosis is established with the following:

1. **Blood tests:** The alkaline phosphatase levels are markedly increased, indicating rapid bone turnover.
2. **Radiographs:** Radiographic survey of the affected bone can show enlargement, resorption, and deformities.
3. **Bone scans:** Bone scans can detect changes in bones due to Paget's disease much earlier than standard radiographs. Another advantage is that a bone scan is able to detect all bones affected with the disease.

Complications

The disease progresses slowly. Osteoarthritis, cardiac failure, and osteosarcoma, however, are some of the complications that are associated with Paget's disease.

Treatment

A slowly progressing disease process may not need much care, but a progressive disease may need some or all of the treatments listed in the following sections.

Surgery

Surgical intervention may be needed to correct bone deformity or relieve osteoarthritis-associated joint problems with joint prostheses. Patients with a joint prosthesis will have to be **premedicated for life**, according to the AHA antibiotic premedication guidelines, for all invasive dentistry.

Medical Management

The following medications are used to manage symptoms associated with Paget's disease: NSAIDS, bisphosphonates/anti-resorptive drugs, and calcitonin.

NSAIDS

NSAIDS are given to control the arthritis-associated pain. Refer to the section "NSAIDS" for a detailed discussion.

Bisphosphonates/Anti-resorptive Drugs

Bisphosphonates/anti-resorptive drugs help decrease the bone activity and are the **main** class of drugs used in the management of Paget's disease. Refer to Chapter 41 for a detailed discussion on bisphosphonates/anti-resorptive drugs.

Calcitonin

Calcitonin is given to patients who have Paget's disease and associated renal disease when bisphosphonates/anti-resorptive drugs are contraindicated. Thus, it serves as an **alternate** drug in the management of Paget's disease. Calcitonin (Miacalcin) regulates calcium and bone metabolism. Refer to Chapter 41 for a detailed discussion on calcitonin.

Paget's disease alert: Paget's disease is associated with increased vascularity in the affected areas. Any one of these two medications, when given for some time prior to surgery, will help reduce the number of blood vessels in the area and associated bleeding with surgery.

SUGGESTED DENTAL GUIDELINES FOR PAGET'S DISEASE

Follow these guidelines during dentistry:

1. Prior to treatment, obtain the CBC with platelets and WBC differential, serum creatinine, and LFTs. Calculate the ANC and implement the ANC guidelines when the WBC count is decreased. Assess the status of the liver and kidney and implement appropriate guidelines when either or both organs are compromised.
2. In the early osteolytic stage, bone resorption predominates and there may be increased bleeding because of greatly increased vascularity in the affected tissue during this stage.
3. In the later sclerotic stage, the affected bones become enlarged and dense, and because of poor blood supply to the bones, surgery in this stage can predispose to suppurative osteomyelitis. Antibiotic coverage **prior** to surgery will prevent infection and promote the healing process.
4. The maxilla is more affected than the mandible, but jaw involvement is less in general with Paget's disease.
5. Dentures frequently have to be replaced in patients with Paget's disease because the alveolar bone resorption continues over time and proper fitting of the dentures becomes an issue.
6. Patients with joint prosthesis need to be premedicated prior to all invasive procedures. Amoxicillin does not have as good a bone penetration when compared to all the other antibiotics on the AHA list. It is better to use cephalosporins, clindamycin, azithromycin, or clarithromycin instead because all these antibiotics have excellent bone penetration.
7. Occasionally, steroids may also be prescribed, and you have to consider "the rule of twos" prior to major surgery.
8. Patients on bisphosphonates/anti-resorptive drugs must be educated about maintaining a healthy dental status and have more frequent hygiene recalls to prevent any adverse side effects from the drug. All infections must be aggressively treated with antibiotics and pain medications in the presence of bisphosphonates/anti-resorptive drugs.

DISEASES AFFECTING MUSCLES: MALIGNANT HYPERTHERMIA

Malignant hyperthermia (MH) is an autosomal dominant disorder that causes severe muscle contractions upon exposure to specific general anesthetics and a sudden sharp rise in body temperature. Once a patient is diagnosed with MH, all family members are considered to have MH.

Pathophysiology

The basic defect is an inability of the skeletal muscles to regulate calcium. **Reuptake** of calcium is necessary for the **termination** of skeletal muscle **contraction,** and with MH there is a **reduction in the reuptake** of calcium by the sarcoplasmic reticulum. The skeletal muscle contraction is thus sustained, causing a rapid rise in body temperature. With the associated hypermetabolic crisis there is a constant demand for oxygen by the skeletal muscles. Initially, the body tries to compensate, but eventually the patient experiences a circulatory collapse.

Causative Factors

Malignant hyperthermia patients become symptomatic **within one hour** when exposed to the following:

1. Succinylcholine: a depolarizing muscle relaxant.
2. Specific volatile anesthetics: halothane, desflurane, enflurane, isoflurane, and sevoflurane.

Diagnostic Tests

The two muscle biopsy-associated tests that aid in MH diagnosis are:

1. The in vitro contracture test (IVCT)
2. The caffeine-halothane contracture test

Symptoms and Signs

MH is characterized by a rapid rise in body temperature with associated skeletal muscle rigidity, lockjaw, tachycardia, cardiac arrhythmias, hypotension, hypoxemia (low oxygen in the blood), hypercarbia (increased carbon dioxide in the blood), respiratory and metabolic acidosis, and skeletal muscle breakdown in the blood.

Treatment

Treatment must be immediate and consists of the following:

1. **Call for help immediately.**
2. Hyperventilate the patient with 100% oxygen.
3. Cool down the patient with cold blankets.
4. Give **cold** intravenous (IV) fluids 15 cc/kg.
5. Inject IV Dantrolene immediately.

Dantrolene

Dantrolene is a muscle relaxant that works directly on the ryanodine receptor and prevents the release of calcium. Listed are the bolus, follow-up, and maintenance doses of dantrolene:

1. **Dantrolene bolus dose:** Give dantrolene 2.5 mg/kg IV stat.
2. **Dantrolene follow-up dose:** Give dantrolene 2 mg/kg every five minutes, until the patient is stable.
3. **Dantrolene maintenance dose:** The patient is maintained on dantrolene at a rate of 1–2 mg/kg/h.

Suggested Safe Drugs for Use in Dentistry

1. **Anxiety-relieving medications:** lorazepam (Ativan), diazepam (Valium), triazolam (Halcion), and midazolam (Versed).
2. **Barbiturates/intravenous anesthetics:** diazepam (Valium), methohexital (Brevital), and midazolam (Versed).
3. **Inhaled nonvolatile general anesthetics:** nitrous oxide.
4. **Local anesthetics:** bupivicaine (Marcaine), lidocaine (Xylocaine), mepivicaine (Carbocaine), prilocaine (Citanest), and septocaine (Articaine).
5. **Narcotics (opioids):** codeine (Methyl Morphine), fentanyl (Sublimaze), hydromorphone (Dilaudid), meperidine (Demerol), methadone (Dolophine), morphine, naloxone (Narcan), and oxycodone (Percocet).
6. **Antibiotics:** All antibiotics used in the dental setting are safe with MH.
7. **Analgesics/antipyretics:** All analgesics-antipyretics used in the dental setting are safe with MH.

DISEASES AFFECTING MUSCLES: POLYMYOSITIS AND DERMATOMYOSITIS

Polymyositis

Polymyositis is an inflammatory myopathy that is considered to be an autoimmune disease. The exact etiology is not clear. It is thought to occur secondary to a viral or bacterial infection. It is more common in the black population compared to the white population, and women are more frequently affected than men. Patients are usually 40–50 years old at the onset of the disease.

Polymyositis Symptoms and Signs

The symptoms of polymyositis are gradual in onset. The patient usually experiences weakness in the hip and shoulder muscles making it difficult for the patient to get in and out of bed or a chair. Mild joint pains, muscle tenderness, fatigue, generalized malaise, and difficulty swallowing are also experienced.

Dermatomyositis Symptoms and Signs

Dermatomyositis is associated with specific skin lesions, commonly a butterfly rash, **and** all the symptoms and signs associated with polymyositis. Etiology for dermatomyositis is the same as the etiology for polymyositis.

Dermatomyositis usually affects patients 50–60 years old, and females are more frequently affected than males. Other collagen vascular disorders can also be associated with dermatomyositis.

Polymyositis and Dermatomyositis Diagnosis

Diagnosis of both disease states is made as follows:

1. **Medical history:** The classic presentation is often very suggestive of either of the two diseases.
2. **Muscle biopsy:** Muscle biopsy may reveal muscle changes suggestive of the disease.
3. **Electromyography:** Different muscles are tested with electromyography to reveal the underlying disease state.
4. **Blood tests:** Blood tests show increased levels of creatinine kinase and aldolase, indicating muscle damage.

Polymyositis and Dermatomyositis Complications

Polymyositis and Dermatomyositis are often associated with other connective tissue disorders. These patients can also have associated heart disease, cardiac arrhythmias, heart failure, and interstitial lung disease with fibrosis.

Polymyositis and Dermatomyositis Management

Medical management frequently involves medications in addition to physical therapy. Physical therapy is provided to tone and loosen the muscles and joints. The following drugs are most often prescribed:

1. **Corticosteroids and bisphosphonates:** Steroids are given long term and bisphosphonates are often prescribed along with the steroids to counteract the steroid-associated osteoporosis.
2. **Immunosuppressants:** Azathioprine (Imuran) or methotrexate (Rheumatrex) is prescribed as alternates if steroids are ineffective or not well tolerated by the patient.

Polymyositis and Dermatomyositis Suggested Dental Alerts

The following are dental alerts:

1. Follow the suggested guidelines outlined for the earlier section "Classic Rheumatic Diseases."
2. Take into consideration the associated anemia, collagen-vascular abnormalities, and corticosteroid or immunosuppressant therapy.
3. These patients benefit when given shorter appointments as this prevents undue exhaustion.

DISEASES AFFECTING MUSCLES: PARKINSON'S DISEASE

Parkinson's disease (PD) is a motor system disorder, caused by loss of dopamine-producing brain cells in the basal ganglia. This results in localized deficiency of dopamine. Parkinson's disease is also called **paralysis agitans** and it usually affects patients in their 50s.

Some patients progress slowly with the disease whereas others progress rapidly. It is not uncommon for these patients to experience infrequent blinking, drooling due to poor swallowing, emotional and sleep disturbances, and bowel and bladder control problems.

Presentation

Parkinson's disease primarily presents in one of four ways:

1. **Tremors:** The patient experiences trembling in the hands, arms, legs, jaw, and face when Parkinson's presents as tremors. Hands and arm tremors cause a pin-rolling movement pattern and the tremors are worst at rest.
2. **Rigidity:** There is stiffness of the limbs and trunk when Parkinson's presents with rigidity. The patient's arms are flexed and held to the sides. Cogwheel rigidity is seen during movement of the limbs, and a stooping posture occurs because of rigidity.
3. **Bradykinesia:** There is slowness of movement in this form of Parkinson's presentation and slowness in initiation and execution of movements, and the patient often shuffles when walking.
4. **Postural instability:** Another form of presentation is when the patient experiences impairment of balance and coordination.

Diagnosis

Diagnosis of Parkinson's disease is made:

1. Through evaluation of the medical history.
2. Through a thorough neurological examination.

Management

Parkinson's disease is managed as follows:

1. **Anticholinergics:** benztropine (Cogentin), hyoscyamine sulfate (NuLev), and trihexyphenidyl.
2. **Catechol o-methyl transferase (COMT) inhibitors:** entacapone (Comtan) and tolcapone (Tasmar).
3. **Cholinesterase Inhibitors:** rivastigmine (Exelon).
4. **DOPA-decarboxylase inhibitor:** carbidopa (Lodosyn).
5. **DOPA-decarboxylase inhibitor + dopamine precursor:** carbidopa/levodopa (Parcopa/Sinemet) and carbidopa/levodopa CR (Sinemet CR) Sust-rel tabs.
6. **Dopamine agonists:** amantadine (Symmetrel), apomorphine (Apokyn), bromocriptine (Parlodel), pramipexole (Mirapex; Mirapex ER/Ext-rel tabs), and ropinirole (Requip; Requip XL/Ext-rel tabs). Pramipexole and popinirole are first line treatment drugs for Parkinson's disease.

7. **DOPA-decarboxylase inhibitor + dopamine precursor + catechol o-methyl transferase inhibitors combination:** carbidopa/levodopa + entacapone (Stalevo).
8. **Monoamine oxidase-B inhibitors:** rasagiline (Azilect) and selegiline (Eldepryl/ Zelapar).
9. **Deep brain stimulation (DBS):** Electrodes implanted into the brain are connected to a small electrical device that is externally programmed. DBS helps decrease tremors, slowness of movements, gait problems, and the need for medications.

Suggested Dental Guidelines

The following are the suggested dental guidelines to use with patients with Parkinson's disease:

1. Follow the suggested dental guidelines outlined for "Classic Rheumatic Diseases."
2. Additionally, a Parkinson's patient with mild tremors may need to be strapped in the chair with a Velcro belt so the head can be stable during treatment.
3. Patients experiencing significant tremors will need to be sedated for dentistry. Low-dose sedation should be used to minimize the additive sedation with anti–Parkinson's disease drugs.
4. Minimize the amount of epinephrine use in the patient on COMT inhibitors and use local anesthetics with 1:200,000 epinephrine or without epinephrine, maximum two carpules. Avoid using the 4% LAs.
5. Avoid clarithromycin, tetracycline, doxycycline, and azole antifungals with the dopamine antagonist drugs.

DISEASES AFFECTING MUSCLES: MYASTHENIA GRAVIS

Myasthenia gravis is a condition associated with muscle weakness due to poor response of the muscle receptor to the neurotransmitter acetylcholine. Autoantibodies to the acetylcholine receptor protein are often found in many cases. The weakness and fatigue of affected muscles is gradual or insidious in onset. The weakness may be localized, or more generalized when several muscles are affected. It is often unmasked and/or exacerbated by certain stress factors such as infection, pregnancy, or menstrual periods. Muscle weakness becomes more pronounced as the day progresses.

Myasthenia gravis can occur at all ages, but it is most common in young females who have the HLA-DR3 gene. Myasthenia gravis can occasionally be associated with other conditions such as SLE, RA, thyrotoxicosis, or thymoma. Myasthenia gravis affects men more commonly in their 60s when the disease is present along with thymoma.

Symptoms and Signs

The symptoms experienced are associated with the muscles involved: involvement of the ocular muscles results in ptosis and vision problems; involvement of the muscles of mastication and pharyngeal muscles causes the patient to complain of difficulty chewing and swallowing. A very lax jaw can be found on physical examination. Involvement of the respiratory muscles results in breathing impairment, and involvement of the muscles in the extremities causes weakness in the limbs. There is difficulty supporting the neck when the neck muscles are affected. The gag reflex can be absent or poor, and the ability to cough may be compromised in the myasthenia gravis patient, causing an increased risk of aspiration.

Diagnostic Tests

The following tests help diagnose myasthenia gravis:

1. **Endrophonium (Tensilon) injection test:** The diagnosis of myasthenia gravis is confirmed by demonstration of improved patient response to IV endrophonium, a short-acting anticholinesterase.
2. **Acetylcholine receptor antibody test:** Blood tests showing elevated levels of circulating acetylcholine receptor antibodies confirms the diagnosis of myasthenia gravis.

Treatment

Myasthenia gravis treatment considerations are as follows:

1. **Anticholinesterases, neostigmine, and pyridostigmine:** Anticholinesterases increase the amount of available acetylcholine (ACh) at the myoneural junction by inhibiting the degradation of ACh.
2. **Neostigmine (Prostigmin)** and **pyridostigmine (Mestinon):** These drugs are used alone or in combination and provide symptomatic relief by enhancing neuromuscular transmission, but they do not affect the course of the disease.
3. **Corticosteroids or cyclosporine (Sandimmune) or azathioprine (Imuran):** Occasionally, the treatment is supplemented with corticosteroids or cyclosporine or azathioprine, to suppress the abnormal antibody production and provide symptomatic relief.
4. **Surgery:** Surgical removal of a myasthenia-associated thymoma causing significant symptoms can result in disease remission, post surgery.

Suggested Dental Guidelines

Follow these guidelines for dentistry:

1. Always confirm the extent of disease affecting the entire body and particularly the head and neck region.
2. Check for the gag reflex plus the ability to cough, and confirm that both are adequate before you begin treatment.
3. Anticholinesterases increase salivation, and you may often have to provide active suction during dental treatment.
4. Morning appointments are recommended because the weakness is least in the morning and worsens as the day progresses.
5. Follow the rule of twos.
6. Any form of infection or emotional stress and certain medications can worsen the status of the disease. Explain the procedure for the day to help the patient relax and decrease any anxiety.
7. Avoid all types of muscle relaxants.

8. Use a minimal dose of local anesthesia, limit it to two carpules only, plus avoid lidocaine and the 4% LAs.
9. Avoid macrolides, tetracycline, aminoglycosides, and fluoquinolones diazepam (Valium), lorazepam (Ativan), and general anesthesia because these drugs can aggravate myasthenia gravis symptoms.

DISEASES AFFECTING MUSCLES: MULTIPLE SCLEROSIS

Multiple sclerosis (MS), a central nervous system disease, is considered to be an autoimmune condition that causes progressive antibody-mediated damage of the nerve fibers in the brain and spinal cord. Antibodies are directed against the myelin-producing cells causing inflammation of the myelin sheaths. Multifocal plaques of demyelination occur in the CNS causing patchy areas of sclerosis with resultant motor and sensory dysfunction. The demyelination causes decreased nerve conduction velocity, a differential rate of impulse transmission, partial conduction blocking, or complete failure of impulse transmission.

The exact cause of MS is not known, but viruses (most often, the Epstein-Barr virus) have often been implicated as either triggering the onset of the disease or triggering an exacerbation of the disease. Pregnancy is also known to worsen the disease. The disease can be progressive and debilitating; however, spontaneous remission is known to occur in some patients.

Multiple Sclerosis Types

The disease can present in one of four ways:

1. **Relapsing-remitting:** Most patients give a history of frequent flare-ups that last weeks, followed by phases of remission.
2. **Primary progressive:** A few patients, especially those that experience initial symptoms after age 40, can have progressively deteriorating symptoms as a primary form of presentation.
3. **Secondary progressive:** A small number of the relapsing-remitting patients can ultimately go on to develop progressively deteriorating symptoms, and this form of the disease is the secondary progressive form of MS.
4. **Progressive relapsing:** This is a variant of primary progressive MS. The patient experiences periodic flare-ups exacerbating existing symptoms or causing new symptoms.

Age of Onset

MS primarily affects patients between the ages of 20 and 40. Females are more affected than males.

Symptoms and Signs

The wide range of symptoms experienced depends on the neurological areas affected and the severity of the disease. Excessive fatigue, vision problems, and problems with gait are the common initial symptoms experienced.

However, the specific symptoms that may be experienced are blurring of vision; colored halos; impaired vision; unilateral blindness; paresthesias and "pins and needles" sensations in the extremities; tremors and dizziness; hearing loss; speech problems; progressive muscle weakness affecting the limbs; impaired coordination and balance; impaired walking; partial or complete paralysis; impairment of the bowel and bladder function; depression; and difficulty with concentration, memory, and judgment.

Diagnosis

The diagnosis of MS can be established as follows:

1. **Medical history:** There are no specific tests that can diagnose MS, but a thorough medical history can unearth the motor and sensory deficits, neuromuscular symptoms affecting the extremities, vision problems, and problems with gait or coordination.
2. **Magnetic resonance imaging (MRI):** MRI will help detect areas of sclerosis or evidence of plaques in the brain.
3. **Spinal tap:** A spinal tap is done only when the diagnosis is questionable. The CSF will show elevated levels of proteins and mononuclear WBCs.

Treatment

There is no known effective treatment that can eradicate the disease. There are, however, two basic forms of MS therapies:

1. Drugs used to slow the progression of MS
2. Treatment modalities for symptoms associated with MS

Drugs Used to Slow the Progression of Multiple Sclerosis

The following drugs are used to slow the progression:

1. **Beta interferon:** Beta interferon preparations decrease exacerbations or severity of symptoms and slow the progression of MS. They help fight viral infections and enhance the immune system. FDA-approved beta interferons available for the management of MS are:
   a. Interferon beta-1a injection (Avonex or Rebif)
   b. Interferon beta-1b injection (Betaseron)
2. **Copolymer 1/glatiramer acetate (Copaxone):** Copolymer I (Copaxone) injection, a synthetic form of basic myelin protein, decreases the relapse rate by one-third. This drug prevents the immune system from attacking myelin.
3. **Mitoxantrone injections (Novantrone):** Mitoxantrone (Novantrone), an immunosuppressive drug, is used short term (2–3 years) for the treatment of advanced progressive MS.

Treatment Modalities for Symptoms Associated with Multiple Sclerosis

Treatment modalities for MS are:

1. **Steroids:** Steroids, when given, are used to reduce the severity and duration of attacks. Occasionally, a patient experiencing troublesome optic symptoms can benefit from a short course of IV methylprednisolone (Solu-Medrol) followed by oral steroids.
2. **Muscle relaxants:** Beclofen (Lioresal) and tizanidine (Zanaflex) muscle relaxants are dispensed for the treatment of muscle stiffness, muscle spasms, and increased muscle tone. Be aware that these drugs can cause **drowsiness and xerostomia.**
3. **Anticonvulsants:** The patient may be on carbamazepine (Tegretol) or phenytoin sodium (Dilantin) for the treatment of trigeminal neuralgia or neuropathy. Refer to Chapter 43 for suggested dental guidelines.
4. **Antidepressant medications:** Tricyclic antidepressants are often prescribed to overcome the associated depression.
5. **Physical therapy and exercise:** Physical therapy and exercise is provided to help maintain muscle function and mobility.

SUGGESTED DENTAL ASPECTS AND GUIDELINES FOR MULTIPLE SCLEROSIS

Follow these guidelines for dentistry:

1. Patients with severe MS will need shorter appointments because they are unable to keep their mouth open for a longer duration.
2. It is best to treat these patients during morning appointments because fatigue experienced is more pronounced in the afternoon.
3. These patients may need assistance with transfer from the wheelchair to the dental chair.
4. Evaluate the CBC, serum creatinine, and LFTs prior to the start of dental treatment.
5. The patient can experience abnormal facial pain or intraoral pain and discomfort that may be localized or generalized. The patient must be thoroughly evaluated to determine the cause and be referred to the medical side for further evaluation. Incomplete assessment could lead to unnecessary extractions or endodontic treatment.
6. MS can trigger the development of trigeminal neuralgia that is often **bilateral**. It causes paroxysmal pain that simulates electrical shocks, and it can be brought on by chewing or stroking of the cheek. The pain, when it occurs, is severe and recurring.
7. The trigeminal sensory neuropathy-associated parasthesia is progressive and the maxillary and mandibular divisions of the trigeminal nerve are frequently affected.
8. Significant facial anesthesia can also occur in severe cases of MS.
9. Numbness of the lower lip and chin with or without pain can occur if the mental nerve is involved.
10. A significant number of patients may be affected with facial palsy, which occurs later in the disease.
11. Severe respiratory problems can occur when the respiratory muscles are affected. The gag reflex may be lacking or impaired. These patients can also suffer from vertigo, which can worsen in the lying-down position. For all these reasons the patient should be treated in a semi-sitting position. The rubber dam should be used only if the patient can adequately breathe through the nose.

12. There is a higher incidence of caries in patients with MS because there is significant xerostomia.
13. It is not uncommon to find stomatitis, ulcerations, gingivitis, herpes infection, candidiasis, and parotid gland enlargement in addition to the xerostomia.
14. Dentistry for severe cases may have to be done under general anesthesia in a hospitalized setting.
15. Interferon and many of the immunosuppressant drugs can cause changes in the CBC affecting the WBCs (neutropenia and/or lymphopenia), hemoglobin, hematocrit, and platelets. Always evaluate the CBC prior to dentistry and stringently implement the ANC guidelines when indicated. All infections should be aggressively treated because infections can worsen the status of the disease. Also, adequately compensate for thrombocytopenia, when present.
16. Interferon beta-1a (Avonex/Rebif) causes leukopenia, anemia, thrombocytopenia, and alteration of the LFTs. All hepatotoxic drugs must be avoided with Avonex/Rebif.
17. Interferon beta-1b (Betaseron) causes significant lymphopenia and neutropenia.
18. Copolymer-1/Glatiramer acetate (Capoxone) can cause enlargement of the parotid glands and severe stomatitis.
19. Mitoxantrone (Novantrone) can cause changes in the LFTs plus significant pancytopenia, stomatitis, and mucositis.
20. Evaluate the oral cavity for candida infection in patients on steroids and treat appropriately if present.
21. Follow "the rule of twos" during major dentistry if the patient is currently on steroids or has been on steroids for two weeks or longer within the past two years. Always provide antibiotic coverage for five days following major dentistry, to prevent any post-op infection.
22. Steroids mask the symptoms and signs of infection; so be extra vigilant. Carefully examine and treat any infection found in the oral cavity.

Multiple Sclerosis and Anesthetics

Follow these guidelines for dentistry:

1. Limit the anesthetic to a maximum of two carpules per visit.
2. Avoid articaine (Septocaine) and prilocaine (Citanest) because both these local anesthetics are known to cause parasthesias.
3. Avoid epinephrine-containing local anesthetics in the presence of tricyclic antidepressants.

Multiple Sclerosis and Analgesics

Follow these guidelines for dentistry:

1. Avoid aspirin and NSAIDS because these drugs can promote gastric ulceration.
2. Meperidine (Demerol) and propoxyphene (Darvon) should be avoided because the MS drugs affect the LFTs.
3. Follow the liver dosing guidelines when prescribing acetaminophen, acetaminophen + codeine (Tylenol #3), oxycodone + acetaminophen (Percocet), or hydrocodone + acetaminophen (Vicodin) in the presence of abnormal liver enzymes.

4.   Use regular-strength acetaminophen (Tylenol) in the presence of antiseizure medications.

Multiple Sclerosis and Antibiotics

No specific antibiotic contraindication exists; however, avoid antibiotics metabolized and cleared by the liver if the LFTs are affected.

XVIII

Oncology: Head and Neck Cancers, Leukemias, Lymphomas, and Multiple Myeloma

Head and Neck Cancers and Associated Dental Management Guidelines

ONCOLOGY OVERVIEW

Cancers of the mouth, salivary glands, sinuses, nose, throat, and lymph nodes in the neck are designated head and neck cancers. Difficulty swallowing, hoarseness, lesions in the oral cavity, and lymph node enlargements in the neck are frequently how head and neck cancers present.

The dentist plays a very important role in the detection of head and neck cancers because oral cancer screening is a routine part of patient examination, and patients visit dentists more frequently than physicians.

Cancer care is multifaceted and multidisciplinary. This chapter discusses cancer terminology, cancer staging, cancer treatment principles and goals, cancer treatment options, and treatment response definitions. This information will enable the reader to understand and participate in the cancer patient's care.

HEAD AND NECK CANCER DETECTION AND THE DENTIST

The dentist might be the first provider to track and follow through with a patient experiencing difficulty swallowing. The dentist can also identify hoarseness that is of concern and request further evaluation; the dentist can identify suspicious oral lesions because of their color, shape, or size, and refer the patient for biopsy.

The dentist can focus on lesions associated with poor healing and triage the patient to a physician for further assessment. The dentist can find lymph node enlargements that do not fit the picture of infection-associated enlargements, but rather have cancer-associated features. Thus, the dentist is often the first provider to refer the patient to the medical side for further evaluation.

A dentist can also aid in the diagnosis of leukemias and lymphomas by detecting the following:

1. Enlargement of the lymph nodes in the head and neck region associated with sudden onset of systemic symptoms.

Dentist's Guide to Medical Conditions, Medications, and Complications, Second Edition. Kanchan M. Ganda.
© 2013 John Wiley & Sons, Inc. Published 2013 by John Wiley & Sons, Inc.

2. Oral findings that frequently accompany lymphomas and leukemias from associated acute deficiency of RBCs and platelets.
3. Oral findings due to lack of normal functioning WBCs, RBCs, and platelets.

NEOPLASMS OF THE ORAL CAVITY

To understand cancer growth one has to understand tumor biology. One malignant cell creates 10^9 cells. These cancer cells grow faster than normal cells and have unstable DNA that cannot be repaired.

Head and neck cancers account for 6% of all cancers, and of these, 30% of the cancers occur in the oral cavity. Males are more often affected than females. The patients are usually in their 40s or 50s. The most common tumor of the oral cavity is a squamous cell carcinoma in the upper aero digestive tract.

NEOPLASMS OF THE NASAL CAVITY

Neoplasms of the nasal cavity are rare. There are two types of neoplasms:

1. **Juvenile nasopharyngeal angiofibroma:** Juvenile nasopharyngeal angiofibroma can sometimes affect adolescent males. It is often benign and the patient frequently experiences recurrent epistaxis.
2. **Nasopharyngeal carcinoma:** Nasopharyngeal carcinoma can be due to exposure to hardwood or heavy chemicals, particularly metals. Nasopharyngeal carcinoma is frequently encountered in males from the Canton Province of China.

HEAD AND NECK CANCER SYMPTOMS AND SIGNS

Symptoms and signs frequently experienced are localized pain, odynophagia (pain on swallowing), dysphagia (difficulty swallowing), hoarseness, dyspnea (shortness of breath), coughing up blood, and referred pain to the ear from the upper digestive tract, especially in patients with alcohol and tobacco use.

LYMPH NODES OF THE HEAD AND NECK

A dentist needs to know about cancers of the head and neck region **and** the associated lymphatic drainage so the two can be correlated to assist in the diagnosis, treatment, and follow-up of benign or malignant tumors. The lymph nodes surrounding the base of the skull and the cervical chains of lymph nodes are **the** nodes of great importance for head and neck tumors. A dentist should have a clear understanding of what specific areas each set of nodes drains. Thus, when a lesion is detected during physical examination, the appropriate lymph nodes should be palpated to determine the extent of involvement.

Lymph Nodes Surrounding the Base of the Skull

These nodes include the following:

- The preauricular or superficial parotid node
- The postauricular nodes

- The occipital nodes
- The deep parotid nodes
- The retropharyngeal nodes
- The submandibular nodes
- The submental nodes
- The tonsilar/jugulodigastric node
- The juguloomohyoid node
- The para-tracheal and pre-tracheal nodes

The Cervical Chain of Lymph Nodes

These nodes include the following:

- The superficial cervical chains
- The deep cervical chains

The Superficial Cervical Chains

The superficial cervical chains receive drainage from the preauricular, postauricular, and occipital nodes. The superficial cervical chains, in turn, drain into the deep cervical chains.

The Deep Cervical Chains

The deep cervical nodes receive drainage from the salivary glands, thyroid gland, tongue, tonsils, nose, pharynx, and larynx (Table 51.1). On the left side, the deep cervical chain drains into the thoracic duct. On the right side, the deep cervical chain drains into the right lymphatic duct, or the internal jugular, subclavian, or brachiocephalic veins.

GENERAL CANCER RISK FACTORS AND PREVENTION

The general risk factors for cancer are **smoking tobacco, alcohol consumption, and miscellaneous other causes.**

Smoking as a Cancer Factor

Smoking tobacco accounts for 170,000 deaths each year. Of all cancers, 30% are due to tobacco and 80% of all lung cancers are due to smoking.

Examples of Tobacco-Related Cancers

Tobacco-associated cancers include lung, mouth, and pharynx cancers; esophageal cancers; pancreatic cancer; uterus, cervix, kidney, and bladder cancers; oral cancer from chewing tobacco; and lung, oral, larynx, and esophageal cancers from cigar smoking.

Table 51.1. Head and Neck Lymph Nodes Identifying Tissues Drained and Specifying Direct or Indirect Drainage into the Deep Cervical Chains

Lymph Nodes	Areas Drained	Drainage
Pre-auricular or Superficial Parotid Nodes:	Drain the external ear canal, front of auricle, and the adjacent scalp	**Indirect drainage** from Superficial Cervical to Deep Cervical nodes
Post-auricular Nodes:	Drain the external ear canal, back of the auricle and the adjacent scalp	**Indirect drainage** from Superficial Cervical to Deep Cervical nodes
Occipital Nodes:	Drain the posterior part of scalp and adjacent region of neck	**Indirect drainage** from Superficial Cervical to Deep Cervical nodes
Deep Parotid Nodes:	Drain the anterior half of scalp, infra-temporal region, orbit, lateral eyelids, maxillary molar teeth, external ear canal, and the parotid gland	**Direct drainage:** Deep Parotid nodes directly drain into the Deep Cervical nodes
Retropharyngeal Nodes:	Drain the upper part of the pharynx and adjoining structures	**Direct drainage:** These nodes drain directly into the Deep Cervical nodes
Submandibular nodes:	Drain the anterior nasal cavities, tongue, teeth, gums, submandibular and sublingual glands, and all of the face except the lateral eyelids and medial lower lip and chin	**Direct drainage:** These nodes drain directly into the Deep Cervical nodes
Submental nodes:	Drain the tip of the tongue, floor of the mouth, and the lower lip and chin	**Direct drainage:** These nodes drain directly into the Deep Cervical nodes
Tonsilar/Jugulo-digastric Nodes:	Drain the tonsils and lateral part of the tongue	**Direct drainage:** These nodes drain directly into the Deep Cervical nodes
Jugulo-Omohyoid Nodes:	Drain the tongue via the submental and submandibular nodes	**Direct drainage:** These nodes drain directly into the Deep Cervical nodes
Para Tracheal and Pretracheal Nodes:	Drain the trachea and thyroid gland. These nodes drain into the tracheo-bronchial nodes in the mediastinum	**Direct drainage:** These nodes drain directly into the Deep Cervical nodes

Alcohol as a Cancer Factor

Alcohol accounts for 19,000 deaths per year and alcohol is an important etiological factor for many cancers, especially cancers of the head and neck. Oral cancer risk is highest in patients using both alcohol and tobacco, compared with those using just one or the other.

Miscellaneous Risk Factors

Other risk factors for head and neck cancers are obesity, viruses, exposure to ultraviolet light, and immune conditions.

CANCER PREVENTION

The risk of cancer can be lowered with smoking cessation, screening tests, sunscreen use, diet modification, and healthy lifestyle.

SCREENING TESTS FOR CANCER DETECTION AT SPECIFIC BODY SITES

A dentist has to be very familiar with oral cancer screening, and as a health-care provider, the responsibility extends to knowing other forms of cancer screenings too. Your patient may provide information about having had specific tests or may question you about other screening methods or tests, so it is important to be knowledgeable. Common cancer screening tests are:

1. **Breast:** Screening is done by self-exam and mammogram.
2. **Testicular:** Screening is done by self-exam.
3. **Cervix:** Screening is done by Pap smear.
4. **Colon:** Screening is done by colonoscopy and fecal occult blood test.
5. **Skin:** Screening is done by dermatological examination.
6. **Oral:** Screening is done by oral examination.
7. **Prostate:** Screening is done by digital rectal examination.
8. **Lungs:** There is no good screen as yet for lung cancer.

CANCER MANAGEMENT

Cancer management is multi-tiered and consists of the following:

1. Cancer diagnostic aids
2. Cancer staging
3. Cancer treatment

CANCER DIAGNOSTIC AIDS

To confirm cancer pathology, tissue samples can be obtained using any of the following options; biopsy of suspect tissue, bone marrow aspiration, blood sample, assessment of cell surface markers, and cytogenics or DNA analysis.

CANCER STAGING

Tumor staging can be done using the Broder's classification and/or the TNM staging system.

Broder's Classification

Tumor grading using the Broder's classification (Tumor Grade [G]), is as follows:

G1: Tumor that is well differentiated
G2: Tumor that is moderately well differentiated
G3: Tumor that is poorly differentiated
G4: Tumor that is undifferentiated

The TNM Staging System

The TNM staging system is a clinical staging system that helps estimate the extent of disease *prior* to treatment. The staging process helps determine the treatment choice, the predictive treatment response, and survival. The tumor and nodes are assessed by inspection and palpation when possible. The status of the tumor must be confirmed histopathologically before treatment options are explored. Additional tests that help with the staging process are biopsy, x-ray, CT scan, MRI, nuclear study, or surgery.

For detection and localization of head and neck tumors, magnetic resonance imaging (MRI) is a better option compared with CT scans. MRIs are also better than CT scans in distinguishing lymph nodes from blood vessels in the assessment of head and neck cancers. In the event of a relapse, restaging of the cancer is done to determine appropriate additional treatment that will be required.

American Joint Committee on Cancer (AJCC) TNM Classification

TNM staging is done using these definitions for tumor, lymph nodes, and metastasis:

1. **Tumor definitions:**
   - Primary tumor (T) represents the extent of the primary tumor
   - TX: Primary tumor cannot be assessed
   - T0 (T zero): No evidence of primary tumor
   - TIS: Carcinoma in situ
   - T1: Tumor ≤2cm in its greatest dimension
   - T2: Tumor >2cm but ≤4cm in its greatest dimension
   - T3: Tumor >4cm in its greatest dimension
   - T4: Invasive tumor
2. **Regional lymph nodes (N) definitions:**
   - N represents the degree of lymph node involvement
   - NX: Regional lymph nodes cannot be assessed
   - N0 (N zero): No regional lymph node metastasis present
   - N1: Metastasis present in a single ipsilateral (same side) lymph node, ≤3cm in its greatest dimension
   - N2a: Metastasis in a single ipsilateral (same side) lymph node >3cm but ≤6cm in dimension
   - N2b: Metastasis in multiple ipsilateral lymph nodes, ≤6cm in greatest dimension
   - N2c: Metastasis in bilateral or contralateral (on the opposite side) lymph nodes, ≤6cm in greatest dimension
   - N3: Metastasis in a lymph node >6cm in greatest dimension
3. **Distant Metastasis (M) Definitions:**
   - M represents the presence of metastasis
   - MX: Distant metastasis cannot be assessed
   - M0 (M zero): No distant metastasis present
   - M1: Distant metastasis present

The TNM Stages

The TNM stages are as follows:

Stage 1: Primary tumor
Stage 2: Large primary tumor with or without lymph node involvement
Stage 3: Primary tumor plus lymph node involvement
Stage 4: Indicates metastasis

American Joint Committee on Cancer (AJCC) Stage Groupings

The stage groupings indicate the TNM definitions associated with each of the TNM stages:

Stage 0: TIS, N0, M0
Stage I: T1, N0, M0
Stage II: T2, N0, M0
Stage III: T3, N0, M0; T1, N1, M0; T2, N1, M0 **or** T3, N1, M0
Stage IVA: T4a, N0, M0; T4a, N1, M0; T1, N2, M0; T2, N2, M0; T3, N2, M0 **or** T4a, N2, M0
Stage IVB: Any T, N3, M0 or T4b, any N, M0
Stage IVC: Any T, any N, M1

The Eastern Cooperative Oncology Group Scale

The Eastern cooperative oncology scale helps decide which patients can receive treatment. It does so by classifying the patient's level of activity with the associated cancer. According to the scale, it is appropriate to treat only Stage 2 or better because the patient loses one level during treatment. The following are the stages according to the Eastern Cooperative Oncology Scale:

Stage 0: This scale represents working full time.
Stage 1: This scale represents working part time.
Stage 2: This scale represents a patient disabled with cancer therapy and spending <50% time in bed or a chair.
Stage 3: This scale represents a patient who spends >50% time in bed or a chair.
Stage 4: This scale represents a bedridden patient.

CANCER TREATMENT

Cancer treatment entails establishment of the following:

1. Cancer treatment options and goals
2. Principles of treatment
3. Treatment response definitions
4. Head and neck cancer treatment options

Treatment Options and Goals

Cancer treatment options and their respective goals are as follows:

1. **Curative:** This option completely gets rid of the cancer.
2. **Adjuvant:** This option prevents relapse once the cancer is removed.

3. **Palliative:** With this option, although the cancer cannot be gotten rid of, disease progression is prevented.
4. **Supportive care:** Supportive care is needed for side effects associated with cancer treatment, such as nausea, anorexia, weight loss, and so on.
5. **Hospice:** When the cancer cannot be controlled, hospice care treats the pain and suffering to make the end stage comfortable for the patient.

Treatment Principles

Cancer treatment options depend on the invasiveness of the cancer; the options offered are:

1. **Localized cancer:** The treatment option for localized cancer is surgery and/or radiation.
2. **Systemic cancer:** The options for systemic cancer are chemotherapy, radiation, hormonal therapy, or immunotherapy.

Treatment Response Definitions

The dentist plays a very important role in managing and maintaining the oral health status of the cancer patient during chemotherapy and/or radiotherapy. The treating oncologist can sometimes forward the patient's records to the dental provider to assist with the care. Familiarity with the treatment response definitions often used by the treating oncologists is thus helpful in evaluating the records and assessing the patient's status. Common treatment response definitions used are:

1. **CR:** Complete remission
2. **PR:** Partial remission
3. **SD:** Stable disease and one that is not progressing
4. **DP:** Disease progression
5. **Relapse:** Disease occurrence after complete remission (CR)
6. **Refractory:** Disease never in complete remission (CR)

Head and Neck Cancer Treatment Options

The treatment options for cancer care are:

1. Surgery
2. Radiation therapy
3. Chemotherapy
4. Chemotherapy plus radiation

Stage I and Stage II cancers are highly curable by surgery or radiation therapy. Stage III or Stage IV cancer patients are candidates for treatment by a combination of surgery and radiation therapy. They should also be considered for a combination of chemotherapy with surgery and/or radiation therapy to improve local control and to decrease the frequency of distant metastases.

HEAD AND NECK CANCER TREATMENT

Surgery

Advantages of Surgical Therapy

Surgical therapy is curative and ideal for early-stage cancer with limited involvement.

Risks of Surgical Therapy

Risks are limited to what can be removed, the microscopic disease status, and the operating room risks. Surgery is not a useful choice in widespread disease.

Radiation Therapy

Advantages of Radiation Therapy

Radiation works differently in different cancers but is a good choice for tumors that cannot be removed. The mechanism of action of radiotherapy is different than that for chemotherapy. The response is fast and with minimal side effects.

Risks of Radiotherapy

Radiotherapy damages the surrounding normal tissues and it is useless in widespread cancers.

Radiation Therapy Options

A dentist should be familiar with all forms of radiation therapy to the head and neck region and **know the amount** of radiation the patient has received during cancer care. Radiation options available are:

1. **External-beam radiation therapy:** This is the treatment option for large tumors. The area radiated includes the tumor and regional lymph nodes, even if they are not clinically involved.
2. **Interstitial implantation radiation therapy:** Interstitial implantation alone is a treatment option for small superficial cancers.
3. **Both external-beam and interstitial implantation radiation therapy:** This form of combined radiation is needed for large primary tumors and/or bulky nodal metastases.

Chemotherapy

Knowledge of the following chemotherapy-associated topics is important for optimal patient care:

1. Chemotherapy schedules
2. Chemotherapy vascular access
3. Chemotherapy choices

Chemotherapy Schedules

For provision of dental care during chemotherapy, it is always important to know the patient's chemotherapy schedule and the terms used to describe the schedules. Some of the terms used are:

1. **Chemotherapy cycle:** A chemotherapy cycle represents one treatment. Usually the treatment consists of multiple cycles.
2. **Chemotherapy frequency:** Frequency defines the rate at which chemotherapy is given. The frequency can be monthly, weekly, or continuous.

Chemotherapy Vascular Access

Multiple (four in all) vascular accesses are established **prior** to the start of chemotherapy. The reason multiple accesses are established is that if one line gets infected, it has to be removed and another line gets inserted. To create a new access during chemotherapy is not possible because of tissue scarring. Two jugulars and two subclavial vascular lines are needed for blood draws. Presence of a vascular access requires the dentist to premedicate the patient prior to dental treatment.

Chemotherapy Choices

Chemotherapeutic choices are determined by identifying the cycle specificity and the phase specificity:

1. **Cycle nonspecific choice:** Corticosteroid is the cycle nonspecific choice drug.
2. **Cycle-specific, phase-nonspecific:** Alkylating agents are the cycle-specific, phase-nonspecific choices.
3. **Cycle-specific, phase-specific:** Antimetabolites are the cycle- and phase-specific choices.

BONE MARROW TRANSPLANT

Bone marrow transplant (BMT) is another option available for cancer care. High-dose chemotherapy, usually ten times the normal dose, is needed for BMT. Stem cells used are taken from the patient or from a donor. In donor cells BMT, one can get a host-graft in which the donor cells see the cancer cells as bad and attack it. Post-transplant immune suppression is always needed to prevent rejection.

Bone Marrow Transplant Complications

Significant complications associated with bone marrow transplantation are: xerostomia; mucositis; fungal, viral, or bacterial infections; and graft versus host disease.

Graft versus host disease is an adverse reaction wherein donor cells attack the healthy cells of the host. The right thing to happen with BMT is for donor cells to see tumor cells as bad and attack them. This is the graft versus tumor attack.

IMPORTANT HEAD AND NECK CANCER FACTS

Most head and neck cancers are of the squamous cell variety. Patient factors and local expertise influence the choice of treatment. When the tumor invades the vasculature, the prognosis is bad. Leukoplakia is a descriptive term that indicates a white patch that does not rub off. Early cancers of the buccal mucosa are equally curable by radiation therapy or by adequate excision. The treatment options for lip and oral cavity cancer may be surgery alone, radiation therapy alone, or a combination of surgery, radiation, and chemotherapy.

Larger cancers require composite resection with reconstruction of the defect by pedicle flaps. Moderate excisions of tongue, even hemiglossectomy, often results in little speech disability. With extensive tongue resection there can be problems with aspiration, difficulty swallowing, and speech difficulties.

Patients who **smoke** while on radiation therapy have **lower** response and survival rates, and such patients should be counseled to stop smoking before starting radiation therapy. Additionally, poor oral hygiene and tobacco or alcohol use during radiation can accelerate the onset of osteoradionecrosis (ORN). Be aware that patients with head and neck cancers have an **increased incidence** of developing a **second** primary tumor of the upper aerodigestive tract.

Surgery for parotid tumor can lead to **facial paralysis** because the facial nerve goes through the gland. Dental status evaluation should be performed **prior** to radiation or chemotherapy. Prosthodontic rehabilitation post treatment is implemented for better quality of life.

Localized and Systemic Complications Associated with Head and Neck Cancer Therapy

Localized and systemic complications associated with head and neck cancer therapy are mucositis, xerostomia, xerostomia-associated rampant caries and periodontal disease, infection (viral, fungal, and bacterial), pain, nausea and vomiting, malnutrition, deformity, trismus, microvascular injury, osteoradionecrosis (ORN), bone marrow suppression, and death.

HEAD AND NECK CANCERS AND DENTISTRY

Dentistry in a patient with a current or past history of head and neck cancer has to be a well-thought-out, planned process. Several aspects associated with the cancer care have to be evaluated **prior** to implementation of dentistry. Head and neck radiation therapy causes short-term and long-term side effects. Short-term side effects associated with radiation therapy are:

1. Mucositis and mucosal infections
2. Altered salivary gland function

Mucositis usually begins by the **third week** of radiation and it presents as an inflammation or ulceration of the oral mucosa. Patients suffering from mucositis often benefit from using a mouthwash prepared as follows: Mix 2tsp salt and 2tsp baking soda in 8oz cold water. The patient should gargle and **expectorate** the mixture.

Altered salivary gland function causes xerostomia, and xerostomia in turn leads to oral candidiasis and caries. It is absolutely necessary to avoid alcohol-based mouth rinses at this time because further drying of the oral mucosa can occur.

The long-term side effects of radiation occur because of progressive vascular and cellular changes in the bones and soft tissue. There is slow remodeling of the bone and soft tissue, and this leads to necrosis and an increased rate of infection. Salivary gland damage and increased fibrosis also occurs. The hallmark features of long-term radiation-associated side effects are hypoxic, hypovascular, and hypocellular tissues, the classic "3H's." These side effects **worsen with time**, and this fact **must always** be factored in and appropriately addressed during patient care. Provide antibiotic coverage starting one hour prior to dentistry and prescribe penicillin VK or clindamycin for five days post-op to promote the healing process in such patients and prevent the occurrence of any infection.

OSTEORADIONECROSIS

Osteoradionecrosis (ORN) is a serious consequence of radiation to the head and neck region. **Lifelong** risk exists with high doses of radiation, and invasive surgical procedures such as extractions and periodontal surgery should be avoided with high doses of radiation. Necrosis is **more pronounced** and the healing is **more depressed** as the postradiation time interval increases. The bone becomes susceptible to infection and the ability to repair is compromised.

The mandible is most commonly affected because the bone density is high and the vascularization is poor. Patients receiving radiation for tumors anatomically related to the mandible develop necrosis five times more frequently than patients with tumors at other sites. ORN is more common in the anterior part of the mandible due to limited vascular supply. ORN of the maxilla is rare.

Radiation by implants is more often associated with ORN compared with radiation from an external source. Therefore, consultation with the radiologist **prior** to dentistry is a must to determine the duration and type of radiation planned or given. The radiologist will inform you if radioactive implant or external beam radiotherapy is planned or was used. The consult will also provide the location and size of the treatment fields plus the total radiation dose.

When the radiation dose has been <6,500 RADS, extractions, when required post radiation, should be done **one year after radiation**, using antibiotic coverage. Usually penicillin or clindamycin can be given for five days to promote the healing process.

A radiation dose >6,500 RADS/65Gy is associated with an increased incidence of osteoradionecrosis. If a patient has to have extractions after having undergone radiation to the head and neck region using doses >**6,500** RADS, then hyperbaric O_2 therapy is strongly suggested. The patient has to have hyperbaric O_2 dives or treatment cycles during the pre-op and post-op time period. 100% O_2 is provided at 2–2.5 atmospheres of pressure for 90 minutes per dive to prevent ORN. The patient needs up to 20 dives prior to surgery and 10 dives after surgery for a good outcome.

Hyperbaric O_2 treatment stimulates tissue angiogenesis in the hypovascular irradiated tissue. Intermittent high O_2 tissue levels stimulate fibroblasts to secrete a collagen matrix, which capillaries follow during angiogenesis, and this leads to more fibroblastic activity. The cost for each dive is $500–$700.

It should be quite evident that to prevent problems post radiation, non-restorable teeth should be extracted at least **two weeks prior** to radiation so healing can occur.

CHEMOTHERAPY-ASSOCIATED LOCALIZED AND SYSTEMIC SIDE EFFECTS

Chemotherapy-associated side effects are discussed in the following sections.

Myelosuppression

Myelosuppression occurs for 10–14 days following chemotherapy when there is a **drop** in the blood counts. As previously discussed, this pattern of myelosuppression also occurs with radiotherapy. Low WBC count increases the potential for infection, low RBC count leads to developing anemia, and low platelets are associated with easy bruising and bleeding. Thus, dental intervention is **not** recommended during the first two weeks following chemotherapy/radiotherapy.

Fever and Oral Infections

Fever may have an oral origin in chemotherapy patients. Immune-suppressed patients usually have less swelling, pain, and fever, so it makes it harder for the clinician to detect an infection. Always be vigilant, and once detected, treat all infections aggressively and completely.

As previously mentioned, conventional symptoms and signs associated with infections are usually absent because of decreased immunity during chemotherapy. Oral flora is different compared with the normal patient, and anaerobic organisms abound. Broad-spectrum systemic antibiotics are usually administered when needed. Generally, carbenicillin, a semi-synthetic penicillin, is used. Carbenicillin 1–2 tablets q6h for five days, or aminoglycosides, gentamycin, or tobramycin, are prescribed.

Graft Versus Host Disease

Graft versus host disease is seen more often if the patient has periodontal disease, and it can last for years in severe cases.

Organ Damage

Chemotherapeutic drug toxicity can sometimes adversely affect the liver and the kidneys.

Neurotoxicity

Neurotoxicity can cause the patient to experience persistent deep aching and burning pain. A certain class of drugs, vancomycins and alkaloids, are more commonly associated with these side effects. Benzodiazepines are usually prescribed, when possible, to control the discomfort.

Integument Involvement

Integument involvement results in mucositis, diarrhea, nausea, vomiting, and alopecia. Mucositis, when present, should be treated with lidocaine + Benadryl + Maalox rinse. An antifungal rinse should also be given to prevent superinfection.

Toothache

The patient can experience dental discomfort that **mimics** a toothache. Therefore, it is important to evaluate and treat the patient's dental needs **before** starting chemotherapy.

SUGGESTED DENTAL GUIDELINES FOR THE CHEMOTHERAPY- AND/OR RADIOTHERAPY-TREATED HEAD AND NECK CANCER PATIENT

Follow these guidelines in the dental setting:

1. The dentist must intervene in the chemotherapy/radiotherapy schedule with minimal disruption and work as a team with the patient's oncologist.
2. The dentist must consult with the oncologist and do so frequently if needed.
3. Chemotherapy is given in cycles, and one cycle equals one treatment. The treatment can be continuous, weekly, or monthly. Determine the patient's chemotherapy schedule and plan the dental treatment during weeks 3 and 4.
4. The majority of cancer patients receiving chemotherapeutic drugs have an **Infusaport or a Hickmann Venous access** for administration of the drugs. Use AHA **SBE prophylaxis** when providing dental treatment in these patients.
5. All head and neck radiation patients **and** 75% of the blood and bone marrow transplant patients are at risk for oral complications. Of chemotherapy patients, 40% have a higher rate of myelosuppression.
6. Bone marrow transplant (BMT) patients have an increased incidence of host versus graft disease if periodontal disease is present. Transplant patients must have dental assessment and care **before** transplant.
7. Always determine the platelet count and the absolute neutrophil count (ANC) prior to dentistry in these patients. Calculate the ANC and follow the ANC guidelines if the WBC count is $\leq$3,500 cells/mm^3. Counts are highest prior to the next cycle so obtain blood tests **within 24 hours** of providing treatment.

    You can treat a patient with an ANC as low as 500 cells/mm^3 in the outpatient dental setting with adequate antibiotic use. Patients with an ANC <500 cells/mm^3 need to be hospitalized. You can treat a patient with platelets as low as 50K.
8. The WBC count can decrease with radiation/chemotherapy, and the count is lowest during the first two weeks after treatment. The counts begin to rise during weeks 3–4 of the post-treatment period. Any emergent dental work, when needed, should therefore be done in weeks 3–4, post treatment.
9. Educate the patient about the importance of hygiene and good home care. Treat all sources of oral infection **prior** to chemotherapy, radiotherapy, or bone marrow transplant. It is critical to treat periodontal disease early and conservatively. To minimize complications, do not introduce new practices.
10. Before chemotherapy or radiation therapy, do caries controls, control all lesions, complete all dental needs, and provide fluoride trays.

11. **Fluoride care:** Prescription-strength fluoride toothpastes and varnish are better than rinses during chemotherapy or radiotherapy, but there is low patient compliance with these products. Fewer root caries occur with fluoride use. Fluoride increases mineralization and this decreases mucositis associated with chemotherapy or radiotherapy.

12. Dental extractions in the field of radiation should be done **prior** to radiation if the teeth are non-restorable, need excessive restoration, or need periodontal or endodontic treatment. Also, prior to radiation remove orthodontic bands when present.

13. Treat pericoronitis or deep periodontal pockets immediately. Do scaling and root planing and prescribe metronidazole (Flagyl) treatment for five days to eradicate all existing anaerobic organisms.

14. For deep pockets, dental minocycline (Arestin) is placed in the pockets and repeated weekly until the condition resolves.

15. Prescribe the nonalcoholic (alcohol prevents mucositis from healing) chlorhexidine rinse bid, to de-germ the oral cavity and also schedule frequent recalls. Also have the patient use a nonalcoholic mouth rinse prior to treatment.

16. **Trismus:** Fibrosis around the muscles of mastication can cause trismus. The patient must be advised to open and close the mouth frequently during the entire radiation period.

17. **Sedation:** The patient should be provided with sedation for dental procedures.

18. **Analgesics:** The following pain-management options should be used when needed: codeine alone or in combination with Tylenol can be given q4–6h. Additionally morphine, meperidine (Demerol), or a fentanyl patch may also be used.

19. **Vomiting during chemotherapy:** Advice the patient to rinse with the following mixture: Add 1/4 tsp baking soda and 1/8 tsp salt to 1c warm water and rinse several times a day. Each mixture use should be followed by rinsing with plain water.

ORAL LESIONS AND SIDE EFFECTS ASSOCIATED WITH CHEMOTHERAPY AND RADIOTHERAPY, AND SUGGESTED MANAGEMENT GUIDELINES

See Table 51.2 for an overview of the following sections.

Mucositis

Overview

Mucositis is associated with white ropy thickening of the mucosa and formation of a pseudomembrane. When this membrane sloughs off, large areas of raw underlying tissue are exposed causing extreme pain that needs IV morphine for control. Burned tissue from radiation appears red, and tissue turnover occurs every five days.

There can be DNA injury from chemotherapy or radiation. This leads to clonogenic cell death associated with destruction of the tissues, which then become an open window for infection. Ragged restorations and sharp teeth can cut the mucosa. Oral bleeding because of low platelets can occur from chemotherapy or bone marrow transplant.

Table 51.2.   Summary of Chemotherapy or Radiotherapy Associated Oral Lesions or Side Effects and Suggested Management Guidelines

Oral Side Effects	Prescriptions
Mild Mucositis:	• **Alkaline saline:** Use 2% sodium bicarbonate in Normal Saline as mouth rinse q4h. • **Hydrogen Peroxide (Peroxyl) rinse:** In the presence of dried mucus, rinse with 1.5% H_2O_2 in mint base. Use Peroxyl **first** and then alkaline saline rinse. • **Mouthwash mixture for Mucositis:** Swish with 5cc of a mouthwash mixture consisting of 4oz diphenhydramine (Benadryl) elixir + 1oz Nystatin + 1,500mg Tetracycline + 60mg Hydrocortisone + 7oz Water. • Add 10cc **Nystatin (Nilstat)** PO tid if thrush is present, and avoid spicy foods.
Moderate Mucositis: The patient has ulcers but can eat	• **Hydrogen Peroxide (Peroxyl) rinse:** Use hydrogen peroxide (Peroxyl) rinse diluted 1:1 followed with copious amounts of alkaline saline rinses for general care. • **Phenol (Ulcerease):** Swish and hold 5–10cc topical Phenol mouth rinse (Ulcerease) for 30 second PRN, to alleviate ulcer pain. Follow with "mouthwash mixture for Mucositis" as specified under mild mucositis.
Severe Mucositis: The patient has severe ulcerations and is not able to eat	• Treatment is the same as with moderate mucositis. • **Calcium Carbonate/Magnesium Carbonate (Mylanta)-Lidocaine-Diphenhydramine (Benadryl) Paste:** A paste consisting of: 3 parts calcium carbonate/magnesium carbonate (Mylanta), 2% viscous lidocaine and 1 part diphenhydramine (Benadryl) can be applied over the ulcers • **Consider IV nutrition** supplementation if unable to eat.
Xerostomia Treatment: Refer to Chapter 48 for more complete prescription details.	• **Give sialogogues** 1 hour prior to radiotherapy to spare some of the salivary glands. • **Xylitol:** Xylitol is a natural sugar substitute that increases saliva flow and does not promote caries. Xylitol actually decreases caries. Use xylitol following meals after rinsing 3–5 times/day and use it in place of chewing gum or candy. • **Mouth guards and sonic toothbrush:** Recommend mouth guards and sonic toothbrush use as it increases saliva flow. • **Chlorhexidine (Peridex) rinse:** Rinse and expectorate with nonalcoholic, 0.12% chlorhexidine (Peridex) gargles bid. This helps tremendously and de-germs the oral cavity. • **Lubricants:** Saliva flow can also be increased with lubricants like vitamin E or borage seed oil to decrease discomfort. • **Gene therapy:** Gene therapy associated insertion of Aquoporin-1 helps increase saliva flow and overcome xerostomia.
Herpes Simplex/Herpes Zoster: Refer to Chapter 48 for more complete prescription details.	• Provide prophylactic treatment with antiviral medications **valacyclovir (Valtrex), famciclovir (Famvir), or acyclovir (Zovirax)** to prevent complications during treatment.

Table 51.2. Summary of Chemotherapy or Radiotherapy Associated Oral Lesions or Side Effects and Suggested Management Guidelines (*Continued*)

Oral Side Effects	Prescriptions
Oral/esophageal Candidiasis: Refer to Chapter 48 for more complete prescription details.	Topical antifungal Therapy: • **Clotrimazole cream:** Clotrimazole cream is good for angular chelitis. • **Nystatin oral suspension:** Nystatin rinse is preferred as the mouth is dry during cancer treatment and Nystatin has no DDIs with other medications. • **Clotrimazole troche:** Clotrimazole troche is **not** the first drug of choice, as it does not dissolve well in a dry mouth. Systemic Antifungal Therapy: 1. **Fluconazole:** Consider fluconazole if the patient is unable to keep up with home care. It should not be the first choice because Fluconazole can affect the liver, and the patient can develop resistance to the drug. 2. **Itraconazole (Sporanox):** 20mL of Sporanox liquid or 200mg bid, Sporanex capsules. 3. **Amphotericin B IV:** If all else fails, use IV amphotericin B.
Trismus:	Teach stretching exercises, provide mechanical devices like Therabite or stacked Popsicle sticks.
Vomiting with Chemotherapy:	Add 1/4tsp of baking soda and 1/8tsp salt to 1 cup of warm water, and rinse followed by expectorate, several times a day. Then rinse with plain water, each time.

Mild Mucositis

The patient has erythematous areas of burn or white plaques that can be treated as follows: **Mild mucositis prescriptions:**

1. **Alkaline saline rinse:** Use 2% sodium bicarbonate in normal saline (NS) as mouth rinse q4h.
2. **Hydrogen peroxide (Peroxyl) rinse:** With the presence of dried mucus, rinse with 1.5% H_2O_2 hydrogen peroxide (Peroxyl) in mint base **first** and then use the alkaline saline rinse.
3. **Prepared mouthwash for mucositis:** Swish with 5cc of the following mouthwash mixture. Mix 4oz diphenhydramine (Benadryl) elixir **plus** 1oz nystatin **plus** 1,500mg tetracycline **plus** 60mg hydrocortisone **plus** 7oz water. Add 10cc nystatin (Nilstat) liquid PO tid if thrush is present, and avoid spicy foods.

Moderate Mucositis

With moderate mucositis the patient has ulcers but can eat.
Moderate mucositis prescriptions:

1. **Hydrogen peroxide (Peroxyl) rinse:** Use hydrogen peroxide (Peroxyl) diluted 1:1 followed with copious amounts of alkaline saline rinses for general care, as with mild mucositis.

2. **Phenol (Ulcerease) mouth rinse:** Have the patient swish and hold 5–10cc of topical phenol mouth rinse (Ulcerease) for 30sec PRN to alleviate pain from ulcers.
3. **Prepared mouthwash for mucositis:** Follow with use of prepared mouthwash mixture specified under mild mucositis.

Severe Mucositis

The patient with severe mucositis has severe ulcerations and is **not** able to eat.
   Severe mucositis prescriptions:

1. Treatment for severe mucositis is the same as for moderate mucositis.
2. **Calcium carbonate/magnesium carbonate (Mylanta) lidocaine-diphenhydramine (Benadryl) paste:** The paste is applied over the ulcers to numb the pain and it is prepared by mixing the following: Mix three parts calcium carbonate/magnesium carbonate (Mylanta) **plus** 2% viscous lidocaine **plus** one part diphenhydramine (Benadryl).
3. **IV nutrition:** Consider IV nutrition supplementation in cases where the patient is unable to eat because of the severe mucositis.

Xerostomia

Saliva and Xerostomia Facts

Saliva is medically necessary for optimal health of the oral cavity. Severe abrasion and attrition of tissues can occur with xerostomia. Patients can have toothbrush abrasion and caries at the same time because of xerostomia.
   Provide treatment with fluoride, lubrication, or sialogogues to prevent adverse effects associated with xerostomia. Fluoride acts as a catalyst for remineralization.

Consequences of Reduced Saliva

Reduced saliva flow can be associated with the following:

1. There is increased incidence of infection: candidiasis, periodontal disease, or both.
2. Loss of remineralization is responsible for the very high incidence of caries in these patients compared with the normal population.
3. Decreased lubrication causes difficulty speaking and trouble swallowing.
4. Xerostomia creates an acidic environment.
5. There is poor stability of dentures.
6. Poor salivation is also associated with mucositis, ulcerations, halitosis, altered taste, and sleeping problems.

Xerostomia Prevention During Radiotherapy

Prevention can be achieved with the following:

1. Use of computer-assisted 3D confocal radiation (IMRT) during radiotherapy helps reduce destruction of the salivary glands as it varies the shape and intensity of radiation.

2. Give sialogogues **one hour prior** to radiotherapy to spare some of the salivary glands from destruction. Once the glands are destroyed they cannot regenerate.

Xerostomia Prescriptions

Chemotherapy- or radiotherapy-associated xerostomia can be corrected using the following:

1. **Xylitol:** Xylitol is a natural sugar substitute that increases saliva flow and does not promote caries. Xylitol actually decreases caries. Use Xylitol following meals after rinsing, 3–5 times/day, and use it in place of chewing gum or candy.
2. **Mouth guards and sonic toothbrush:** Recommend mouth guards and sonic toothbrush use because they increase saliva flow.
3. **Chlorhexidine (Peridex) rinse:** Rinse and expectorate with nonalcoholic, 0.12% chlorhexidine (Peridex) gargles bid. This helps tremendously and de-germs the oral cavity.
4. **Lubricants:** Saliva flow can also be increased with lubricants such as vitamin E or borage seed oil to decrease discomfort.
5. **Gene Therapy:** Gene therapy–associated insertion of Aquoporin-1 helps increase saliva flow and overcome xerostomia.

Infections

Herpes Simplex/Herpes Zoster

The virus can be reactivated during radiation and shows up in unusual places. It is best to provide prophylactic treatment with antiviral medications, famciclovir (Famvir), valacyclovir (Valtrex), or acyclovir (Zovirax), to prevent complications during treatment.

Candidiasis

Candidiasis can be treated with many presentations, and if caught early it is easier to treat. In the neutropenic patient, systemic spread of candidiasis can lead to death.

Topical Antifungal Therapy

Use the following for topical antifungal therapy:

1. **Clotrimazole cream:** Clotrimazole cream is good for angular cheilitis.
2. **Nystatin oral suspension:** Nystatin rinse is **preferred** because the mouth is dry during cancer treatment.
3. **Clotrimazole troche:** Clotrimazole troche is **not** the first drug of choice because it does not dissolve well in a dry mouth.

Systemic Antifungal Therapy

Use the following for systemic therapy:

1. **Fluconazole:** Fluconazole is an option to consider if the patient is unable to keep up with home care. It should not be the first choice, because fluconazole can affect the liver and the patient can develop resistance to the drug.
2. **Itraconazole (Sporanox):** 20mL of Sporanox liquid or 200mg Sporanex capsules is dispensed bid.
3. **Amphotericin B IV:** If all fails, the patient is put on IV amphotericin B.

With all three preparations, continue treatment for at least two weeks until the condition is eradicated. The infection is very hard to treat and comes back easily when the patient does not have proper saliva. If the saliva is low, infections can get precipitated in the salivary ducts causing stones and blockage. The patient is treated with doxycycline when this occurs.

Trismus

Definition

Trismus is restricted opening of the mouth, and it often is secondary to surgery. Fibrosis due to radiation treatment has an effect on the muscles of mastication and it occurs 6–12 months after radiation. Trismus causes problems with chewing, and it is difficult to do dentistry in the presence of trismus.

Treatment

Treatment consists of teaching stretching exercises and providing mechanical devices such as Therabite or stacked Popsicle sticks.

LEUKEMIA

Leukemia or liquid cancer of the blood and bone marrow can present as acute lymphoblastic/lymphocytic leukemia, chronic lymphocytic leukemia, acute myelocytic leukemia, or chronic myelocytic leukemia.

Acute Leukemias Overview

The acute forms of leukemia are associated with rapid accumulation of dysfunctional immature cells in the blood and the bone marrow, and an associated reduction in the number of normal, functioning, mature white blood cells.

In addition to the inadequate number of normal white blood cells, there is often an associated reduction in the number of red blood cells and platelets. Thus, increased susceptibility to infection, anemia, and platelet deficiency–associated bleeding, bruising, and petechiae are often seen in patients suffering from the acute forms of leukemia.

Chronic Leukemias Overview

The chronic forms of leukemia progress slowly, and consequently, the bone marrow is able to produce more mature functional cell lines. The patient is less symptomatic and it is not uncommon for the leukemia to be accidentally detected on routine examination.

Prevalence

Leukemia affects males more than females, and patients of African descent are more likely to be affected, compared with those of European descent.

Acute lymphoblastic leukemia (ALL) is the most common form of leukemia affecting children ages 0–19 years, and ALL is now considered a curable cancer in the majority of patients affected by the disease.

Acute myelogenous leukemia (AML) and chronic lymphocytic leukemia (CLL) are the most common forms of leukemia affecting adults. Chronic myelogenous leukemia (CML) affects people above age 60. AML, CML, and CLL are most common in the seventh, eighth, and ninth decades of life. Leukemias thus occur more commonly in the elderly, after age 60.

Symptoms and Signs

Symptoms and signs associated with acute leukemia reflect the lack of normal levels of WBCs, RBCs, and platelets. The patient experiences anemia-associated fatigue, pallor, and decreased ability to perform routine chores. This is In addition to platelet deficiency–associated mucosal bleeding, petechiae, easy bruising, easy bleeding, and increased susceptibility to infection and poor wound healing due to the decreased number of mature, normal, functioning WBCs. Chronic leukemia in many patients is often asymptomatic and is an accidental discovery during routine medical examination.

Diagnosis

Leukemia diagnosis is made by pathological examination of the peripheral smear and the bone marrow aspirate.

Treatment Terminology

A dental provider helps manage the oral side effects associated with leukemia and also helps maintain ongoing oral health for optimal outcome. Thus, it becomes important to clearly understand leukemia remission and leukemia relapse, as discussed in the following sections.

Leukemia Remission

With remission, treatment leads to complete recovery of the blood and bone marrow to normal, and the patient becomes fully functional. Palliative and supportive dental intervention is done during the acute stage, and subsequently the patient is kept on 4–6 months maintenance recall to access ongoing status.

Leukemia Relapse

Relapse is a return of the leukemia, and abnormal cells are seen again in the circulation and the bone marrow. Palliative and supportive dental intervention is done during the acute and relapse stages, and maintenance is provided if recovery occurs subsequently after the relapse.

Leukemia Treatment

When there is **complete remission for five years** after treatment, the acute forms of leukemia are said to be cured. The five-year survival rate has improved for all forms of leukemia.

Treatment Protocols

Discussed in the next sections are treatment protocols for the following leukemias:

1. Acute lymphoblastic leukemia (ALL)
2. Acute myeloid leukemia (AML)

ACUTE LYMPHOBLASTIC LEUKEMIA (ALL) TREATMENT PROTOCOL

Treatment options offered for ALL depends on the patient's age and the health status at the time of diagnosis.

The treatment protocol for ALL is a **three-step** process:

1. Induction chemotherapy
2. Consolidation chemotherapy
3. Maintenance chemotherapy

Induction Chemotherapy

Induction chemotherapy is usually done with daunorubicin, vincristine, prednisone, asparaginase, and occasionally cyclophosphamide (Cytoxan). Neupogen, red cell, and/or platelet transfusion are often used as adjunct supports to compensate for the associated lack of functioning WBCs, RBCs, and platelets.

Consolidation Chemotherapy

The consolidation chemotherapy follows the induction chemotherapy. The patient is given multiple cycles of intensive chemotherapy for a period of 6–9 months.

Maintenance Chemotherapy

The third step of ALL care is the maintenance chemotherapy that is done with oral chemotherapeutic drugs for a period of 18–24 months.

ACUTE MYELOID LEUKEMIA (AML) TREATMENT PROTOCOL

Treatment of AML consists of the following:

1. Remission induction
2. Consolidation

Remission Induction Therapy

Intensive chemotherapy is provided over one week, to induce remission with two chemotherapy drugs, Cytarabine (ara-C) and daunorubicin/idarubicin (Daunomycin, Idamycin). Occasionally, a third drug, 6-Thioguanine, may be added.

Consolidation Therapy

Consolidation therapy follows remission induction therapy. It is provided with using multiple cycles of the drug Cytarabine (ara-C). This form of therapy is used to destroy any remaining leukemia cells and prevent relapse.

Leukemia and Suggested Dental Guidelines

Follow the same guidelines as those discussed under head and neck cancers.

HODGKIN'S LYMPHOMA

Overview

Hodgkin's and non-Hodgkin's lymphomas are common cancers of the lymphatic system; Hodgkin's lymphoma is less common in occurrence than non-Hodgkin's lymphoma. Early diagnosis and excellent treatment options available are responsible for the significantly lower death rates today with Hodgkin's lymphoma. Hodgkin's lymphoma is now considered a highly treatable disease.

Pathophysiology

B cell dysfunction results in accumulation of abnormal B cells. The abnormal B cells, also called **Reed-Sternberg cells**, are responsible for the occurrence of the malignancy.

Risk Factors

Risk factors associated with Hodgkin's lymphoma are:

1. **Sex:** Males are more affected than females.
2. **Age:** Patients age 15–40 years and beyond 55 are more prone to develop the malignancy.
3. **Immune status:** Reduced immunity from HIV/AIDS, chemotherapy, radiotherapy, or organ transplant increases the susceptibility to Hodgkin's lymphoma.
4. **Family history:** Family history of Hodgkin's lymphoma increases the risk for Hodgkin's in another member of the family.
5. **Infection:** Past history of infectious mononucleosis can predispose to the development of Hodgkin's lymphoma.

Symptoms and Signs

The patient usually presents with tiredness, weakness, fatigue, night sweats, anorexia, weight loss, and flulike symptoms. These symptoms are associated with an **organized,** progressive, **painless** enlargement of the lymph glands in the visible areas of the body, such as the neck, axilla, or groin. Lymph glands in the non-visible areas, such as the thoracic cavity and the abdomen, can also be affected.

Diagnosis

Diagnosis is confirmed with demonstration of the Reed-Sternberg cells on examination of a lymph node biopsy specimen. Complete blood count (CBC), bone marrow biopsy, computerized tomography (CT) scan, radiographs, magnetic resonance imaging (MRI), and positron emission tomography (PET) scans are additional tools that can assist with the diagnosis of Hodgkin's lymphoma.

Staging

The extent of tissue involvement or spread of Hodgkin's lymphoma defines the disease stage. The I–IV staging helps with determination of treatment options available for the patient. Stage I and Stage II have the best ten-year survival rates.

Stage I: Only one set of lymph nodes are involved with this stage.
Stage II: Two sets of lymph nodes in one given area, either above or below the diaphragm, are affected during this stage.
Stage III: Lymph nodes above and below the diaphragm are affected with total sparing of all organ involvement.
Stage IV: This stage has all the findings of Stage III plus involvement of the liver and/or the bone marrow.

Treatment

Treatment options include:

1. **Radiation therapy:** Radiation therapy alone is reserved for Stage I Hodgkin's lymphoma. More commonly, however, radiation in combination with chemotherapy is used to completely eradicate the cancer.
2. **Combined chemotherapy:** Combined chemotherapy is the best option for progressive disease and the preferred treatment of choice is mechlorethamine, oncovin, procarbazine, and prednisone (MOPP).
3. **Bone marrow transplant (BMT):** BMT is an option used for recurrent cases of Hodgkin's lymphoma.

Suggested Dental Guidelines

The suggested dental guidelines for Hodgkin's lymphoma are the same as those discussed collectively for head and neck cancers.

NON-HODGKIN'S LYMPHOMA (NHL)

Pathophysiology

NHL can be a B or T cell-associated cancer, and more than 30 different types of non-Hodgkin's lymphomas have been identified. NHL can be aggressive or of the slow-growing type. NHL has a greater tendency to go toward extranodal sites, compared with Hodgkin's lymphoma. Thus, the treatment options and outcomes of care depend on the aggressive or nonaggressive nature of the cancer. Aggressive NHLs occur more commonly in the HIV/AIDS patients, and Burkitt's lymphoma is an example of a B cell lymphoma.

Etiology

Non-Hodgkin's lymphoma can occur at any age, but it is more common in individuals above age 60. Infectious mononucleosis, H. pylori infection, malaria, and decreased immunity from HIV/AIDS or organ transplant are all risk factors increasing the incidence of non-Hodgkin's lymphoma.

Symptoms and Signs

Symptoms and signs associated with NHL are the same as with Hodgkin's lymphoma.

Diagnosis

The diagnostic criteria (x-rays, scans, and biopsy) are also the same as with Hodgkin's lymphoma.

Staging

NHL staging is also the same as with Hodgkin's lymphoma.

Treatment

There are two NHL Treatment options available:

1. Treatment as outlined for Hodgkin's lymphoma
2. Newer forms of NHL treatment

Treatment as Outlined for Hodgkin's Lymphoma

As with Hodgkin's lymphoma, radiation therapy is the option for early, slow-growing/low-grade tumors. Combination chemotherapy is the option for high-grade, aggressive tumors, and bone marrow transplant is the option for recurrent cancers. Radiation and combination chemotherapy, when instituted immediately, can also improve the survival rate in affected patients with early-detected aggressive NHLs. Early-detected low-grade, nonaggressive Stage I and II tumors have the best ten-year survival rates.

Newer Forms of NHL Treatment

The newer forms of NHL treatment are:

1. **Biological treatment:** Rituximab (Rituxan), a type of monoclonal antibody, is used in combination with chemotherapy.
2. **Radioimmunotherapy:** Radioimmunotherapy with ibritumomab (Zevalin) and tositumomab (Bexxar) is used for aggressive and recurrent NHLs.

NHL and Suggested Dental Guidelines

The suggested dental guidelines for NHL are the same as those discussed collectively under head and neck cancers.

MULTIPLE MYELOMA

Multiple Myeloma (MM) is a form of cancer that is associated with a proliferation of malignant plasma cells, resulting in an overabundance of monoclonal paraprotein. The exact cause for MM is not known, but genetic predisposition, viruses, chemicals, and exposure to radiation have been implicated as precipitating factors.

To better understand MM, it is important first to discuss the **normal** bone and immunoglobulin production cycles, the **normal** immunoglobulins, and then the pathophysiology associated with MM.

Normal Bone Cell Activity

Osteoclasts normally function with bone-forming cells or osteoblasts to rebuild areas of bone that are wearing out. This process is called **bone remodeling**, and healthy bone is continuously being remodeled. During the normal bone-remodeling process, osteoclasts are attracted to the area of fatigued bone. There they remove the worn out bone by breaking it down and creating a cavity in the bone. Osteoblasts get attracted to the cavity in the bone. They fill in the cavity with a matrix or framework and eventually new bone forms. Normally, the activity of the osteoclasts and osteoblasts is well balanced. The osteoclasts clear out the fatigued bones and the osteoblasts begin the rebuilding of new bones immediately.

In patients with multiple myeloma, bone resorption by the osteoclasts is **increased and exceeds** bone formation. Calcium lost from the bones appears in increasing amounts in the patient's serum and urine. This increase in bone resorption can result in pain, bone fractures, spinal cord compression, and hypercalcemia.

Normal Immunoglobulin Production Cycle

Stem cells from the bone marrow develop into B and T lymphocytes. B cells go on to mature in the lymph nodes and then travel throughout the body. When foreign substances or antigens enter the body, B cells develop into plasma cells that produce immunoglobulins or antibodies that help fight infection and disease. Plasma cells therefore develop from B cells, and it is the **plasma cells** that **produce the antibodies** that help fight infections or diseases.

Immunoglobulins

Every infection or disease triggers its own specific antibody production. With time, the plasma cells produce many different immunoglobulins in the body. Antibodies or immunoglobulins are made up of two long protein chains called **heavy chains** and two shorter chains called **light chains**. Immunoglobulin light chains are labeled as kappa (κ) or lambda (λ).

Immunoglobulin Types

The five major classes of antibodies or immunoglobulins made by the plasma cells are gamma (IgG), alpha (IgA), mu (IgM), epsilon (IgE), and delta (IgD). IgG is normally present in the largest amounts in blood, followed by IgA and IgM, IgD and IgE. The rest (other than IgG), are present in very small amounts in the blood.

Malignant Plasma Cells Formation Cycle and Associated Pathophysiology

Multiple genetic abnormalities transform a normal B cell into a malignant plasma cell that continues to divide unchecked, generating more malignant plasma cells or myeloma cells. The myeloma cells collect in the bone marrow via the blood and cause permanent damage to healthy tissue. Myeloma plasma cells target the stromal cells of the bone marrow and this triggers an unchecked growth of the myeloma cells.

The myeloma and stromal cells produce cytokines that stimulate the growth of myeloma cells and inhibit natural cell death, or apoptosis, causing excess production of MM cells that ultimately cause bone destruction. Myeloma cells also produce growth factor that promotes angiogenesis or new blood vessel formation. These new blood vessels provide the nutrition that promotes tumor growth.

Mature myeloma cells often produce substances that decrease the body's normal immune response, and when the defense is down, the cells grow unchecked. The myeloma cells affect all the large bones of the body, forming multiple small lesions. Myeloma cells produce an abnormal immunoglobulin protein called **monoclonal** or **M protein**, and these M proteins show up as a spike during electrophoresis.

In addition to the abnormal plasma cells that overwhelm the bone marrow, MM is also associated with an overproduction of Bence Jones proteins that are free monoclonal κ and λ light chains. The malignant cells lack normal function and cause excess production of immunoglobulins of a single type and reduced numbers of normal immunoglobulins. The abnormal antibody production leads to impaired humoral immunity and this leads to an increased incidence of infections. The overproduction of these antibodies may also lead to hyperviscosity, amyloidosis, and renal failure. The malignant plasma cells additionally cause leucopenia, anemia, and thrombocytopenia.

Multiple Myeloma Prevalence

Multiple myeloma is the second most common blood cancer after non-Hodgkin's lymphoma, and it occurs more frequently in men than women. It occurs most commonly around age 60 and older, but some cases do occur in patients under age 40. The median age of occurrence is 68 years for men and 70 years for women. It is more prevalent in

African Americans and Native Pacific Islanders compared with Asians. Myeloma is one of the leading causes of cancer deaths among African Americans.

Multiple Myeloma Clinical Features

Multiple myeloma can be asymptomatic or insidious in onset. It may be discovered accidentally during routine blood testing because symptoms are uncommon in the early stages of myeloma. When symptoms are present, however, they are often vague and simulate those caused by many other conditions.

Symptoms and Signs

Amyloid Deposits

Amyloidosis is a rare complication that occurs in patients with light chain myeloma because the light chains can combine with other serum proteins to produce amyloid. Macroglossia is a common finding in patients with amyloidosis. Bilateral swelling of the shoulder joints secondary to amyloid deposition can cause the shoulder pad sign. The swelling is hard and rubbery.

The amyloid protein may be deposited in the nerves, kidneys, liver, and heart, disrupting the organ's normal functions. Amyloid can also stick to the walls of blood vessels, causing them to lose their elasticity; the patient is then unable to maintain the blood pressure. Hence, amyloidosis can produce neuropathies, low blood pressure, and kidney, heart, or liver failure.

Alert: Avoid extra-strength Tylenol, aspirin, NSAIDS, meperidine, and propoxyphene in the presence of kidney disease.

Anemia and Ecchymosis

Excess production of abnormal plasma cells causes decreased production of normal RBCs, WBCs, and platelets. Patients can present with pallor, ecchymoses, or purpura resulting from thrombocytopenia. A complete blood count (CBC) will confirm the presence of anemia, thrombocytopenia, or leucopenia.

Fatigue

Anemia causes tiredness, weakness, fatigue, and pallor. Anemia, when present, is treated with erythropoietin and/or transfusions.

Infection

Impaired production of normal immunoglobulins results in an increased susceptibility to viral and bacterial infections. Aggressive treatment is provided with antivirals, antibiotics, and IV immunoglobulin therapy.

Clotting Factor Deficiency–Associated Bleeding

In some patients the monoclonal protein can occasionally absorb the clotting factors and cause bleeding. Monitor the PT/INR prior to dentistry in such cases.

Blood Hyperviscosity

High protein concentration in the blood causes the blood to become very thick and sticky. This can cause the patient to experience shortness of breath, confusion, and chest pain.

Bone Pain

MM patients experience pain in the ribs or lower back due to tiny fractures of bones weakened with plasma cell infiltration. Physical therapy, surgical correction of fractures, radiation, and bisphosphonates/anti-resorptive agents are treatment options for patients experiencing bone pains.

Osteoporosis

Diffuse osteoporosis involves the pelvis, spine, ribs, and skull.

Hypercalcemia

Excessive bone breakdown causes elevated calcium levels in the blood. The patient can experience tiredness, weakness, fatigue, anorexia, confusion, nausea, vomiting, constipation, increased thirst, and excessive urination. Hypercalcemia is usually treated with steroids, furosemide (Lasix), and bisphosphonates/anti-resorptive agents.

Renal Damage

The MM patient can experience kidney disease, renal failure, or hypercalcemia-associated renal symptoms. Additionally, the Bence Jones protein deposits in the kidney cause kidney damage and consequent renal failure.

Cryoglobulinemia

Cryoglobulinemia occurs when the abnormal protein comes out of the solution as particles on exposure to cold temperatures. These particles can block small blood vessels and cause pain, tingling, and numbness in the fingers and toes in cold weather.

Neurological Deficits

Neurologic findings may include sensory changes due to spinal cord compression, weakness, or carpal tunnel syndrome. Nerve impingement associated with collapsing bones is not uncommon with this disease.

Plasmacytomas

Plasmocytomas are soft tissue masses of plasma cells and they are a common finding in myeloma patient.

Skin Lesions

Wax papules or nodules may occur on the back, the ears, or the lips, and the papules are painful.

Multiple Myeloma Types

Overview

The most common types of myeloma are the IgG and IgA types. IgG myeloma accounts for about 60–70% of all cases of myeloma, and IgA accounts for about 20% of cases. A few cases of IgD and IgE myeloma have also been reported.

Classification

The three types of multiple myeloma are:

1. **The M protein myeloma:** This is the classic or the most common type of myeloma that is associated with a high level of M protein in the blood.
2. **Light chain or Bence Jones myeloma**: A small percentage of patients have only the light chain portion of the immunoglobulin called the *Bence Jones proteins*. Bence Jones proteins in these patients are detected by immunoelectrophoresis of the urine.
3. **Nonsecretory myeloma:** This is a rare form of myeloma that affects an extremely small percentage of myeloma patients. The plasma cells in this form **do not** produce M protein or light chains.

Multiple Myeloma Diagnosis

Diagnosis is made with medical evaluation/assessment and bone studies.

Medical Evaluation/Assessment

The presence of anemia and a high serum protein can alert the physician to further evaluate the patient. A diagnosis of multiple myeloma is difficult to make on the basis of any single laboratory test result. Currently, the diagnosis requires one major **and** one minor criterion **or** three minor criteria.

Major Criteria Associated with Multiple Myeloma

The findings classified as major criteria for MM are:

1. A biopsy confirming plasmacytoma
2. A bone marrow aspiration showing 30% plasma cells
3. Elevated monoclonal immunoglobulin levels in the blood or urine

Minor Criteria Associated with Multiple Myeloma

The findings classified as minor criteria for MM are:

1. A bone marrow sample showing 10–30% plasma cells.

2. Minor monoclonal immunoglobulin levels in blood or urine.
3. Imaging studies showing holes in bones due to tumor growth.
4. Normal antibody levels that are abnormally low in the blood.
5. Detection of serum levels of beta-2 microglobulin (β2-M) that reflect the tumor mass and are a standard measure of tumor burden.
6. Detection of C-reactive protein that is a surrogate marker for IL-6, a growth factor for myeloma cells.
7. **Quantitive immunoglobulins (QIGs):** QIGs measure the levels of different types of antibodies—IgG, IgA, and IgM.
8. **Serum protein or urine protein electrophoresis (EP):** serum/urine protein EP measures the levels of various proteins in the blood or urine, respectively.
9. **Immunoelectrophoresis (IEP):** IEP also detects the presence of abnormal antibody M protein. IEP helps track the progression of myeloma disease and response to treatment. M protein appears as a spike on electrophoresis.
10. **Twenty-four-hour urine protein:** Twenty-four-hour urine protein determination helps stage the patient's status and assess the progression of the disease and the patient's response to treatment.
11. **The FREELITE test:** The new serum-based assay FREELITE helps detect and quantify free light chains.

Bone Studies

The following tests performed on the bone aid the diagnosis of MM:

1. X-rays of affected bone
2. Total body bone survey
3. Magnetic resonance imaging (MRI)
4. Computerized axial tomography
5. Bone marrow biopsy taken from the hip

Multiple Myeloma Treatment

Overview

The patient can be asymptomatic, minimally symptomatic, or significantly symptomatic with MM. Chemotherapy is the ultimate treatment for MM, and chemotherapy has its own significant side effects. Determination of how debilitating the MM symptoms are for the patient is therefore one way to decide when to begin chemotherapy.

In the initial stages some patients decide to get bisphosphonates/anti-resorptive therapy for the associated osteoporosis; others prefer supportive care for symptoms and complications. In all these cases, postponing therapy may help avoid the risk of complications associated with chemotherapy and may also delay development of resistance to chemotherapy.

Treatment Classification

For decisions on treatment, MM patients are classified into one of three myeloma categories:

1. The Monoclonal Gammopathy of Undetermined Significance (MGUS) Category
2. The Asymptomatic Category
3. The Symptomatic Category

The Monoclonal Gammopathy of Undetermined Significance (MGUS) Category

The MGUS category is a common finding among patients suspected of having MM. Patients in this category demonstrate the presence of a monoclonal protein but **no cause** for the increased protein can be identified. There are **no symptoms,** and other criteria for myeloma diagnosis are absent. MGUS occurs in about 1% of the general population and in about 3% of normal individuals over 70 years of age. MGUS by itself is harmless, but after many years approximately 16% of patients with MGUS progress toward a malignant plasma cell disorder.

Asymptomatic Multiple Myeloma

Patients with asymptomatic multiple myeloma have a monoclonal protein and slightly increased numbers of plasma cells in the bone marrow. They may have mild anemia and/or a few bone lesions, but they do not exhibit the renal failure and frequent infections that characterize active multiple myeloma. In these patients the myeloma is static and may not progress for months or years.

Symptomatic Multiple Myeloma

Patients who present with symptoms typically have a monoclonal protein and increased numbers of plasma cells in the bone marrow. They also have anemia, kidney failure, and hypercalcemia or bone lesions. Patients with symptomatic myeloma require immediate treatment.

Treatment Options

Although patients benefit from treatment, currently there is no cure. The currently available therapies for multiple myeloma are:

1. **Chemotherapy:** When therapy is indicated, the patient typically receives chemotherapy. Chemotherapeutic agents are used to reduce the disease burden. Trimethoprim-sulfamethoxazole is commonly used as prophylaxis for P. carinii pneumonia during chemotherapy. The chemotherapy choices offered are:
   a. Melphalan and prednisone (M and P): **This is the most commonly used regimen.**
   b. Vincristine, bischloroethylnitrosourea, melphalan, cyclophosphamide, and prednisone.
   c. Vincristine, doxorubicin (Adriamycin), and dexamethasone (VAD).
   d. Vincristine, bischloroethylnitrosourea, doxorubicin, and prednisone
2. **Radiotherapy**
3. **Stem cell transplantation**
4. **Thalidomide (Thalomid):** Thalidomide is now often used as first-line therapy either as a single agent or in combination with steroids.

5. **Bisphosphonates:** Zoledronic acid (Zometa) is a very potent bisphosphonate and is commonly used in MM patients.
6. **Erythropoietin:** Erythropoietin corrects the anemia resulting from either myeloma alone or from chemotherapy and has been shown to improve the patient's quality of life.

Multiple Myeloma Suggested Dental Guidelines

Follow these guidelines in the dental setting:

1. Thoroughly assess the patient and note significant medical history and physical examination findings.
2. Communicate with the patient's physician to understand the extent of the disease.
3. Evaluate the CBC with differential and platelet counts, PT/INR, serum creatinine, and LFTs, and note vital organ status.
4. Specifically determine the patient's cardiac status by communicating with the patient's physician.
5. Incorporate the suggested anemia, thrombocytopenia, ANC, serum creatinine, PT/INR, and LFT guidelines when the tests indicate abnormality. In the presence of neutropenia, the patient may need premedication, as per ANC guidelines.
6. Always have the patient use a nonalcoholic mouth rinse prior to every dental visit to de-germ the oral cavity.
7. Follow stringent asepsis guidelines and treat all infections aggressively.
8. Always check if the patient has a porta-catheter or IV line or Hickman line for chemotherapy. Premedication prophylaxis should be provided when present.
9. Check if the patient is on bisphosphonates and for how long. Review and follow the bisphosphonates associated guidelines as outlined in Chapter 41.
10. Significant osteoporosis can cause jaw pains and frequent denture adjustments.
11. Significant neuropathies can shorten chair time or may require adaptation of proper positioning in the chair.
12. **Anesthetics:** The local anesthetic use will be dictated by the extent of anemia or kidney, liver, or cardiac diseases, when present. Avoid the 4% LAs in the presence of neuropathies and anemia and/or kidney disease associated hypoxia.
13. **Analgesics:** Avoid extra-strength Tylenol, aspirin, NSAIDS, meperidine, and propoxyphene because of the anemia, kidney disease, and/or associated liver disease.
14. **Antibiotics:** The antibiotic use will be dictated by the extent of anemia, kidney disease, or liver disease when present, and by the PCP prophylaxis, when used. When the patient is on PCP prophylaxis, determine if the antibiotic used is a cidal or a static antibiotic. The antibiotic you prescribe should match the PCP antibiotic type (cidal with cidal, static with static). Maintain an interval of six hours when the two antibiotics are different.

XIX

Psychiatry

Psychiatric Conditions: Assessment of Disease States and Associated Dental Management Guidelines

ANXIETY DISORDERS

Anxiety is a normal, healthy reaction to stress and it helps a patient deal with stressful situations. When anxiety becomes excessive or irrational it becomes a disabling disorder. The intensity of symptoms is directly related to the patient's ability to cope.

Anxiety Disorder Classification

The five major types of anxiety disorders are:

1. Generalized anxiety disorder
2. Obsessive-compulsive disorder (OCD)
3. Panic disorder
4. Posttraumatic stress disorder (PTSD)
5. Social phobia, or social anxiety disorder

Generalized Anxiety Disorder (GAD)

GAD is associated with excessive, unrealistic anxiety that lasts six or more months. These patients also experience trembling, muscle aches, insomnia, bowel movement upsets, dizziness, and irritability.

Obsessive-Compulsive Disorder (OCD)

The OCD patient is plagued by obsessions due to increased anxiety or fears. The obsessions lead the patient to perform a ritual to relieve the anxiety caused by the obsession.

Dentist's Guide to Medical Conditions, Medications, and Complications, Second Edition. Kanchan M. Ganda.
© 2013 John Wiley & Sons, Inc. Published 2013 by John Wiley & Sons, Inc.

Panic Disorder

Patients with panic disorders go through a phase of extreme anxiety when faced with a specific situation—for example, fear of heights or closed spaces. They experience severe palpitations, chest discomfort, sweating, trembling, tingling sensations, feeling of choking, fear of dying, and fear of losing control.

Posttraumatic Stress Disorder (PTSD)

PTSD can follow an exposure to a traumatic event, such as an assault of any kind, unexpected death of a family member/spouse, or experiencing a natural disaster. The patient relives the traumatic event by experiencing flashbacks and nightmares. The patient avoids places related to the trauma and becomes emotionally detached from others. The patient also experiences difficulty sleeping, irritability, and poor concentration. Internal or external stimuli can trigger an attack of PTSD. Drug and alcohol abuse is a **common** occurrence with PTSD.

Social Anxiety Disorder (SAD)

SAD is associated with extreme anxiety about being judged by others or having extreme anxiety about behaving in a way that might cause embarrassment or ridicule. The patient experiences blushing, palpitations, and sweating. Good history-taking will show that the patient starts to avoid situations that will cause SAD.

Treatment of Anxiety Disorders

Anxiety disorders are treated as follows:

1. Psychosocial therapies
2. Medications
3. Both psychosocial therapies and medications

Anxiety Medications

Combination therapies are often utilized in the management of anxiety. Drugs used to treat anxiety disorders are:

1. Benzodiazepines
2. Beta-blockers
3. Monoamine oxidase inhibitors (MAOIs): an antidepressant with anxiolytic effects
4. Selective serotonin reuptake inhibitors (SSRIs): antidepressants with anxiolytic effects
5. Tricyclic antidepressants: antidepressants with anxiolytic effects

Anxiety Disorders and Alcohol Abuse

Patients with anxiety and alcohol abuse could present with the following complications:

1. These patients often have poor treatment compliance.
2. They have an increased risk of relapse into alcohol abuse following detoxification.

3. They can have severe drug interactions between prescription medication and alcohol.
4. Patients with social anxiety disorder (SAD), posttraumatic stress disorder (PTSD), generalized anxiety disorder (GAD), and panic disorder often abuse alcohol.
5. Substance abuse or alcohol abuse is treated with individual therapy or group therapy that utilizes the twelve-step programs birthed by Alcoholics Anonymous.
6. SSRIs are often prescribed in conjunction with therapy to assist with the recovery process. Common SSRIs prescribed are fluoxetine (Prozac), sertraline (Zoloft), fluvoxamine (Luvox), paroxetine (Paxil), citalopram (Celexa), and escitalopram (Lexapro).
7. Benzodiazepines should be avoided in these patients as they can increase the risk of abuse, tolerance, and physical dependence.

Anxiety Disorders and Suggested Dental Alerts

The following are dental alerts for anxiety disorders:

1. The anxious individual will tend to be very alert, quite hyperactive, and fidgety in the dental environment. It is best to address the anxiety with the patient before you begin treating the patient.
2. Always establish good communication and trust with these patients. Show genuine concern and offer stress management.
3. $O_2 + N_2O$ or benzodiazepines can be used to control the anxiety with the following precautions: Use benzodiazepines for stress management **only** if approved by the patient's physician, the patient is **not** on any medications to control the anxiety, or the patient is already on benzodiazepines to control the anxiety. Use $O_2 + N_2O$ for patients on antidepressant medications.
4. An occasional physician may allow the use of low-dose benzodiazepines in conjunction with the patient's anti-anxiety or antidepressant medications. You are advised, therefore, to always check with the patient's MD.
5. Benzodiazepine use is contraindicated in the pregnant patient, the elderly patient, the obese patient, the alcoholic patient, the patient on centrally acting drugs, and the patient on H_2 blockers for GERD, peptic ulceration, or gastritis. When benzodiazepines have to be used in the presence of H_2 blockers, keep an interval of **two hours** between both the medications.
6. **Anesthetics:** Avoid epinephrine in the local anesthetic and epinephrine cords in the presence of TCAs and MAOIs. Epinephrine is not contraindicated with the SSRIs.
7. Patients suffering from anxiety often experience aphthous ulcerations, ulcerative gingivitis, TMJ problems, lichen planus, geographic tongue, and myofacial pain. These conditions should also be additionally addressed in the dental setting.
8. Xerostomia is a genuine concern in patients taking all kinds of psychiatric medications. Follow the suggested xerostomia management guidelines in Chapter 48.
9. Psychiatric medications cause postural hypotension. Assist the patient out of the chair to prevent a fall or collapse.

Anesthetics, analgesics, and stress management summary: Avoid sedatives, epinephrine (except with SSRIs), narcotic analgesics, sedating antihistamines, and epinephrine cords with psychiatric medications.

MOOD DISORDERS: DEPRESSION

Depression is a condition where a patient feels sad, hopeless, and/or disinterested in life in general. Depression is an illness that affects the way a person thinks, feels, behaves, and functions. When these feelings last for more than two weeks and when the feelings interfere with daily living, it is called a **major depressive episode**.

Major Depressive Episode Symptoms

Symptoms experienced are persistent sadness, hopelessness, pessimism, worthlessness, decreased energy, fatigue, difficulty concentrating and making decisions, insomnia, early-morning awakening or oversleeping, decreased appetite and/or weight loss, overeating and weight gain, thoughts of death or suicide, suicide attempts, restlessness, and irritability. The patient experiences persistent physical symptoms such as headaches, digestive disorders, and pain for which no other cause can be determined. The patient does not respond to treatment for any of these symptoms.

Depression Disorder Classification

The three main types of depressive disorders can occur with any of the major anxiety disorders:

1. Major depression
2. Dysthymia/chronic depression
3. Bipolar disorder

Major Depression

Major depression is diagnosed when the patient is symptomatic for a two-week period. Major depressive episodes may occur once or twice in a lifetime, or may recur frequently throughout life. They may occur spontaneously and some patients may attempt suicide.

Dysthymia/Chronic Depression

Dysthymia is a less severe and more chronic form of depression. The patient mainly experiences decreased energy, poor appetite or overeating, insomnia or oversleeping, and extreme pessimism.

Bipolar Disorder/Manic-Depressive Psychosis

Understanding Bipolar Disorder

Bipolar disorder/manic-depressive illness causes extreme mood swings with episodes of mania and depression, or a mixture of both. People with depression may feel sad or have difficulty with activities of daily living.

The classic signs of depression include:

- Alterations of sleep, difficulty falling or staying asleep, or sleeping too much.
- Little or no interest in any activity previously found to be pleasurable.
- Alterations in appetite, loss of appetite, or eating too much.
- A low threshold for becoming irritated.

- Fatigue, loss of energy, or sluggishness.
- Feelings of worthlessness or guilt.
- Difficulty concentrating and making decisions.
- Recurring thoughts of death or suicide.

A patient in the manic phase may demonstrate a period of abnormally elevated or irritable mood for at least four days (for hypomania) to seven days (for mania) and display these symptoms:

- Rapid, pressured speech; patient is more talkative.
- Inflated ego or grandiosity.
- Flight of ideas or complaints of racing thoughts.
- Decreased need for sleep, such as two to three hours of sleep.
- Distraction that occurs easily.
- Psychomotor agitation or increase in goal-directed activity, like social or occupational activity.
- Hypersexuality.
- Overindulgence in pleasurable activities like sexual indiscretions, buying sprees, unwise business decisions.

A "mixed" episode is characterized by a period of a week or more in which the symptoms of both a major depressive episode and a manic episode are present daily. These episodes may last from a week to a few months. The patient may experience mixed episodes, manic, and/or depressive episodes over the course of the illness. A mixed episode may evolve from a manic or a major depressive episode, or it may emerge on its own. Besides extreme mood swings, patients with bipolar disorder can experience anger, panic attacks, agitation, anxiety, restlessness, suicidal thoughts, persecutory delusions, hallucinations, and confusion.

Bipolar Subtypes

Subtypes of bipolar disorder include:

- **Bipolar I Disorder:** At least one episode of mania alternates with major depression. Mania may also include symptoms of psychosis.
- **Bipolar II Disorder:** Episodes of hypomania alternate with major depression. This form of bipolar disorder, which is not as severe as bipolar I disorder, often increases the patient's functioning when in the hypomanic state. Hypomania is a milder form of mania that lasts for at least four days at a time but tends not to interfere with the patient's daily activities. The patient with hypomania tends to be euphoric, but suicidal tendencies are a particular risk for patients experiencing major depression.
- **Cyclothymia:** Patients alternate between hypomania and minor depression for a period of at least two years.
- **Bipolar disorder not otherwise specified:** Patients experience episodes of hypomania without major depression.

Bipolar Disorder Treatment

Treatment of bipolar disorder is very patient-specific. Health-care providers must use their expertise, time, and patience to find the correct combination of medications to attain satisfactory results.

The Role of Psychotherapy

After a patient is no longer in a state of mania, psychotherapy may be used to help the patient cope more adaptively to stressors and decrease the possibility of relapse. Pharmacology and psychotherapy are considered crucial during the continuation and maintenance phases of bipolar disorder.

Interpersonal and social rhythm therapy is another formalized therapy that has been tested in combination with pharmacologic interventions in randomized clinical trials as treatment for patients who are in the maintenance phase of bipolar disorder. This therapy focuses on factors that are related to recurrence of symptoms, including nonadherence, stress reduction, and support systems.

Lithium

Lithium is a psychotropic agent with an established record of efficacy for treating acute manic episodes of bipolar I disorder, in addition recurrent manic and depressive episodes. It inhibits 80% of acute manic and hypomanic episodes within 10–21 days of the start of treatment. Lithium is not as effective for symptoms of mixed mania or for rapid cycling.

Lithium mechanism of action (MOA): MOA of lithium is not completely understood. Chemically similar to sodium and potassium, lithium is a positively charged ion that seems to affect electrical conductivity in neurons. According to one theory, bipolar disorder is caused by an overexcitement of neurons in certain parts of the brain; lithium interacts with sodium and potassium at the cell membrane to stabilize electrical activity.

Lithium improves mood in patients with bipolar disorder who are depressed, and it augments antidepressant therapy when antidepressants alone fail to improve mood in patients who are depressed. Lithium is also effective as prophylaxis against recurrent depression in patients with bipolar disorders.

Because lithium must reach a therapeutic blood level, it can take up to three weeks to control symptoms in patients with mania. Generally, the target serum level for acute treatment in adults is between 0.8 and 1.4mEq/L, and slightly lower levels (0.6–1.2mEq/L) are suggested for older adults, due to decreased renal clearance.

Adverse DDIs associated with Lithium

- **Drugs that decrease lithium levels by increasing lithium excretion:** acetazolamide, alcohol, sodium bicarbonate, caffeine, urea, and xanthine derivatives.
- **Drugs that increase lithium levels and associated toxicity by increasing sodium excretion:** angiotensin-converting enzyme (ACE) inhibitors and diuretics.
- **Calcium channel blockers (CCBs):** CCBs and carbamazepine increase neurotoxicity in combination with lithium.
- **Fluoxetine:** Fluoxetine may increase or decrease lithium levels.
- **Metronidazole:** Metronidazole may cause lithium toxicity by reducing renal clearance of lithium.
- **NSAIDS:** NSAIDS increase lithium levels by reducing renal clearance of lithium.

Lithium Side Effects

Fine hand tremors, polyuria, and mild thirst are common adverse reactions during initial treatment. The patient may also experience transient mild nausea and general discomfort during the first few days of lithium administration. These adverse reactions should subside shortly after initiation of treatment, but if they persist, a reduced dosage or cessation of therapy is indicated.

Lithium Toxicity Concerns

Lithium has a very narrow therapeutic window, so always be concerned about possible toxicity. Because of the risk for toxicity, serum lithium levels must be checked regularly throughout treatment. Serum lithium levels greater than 1.5mEq/L carry a greater risk of toxicity than lower levels. When signs and symptoms of toxicity appear, the patient must contact the health-care provider, withhold the medication, and obtain a lithium level as prescribed. The health-care provider can then reevaluate the dosage.

Early signs and symptoms of toxicity include nausea, vomiting, diarrhea, thirst, polyuria, lethargy or drowsiness, slurred speech, muscle weakness, incoordination, and fine hand tremor.

With serum levels between 1.5–2.0mEq/L (advanced toxicity), patients begin to experience coarse hand tremors, persistent gastrointestinal (GI) upset, mental confusion, muscle hyperirritability, electroencephalographic changes, incoordination, and sedation.

The patient may display ataxia, giddiness, serious electroencephalographic changes, tinnitus, and blurred vision, when serum lithium levels are between 2.0–2.5mEq/L (severe toxicity). Other signs include clonic movements, large output of dilute urine, seizures, stupor, severe hypotension, and coma. Severe toxicity may be fatal; death is usually secondary to pulmonary complications.

Lithium is not typically given to women who are pregnant due to the potential for harm to the fetus. Lithium is categorized as a Category **D** drug because of evidence of human fetal risk, but it may be used in the event of a life-threatening risk to the mother or threat of serious illness. Lithium is also contraindicated in women who are breast-feeding.

Lithium Alerts for Patients

Missing doses of lithium may increase the risk for a relapse in mood symptoms. Lithium may make the patient drowsy. Driving or operating machinery should be avoided particularly during the start of therapy. Avoid alcohol or recreational drugs while taking lithium.

The loss of too much water or salt from the body can lead to serious adverse reactions because of lithium. The patient must drink enough water at all times, especially during phases of vomiting and/or diarrhea. Taking lithium with food can help decrease or avoid stomach upset. A low-salt diet, leading to low sodium blood levels, can increase the risk of lithium toxicity.

Antiepileptic Drugs

Although classified as anti-seizure medications, antiepileptic drugs (AEDs) are also used to treat bipolar disorder. Under certain circumstances, AEDs such as valproate and carbamazepine are now being used as mood stabilizers.

Valproate

Valproate products that are FDA-approved to treat manic or mixed episodes associated with bipolar disorder include valproate sodium (Depacon), valproic acid (Depakene), and divalproex sodium (Depakote). Divalproex is a formulation of valproate that can minimize gastrointestinal (GI) distress.

Valproate is believed to decrease the firing rate of very-high-frequency neurons in the brain. This membrane-stabilizing effect may account for its ability to decrease mood swings in patients with bipolar disorder. Valproate may also increase levels of gamma-aminobutyric acid, an inhibitory neurotransmitter in the brain.

Carbamazepine

Carbamazepine (Tegretol), another AED, is an effective alternative to both lithium and valproate for treating bipolar disorder in some patients. The exact mechanism of action of carbamazepine is unknown. Carbamazepine may cause life-threatening dermatologic reactions including Stevens-Johnson syndrome (SJS) and toxic epidermal necrolysis (TEN). These reactions may cause severe damage to the skin and internal organs. The risk of SJS or TEN is highest in people of Asian ancestry who have a genetic risk factor. Patients should contact their health-care provider immediately if they develop a rash, blisters, or a fever during their treatment with carbamazepine. SJS or TEN usually occurs during the first few months of treatment with carbamazepine.

Adverse Reactions Associated with AEDs

- **Divalproex, valproate sodium and valproic acid:** These drugs commonly cause gastrointestinal (GI) upset, dizziness, tremors, sleepiness, weight gain, and temporary hair loss. Less common but serious side effects are thrombocytopenia, pancreatitis, and hepatotoxicity.
- **Carbamazepine:** This drug commonly causes nausea, vomiting, anorexia, sedation, poor coordination, skin reactions, and hyponatremia. Less common but serious side effects include, thrombocytopenia, leucopenia, anemia, agranulocytosis, Stevens-Johnson syndrome, and toxic epidermal necrolysis.
- **Lamotrigine:** This drug commonly causes weight gain, gastrointestinal (GI) upset, increased appetite, sedation, tremors, ataxia and hypotension. Less common but serious side effects associated with lamotrigine are serious skin rashes including Stevens-Johnson syndrome.

Dental alert: Because carbamazepine can cause blood dyscrasias, dentists should monitor CBC results closely. Leukopenia increases the risk of infection, so assess the patient for signs and symptoms of infection, as well as signs and symptoms of bleeding resulting from thrombocytopenia. Carbamazepine induces liver enzymes, causing lower serum concentrations of other drugs given with it. Carbamazepine also interferes with hormonal contraceptives, so the patient has to use barrier protection in addition to the contraception.

Atypical Antipsychotics

In the past few years, atypical antipsychotics, also known as second-generation antipsychotics, have been used as part of a regimen for treating bipolar disorder. Some examples include olanzapine (Zyprexa), quetiapine (Seroquel), risperidone (Risperdal), and ziprasidone (Geodon).

Adverse Reactions Associated with Atypical Antipsychotics

Neuroleptic malignant syndrome (NMS) is a potentially life-threatening situation that can develop after a patient starts treatment with traditional or atypical antipsychotics. Signs and symptoms of NMS include hyperpyrexia, muscle rigidity, altered mental status, and signs of autonomic instability including diaphoresis, cardiac dysrhythmias, and BP changes. Other signs may include myalgia, increased serum creatine kinase, myoglobinuria, and acute kidney injury. **Dental alert:** Avoid the 4% LAs in the presence of these drugs.

Tardive dyskinesia (TD) is a serious, and sometimes permanent, adverse reaction. Patients with TD experience involuntary movements of the face, tongue, and other parts of the body. The risk for developing TD and the chance that it will become permanent are thought to increase the longer a person takes the medication and as the person takes increasing amounts of the medication over time.

Patients taking atypical antipsychotics, especially olanzapine, quetiapine, and risperidone, are at risk for metabolic problems including weight gain, diabetes mellitus, glucose intolerance, and dyslipidemia.

Dental alert: Monitor and assess the patient's weight, BP, and serum glucose and lipid levels prior to dentistry.

Extrapyramidal Side Effects

Extrapyramidal side effects (EPS) often occur after a patient begins therapy with psychotropic medications. Three of these adverse reactions, which are reversible by either reducing the dosage or changing to another medication, include:

Acute dystonic reaction: spasmodic contractions of skeletal muscle throughout the body, including laryngeal spasms.
Akathisia: the inability to stop moving.
Pseudoparkinsonism: symptoms similar to those of Parkinson's disease, such as tremors and shuffling gait.

DEPRESSION AND SUGGESTED DENTAL ALERTS

The following are dental alerts for depression:

1. Poor personal and oral hygiene, decreased salivary flow, increased dental caries, increased periodontal disease, and facial pain syndromes are common in patients suffering from depression.
2. Patients suffering from anxiety or depression often experience aphthous ulcerations, ulcerative gingivitis, TMJ problems, lichen planus, geographic tongue, and myofacial pain. These conditions must also be addressed in the dental setting.
3. Always show empathy toward the patient and try to clearly understand the patient's problems.
4. Injury to the oral cavity may occur during mania. Over-brushing can cause abrasion of the teeth and over-flossing can injure gingival tissue in bipolar patients.
5. Antidepressants have anticholinergic side effects and this can precipitate xerostomia. MAOIs and TCAs induce significant xerostomia. Therefore, patients on antidepressants should use fluoride rinses on a regular basis. Xerostomia is

actually a genuine concern in patients taking all kinds of psychiatric medications. Follow the suggested xerostomia management guidelines outlined in Chapter 48.

6. **Anesthetics with MAOIs:** MAO inhibitors interact with epinephrine. Vasoconstrictors in the local anesthetics are contraindicated with MAOIs, due to the possibility of hypertensive episodes.

7. **Sedatives and narcotic analgesics with MAOIs:** Sedatives and narcotic analgesics are strictly contraindicated in patients on MAOIs.

8. **Anesthetics with TCAs:** Tricyclic antidepressants enhance the effect of catecholamines. Avoid local anesthetics with vasoconstrictors in patients on TCAs. In conclusion, avoid epinephrine in the local anesthetic and epinephrine cords in the presence of TCAs and MAOIs. No epinephrine contraindications exist with the SSRIs.

9. **Sedatives and narcotic analgesics with TCAs:** Sedatives and narcotic analgesics should also be avoided with TCAs.

10. Psychiatric medications cause postural hypotension. Assist the patient out of the chair to avoid collapse.

In conclusion, avoid sedatives, epinephrine (except with SSRIs), narcotic analgesics, sedating antihistamines and epinephrine cords in the presence of psychiatric medications.

DEMENTIA

Dementia is a cognitive disorder and it can be associated with any one of the following conditions:

1. Alzheimer's disease
2. HIV disease
3. Parkinson's disease
4. Vascular causes/stroke

Overview and Facts

Old age, stroke, and Alzheimer's disease are the more common causes of dementia. Aging dementia occurs most commonly in patients 80 years and older and less commonly in patients between the ages of 65–70.

Dementia is not a specific disease. Patients with dementia have serious problems with two or more brain functions, such as memory and language. Memory loss is a common symptom of dementia. A progressive deterioration of intellectual functioning, behavioral and mood changes, and impairment of occupational and social functions occurs with dementia.

Initially, a clinician will observe subtle changes such as social withdrawal, apathy, and lack of spontaneity. As the dementia progresses, the patient is unable to learn or recall new information, is unable to identify family members, has impaired judgment, gets disoriented often, is unable to clothe or feed independently, and often has impairment of sleep pattern. The patient becomes agitated, confused, and delusional. The patient loses the ability to think and ultimately is not able to remember and recognize things or people. There is a definite change in and deterioration of the patient's personality.

Classification

Depending on the severity, dementia can be subdivided into the following categories:

1. **Mild dementia:** At this stage of dementia, the patient's work or social activities are impaired, but the patient's capacity for independent living remains.
2. **Moderate dementia:** During this stage of dementia, independent living becomes hazardous.
3. **Severe dementia:** During this stage of dementia, cognition and function are so impaired that continuous supervision is required.

ALZHEIMER'S DISEASE

Alzheimer's disease (AD) is a progressive degenerative disease that affects cognition, behavior, and the ability to perform activities of daily living. Alzheimer's is the most common cause of dementia. It is the most common degenerative neurologic disorder in older adults. Progressive decline in function and behavior leads to patient dependency, nursing home placement, neuropsychiatric impairments, and eventual death. The exact etiology of Alzheimer's disease is not known, but the disease is familial and associated with old age.

The National Institute on Aging (NIA) and the Alzheimer's Association have established and recently published criteria for the early diagnosis of AD. Biomarkers help establish a diagnosis and play a very important role in the identification of the three phases of AD.

AD Identifying Biomarkers

- **MRI:** MRI shows brain atrophy reflecting neurodegeneration due to AD. MRI shows classic atrophy of the hippocampal regions in a patient with AD.
- **Fluorodeoxyglucose-positron emission tomography (FDG-PET):** FDG is a glucose analog, and reduced metabolism of the brain/brain activity is reflected in FDG-PET reductions.
- **Amyloid PET:** The FDA recently approved Amyvid (Florbetapir F 18 Injection), a radioactive diagnostic agent indicated for brain imaging of beta-amyloid plaques in patients with cognitive impairment who are being evaluated for AD and other causes of cognitive decline. Amyvid binds to amyloid plaques and is detected using PET scan images of the brain.

  It is important to note that a negative Amyvid scan only indicates that few or no amyloid plaques are present in the patient's brain, which may rule out AD but not other forms of cognitive dementia. A positive Amyvid scan firmly establishes only that there are amyloid deposits in the brain.

  Although amyloid plaques are always associated with AD, they may also be present in patients with other types of neurologic conditions, as well as in older people who have normal cognition. AD-associated amyloid deposition that is seen on amyloid imaging initially occurs in the frontal lobes and progresses to the parietal lobes while completely sparing the occipital lobes.
- **Cerebral spinal fluid (CSF):** CSF assessment shows an elevated tau and reduced amyloid β, confirming the clinical diagnosis.

AD Classification

- **The preclinical phase:** Cognitively, the patient is functioning and has no symptoms but has a positive biomarker identifying AD-like amyloid deposits in the brain.
- **The prodromal or mild cognitive impairment (MCI) phase:** MCI is a form of AD where symptoms are present but the patient does not yet meet the criteria for dementia.
- **Alzheimer's disease (AD):** The patient develops Alzheimer's-type dementia.

The clinical criteria for diagnosis are based on a history of gradually progressive symptoms associated with two or more cognitive deficits, progressive worsening of memory and function, and absence of other neurological disorders that can cause progressive cognitive deficits.

The Standardized Mini-Mental State Examination

The standardized mini-mental state examination (MMSE) is used to assess the extent of disease/stages of Alzheimer's dementia:

- **Preclinical AD:** Preclinical AD correlates with a MMSE score greater than 26.
- **Mild functional AD:** Mild functional AD correlates with a MMSE score of 20–26. The patient has mild cognitive impairment leading to some dependency. Patients are alert and sociable, but forgetfulness begins to interfere with daily living.
- **Moderate AD:** Moderate AD correlates with a MMSE score of 10–20. The patient has clinically evident dementia with more immediate dependency, experiencing difficulty with personal and oral hygiene. There is deterioration of intellect, logic, behavior, and function.
- **Severe AD:** Severe AD correlates with a MMSE score less than 10. The patient is completely dependent and needs constant supervision. Patients need complete assistance with washing, eating, and using the bathroom. There is loss of long-term memory and language skills.

AD Pharmacotherapy

The degeneration of cholinergic neurons and declining levels of choline acetyltransferase, the enzyme responsible for acetylcholine synthesis, is associated with diminishing cholinergic transmission in brain areas that are critical for learning and memory. Research shows that the cholinergic deficit in AD worsens with disease progression and that this reduction is inversely proportional to increasing β-amyloid burden in the brain.

Therefore, **cholinesterase inhibitors (ChEIs), such as donepezil (Aricept)**, act by inhibiting the degradation of ACh in the synaptic cleft, leaving more ACh to interact with post-synaptic cholinergic receptors.

Glutamate is an excitatory neurotransmitter that is produced and released by nerve cells in the brain. Once released, glutamate attaches to a receptor on the surface of the cells called the N-methyl-D-aspartate (NMDA) receptor. It is postulated that excessive stimulation of nerve cells by glutamate in the brain may be responsible for the degeneration of nerves that occurs in AD. **Memantine (Namenda), a competitive antagonist of NMDA receptors**, blocks this receptor and thereby decreases the effects of glutamate, thus protecting nerve cells from excess stimulation by glutamate.

Research shows that memantine (Namenda) alone modestly improves cognition, function, and behavior in patients with moderate-to-severe AD, and the drug may slow the rate of decline over time. Memantine is often used in combination with cholinesterase inhibitors; **the combination of memantine and donepezil (Aricept) has been found to offer greater benefit than donepezil (Aricept) alone in patients with moderate-to-severe AD.**

ChEIs and memantine provide symptomatic treatments, slowing the rate of loss of cognitive and functional abilities over time. Patients who respond to AD-specific medications will lose the benefits of treatment when the medication is stopped. In some cases, the benefits may not be regained if the medication is restarted. Only donepezil (Aricept) and memantine (Namenda) are approved for the treatment of moderate-to-severe AD.

FDA-Approved ChEIs for AD Management

Older ChEI: Tacrine (Cognex)

Newer ChEIs are more tolerable and have absence of significant hepatotoxicity, compared to tacrine. They include:

- **Donepezil (Aricept):** Approved to treat mild, moderate, or severe AD.
- **Rivastigmine (Exelon):** Approved to treat mild or moderate AD only.
- **Galantamine (Razadyne):** Approved to treat mild or moderate AD only.

Future Therapies: Gammagard for Alzheimer's Patients

The first long-term treatment with **IVIG/Gammagard** has shown to halt the progression of Alzheimer's disease, although it is still in testing. The Gammagard therapy neutralizes the potential damage of amyloid plaques and appears to halt the damage that inflammation can cause, but Gammagard does not remove plaque.

Gammagard already has FDA approval for treating other immune-disorder associated diseases, but it is extremely expensive. Gammagard is made from plasma donated by healthy people and is it rich in antibodies. It can have side effects, including the transmission of viruses. If the trial is ultimately successful then this will provide a direction for AD treatment. All other already completed research trials have shown that maximum benefit is attained if treatment is started early in patients with Alzheimer's disease.

All current and future studies are targeting amyloid plaques in the brain, because amyloid is suspected to cause damage and eventual killing of neurons.

AD Medication Alerts

- Nausea, vomiting, and diarrhea are the common side effects experienced when treatment is started or following a dose increase. Less frequent side effects associated with ChEI therapy include bradycardia, syncope, muscle cramps, weakness, insomnia, nightmares, exacerbation of asthma symptoms, anorexia, weight loss, peptic ulcer disease, and gastrointestinal (GI) bleeding.
- Memantine is well tolerated, and the most frequently occurring side effects include dizziness, confusion, headache, fatigue, somnolence, and constipation.
- Cholinesterase inhibitors and memantine should not be chewed but can be given with food to decrease the risk of GI side effects.

- Memantine tablets should not be crushed or chewed because this may increase the rate of absorption.
- Memantine is cleared by the kidneys, so it is given at a lower dose in patients with creatinine clearance <30mL/min.
- **Dental alerts:** Avoid nephrotoxic drugs, particularly NSAIDS, in the presence of renal disease and memantine. Concurrent use of NSAIDS should be avoided. Additionally, avoid the use of 4% local anesthetics in patients on AD medications.

ALZHEIMER'S DISEASE SUGGESTED DENTAL GUIDELINES

The following are dental guidelines for Alzheimer's disease:

1. Never leave a dementia or Alzheimer's patient alone in the chair; the patient could walk away because of confusion or anxiety.
2. In the initial stages of the disease, written reminders can help Alzheimer's patients lead a relatively normal life. This is because in the early stages of the disease, they can remember how to do things once they are reminded to do them. It is only later that they lose the ability to perform simple tasks. Therefore, make "to-do" lists and provide notes to the patient. This helps the patient remember things better, experience less anxiety, and have a calmer living situation.
3. Oral injuries that frequently occur in these patients involve the cheeks, tongue, and alveolar mucosa, due to injuries sustained with forks or spoons or during mastication.
4. Poor oral hygiene, increased incidence of caries, and periodontal disease are common findings.
5. Xerostomia often occurs because of the common use of antipsychotic drugs in these patients.
6. **Anesthetics:** Avoid epinephrine in the presence of antipsychotic drugs.
7. **Stress management and analgesics:** Avoid sedatives, hypnotics, narcotic analgesics, and antihistamines in patients with Alzheimer's disease and with all other CNS disorders.
8. Alzheimer's patients do best seeing the same dentist in order to maintain consistency and decrease anxiety. Explain all the action and activities that will occur during a dental appointment. Use short, simple sentences while communicating with the patient.
9. Be aggressive with their dental care. Frequent hygiene recalls (three-to-four month intervals), fluoride gel applications, and adjustments of prosthesis are some of the heightened dental needs of these patients.

SCHIZOPHRENIA

Schizophrenia is a chronic, disabling mental illness that can often be severe. Men and women are equally affected. Schizophrenia is usually diagnosed around the ages of 17–35 years. The illness appears earlier in men than in women and many of the patients are disabled with the disease. Some, however, recover enough with treatment to live a relatively independent life.

Schizophrenia is a disturbance in thinking and perception and a splitting away from reality. These patients are often confused, withdrawn, depressed, and anxious.

Hallucinations and/or delusions are common. They do not show any emotions and speak in monotones. Prior to the start of the treatment the patient may be hyperactive, pacing, stationary, or catatonic.

Genes, infections, stresses, and the neurotransmitters dopamine, serotonin, and glutamate have been implicated as causative factors for schizophrenia.

Symptoms

Schizophrenia is usually associated with the following symptoms:

1. **Delusions**: Delusions are false beliefs held by the patient. These delusions seem very real to the patient.
2. **Hallucinations**: The patient experiences visual, auditory, taste, or smell sensory perceptions or hallucinations. These hallucinations occur in the absence of actual external stimuli.
3. **Disorganized thoughts and behaviors:** These thoughts and behaviors are out of context with reality.
4. **Disorganized speech:** Due to the loss of contact with reality, the patient's speech is in response to hallucinations experienced.
5. **Catatonic behavior:** The patient may be rigid and unresponsive for hours during the catatonic phase.

Diagnosis

Schizophrenia diagnosis is made when the active symptoms of schizophrenia have been present and untreated for at least six months, or with treatment for only one month.

Treatment

Schizophrenia management is done with neuroleptics and atypical psychotics.

Neuroleptics

These comprise the older class of drugs that control acute symptoms well but are not that effective in correcting lack of emotional expression and decreased motivation. Drugs that belong to this class include chlorpromazine (Thorazine), fluphenazine (Prolixin), haloperidol (Haldol), molindone (Moban), mesoridazine (Serentil), perphenazine (Trilafon), thioridazine (Mellaril), thiothixene (Navane), and trifluoperazine (Stelazine).

Neuroleptics Side Effects

Hypotension, xerostomia, tachycardia, arrythmia, thrombocytopenia, and leucopenia, are side effects of neuroleptics.

Atypical Antipsychotics

The atypical antipsychotics are newer drugs that have minimal or no neurological side effects. These medications have successfully treated affected patients who have become active members of society. Drugs in this category include aripiprazole (Abilify), clozapine (Clozaril), olanzapine (Zyprexa), quetiapine (Seroquel), risperidone (Risperdal), and ziprasidone (Geodon).

Atypical Antipsychotics Side Effects

These drugs cause **severe** agranulocytosis. The **CBC** must be monitored weekly during the first six months of treatment and then every two weeks to detect the agranulocytosis.

SCHIZOPHRENIA SUGGESTED DENTAL GUIDELINES

Follow these guidelines in the dental setting:

1. **Anesthetics:** Do not use topical epinephrine or epinephrine-containing local anesthetics with any of the drugs used to treat schizophrenia.
2. **Stress management and analgesics:** Sedative hypnotics, epinephrine, atropine, antihistamines, and narcotics are all contraindicated with psychiatric drugs or CNS-acting drugs. Sedating antihistamines are contraindicated because they enhance sedation.
3. Monitor the CBC and calculate the ANC count in patients on neuroleptics and atypical antipsychotics. Follow the ANC guidelines in patients with leucopenia.
4. Oral side effects and management of the oral lesions are the same as those discussed in the section "Depression and Suggested Dental Alerts."

EATING DISORDERS

Eating disorders are associated with serious disturbances in eating behavior. There is an extreme, distorted concern and anxiety about the body shape or size thus triggering a severe, unhealthy under-eating or overeating pattern. Once established, the pattern is difficult to break.

Eating disorders are true medical illnesses that commonly affect adolescent or young adults, and females outnumber males in being affected with the disease. Anxiety, depression, suicide attempts, low self-esteem, and alcohol and/or substance abuse often coexist with the eating disorders. Eating disorders, particularly anorexia nervosa, can adversely affect the heart causing renal failure, cardiac arrhythmia, and sudden death in the process.

Eating Disorder Classification

The three most common eating disorders are anorexia nervosa, bulimia, and binge eating.

Anorexia Nervosa

The patient is very afraid of gaining weight despite being extremely thin and grossly underweight. There is true opposition to maintaining ideal body weight. There is a distorted perception of one's own body shape or size and denial that a weight problem exists. This type of patient obsessively goes to extremes to lose more weight.

The patient picks at food, often eating only select food items and eating infrequently or in small portions. Purging and laxative and diuretic abuse are additional ways in which the weight is decreased. Serious weight loss results in loss of menstruation in affected females.

Some patients can recover with proper medical intervention, some can go on to suffer chronically with the disease, and still others may develop serious complications and succumb to the disease because of medical complications or ultimately suicide. Severe electrolyte loss and hypokalemia (decreased potassium) caused by the purging and undereating precipitates cardiac arrhythmia, kidney failure, and death.

Bulimia

The bulimic patient reacts differently to food when compared with the anorexia nervosa patient. The emphasis is on eating uncontrollably (binge eating) over a finite time, and then eliminating the food immediately from the body by forced vomiting. The patient has no control over the eating and eats quickly and excessively to the point of hurting. The patient is secretive about these practices and is ashamed of the behavior, but gets a sense of relief with food elimination by purging.

It is not uncommon for this type of patient to abuse diuretics, laxatives, rigorous exercise, and tools to promote the gag reflex (fingers, throat sticks, spoon, an so on) to assist with vomiting. The patient is usually close to normal body weight but has a distorted perception of her/his own weight.

Bulimia Diagnosis

The patient must have had at least two food-abuse episodes/week for three months to be diagnosed with bulimia.

Binge Eating

Binge eating is a variant of bulimia. In binge eating there is an abnormal compulsion to eat large volumes of food in the shortest possible time until it hurts and no more can be eaten. The patient eats in the presence of others and there is tremendous guilt experienced after eating. These patients do not resort to purging or laxative/diuretic abuse. Consequently, many of these patients are overweight rather than underweight. The etiology and treatment protocols for binge eating are the same as with bulimia.

Binge Eating Diagnosis

Binge eating is considered a true disorder when it happens twice/week, for six months.

Eating Disorders Treatment

The patient needs to want to get better, because patient participation and commitment are very important. Treatment for anorexia consists of a number of disciplines coming together to help the patient. It is a true team effort to target and address every factor causing the disorder. The team includes the physician, psychologist, therapist, nutri-tionist, family support, and medications, when needed.

A patient with associated life-threatening conditions is invariably hospitalized whereas others are treated in an outpatient setting. The hospitalized patient's feeds are monitored closely and provided by intravenous therapy. The anorexia patient needs to gain weight, deal with the psychological conditions promoting the disorder, and learn to maintain the weight.

SSRIs are sometimes used after weight improvement to alleviate anxiety, continue with weight maintenance, and help the patient feel good and maintain a positive attitude.

The same kind of team approach previously mentioned is also utilized for the bulimia patient. The patient is encouraged to decrease the meal volume, deal with the underlying psychiatric conditions promoting the eating disorder, develop a healthy attitude toward body shape and size, and take SSRIs to help cope with the recovery process.

EATING DISORDERS SUGGESTED DENTAL GUIDELINES

Follow these guidelines when treating patients who have eating disorders:

1. Always confirm that a patient with an eating disorder is aware of the association of the patient's disease state with enamel erosion, increased incidence of dental caries, and xerostomia. The patient has to "partner" with the dentist in wanting to improve the mouth, reverse the erosion and decay, and maintain the repair. Be aware that continuation of the eating disorder will negatively impact on the expensive dentistry. The patient should be coaxed to follow through with the eating-disorder recovery process.
2. Confirm that the patient has ongoing psychotherapy support to prevent reverting back to the disorder.
3. Thorough history-taking should include assessment of laxative and diuretic use/abuse.
4. Always check for symptoms and signs of hypokalemia in eating disorder patients: muscle cramps, muscle weakness, tingling numbness in the hands and feet, fatigue, and irregular pulse. Delay dental treatment and refer a patient who is symptomatic for hypokalemia to the medical side.
5. Teach the patient to rinse the mouth with water as soon as the acid is felt in the mouth.
6. Treat the xerostomia and candidiasis, when present, according to the protocol dis-cussed in Chapter 48.
7. **Anesthetics:** Avoid epinephrine use in a patient complaining of palpitations or irregular pulse. Epinephrine in the local anesthetic is not contraindicated with the SSRIs.
8. **Stress management, anesthetics, and analgesics:** Epinephrine, sedatives, hyp-notics, narcotics, and sedating antihistamines are contraindicated with all other psy-chiatric medications if being used by the patient (Table 52.1).

Table 52.1. Psychiatric Medications Side Effects and Epinephrine Use in LAs

Psychiatric Drugs Category	Side Eeffects
Anti-Anxiety Drugs:	
– Benzodiazepines: Epinephrine can be used	– Xerostomia
– Beta-blockers: Limit epinephrine to 2 carpules	– Postural
Anti-depressants with anti-anxiety effects:	– Hypotension
– Monoamine oxidase inhibitors (MAOIs): Avoid epinephrine	
– Selective Serotonin Reuptake Inhibitors (SSRIs): Epinephrine can be used	
– Tricyclic antidepressants: Avoid epinephrine	
Anti-Depressant Drugs:	
Tricyclic anti-depressants (TCAs):	
– Amytriptyline (Elavil)	– Postural hypotention
– Imipramine (Tofranil/Norpramine)	– Tachycardia
– Nortriptyline (Aventyl)	– Arrythmia
– Doxepin (Sinequan)	– Xerostomia
Avoid epinephrine	
Mono amine oxidase inhibitors (MAOIs):	
– Phenelzine (Nardil)	– Postural hypotention
– Isocarboxazid (Marplan)	– Xerostomia
– Tranylcypromine (Parnate)	
Avoid epinephrine	
Selective Serotonin reuptake inhibitors (SSRIs):	– Postural hypotension
– Paroxetin (Paxil)	– Xerostomia
– Fluoxetin (Prozac)	
– Sertraline (Zoloft)	
– Citalopram (Celexa)	
Epinephrine can be used.	
Lithium: Avoid epinephrine	– Tremors
	– Anxiety
	– Memory impairment
	– Skin rash
	– Impairment of the renal function
	– Excessive loss of potassium
	– Xerostomia
	– Stomatitis
Treatment for Bipolar or Manic-Depressive Psychosis:	– Tremors
– Lithium Carbonate (Lithane or Lithobid or Lithonate or Eskalith)	– Anxiety
	– Memory impairment
– Carbemazepine (Tegretol)	– Skin rash
– Valproic Acid (Depakote)	– Impairment of the renal function
Avoid Epinephrine with these drugs	– Excessive loss of potassium
	– Xerostomia
	– Stomatitis
	– Leukopenia and thrombocytopenia with Valproic acid

(continued)

Table 52.1.   Psychiatric Medications Side Effects and Epinephrine Use in LAs (*Continued*)

Psychiatric Drugs Category	Side Eeffects
Anti-Schizophrenic Drugs: **Neuroleptics:** – Chlorpromazine (Thorazine) – Fluphenazine (Prolixin) – Haloperidol (Haldol) – Molindone (Moban) – Mesoridazine (Serentil) – Perphenazine (Trilafon) – Thioridazine (Mellaril) – Thiothixene (Navane) – Trifluoperazine (Stelazine) **Avoid epinephrine with these drugs**	– Hypotention – Xerostomia – Tachycardia – Arrythmia – Thrombocytopenia – Leukopenia
Atypical Anti-Psychotics: – Aripiprazole (Abilify) – Clozapine (Clozaril) – Olanzapine (Zyprexa) – Quetiapine (Seroquel) – Risperidone (Risperdal) – Ziprasidone (Geodon) **Avoid epinephrine with these drugs**	– They cause severe agranulocytosis – Monitor CBC weekly in the first six months of care, then every two weeks to detect agranulocytosis
Alzheimer's Drugs: **Acetylcholinesterase Inhibitors:** – Donepezil (Aricept): Acetylcholinesterase inhibitor – Galantamine (Reminyl): Acetylcholinesterase inhibitor – Rivastigmine (Exelon): Acetylcholinesterase and Butyrylcholinesterase inhibitor – Tacrine (Cognex): Acetylcholinesterase inhibitor **Avoid epinephrine with these drugs**	– Nausea – Vomiting – Diarrhea – Weight loss

XX Transplants

Organ Transplants, Immunosuppressive Drugs, and Associated Dental Management Guidelines

ORGAN TRANSPLANTS OVERVIEW AND FACTS

Organ transplantation has come a long way from the first transplant done in the early 1950s. Most organ transplants initially had been allografts or tissues from genetically nonidentical donors. This accounted for the less-than-satisfactory outcomes with organ transplants. Now, with newer trends, the live, related-donor rates have increased, accounting for an improved outcome and greater hope for organ transplantations. The success rates for organ transplants have also increased tremendously with the discovery of immunosuppressants cyclosporine and tacrolimus (Prograf). These drugs have improved the survival rates in transplanted patients.

Care post organ transplant has also seen some changes in the way the patients are managed. The trend now is to keep the patient's immunity at a specific optimal level, such that the need for immunosuppression drugs is decreased. This improves the recipient's immune system response in helping to ward off infections or deal with infections. Some transplant centers are now providing the patient with steroid-free and calcineurin-inhibitor–free immunosuppressions. The short-term results with these new strategies have been promising thus far, but the long-term outcome data need to show that this process is truly a move in the right direction. The physician now can utilize **Immu-Know**, an assay to assess immune system function from a single blood drop. The test measures the vitality of the patient's immune system, thus allowing the physician to better manage the patient's response to infection thereby personalizing the care to prevent organ rejection. These newer methods of care will definitely lower the cost of medications in the future and prolong the organ recipient's life. The major organs transplanted today are bone marrow, heart, lungs, pancreas, liver, and kidneys.

Kidney Transplant Facts

Dialysis is a very expensive option in the long run for renal failure patients. A kidney transplant is also expensive at first, but overall it has a lower yearly maintenance cost

---

Dentist's Guide to Medical Conditions, Medications, and Complications, Second Edition. Kanchan M. Ganda.
© 2013 John Wiley & Sons, Inc. Published 2013 by John Wiley & Sons, Inc.

compared with dialysis. With kidney transplant, the quality of life improves for the patient and there is also an improvement of uremia, anemia, peripheral neuropathy, and autonomic neuropathy. A kidney transplant can double the life span of kidney failure patients.

The transplanted kidney can be obtained from a cadaver—50% of transplants utilize this source—a live related donor, or a live distant/unrelated donor. Kidneys obtained from a live donor are much better than those obtained from a nonliving or cadaveric donor.

Liver Transplant Facts

A liver transplant is much more complicated than a kidney transplant because of the complexity of the surgical procedure. To prioritize a patient on the liver transplant list, the severity of a liver failure patient's status is assessed using the model of end-stage liver disease (MELD) criteria. The MELD criteria evaluate the following tests: bilirubin, PT/INR, and serum creatinine. The serum creatinine is the most sensitive mortality-risk indicator of liver failure.

Cells Responsible for Prevention of Organ Rejection

The following cells constitute the cell-mediated defenses for the prevention of organ rejection:

1. T cells: the most important cells
2. Antigen-presenting cells
3. Natural killer cells
4. Monocytes

TYPES OF IMMUNOSUPPRESSION

Post-transplant immunosuppression includes the giving of a combination of drugs to prevent rejection of the transplanted organ, but how and when these drugs are given is based on a patient's individual situation. Depending on these factors, the approaches could include:

- Induction immunosuppression
- Maintenance immunosuppression
- Anti-rejection immunosuppression

Induction Immunosuppression

In this approach, all medications are given in very high doses immediately after transplantation as to prevent any acute rejection. The drugs may be continued for the first 30 days after transplant, but they are not used long term for immunosuppressive maintenance. Medications often used for this type of immunosuppression include methylprednisolone, atgam, thymoglobulin, OKT3, basiliximab, or daclizumab.

Maintenance Immunosuppression

In maintenance immunosuppression, all immunosuppressive medications are given before, during, or after transplant with the intention to maintain their use long term. Drugs often used for this type of immunosupression include prednisone, cyclosporine, tacrolimus, mycophenolate mofetil, azathioprine, or rapamycin.

Anti-Rejection Immunosuppression

In this approach, all immunosuppressive medications are given to treat an acute rejection episode during the initial post-transplant period or during a specific follow-up period, usually up to 30 days after the diagnosis of acute rejection. Medications used include methylprednisolone, atgam, OKT3, thymoglobulin, basiliximab, or daclizumab.

IMMUNOSUPPRESSANT DRUGS

Immunosuppressants currently available are azathioprine, basiliximab, cyclosporine, daclizumab, muromonab-CD3, mycophenolic acid, mycophenolate mofetil, prednisone, sirolimus, and tacrolimus. These drugs do cause side effects, but the physician may control these adverse effects by changing doses or switching medications. The maintenance immunosuppression drugs will be discussed because they are the most commonly used of all the anti-rejection drugs. The drugs discussed are:

1. Azathioprine (Imuran)
2. The calcineurin inhibitors: tacrolimus (Prograf/FK506) and cyclosporine (Sandimmune)
3. Prednisone
4. Mycophenolate mofetil (Cellcept)
5. Sirolimus (Rapamune)

AZATHIOPRINE (IMURAN)
Mechanism of Action

Azathioprine is an antimetabolite that decreases inflammation and interferes with the growth of rapidly dividing cells. It has a generalized effect on bone marrow and inhibits the production of blood-forming cells, thus preventing rejection. Azathioprine inhibits the white blood cells causing leucopenia and thrombocytopenia. Always **assess** the **CBC prior** to instituting dental treatment in patients on azathioprine (Imuran).

Side Effects

Common side effects experienced by the patient are cold hands and feet; loss of appetite, upset stomach, diarrhea, and vomiting; fever; mouth sores; sore throat; and unusual bleeding or bruising.

CYCLOSPORINE (SANDIMMUNE)

Cyclosporine is used for the management of organ transplants, severe psoriasis, and rheumatoid arthritis.

Mechanism of Action

Cyclosporine decreases the production of interleukins, resulting in decreased replication of helper and killer T cells.

Facts

Cyclosporine is extensively metabolized by the cytochrome P450 enzyme system in the liver. It is not unusual for the BUN and serum creatinine levels to be elevated during therapy if the cyclosporine levels are not kept in check.

Cyclosporine can therefore cause hypertension if the levels are not regulated well. Nephrotoxicity has occurred in patients receiving high doses of cyclosporine. Cyclosporine levels are monitored regularly every four to six weeks. Avoid nephrotoxic drugs in patients on cyclosporine. Cyclosporine is known to cause gingival hyperplasia.

Antibiotics Alert

Macrolides increase cyclosporine toxicity by increasing the intestinal absorption and inhibiting the biliary absorption of cyclosporine.

Antifungal Alert

Fluconazole (Diflucan) also increases cyclosporine toxicity, and the mechanism of action is unknown.

Analgesics Alert

Avoid the use of NSAIDS with cyclosporine because NSAIDS promote nephrotoxicity. Avoid the use of trimethoprim-sulphamethoxazole (Bactrim) with cyclosporine because it also promotes nephrotoxicity. **Note** that Bactrim is ineffective in treating oral infections.

Side Effects

Side effects associated with cyclosporine are diarrhea; increased hair growth; loss of appetite; sinusitis; upset stomach; vomiting; tender, swollen, bleeding gums, and gingival hyperplasia; unusual bleeding or bruising; and sore throat, fever, and/or chills.

Drug Interactions

Avoid the following medications in the dental setting in the presence of cyclosporine: cimetidine (Tagamet), clarithromycin (Biaxin), corticosteroids, erythromycin, fluconazole (Diflucan), itraconazole (Sporanox), and ketoconazole (Nizoral).

TACROLIMUS (PROGRAF), FK506

Tacrolimus is an immunosuppressant that reduces the body's natural immunity in recipients of organ transplants. Tacrolimus (Prograf) is used as an alternate to cyclosporine when cyclosporine cannot be used.

Mechanism of Action

Tacrolimus inhibits cytokine production, including IL-2. It inhibits the expression of IL-2 receptors and blocks cell division.

Side Effects

Side effects associated with tacrolimus are diarrhea; vomiting; difficulty breathing and/or wheezing; itching, skin rash, and/or hives; seizures; sore throat, fever, and/or chills; unusual bleeding or bruising.

Drug Interactions

Avoid the following drugs in the dental setting in the presence of tacrolimus: antacids, cimetidine (Tagamet), clarithromycin (Biaxin), clotrimazole (Mycelex/Lotrimin), drythromycin, fluconazole (Diflucan), itraconazole (Sporanox), ketoconazole (Nizoral), and methylprednisolone (Medrol).

Suggested Dental Alert

Tacrolimus can cause anemia. Avoid nephrotoxic drugs in patients on tacrolimus.

PREDNISONE

Prednisone is an immunosuppressant drug that prevents the body from rejecting a transplanted organ. It is also used to treat certain forms of arthritis, severe allergies, and asthmas, as well as skin, blood, kidney, eye, thyroid, and intestinal disorders.

Mechanism of Action

Prednisone inhibits interluekin-1 secretions, resulting in decreased replication of cytotoxic T cells. It also has a nonspecific anti-inflammatory effect and inhibits the granulocyte function, thus limiting damage to an organ in which the rejection process has already begun.

Side Effects

Side effects associated with prednisone are dizziness; easy bruising; upset stomach; skin rash; swollen face, lower legs, or ankles; osteoporosis; "moon-faced" appearance; and vision problems.

Suggested Dental Facts and Alerts

Be alert to the following:

1. Always determine the current dose of prednisone and the duration for which the patient has been on corticosteroids.
2. Follow "the rule of twos" in patients who are to undergo major dental surgery, by consulting with the patient's MD.
3. Check the oral cavity for candidiasis and treat appropriately, when candidiasis is found.

MYCOPHENOLATE MOFETIL (CELLCEPT)

Cellcept is often combined with cyclosporine, tacrolimus (Prograf), or rapamycin to prevent rejection in organ transplant recipients.

Mechanism of Action

Cellcept lowers the body's immune system by killing the lymphocytes, thus preventing organ rejection.

Side Effects

Common side effects include fever, chills, or flu symptoms; easy bruising or bleeding; bloody, black, or tarry stools; painful or difficulty urinating; and numbness or tingly feeling.

SIROLIMUS (RAPAMYCIN)

Rapamycin is an immunosuppressant drug used to prevent rejection in organ transplantation, and it is typically used in combination with cyclosporine and corticosteroids. It is particularly useful in managing kidney transplants. It prevents activation of T cells and B cells by inhibiting their response to interleukin-2 (IL-2).

Mechanism of Action

The mode of action of sirolimus is to bind the cytosolic protein FK-binding protein 12 (FKBP12) in a manner similar to tacrolimus, and the sirolimus-FKBP12 complex inhibits the mammalian target of rapamycin (mTOR) pathway.

Side Effects

Lung toxicity, cancer risk, high blood pressure, stomach and joint pain, diarrhea, headache, fever, urinary tract infection, low red blood cell count, nausea, low platelet count, and decreased glucose tolerance plus insensitivity to insulin are side effects associated with sirolimus (rapamycin).

OTHER MEDICATIONS

Anti-rejection medications help with the optimal functioning of the new organ and with the prevention of organ rejection. However, as noted previously, these medications often cause side effects that need to be addressed and/or treated with medications. The following are some of the medications a transplant patient has to take, to prevent or control those side effects:

- Antibiotics
- Anti-fungal medications
- Anti-ulcer medications
- Antivirals
- Diuretics
- Statins

Antibiotics

The risk of developing bacterial infections during and after transplant is high, and the standard antibiotics are used to kill or inhibit the growth of any infecting bacteria without causing damage to the transplanted organ.

Anti-Fungal Medications

Anti-fungal medications are used to treat fungal infections of the skin, mouth, throat, intestinal tract or genital area. Topical, oral, or intravenous anti-fungal therapies can be prescribed. These medications should be used exactly as directed and the patient must complete the full course of therapy to minimize recurrence of infections.

Anti-Ulcer Medications

Anti-ulcer medications are used after transplant to treat and prevent the recurrence of ulcers, and to treat excess acid production.

Antivirals

Immunosuppressive drugs make transplant patients susceptible to viral infections, and antivirals are used for the prevention and treatment of those viruses.

Diuretics

Diuretics are used to reduce swelling and fluid retention and control high blood pressure. Because excess amounts of diuretics can cause electrolyte depletion, it is important to monitor electrolytes while the patient is on these medications.

Statins

Because immunosuppressive therapy may aggravate existing cardiovascular disease risk factors or promote the development of new ones, transplant patients are often treated with statins. Statins lower blood cholesterol levels and have known benefits in reducing cardiovascular disease.

TRANSPLANTS AND CANCERS

Cancer is more common in transplant patients than in the general population. Research has shown that it is likely for patients who live for at least ten years after a transplant to develop some type of cancer, including skin cancer. This discussion will focus on the types of cancers associated with transplant recipients and risk factors, prevention, and early detection.

Types of Cancers

There are three different types of transplant-related cancers that may affect transplant recipients:

- Donor related cancers
- Recipient's past history of cancer
- Cancer due to suppression of the immune system

Donor-Related Cancers

Although very rare, cancer can be transmitted through deceased- and living-donor organ, cell, and tissue transplantation. Treatment of donor-related tumors consists of changing, reducing, or stopping immunosuppressive drug therapy, returning to chronic hemodialysis for renal recipients, and possible re-transplantation.

Recipient's History of Cancer

Transplant recipients with a history of preexisting malignancies have a very low incidence of recurrence post transplant. Recurrence rates are obviously affected by the specific type of cancer, the extent of the disease at the time of treatment, the time elapsed since the treatment, and the natural history of the malignancy in the normal population.

Cancer Due to Suppression of the Immune System

In general, transplant recipients have an increased risk of developing new cancers at a rate of 1–2% per year, with a 15–20% higher incidence rate for certain types of cancer. Skin cancer and lymphomas are the most prevalent types of cancer seen post transplantation. The risk of cervical, breast, and colorectal cancers are also increased. In particular, post-transplant patients have a significantly increased risk of developing squamous cell carcinomas, as well as melanoma. A smaller number of transplant recipients develop lymphoma within a year of the surgery. Some lymphomas do respond to lowering the dose of anti-rejection drugs or stopping the drugs temporarily, whereas others will respond to chemotherapy or radiotherapy.

A small number of patients develop solid cancers that are non-skin, and non-lymphoma related cancers. When this occurs, standard cancer treatment options, including surgery, radiotherapy, and chemotherapy must be individualized to the patient. A thorough consideration of the patient's tumor risk, treatment risk, and risk of graft loss is also made during this decision making process.

For renal recipients, immunosuppression may be reduced or stopped even to the point of losing the graft and returning to hemodialysis. For liver recipients with malignancy confined to the transplanted liver, re-transplantation is an option. Switching immunosuppression from a calcineurin inhibitor such as cyclosporine or tacrolimus to a target-of-rapamycin (TOR) inhibitor such as sirolimus, is considered as an option because there are fewer incidences of malignancies associated with TOR inhibitors than calcineurin inhibitors. Also, there have been reports of malignancy regression when immunosuppression has been switched from a calcineurin inhibitor to a TOR inhibitor.

Cancer Risk Factors

The main risk factors contributing to an increased incidence of any cancer is due to suppression of the immune system and duration and intensity of immunosuppression. All types of immunosuppressant medications can increase the risk for certain types of cancer. Other risk factors may include history of cancer, male gender, race, and older age.

Prevention and Early Detection

Early detection of cancer can be helped by monthly breast, testicular, and skin self-examinations and routine medical checkups. PAP smears, breast exams, testicular exams, and skin cancer screening should be done during annual physician visits. Other general measures that should be taken include reduction of sun exposure, cessation of smoking, and proper nutrition and exercise.

SUGGESTED DENTAL GUIDELINES FOR ORGAN TRANSPLANT PATIENTS

Follow these guidelines in the dental setting:

1. Prior to the start of routine dental treatment always obtain laboratory tests to confirm that the transplanted organ is optimally functioning. Never presume that the transplanted organ works well!
2. Obtain a good dental history and perform a thorough dental examination, including full-mouth radiographs.
3. Prioritize the patient's dental problems. Those that are most likely to cause pain, infection, and/or bacteremia in the next 12 months should be taken care of immediately.
4. When treating a **pre-renal transplant** patient, follow the **premedication protocol** for shunts and renal failure anesthetic, analgesic, antibiotic (AAAs) suggested guidelines during dentistry.
5. When treating a **pre-liver transplant** patient, follow the liver failure anesthetic, analgesic, antibiotic (AAAs) suggested guidelines during dentistry.
6. Obtain the CBC and calculate the ANC count in any pre-transplant patient. Provide AHA recommended antibiotic premedication with an antibiotic that is safe in the presence of a failed organ, if the patient has low ANC counts.
7. Premedication should also be provided in the presence of **ascites** in the pre-liver transplant patient.
8. In the patient awaiting a liver transplant, evaluate the PT/INR: fresh frozen plasma (FFP) transfusion will be needed if the PT/INR is prolonged. Also evaluate the platelet count in the patient awaiting a liver transplant. Platelet replacement will be required if the platelet count is <50,000/mm^3.
9. Pre-transplant preparation of the oral cavity is the same as that for patients undergoing chemotherapy or radiotherapy.
10. Routine dentistry should be **deferred for six months**, post organ transplant.
11. If emergency dental treatment is needed within the first six months of an organ transplant, use the AAA guidelines specified for the specific organ during failure (renal failure/cirrhosis).
12. The AAAs used during dentistry will be determined by the current status of the transplanted organ. Obtain appropriate tests to evaluate the status of the transplanted organ and **then** proceed with dentistry.
13. Avoid cimetidine (Tagamet), clarithromycin (Biaxin), corticosteroids, erythromycin, fluconazole (Diflucan), itraconazole (Sporanox), and ketoconazole (Nizoral) in the presence of cyclosporine.
14. Avoid the following drugs in the dental setting in the presence of tacrolimus (Prograf, FK506): antacids, cimetidine (Tagamet), clarithromycin (Biaxin), clotrimazole

(Mycelex), erythromycin, fluconazole (Diflucan), itraconazole (Sporanox), keto-conazole (Nizoral), and methylprednisolone (Medrol).

15. If macrolides are the only antibiotics that can be used in the first six months of the transplant because of allergy to penicillin, communicate with the patient's MD. The MD can assist with temporarily lowering the cyclosporine dose so that the macrolide can be safely used.

16. Bone marrow suppression is a genuine concern post transplant, and there is an increased incidence of infections plus increased susceptibility to infections. Determine the ANC and provide appropriate antibiotics when needed. Treat all infections aggressively.

17. If the patient is on steroids, there could be a need for steroid boost prior to major surgery. Always confirm with the patient's physician.

18. Herpangina occurs commonly post transplant and is very aggressive when it occurs. Treat immediately with valacyclovir (Valtrex) or acyclovir (Zovirax).

19. **Gingival hyperplasia:** Cyclosporine is the leading cause for gingival hyperplasia, post transplant. The patient can be switched to an alternate medication by the MD if the hypertrophy becomes a genuine issue.

20. Potentially, hypertension can occur with cyclosporine use, so always monitor the BP during dentistry.

21. Even if the ANC is normal, consider **premedication** for renal transplant patients that **were** on hemodialysis, but still continue to have the shunt.

22. Consider premedication for any organ transplant patient with decreased immunity as indicated by assessment of the total WBC and the ANC counts. Follow the ANC guidelines if the WBC count is below normal.

23. Always look for oral sores and treat accordingly in patients on Imuran.

24. Tacrolimus (Prograf, FK506) can cause anemia. Follow the anemia AAA suggested guidelines when the CBC indicates anemia.

25. Avoid nephrotoxic drugs in patients on cyclosporine and tacrolimus (Prograf).

XXI

Common Laboratory Tests

Comprehensive Metabolic Panel and Common Hematological Tests

The comprehensive metabolic panel (CMP) is a series of 14 tests done by a medical laboratory using a fasting blood draw from the patient. The CMP is also called the **Chem 12 Panel**. It is often ordered by the physician in order to assess the patient's kidney and liver statuses, electrolytes, proteins, and blood sugar. When the CMP shows any abnormality, the physician then typically orders specific tests to further evaluate the identified disease state.

THE COMPREHENSIVE METABOLIC PANEL COMPONENTS

The CMP includes glucose, calcium, albumin, total protein, sodium, potassium, bicarbonate, chloride, blood urea nitrogen (BUN), creatinine, alkaline phosphatase (ALP), alanine amino transferase (ALT/SGPT), aspartate amino transferase (AST/SGOT), and bilirubin.

COMMON HEMATOLOGICAL TESTS AND DENTISTRY

Common hematological tests reviewed prior to dentistry are:

1. **Complete blood count (CBC):** CBC with platelets and WBC differential and erythrocyte sedimentation rate (ESR) are discussed in Chapter 11.
2. **Coagulation tests:** Prothrombin time (PT)/international normalized ratio (INR), partial thromboplastin time (PTT), and bleeding time (BT) are discussed in Chapter 15.
3. **Renal assessment tests:** Serum creatinine (s.Cr.) and blood urea nitrogen (BUN) are discussed in Chapter 28.
4. **Diabetes assessment tests:** Fasting blood sugar (FBS), postprandial/postmeal blood sugar (PPBS), and hemoglobin A_1C (HbA_1C) are discussed in Chapter 38.
5. **Liver assessment tests:** Hepatic serology and liver function tests (LFTs) are discussed in Chapter 45.

Dentist's Guide to Medical Conditions, Medications, and Complications, Second Edition. Kanchan M. Ganda.
© 2013 John Wiley & Sons, Inc. Published 2013 by John Wiley & Sons, Inc.

6. **Bone assessment tests:** Serum calcium (Ca^{2+}), serum phosphorus (PO_4), and alkaline phosphates (AlkP) are discussed in Chapter 41.
7. **HIV/AIDS assessment tests:** CD_4 count, viral load (HIV RNA), CBC with platelets, WBC differential, LFTs, PT/INR, and serum creatinine; this is discussed in Chapter 47.

THE CMP AND DENTISTRY

The CMP ordered by a physician to monitor a medically compromised patient should also be requested and assessed by the treating dentist using a medical consultation form signed by the patient, who consents to the release of the information. The goal is for the dentist to assess the patient's current medical status and modify the dental management with the appropriate use of AAAs for a successful treatment outcome. The CBC and the CMP, when requested, may occasionally be sent in the standardized lattice format on the medical consultation form itself or in the patient's medical records.

Lattice Pattern Recordings: CBC, PT/INR, and CMP

Figure 54.1 illustrates the blood chemistry profile lattice pattern recording. Also review Figures 12.1, 45.1, and 45.2 for the standardized lattice pattern recordings.

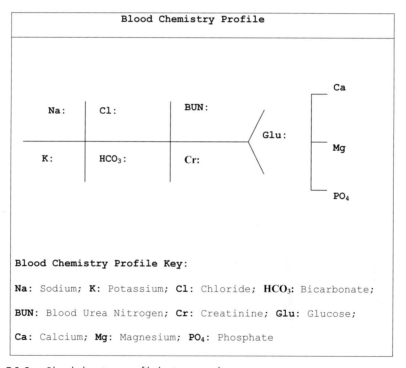

Figure 54.1. Blood chemistry profile lattice recording.

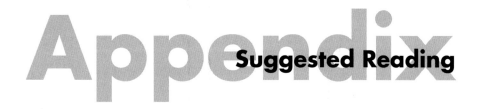

Appendix: Suggested Reading

HISTORY-TAKING AND PHYSICAL EXAMINATION RESOURCES

Bickley LS, Szilagyi PG. Bates' guide to physical examination and history taking. 10th ed. Philadelphia: Wolters Kluwer Health; 2009.

LeBlond R, Brown D, DeGowin R. DeGowin's diagnostic examination, 9th ed. McGraw-Hill Companies, Inc.; 2008.

LOCAL ANESTHETICS RESOURCES

Adewumi A, Hall M, Guelmann M, Riley J. The incidence of adverse reactions following 4% septocaine (articane) in children. Pediatr Dent. 2008;30(5):424–428.

Akerman B, Hellberg IB, Trossvik C. Primary evaluation of the local anaesthetic properties of the amino amide agent ropivacaine (LEA 103) Acta Anaesthesiol Scand. 1988;32:571–578.

Becker DE, Reed KL. Essentials of local anesthetic pharmacology. Anesth Prog 2006;53:98–109.

El-Sharrawy E, Yagiela JA. Anesthetic efficacy of different ropivacaine concentrations for inferior alveolar nerve block. Anesth Prog. 2006;53(1):3–7.

Ernberg M, Kopp S. Ropivicaine for dental anesthesia: a dose-finding study. J Oral Maxillofac Surg 2002;60(9):1004–1010.

Hornke I, Eckert HG, Rupp W. Pharnakokinetik und metabolismus von articain nach intramuskularer injektion am mannlichen probanden. Dtsch Z Mund Kiefer Gesichts Chir 1984;8:67–71.

Kennedy M, Reader A, Beck M, et al. An evaluation of the anesthetic efficacy of .5% ropivacaine with 1 to 200,000 epinephrine in human maxillary local anesthesia infiltration. Oral Surg Oral Med Oral Pathol. 2001;91:406–412.

Kennedy M, Reader A, Beck M, Weaver J. Anesthetic efficacy of ropivacaine in maxillary anterior infiltration. Oral Surg Oral Med Oral Pathol Oral Radiol Endod. 2001;91:406–412.

Dentist's Guide to Medical Conditions, Medications, and Complications, Second Edition. Kanchan M. Ganda.
© 2013 John Wiley & Sons, Inc. Published 2013 by John Wiley & Sons, Inc.

Kirch W, Kitteringham N, Lambers G, et al. Die klinische pharmakokinetik von articain nach intraoraler und intramuskularer application. Schweiz Monatsschr Zahnheilkd 1983;93:713–719.

Malamed SF. Handbook of local anesthesia. 6th ed. St. Louis: Mosby; 2012.

Meechan JG. A comparison of ropivacaine and lidocaine with epinephrine for intraligamentary anesthesia. Oral Surg Oral Med Oral Pathol Oral Radiol Endod. 2002;93:469–473.

Meechan JG. Ropivacaine is equivalent to bupivacaine in maxillary infiltrations. Evidence-Based Dentistry 2002;3:67–68.

Oertel R, Ebert U, Rahn R, Kirch W. Clinical pharmacokinetics of articaine. Clin Pharmacokinet. 1997;33(6):418–420.

Suurkula M, Blomberg S, Sjovall J, Edvardsson N. Central nervous and cardiovascular effects of IV infusions of ropivacaine, bupivacaine and placebo in volunteers. Br J Anaesth. 1997;78:507–514.

US FDA. www.fda.gov/Safety/MedWatch/SafetyInformation/SafetyAlertsforHuman MedicalProducts/ucm250264.htm.

ANALGESICS RESOURCES

Abramowicz M. (Editor). Drug interactions. The Medical Letter. 1999;41:61–62.

Abramowicz M., editor. Drugs for pain: treatment guidelines from The Medical Letter. The Medical Letter on Drugs and Therapeutics. 2007;5:23–32.

American Society of Anesthesiologists Task Force on Acute Pain Management. Practice guidelines for acute pain management in the perioperative setting: An updated report by the American Society of Anesthesiologists Task Force on Acute Pain Management. Anesthesiology 2012;116(2):248–273.

Becker DE. Pain Management: Part 1: Managing Acute and Postoperative Dental Pain. Anesth Prog. 2010;57(2):67–79.

Benson GD, Koff RS, Tolman KG. The therapeutic use of acetaminophen in patients with liver disease. American Journal of Therapeutics 2005;12(2):133–141.

Center for Disease Control. Medication exposures during pregnancy and breast-feeding: Frequently Asked Questions. http://www.cdc.gov/ncbddd/meds/faqs.htm.

Cryer B, Berlin RG, Cooper SA, Hsu C, Wason S. Double-blind, randomized, parallel, placebo-controlled study of ibuprofen effects on thromboxane B2 concentrations in aspirin-treated healthy adult volunteers. Clin Ther. 2005;27:185–191.

Dart RC, Erdman AR, Olson KR, et al. Acetaminophen poisoning: an evidence-based consensus guideline for out-of-hospital management. Clin Toxicol (Phila) 2006;44(1):1–18.

Delaney JA, Opatrny L, Brophy JM, Suissa S. Drug-drug interactions between antithrombotic medications and the risk of gastrointestinal bleeding. CMAJ. 2007; 177:347–351.

Farrell SE. Toxicity, Acetaminophen. eMedicine Journal. January 3, 2006. Available at http://www.emedicine.com/emerg/topic819.htm.

Gislason GH, Rasmussen JN, Abildstrom SZ, et al. Increased mortality and cardiovascular morbidity associated with use of nonsteroidal anti-inflammatory drugs in chronic heart failure. Arch Intern Med. 2009;169:141–149.

Harle DG, Baldo BA, Coroneos NJ, Fisher MM. Anaphylaxis following administration of papaveretum. Case report: implication of IgE antibodies that react with morphine and codeine, and identification of an allergenic determinant. Anesthesiology. 1980;71:489–494.

Herrlin K, Segerdhal M, Gustafsson LL, Kalso E. Methadone, ciprofloxacin, and adverse drug reactions. Lancet 2000;356:2069–2070.

Hyllested M, Jones S, Pedersen JL, Kehlet H. Comparative effect of paracetamol, NSAIDs or their combination in postoperative pain management: a qualitative review. Br J Anaesth. 2002;88:199–214.

Juhl, GI, Norholt, SE, Tonnesen, E, Hiesse-Provost, O, Jensen, TS. Analgesic efficacy and safety of intravenous paracetamol (acetaminophen) administered as a 2g starting dose following third molar surgery. European Journal of Pain; 2006;10(4):371–377.

Kimmey MB. Cardioprotective effects and gastrointestinal risks of aspirin: maintaining the delicate balance. Am J Med. 2004;117:72s–78s.

Larson AM, Polson J, Fontana RJ, et al. Acetaminophen-induced acute liver failure: results of a United States multicenter, prospective study. Hepatology 2005;42(6):1364–1372.

Lichtor JL, Schwartz AJ, Abouleish A, et al. Practice guidelines for acute pain management in the perioperative setting: an updated report by the American Society of Anesthesiologists Task Force on Acute Pain Management. Anesthesiology. 2012;116(2):248–273.

MacDonald TM, Wei L. Effect of ibuprofen on cardioprotective effect of aspirin. Lancet. 2003;361:573–574.

Moore PA, Crout RJ, Jackson DL, et al. Tramadol hydrochloride: analgesic efficacy compared with codeine, aspirin with codeine, and placebo after dental extraction. J Clin Pharmacol. 2003;38:554–560.

Patel TN, Goldberg KC. Use of aspirin and ibuprofen compared with aspirin alone and the risk of myocardial infarction. Arch Intern Med. 2004;164:852–856.

Pergolizzi, JV, Raffa, RB, Tallarida, R, Taylor, R, Labhsetwar, SA. Continuous multimechanistic postoperative analgesia: A rationale for transitioning from intravenous acetaminophen and opioids to oral formulations. Pain Practice 2011;12(2):159–173.

Pinto A, Farrar JT, Hersh EV. Prescribing NSAIDs to patients on SSRIs: possible adverse drug interaction of importance to dental practitioners. Compend Contin Educ Dent. 2009;30:142–151, quiz: 152, 154.

Prasanna N, Subbarao CV, Gutmann JL. The efficacy of pre-operative oral medication of lornoxicam and diclofenac potassium on the success of inferior alveolar nerve block in patients with irreversible pulpitis: a double-blind, randomised controlled clinical trial. Int Endod J. Apr 2011;44(4):330–6.

Shapiro LE, Shear NH. Drug interactions: Proteins, pumps, and P450s. J Am Acad Dermatol 2002;47:467–484.

Smilkstein MJ, Knapp GL, Kulig KW, Rumack BH. Efficacy of oral N-acetylcysteine in the treatment of acetaminophen overdose. Analysis of the national multicenter study (1976 to 1985). 1988;319(24):1557–1562.

Smith HS. Opioid metabolism. Mayo Clin Proc. 2009;84:613–624.

US FDA. Questions and Answers: FDA Regulatory Actions for the COX-2 Selective (includes Bextra, Celebrex, and Vioxx) and Non-Selective Non-Steroidal Antiinflammatory Drugs (NSAIDs). www.fda.gov/cder/drug/infopage/cox2.

US FDA. http://www.fda.gov/NewsEvents/Newsroom/PressAnnouncements/ucm310870.htm.

Van Dyke T, Litkowski LJ, Kiersch TA, Zarringhalam NM, Zheng H, Newman K. Combination oxycodone 5mg/ibuprofen 400mg for the treatment of postoperative pain: a double-blind, placebo- and active-controlled parallel-group study. Clin Ther. 2004;26:2003–2014.

Weiss ME, Adkinson NF, Hirshman CA. Evaluation of allergic drug reactions in the perioperative period. Anesthesiology. 1989;71:483–486.

Whitcomb DC, Block GD. Association of acetaminophen hepatotoxicity with fasting and ethanol. JAMA. 1994;272:1845–1850.

White WB. Defining the problem of treating the patient with hypertension and arthritis pain Am J Med 2009;122(5 suppl):S3–S9.

Wu CL, Raja, SN. Treatment of acute postoperative pain. The Lancet 2011; 377(9784):2215–2225.

www.pharmacist.com.

www.uptodate.com.

Yeh SY, Krebs HA, Changcht A. Urinary excretion of meperidine and its metabolites. J Pharm Sciences. 2006;70:867–870.

Yuan Y, Tsoi K, Hunt RH. Selective serotonin reuptake inhibitors and risk of upper GI bleeding: confusion or confounding? Am J Med. 2006;119:719–727.

Zed and Krenzelok. Treatment of acetaminophen overdose. Am J Health Syst Pharm 1999;56:1081–1091.

ANTIBIOTICS RESOURCES

Alliance for the Prudent Use of Antibiotics. Consumer Information. http://www.tufts.edu/med/apua/Patients/patient.html.

Ballow CH, Amsden GW. Azithromycin: the first azalide antibiotic. Ann. Pharmacother. 1992;26(10):1253–1261.

CDC. Clostridium difficile infection: Centers for Disease Control and Prevention, 2008.

Chu SY, Granneman GR, Pichotta PJ, et al. Effect of moderate or severe hepatic impairment on clarithromycin pharmacokinetics. J Clin Pharmacol. 193;33(5):480–485.

Falagas ME, Karageorgopoulos DE. Adjustment of dosing of antimicrobial agents for bodyweight in adults. Lancet 2010;375:248–251.

Golub LM, Ciancio S, Ramamamurthy NS, Leung M, McNamara TF. Low-dose doxycycline therapy: effect on gingival and crevicular fluid collagenase activity in humans. J Periodontal Res. 1990 Nov;25(6):321–30.

Hardy DJ, Guay DR, Jones RN. Clarithromycin, a unique macrolide: a pharmacokinetic, microbiological, and clinical overview. Diagn Microbiol Infect Dis. 1992;15(1): 39–53.

Leekha S, Terrell CL, Edson RS. General principles of antimicrobial therapy. Mayo Clin Proc. Feb 2011;86(2):156–67.

Mazzei T, Surrenti C, Novelli A, et al. Pharmacokinetics of azithromycin in patients with impaired hepatic function. J Antimicrob Chemother 1993; 31 Suppl E:57–63.

MEDLINEplus Drug Information. US National Library of Medicine. Accessed May 22, 2001.

Moellering RC, Jr. Linezolid: Summaries for patients. Annals of Internal Medicine 138 (January 21, 2003):I–44.

Portnof JE, Israel HA, Brause BD, Behrman DA. Dental premedication protocols for patients with knee and hip prostheses. N Y State Dent J 2006 Apr–May;72(3):20–25. PMID 16774168.

Ray WA, Murray KT, Hall K, Arbogast PG, Stein CM. Azithromycin and the risk of cardiovascular death. N Engl J Med. 2012 May 17;366(20):1881–90.

Simoes JA, et al. Antibiotic resistance patterns of group B streptococcal clinical isolates. Infect Dis Obstet Gynecol 2004;12,1:1–8.

Skidmore R, Kovach R, Walker C, Thomas J, Bradshaw M, Leyden J, Powala C, Ashley R. Effects of subantimicrobial-dose doxycycline in the treatment of moderate acne. Arch Dermatol. 2003 Apr;139(4):459–64.

Thiboutot DM, Shalita AR, Yamauchi PS, Dawson C, Arsonnaud S, Kang S. Combination therapy with adapalene and doxycycline for severe acne vulgaris. Skin Med. 2005 May–Jun;4(3):138–46.

Westphal JF, Macrolide-induced clinically relevant drug interactions with cytochrome P-450A (CYP) 3A4: an update focused on clarithromycin, azithromycin and dirithromycin. Br J Clin Pharmacol. 2000;50(4):285–295.

Wynn RL, Bergman SA, Meiller TF, et al. Antibiotics in treating oral-facial infections of odontogenic origins: An Update. Gen Dent 2001;49(3):238–240,242,244 passim. http://www.medscape.com/viewarticle/569858.

Zuckerman JM, Qamar F Bono BR. Antibacterial therapy and newer agents: review of macrolides (azithromycin, clarithromycin), ketolids (telithromycin) and glycylcyclines (tigecycline). Medical Clinics of North America. 2011;95(4):761–791.

ANTIFUNGALS RESOURCE

Medline Plus. Drug information. Accessed from http://www.nlm.nih.gov/medlineplus/druginformation.

ANTIVIRAL RESOURCES

Andrei G, Snoeck R. Emerging drugs for varicella-zoster virus infections. Rega Expert Opin Emerg Drugs. 2011;16(3):507–535.

Bruxelle J, Pinchinat S. Effectiveness of antiviral treatment on acute phase of herpes zoster and development of post herpetic neuralgia: Review of international publications. Med Mal Infect. 2011;42(2):53–58.

Boivin G, Jovey R, Elliott CT, Patrick DM. Management and prevention of herpes zoster: A Canadian perspective. Can J Infect Dis Med Microbiol. 2010;21(1):45–52.

Chen N, Li Q, Zhang Y, et al. Vaccination for preventing postherpetic neuralgia. Cochrane Database Syst Rev. 2011;(3):CD00779.

Johnson RW, Bouhassira D, Kassianos G, et al. The impact of herpes zoster and post-herpetic neuralgia on quality-of-life. BMC Med. 2010;8:37.

Moon JE. Herpes zoster: Medscape Reference. http://emedicine.medscape.com/article/218683-overview. Accessed April 30, 2012.

Mortensen GL. Perceptions of herpes zoster and attitudes towards zoster vaccination among 50–65-year-old Danes. Dan Med Bull. 2011;58(12):A4345.

MedLine Plus Drug informationfor acyclovir and valacyclovir: www.nlm.nih.gov/medlineplus/druginfo/medmaster/a681045.html.

www.drugs.com/acyclovir.html.
www.drugs.com/valacyclovir.html.

CYTOCHROME ENZYME SYSTEM RESOURCES

Bressler A. Principles of drug therapy for the elderly patient. Mayo Clin Proc. 2003;78:1564–1577.

Bailey DG, Dresser GK. Interactions between grapefruit juice and cardiovascular drugs. Am. J. Cardiovasc. Drugs. 2004;4:281–297.

Classification of in vivo inhibitors of CYP enzymes. http://www.fda.gov/Drugs/DevelopmentApprovalProcess/DevelopmentResources/DrugInteractionsLabeling/ucm080499.htm2. Accessed July 28, 2011.

Eberl S, Renner B, Neubert A, et al. Role of P-glycoprotein inhibition for drug interactions: evidence from in vitro and pharmacoepidemiological studies. Clin Pharmacokinet. 2007;46(12):1039–1049.

Gurley BJ, Swain A, Williams DK, Barone G, Battu SK. Gauging the clinical significance of P-glycoprotein-mediated herb-drug interactions: comparative effects of St. John's wort, Echinacea, clarithromycin, and rifampin on digoxin pharmacokinetics. Mol Nutr Food Res. 2008;52(7):772–779.

Hughes J, Crowe A. Inhibition of P-glycoprotein-mediated efflux of digoxin and its metabolites by macrolide antibiotics. J Pharmacol Sci.2010;113(4):315–24.

Kim RB. Drugs as P-glycoprotein substrates, inhibitors, and inducers. Drug Metab. Rev. 2002;34:47–54.

Mieles L, Venkataramanan R, Yokoyama I, et al. Interaction between FK506 and Clotrimazole in a liver transplant recipient. Transplantation. 1991;52:1086–1087.

Rengelshausen J, Goggelmann C, Burhenne J, et al. Contribution of increased oral bioavailability and reduced nonglomerular renal clearance of digoxin to the digoxin-clarithromycin interaction. Br J Clin Pharmacol. 2003;56(1):32–38.

US FDA. http://www.fda.gov/Drugs/default.htm.

Vasquez EM, Shin GP, Sifontis N, Benedetti E. Comcomitant Clotrimazole therapy more than doubles the relative oral bioavailability of Tacrolimus. Ther Drug Monit. 2005;27:587–591.

Wang JS, Backman JT, Wen X, Taavitsainen P, Neuvonen PJ, Kivistö KT. Fluvoxamine is a more potent inhibitor of lidocaine metabolism than ketoconazole and erythromycin in vitro. Pharmacol Toxicol. 1999 Nov;85(5):201–5.

Zhou S, Yung Chan S, Cher Goh B, Chan E, Duan W, Huang M, McLeod HL. Mechanism-based inhibition of cytochrome P450 3A4 by therapeutic drugs. Clin Pharmacokinet. 2005;44(3):279–304.

PRESCRIPTION-WRITING RESOURCES

Materia Medica, Pharmacology, Therapeutics and Prescription Writing: www.pubmedcentral.nih.gov/articlerender.fcgi?artid=1640934.
www.americanpregnancy.org/pregnancyhealth/fdadrugratings.html.
www.mrm.uci.edu/DEADrugSchedules.doc.
www.perinatology.com/exposures/Drugs/FDACategories.htm.
www.usdoj.gov/dea/pubs/csa.html.

MEDICAL EMERGENCIES RESOURCES

Atkin, PA. Management of medical emergencies: For the dental team. British Dent J 2006;200(9):532.

Bochner BS, Lichenstein LM. Anaphylaxis. N Eng J Med 1991;324:1785–1790.

Boyce JA, Assa'ad A, Burks AW, et al. Guidelines for the diagnosis and management of food allergy in the US: Summary of the NIAID-Sponsored expert panel. J Allergy Clin Immunol Dec 2010;1105–1116.

Brackenridge A, Wallbank H, Lawrenson RA, Russell-Jones D. Emergency management of diabetes and hypoglycaemia. Emerg Med J 2006;23:183–185. doi:10.1136/emj.2005.026252.

DeShazo RD, et al. Allergic reactions to drugs and biological agents. JAMA 1997; 278:1895–1906.

Fenton AM, et al. Vasovagal syncope. Ann Intern Med November 7, 2000;133:714–725.

Field JM, et al. 2010 American Heart Association guidelines for cardiopulmonary resuscitation and emergency cardiovascular care. Circulation. 2010;122[suppl 3]:S640-S656.

Garza AG, Gratton MC, Salomone JA, et al. Improved patients survival using a modified resuscitation protocol for out-of- hospital cardiac arrest. Circulation. 2009;119:2597–2605.

Goldstein DS, Spanarkel M, Pitterman A, Toltzis R, Gratz E, Epstein S, et al. Circulatory control mechanisms in vasodepressor syncope. Am Heart J 1982;104:1071–1075.

Hass, DA. Management of medical emergencies in the dental office: conditions in each country, the extent of treatment by the dentist. Anesth Prog 2006 Spring;53(1):20–24.

Huang F, Chawla K, Jarvinen KM, Nowak-Wegrzyn A. Anaphylaxis in a New York City pediatric emergency department: triggers, treatments, and outcomes. J Allergy Clin Immunol 2012;129:162–168.e3.

Joint Committee on Allergy, Asthma and Immunology. Practice parameters: The investigation and management of anaphylaxis. J Allerg Clin Immunol 1998;101(6):S465–S528.

Kapoor WN. Syncope. N Engl J Med December 21, 2000;343:1856–1862.

Lott C, Hennes HJ, Dick W. Stroke, A medical emergency. J Accid Emerg Med 1999;16(1):2–7.

Low PA, Opfer-Geheking TL, McPhee BR, et al. Prospective evaluation of clinical characteristics of orthostatic hypotension. Mayo Clin Proc 1995;70(7):617–622.

Mackenzie R, Sutcliff RC. Immediate assessment and management of acute medical emergencies. J Royal Army Med Corps 2004;150,3(SUPP/2):107–118.

Malamed, SF. Managing medical emergencies. J Am Dent Assoc 124(8):40–53.

Manolis AS, Linzer M, Salem D, Estes NA III. Syncope: current diagnostic evaluation and management. Ann Intern Med 1990;112:850–863.

Mattu, A. The 2010 AHA Guidelines: The 4 Cs of cardiac arrest care. Circulation. 2010;122:S640–S656.

Sclater A, Alagiakrishnan K. Orthostatic hypotension. A primary care primer for assessment and treatment. Geriatrics 2004;59(Aug):22–27.

Simons FER, Ardusso LRF, Bilo MB, et al. World Allergy Organization guidelines for the assessment and management of anaphylaxis. J Allergy Clin Immunol 2011;127:593.e22.

Simons FER, et al. World Allergy Organization guidelines for anaphylaxis management. Curr Opin Allergy Clin Immunol. 2012;12(4):389–399.

Toback SL. Medical emergency preparedness in office practice. Am Fam Phys 2007;75:1679–1684, 1686.

CONSCIOUS SEDATION RESOURCES

ADA.org. ADA Statement on The Use of Conscious Sedation, Deep Sedation and General Anesthesia in Dentistry. J Am Dent Assoc 2002;133;364–365. www.ada.org/prof/resources/positions/statements/useof.asp.

ADA Council on Scientific Affairs: The American Dental Association's Guidelines for the Use of Conscious Sedation, Deep Sedation and General Anesthesia for Dentists. jada.ada.org/cgi/reprint/133/3/364.pdf.

Aldrete JA. The post-anesthesia recovery score revisited. J Clin Anesth 1995;7:89–91.

Dental Sedation Teachers Group. Sedation in dentistry. The competent graduate. 2000.

Department of Health. Conscious Sedation in the Provision of Dental Care. Report of an Expert Group on Sedation for Dentistry. Commissioned by the Department of Health. 2003. www.dh.gov.uk.

Society for the Advancement of Anaesthesia in Dentistry. Standards for conscious sedation. Report of an Expert Working Group Convened by the Society for the Advancement of Anaesthesia in Dentistry. October 2000.

Society for the Advancement of Anaesthesia in Dentistry and Dental Sedation Teachers Group. Conscious sedation. A referral guide for dental practitioners. September 2001.

White PF, Song D. New criteria for fast-tracking after outpatient anesthesia: A comparison with the modified Aldrete's Scoring System. Anesth Analg 1999;88:1069–1072.

TOP 150 DRUGS RESOURCES

ADA/PDR Guide to Dental Therapeutics, Fourth Edition. American Dental Association, 2006.

http://www.rxlist.com.

http://www.drugs.com.

ANEMIA RESOURCES

Anderson GJ, Frazer DM, McLaren GD. Iron absorption and metabolism. Curr Opin Gastroenterol. 2009;25:129–135.

Benjamin LJ, Swinson GI, Nagel RL. Sickle cell anemia day hospital: an approach for the management of uncomplicated painful crises. Blood 2000;95:1130–1136.

Breymann C. Iron deficiency and anemia in pregnancy: modern aspects of diagnosis and therapy. Blood Cells, Molecules, and Diseases. Nov/Dec 2002.

Clark SF. Iron deficiency anemia: diagnosis and management. Curr Opin Gastroenterol. 2009;25:122–128.

Fleming RE, Bacon BR. Orchestration of iron hemostasis. N Engl J Med. 2005;352:1741–1744.

MedlinePlus. Sickle cell anemia. www.nlm.nih.gov/medlineplus/sicklecellanemia .html.

MedlinePlus. Thalassemia. www.nlm.nih.gov/medlineplus/thalassemia.html.

Nemeth E. Iron regulation and erythropoiesis. Curr Opin Hematol. 2008;15:169–175.

WHO Scientific Group on Nutritional Anaemias. Nutritional anaemias. Report of a WHO Scientific Group (meeting held in Geneva from March 13–17, 1967). World Health Organization. Geneva, 1968.

POLYCYTHEMIA RESOURCES

Anía B, Suman V, Sobell J, Codd M, Silverstein M, Melton L. Trends in the incidence of polycythemia vera among Olmsted County, Minnesota residents, 1935–1989. Am J Hematol 1994;47(2):89–93. PMID 8092146.

Berlin NI. Diagnosis and classification of polycythemias. Semin Hematol 1975;12:339.

Fjellner B, Hägermark O. Pruritus in polycythemia vera: treatment with aspirin and possibility of platelet involvement. Acta Derm Venereol 1979;59(6):505–512. PMID 94209.

Passamonti F, Malabarba L, Orlandi E, Baratè C, Canevari A, Brusamolino E, Bonfichi M, Arcaini L, Caberlon S, Pascutto C, Lazzarino M. Polycythemia vera in young patients: a study on the long-term risk of thrombosis, myelofibrosis and leukemia. Haematologica 2003;88(1):13–8. PMID 12551821.

Torgano G, Mandelli C, Massaro P, Abbiati C, Ponzetto A, Bertinieri G, Bogetto S, Terruzzi E, de Franchis R. Gastroduodenal lesions in polycythaemia vera: frequency and role of Helicobacter pylori. Br J Haematol 2002;117(1):198–202. PMID 11918555.

HEMOCHROMATOSIS RESOURCES

Alexander J, Kowdley KV. Hereditary hemochromatosis: genetics, pathogenesis, and clinical management. Ann Hepatol 2005;Oct–Dec;4(4):240–247.

Beutler E. Hemochromatosis: genetics and pathophysiology. Annu Rev Med 2006;57:331–347.

Kumar V, Abbas AK, Fausto N. Robbins and Cotran Pathologic Basis of Disease. 7th ed. St. Louis: W.B. Saunders; 2005:908–910, 915–917.

Olynyk JK, et al. A population-based study of the clinical expression of the hemochromatosis gene. N Engl J Med 1999 September;341(10):75. PMID 10471457.

BLEEDING DISORDERS RESOURCES

Alexander JH, Becker RC, Bhatt DL, et al. Apixaban, an oral, direct, selective factor Xa inhibitor, in combination with antiplatelet therapy after acute coronary syndrome: results of the Apixaban for Prevention of Acute Ischemic and Safety Events (APPRAISE) trial. Circulation 2009;119:2877–2885.

Ball JH. Management of the anticoagulated dental patient. Compend Contin Educ Dent 1996;17:1100–1102,1104,1106 passim.

Blinder D, Manor Y, Martinowitz U, Taicher S, Hashomer T. Dental extractions in patients maintained on continued oral anticoagulant: comparision of local hemostatic modalities. Oral Surg Oral Med Oral Pathol Oral Radiol Endod 1999;88:137–140.

Connolly SJ, Eikelboom J, Joyner C, et al. Apixaban in patients with atrial fibrillation. N Engl J Med 2011;364:806–817.

Connolly SJ, Ezekowitz MD, Yusuf S, et al. Dabigatran versus warfarin in patients with atrial fibrillation. N Engl J Med 2009;361:1139–1151.

Connolly, SJ, et al. Dabigatran versus warfarin in patients with atrial fibrillation. N Engl J Med 2009;361:1139–1151.

Crowther MA, Donovan D, Harrison L, McGinnis J, Ginsberg J. Low dose oral vitamin K reverses over-anticoagulation due to warfarin. Thromb Haemost 1998;79:1116–1118.

Devani P, Lavery KM, Howell CJ. Dental extractions in patients on warfarin: is alteration of anticoagulant regime necessary? Br J Oral Maxillofac Surg 1998;36:107–111.

Eerenberg ES, Kamphuisen PW, Sijpkens MK, Meijers JC, Buller HR, Levi M. Reversal of rivaroxaban and dabigatran by prothrombin complex concentrate: a randomized, placebo-controlled, crossover study in healthy subjects. Circulation 2011;124:1573–1579.

Eisert WG, Hauel N, Stangier J, Wienen W, Clemens A, van Ryn J. Dabigatran: an oral novel potent reversible nonpeptide inhibitor of thrombin. Arterioscler Thromb Vasc Biol 2010;30:1885–1889.

Ezekowitz MD, et al. Rationale and design of RE-LY: randomized evaluation of long-term anticoagulation therapy, warfarin, compared with dabigatran. American Heart Journal. 2009;157:805–810.

Ferreira J, et al. Dabigatran compared with warfarin in patients with atrial fibrillation and symptomatic heart failure: A Subgroup Analysis Of the RE-LY Trial. AHA 2011 abstract.

Forbes CD, Barr RD, Reid G, et al. Tranexamic acid in control of haemorrhage after dental extraction in haemophilia and Christmas disease. BMJ 1972;2:311–313.

Gasper R, Brenner B, Ardekian L, Peled M, Laufer D. Use of tranexamic acid mouthwash to prevent postoperative bleeding in oral surgery patients on anticoagulant medication. Quintessence Int 1997;28:375–379.

Gibson CM, Mega JL, Burton P, et al. Rationale and design of the Anti-Xa therapy to lower cardiovascular events in addition to standard therapy in subjects with acute coronary syndrome-thrombolysis in myocardial infarction 51 (ATLAS-ACS 2 TIMI 51) trial: a randomized, double-blind, placebo-controlled study to evaluate the efficacy and safety of rivaroxaban in subjects with acute coronary syndrome. Am Heart J 2011;161:815–821.e6.

Granger CB, Alexander JH, McMurray JJV, et al., for the ARISTOTLE Committees and Investigators. Apixaban versus warfarin in patients with atrial fibrillation. N Engl J Med 2011;365:981–92.

Hamm CW, Bassand JP, Agewall S, et al. ESC guidelines for the management of acute coronary syndromes in patients presenting without persistent ST-segment elevation: The Task Force for the management of acute coronary syndromes (ACS) in patients presenting without persistent ST-segment elevation of the European Society of Cardiology (ESC). Eur Heart J 2011;32:2999–3054.

Healey, JS, et al. The risk of peri-operative bleeding with warfarin compared to two doses of dabigatran: results from the RE-LY Trial. AHA 2011 abstract.

Hirsh J, Dalen J, Anderson DR, et al. Oral anticoagulants: mechanism of action, clinical effectiveness, and optimal therapeutic range. Chest 2001;119(suppl 1):85–215.

Hohnloser SH, Oldgren J, Yang S, et al. Myocardial ischemic events in patients with atrial fibrillation treated with dabigatran or warfarin in the RE-LY (Randomized Evaluation of Long-Term Anticoagulatoin Therapy) Trial. Circulation 2012;125:669–76.

Hylek EM, Heiman H, Skates SJ, Sheehan MA, Singer DE. Acetaminophen and other risk factors for excessive warfarin anticoagulation. JAMA 1998;279:657–662.

Jaffer A, Brotman D, Chukwumerije N. When patients on warfarin need surgery. Cleveland Clinic J of Med 2003;70(11):973–984.

Jiang J, Hu Y, Zhang J, et al. Safety, pharmacokinetics and pharmacodynamics of single doses of rivaroxaban—an oral, direct factor Xa inhibitor—in elderly Chinese subjects. Thromb Haemost 2010;103:234–241.

Johnson-Leong C, Rada RE. The use of low-molecular-weight-heparins in outpatient oral surgery for patients receiving anticoagulation therapy. JADA 2002;1083–1087.

Lack of a scientific basis for routine discontinuation of oral anticoagulation therapy before dental treatment. JADA 134:Nov 2003. www.dental.ufl.edu:1180/Offices/Endo/S04_07.doc.

Lip, GY, et al. Comparative validation of a novel risk score for predicting bleeding risk in anticoagulated patients with atrial fibrillation. J Am Coll Cardiol. 2011;57:173–80.

Martinowitz U, Sponitz WD. Fibrin tissue adhesives. Thromb Haemost 1997;78:661–666.

Mega JL, Braunwald E, Mohanavelu S, et al. Rivaroxaban versus placebo in patients with acute coronary syndromes (ATLAS ACSTIMI 46): a randomised, double-blind, phase II trial. Lancet 2009;374:29–38.

Mega JL, Braunwald E, Wiviott SD, et al. Rivaroxaban in patients with a recent acute coronary syndrome. N Engl J Med 2012;366:9–19.

Nagarakanti R, Ezekowitz MD, Parcham-Azad K, et al. Long-term open label extension of the prevention of embolic and thrombotic events on dabigatran in atrial fibrillation (PETRO-Ex study). Circulation 2008;118:18.

Patel MR, Mahaffey KW, Garg J, et al. Rivaroxaban versus warfarin in nonvalvular atrial fibrillation. N Engl J Med 2011;365:883–889.

Patrono C, Andreotti F, Arnesen H, et al. Antiplatelet agents for the treatment and prevention of atherothrombosis. Eur Heart J 2011;32:2922–2932.

Raffaele De Caterina RD, et al. New oral anticoagulants in atrial fibrillation and acute coronary syndromes ESC working group on thrombosis. Task Force on Anticoagulants in Heart Disease Position Paper. J Am Coll Cardiol. 2012;59(16):1413–1425.

Ruff CT, Giugliano RP, Antman EM, et al. Evaluation of the novel factor Xa inhibitor edoxaban compared with warfarin in patients with atrial fibrillation: design and rationale for the Effective aNticoaGulation with factor xA next GEneration in Atrial Fibrillation-Thrombolysis In Myocardial Infarction study 48 (ENGAGE AF-TIMI 48). Am Heart J 2010;160:635–641.

Stangier J, Eriksson BI, Dahl OE, et al. Pharmacokinetic profile of the oral direct thrombin inhibitor dabigatran etexilate in healthy volunteers and patients undergoing total hip replacement. J Clin Pharmacol 2005;45:555–563.

Steg PG, Mehta SR, Jukema JW, et al. RUBY-1: a randomized, double-blind, placebo-controlled trial of the safety and tolerability of the novel oral factor Xa inhibitor darexaban (YM150) following acute coronary syndrome. Eur Heart J 2011;32:2541–54.

Sindet-Pedersen S, Stenbjerg S. Effect of local antifibrinolytic treatment with tranexamic acid in hemophiliacs undergoing oral surgery. J Oral Maxillofac Surg 1986;44:703–707.

Sindet-Pedersen S. Distribution of tranexamic acid to plasma and saliva after oral admini-stration and mouth rinsing: a pharmacokinetic study. J Clin Pharmacol 1987;27:1005–1008.

Sindet-Pedersen S, Ramstrom G, Bernvil S, Blomback M. Hemostatic effect of tranexamic acid mouthwash in anticoagulant-treated patients undergoing oral surgery. N Engl J Med 1989;320:840–843.

Wallentin L, Yusuf S, Ezekowitz MD, et al. Efficacy and safety of dabigatran compared with warfarin at different levels of international normalised ratio control for stroke prevention in atrial fibrillation: an analysis of the RE-LY trial. Lancet 2010;376: 975–83.

Walsh PN, Rizza CR, Matthews JM, et al. Epsilon-aminocaproic acid therapy for dental extractions in haemophilia and Christmas disease: a double blind controlled trial. Br J Haematol 1971;20:463–475.

Warketin TE, Levine MN, Hirsh J, et al. Heparin-induced thrombocytopenia in patients treated with low-molecular-weight heparin or unfractionated heparin. N Engl J Med 1995;332:1330–1335.

Weibert RT, Le DT, Kayser SR, Rapaport SI. Correction of excessive anticoagulation with low dose oral vitamin K1. Ann Intern Med 1997;126:959–962.

Weitz JI. Factor Xa and thrombin as targets for new oral anticoagulants. Thromb Res 2011;127 Suppl 2:S5–12.

Weitz JI, Connolly SJ, Patel I, et al. Randomised, parallel-group, multicentre, multi-national phase 2 study comparing edoxaban, an oral factor Xa inhibitor, with warfarin for stroke prevention in patients with atrial fibrillation. Thromb Haemost 2010;104:633–41.

Wells PS, Holbrook AM, Crowther NR, Hirsh J. Interactions of warfarin with drugs and food. Ann Intern Med 1994;121:676–683.

CIRRHOSIS AND DECOMPENSATION COAGULOPATHY RESOURCES

Amarapurkar PD, Amarapurkar DN. Management of coagulopathy in patients with decompensated liver cirrhosis. International Journal of HepatologyVolume 2011 (2011), Article ID 695470. doi:10.4061/2011/695470.

Boks AL, Brommer EJ, Schalm SW, van Vliet HH. Hemostasis and fibrinolysis in severe liver failure and their relation to hemorrhage. Hepatology. 1986;(1):79–86.

Caldwell SH, Hoffman M, Lisman T, et al. Coagulation disorder and heamostasis in liver disease: pathophysiology and critical assessment of current management. Hepatology. 2006;44:1039–1046.

Ferro D, Celestini A, Violi F. Hyperfibrinolysis in liver disease. Clin Liver Dis. 2009;13:21.

Hugenholtz GGC, Porte RJ, Lisman T. The platelet and platelet function testing in liver disease. Clinics in Liver Disease. 2009;13(1):11–20.

Lisman T, Bongers T, Adelmeijer J, et al. Elevated levels of von Willebrand factor in cirrhosis support platelet adhesion despite reduced functional capacity. Hepatology. 2006;44(1)53–61.

Lisman T, Caldwell SH, Burroughs AK, et al. Hemostasis and thrombosis in patients with liver disease: the ups and downs. Journal of Hepatology. 2010;53(2)362–371.

Lisman T, Porte RJ. Rebalanced hemostasis in patients with liver disease: evidence and clinical consequences. Blood. 2010;116(6)878–885.

Monroe DM, Hoffman M. The coagulation cascade in cirrhosis. Clin Liver Dis 2009;13:1.

Murad MH, Stubbs JR, Gandhi MJ, et al. The effects of plasma transfusion on the morbidity and mortality: a systematic review and meta-analysis. Transfusion. 2010;50:1370.

Ng VL. Liver disease, coagulation testing and heamostasis. Clinics in Laboratory Medicine. 2009;29(2):265–282.

Senzolo M, Cholongitas E, Thalheimer U, et al. Heparin-like effect in liver disease and liver transplantation. Clinics in Liver Disease. 2009;13(1):43–53.

Smalberg JH, Leebeek FWG. Superimposed coagulopathic conditions in cirrhosis: infection and endogenous heparinoids, renal failure, and endothelial dysfunction. Clinics in Liver Disease. 2009;13(1)33–42.

Stanca CM, Montazem AH, Lawal A, et al. Intranasal desmopressin versus blood transfusion in cirrhotic patients with coagulopathy undergoing dental extraction: a randomized controlled trial. J Oral Maxillofac Surg 2010;68:138.

Stravitz RT, Lisman T, Luketic VA, et al. Minimal effects of acute liver injury/acute liver failure on hemostasis as assessed by thromboelastography. J Hepatol 2012;56:129.

Tripodi A, Anstee QM, Sogaard KK, et al. Hypercoagulability in cirrhosis: causes and consequences. J Thromb Haemost 2011;9:1713.

Tripodi A, Chantarangkul V, Primignani M, et al. The international normalized ratio calibrated for cirrhosis (INRlier) normalizes prothrombin time results for model for end-stage liver disease calculation. Hepatology. 2007;46(2):520–527.

Tripodi A, Primignani M, Lemma L, et al. Detection of the imbalance of procoagulant versus anticoagulant factors in cirrhosis by a simple laboratory method. Hepatology. 2010;52(1)249–255.

Tripodi A, Primignani M, Mannucci PM. Abnormalities of hemostasis and bleeding in chronic liver disease: the paradigm is challenged. Internal and Emergency Medicine. 2010;5(1):7–12.

Tripodi A, Salerno F, Chantarangkul V, et al. Evidence of normal thrombin generation in cirrhosis despite abnormal conventional coagulation tests. Hepatology. 2005;41(3):553–558.

Tripodi A. Mannucci PM. The coagulopathy of chronic liver disease. N Engl J Med 2011;365:147.

Tripodi A. Tests of coagulation in liver disease. Clinics in Liver Disease. 2009;13(1):55–61.

RHEUMATIC FEVER, BACTERIAL ENDOCARDITIS, AND PREMEDICATION RESOURCES

ADA, American Academy of Orthopaedic Surgeons. Advisory statement. Antibiotic prophylaxis for dental patients with total joint replacements. J Am Dent Assoc 1997;128(7):1004–1008.

ADA, American Academy of Orthopaedic Surgeons. Advisory statement. Antibiotic prophylaxis for dental patients with total joint replacement. J Am Dent Assoc 2003;134(7):895–859.

AHA. Prevention of Infective endocarditis. Guidelines from the American Heart Association. A Guideline from the American Heart Association Rheumatic Fever, Endocarditis, and Kaasaki Disease Committee, Council on Cardiovascular Disease in the Young, and the council on Clinical Cardiology, Council on Cardiovascular Surgery and Anesthesia, and the Quality of Care and Outcomes Research Interdisciplinary Working Group. Circulation 2007. doi:10.1161/CIRCULATIONAHA.106.183095.

Dental premedication protocols for patients with knee and hip prostheses. NY State Dent J. 2006;72(3):20–25. PMID 16774168. ime.healthpartners.com/IME/Menu/0,1637,6267,00.html

Ferrieri P. Proceedings of the Jones criteria workshop. Circulation 2002;106:2521–2523.

Jones TD. The diagnosis of rheumatic fever. JAMA 1944;126:481–484.

HYPERTENSION/TIA/CVA/ANGINA/MI/KIDNEY DISEASE RESOURCES

AHA. Clinical investigation and reports: Is pulse pressure useful in predicting risk for coronary heart disease? Circulation 1999;100:354–360. 1999 American Heart Association, Inc.

Albers GW. A review of published TIA treatment recommendations. Albers Neurol 2004;62:S26–S28.

Barnett H, Burrill P, Iheanacho I. Don't use aspirin for primary prevention of cardiovascular disease. BMJ 2010;340:c1805.

Bertges DJ, Muluk V, Whittle J, Kelley M, MacPherson DS, Muluk SC. Relevance of carotid stenosis progression as a predictor of ischemic neurological outcomes. Arch Intern Med 2003;163:2285–2289.

Chobanian AV, Bakris GL, Black HR, et al., and the National High Blood Pressure Education Program Coordinating Committee. The Seventh Report of the Joint National Committee on Prevention, Detection, Evaluation, and Treatment of High Blood Pressure (JNC7). The JNC 7 Report. JAMA 2003;289. doi:10.1001/jama.289.19.2560.

Chobanian AV, Bakris GL, Black HR, et al., and the National High Blood Pressure Education Program Coordinating Committee. The Seventh Report of the Joint National Committee on Prevention, Detection, Evaluation, and Treatment of High Blood Pressure (JNC7). The JNC 7 Report. JAMA 2003;289. doi:10.1001/jama.289.19.2560.

Cushman WC, Ford CE, Cutler JA, Margolis KL, Davis BR, Grimm RH, et al. Success and predictors of blood pressure control in diverse North American settings: the antihypertensive and lipid-lowering treatment to prevent heart attack trial (ALLHAT). J Clin Hypertens (Greenwich) 2002;4:393–405.

Delyani J. Mineralocorticoid receptor antagonists: The evolution of utility and pharmacology. Kidney International 2000;57:1408–1411.

European Society of Cardiology. ESC Guidelines for the diagnosis and treatment of acute and chronic heart failure 2012. Acessed from http://www.escardio.org/guidelines-surveys/esc-guidelines/GuidelinesDocuments/Guidelines-Acute%20and%20Chronic-HF-FT.pdf.

Ezzati M, Lopez AD, Rodgers A, Vander Hoom S, Murray CJ. Selected major risk factors and global and regional burden of disease. Lancet 2002;360:1347–1360.

Gray HH, Henderson RA, de Belder MA, et al. Early management of unstable angina and non-ST-segment elevation myocardial infarction: summary of NICE guidance. Heart 2010;96:1662–1668.

Gumieniak O, Williams GH. Current Hypertension Reports. 2004; 6(4):279–287.

Henderson RA, O'Flynn N. Management of stable angina: Summary of NICE guidance. Heart 2012;98(6):500–507.

Hlatky MA, Boothroyd DB, Bravata DM, et al. Coronary artery bypass surgery compared with percutaneous coronary interventions for multivessel disease: a collaborative analysis of individual patient data from ten randomised trials. Lancet 2009;373:1190–1197.

Hueb W, Lopes N, Gersh BJ, et al. Ten-year follow-up survival of the medicine, angioplasty, or surgery study (MASS II). Circulation 2010;122:949–957.

Janket SJ, Baird AE, Chuang SK, Jones JA. Meta-analysis of periodontal disease and risk of coronary heart disease and stroke. Oral Surg Oral Med Oral Pathol Oral Radiol Endod 2003;95(5):559–569. PMID 12738947.

Josephson SA, Bryant SO, Mak HK, et al. Clinical practice. Transient ischemic attack. N Engl J Med. 2002 Nov 21;347(21):1687–1692. www.postgradmed.com/issues/2005/01_05/comm_gladstone.shtml.

Kappetein AP, Feldman TE, Mack MJ, et al. Comparison of coronary bypass surgery with drug-eluting stenting for the treatment of left main and/or three-vessel disease: three-year follow-up of the SYNTAX trial. Eur Heart J 2011;32:2125–34.

Lee HK, Kim YJ, Jeong JU, et al. Desmopressin improves platelet dysfunction measured by in vitro closure time in uremic patients. Nephron Clin Pract 2010;114:c248.

Levey AS, Bosch JP, Lewis JB, et al. A more accurate method to estimate glomerular filtration rate from serum creatinine: A new prediction equation, Ann Int Med 1999;130:461–470.

Linthorst GE, Avis HJ, Levi M. Uremic thrombocytopathy is not about urea. J Am Soc Nephrol 2010;21:753.

London G, Coyne D, Hruska K, Malluche HH, Martin KJ. The new kidney disease: improving global outcomes (KDIGO) guidelines—expert clinical focus on bone and vascular calcification. Clin Nephrol. Dec 2010;74(6):423–32.

McMurray JV, Adamopoulos S, Anker SD, et al. ESC Guidelines for the diagnosis and treatment of acute and chronic heart failure 2012. European Heart Journal. 2012;33:1787–1847.

Mosca L, Banka CL, Benjamin EJ, et al. Evidence-based guidelines for cardiovascular disease prevention in women: 2007 Update. doi: 10.1161/CIRCULATION-AHA.107.181546

Mosca L, Benjamin EJ, Berra K, Bezanson JL, Dolor RJ, Lloyd-Jones DM, et al. Effectiveness-based guidelines for the prevention of cardiovascular disease in women—2011 update: a guideline from the American Heart Association. J Am Coll Cardiol. 2011;57:1404–1423.

Neal B, MacMahon S, Chapman N. Effects of ACE inhibitors, calcium antagonists, and other blood-pressure-lowering drugs: results of prospectively designed overviews of randomised trials. Blood Pressure Lowering Treatment Trialists' Collaboration. Lancet 2000;356:1955–1964.

Pearson TA, Mensah GA, Alexander RW, et al. Markers of inflammation and cardiovascular disease: application to clinical and public health practice: A statement for healthcare professionals from the Centers for Disease Control and Prevention and the American Heart Association. Circulation 2003;107(3):499–511. PMID 12551878.

Peralta CA, Norris KC, Li S, et al. Blood pressure components and end-stage renal disease in persons with chronic kidney disease: The Kidney Early Evaluation Program (KEEP). Arch Intern Med. Jan 9 2012;172(1):41–47.

Plantinga L, Grubbs V, Sarkar U, et al. Nonsteroidal Anti-Inflammatory drug use among persons with chronic kidney disease in the United States. Ann Fam Med. 2011;9(5):423–430.

Pihlstrom BL, Michalowicz BS, Johnson NW. Periodontal diseases. Lancet 2005; 366(9499):1809–1820. PMID 16298220.

Scannapieco FA, Bush RB, Paju S. Associations between periodontal disease and risk for atherosclerosis, cardiovascular disease, and stroke. A systematic review. Ann Periodontol 2003;8(1):38–53. PMID 14971247.

Shaw LJ, Berman DS, Maron DJ, et al. Optimal medical therapy with or without percutaneous coronary intervention to reduce ischemic burden: results from the Clinical

Outcomes Utilizing Revascularization and Aggressive Drug Evaluation (COURAGE) trial nuclear substudy. Circulation 2008;117:1283–1291.

Skinner JS, Smeeth L, Kendall JM, et al. NICE guidance. Chest pain of recent onset: assessment and diagnosis of recent onset chest pain or discomfort of suspected cardiac origin. Heart 2010;96:974–978.

Spahr A, Klein E, Khuseyinova N, et al. Periodontal infections and coronary heart disease: role of periodontal bacteria and importance of total pathogen burden in the coronary event and periodontal disease (CORODONT) study. Arch Intern Med 2006;166(5):554–559. PMID 16534043.

Stone GW, Rizvi A, Newman W, et al. Everolimus-Eluting versus paclitaxel-eluting stents in coronary artery disease. New Engl J Med 2010;362:1663–74.

Tangri N, Stevens LA, Griffith J, Tighiouart H, Djurdjev O, Naimark D, et al. A predictive model for progression of chronic kidney disease to kidney failure. JAMA. Apr 20 2011;305(15):1553–1559.

Tardif JC, Ponikowski P, Kahan T, et al. Efficacy of the I(f) current inhibitor ivabradine in patients with chronic stable angina receiving beta-blocker therapy: a four-month, randomized, placebo-controlled trial. Eur Heart J 2009;30:540–548.

Task Force on Myocardial Revascularization of the European Society of Cardiology (ESC) and the European Association for Cardio-Thoracic Surgery (EACTS). Guidelines on myocardial revascularization. Eur Heart J 2010;31:2501–2555.

Tucker ME. Medscape medical news: new diabetes guidelines ease systolic blood pressure target. Dec 20, 2012.

Vegter S, Perna A, Postma MJ, et al. Sodium intake, ACE inhibition, and progression to ESRD. J Am Soc Nephrol. 2012;23(1):165–173.

Wilson AM, Ryan MC, Boyle AJ. The novel role of C-reactive protein in cardiovascular disease: risk marker or pathogen. Int J Cardiol 2006;106(3):291–297. PMID 16337036.

Wright RS, Anderson JL, Adams CD, Bridges CR, Casey DE Jr, Ettinger SM, et al. 2011 ACCF/AHA Focused update of the guidelines for the management of patients with unstable angina/non-ST-elevation myocardial infarction (Updating the 2007 Guideline): a report of the American College of Cardiology Foundation/American Heart Association Task Force on Practice Guidelines. Circulation. March 28, 2011.

ATRIAL FIBRILLATION RESOURCES

ACC/AHA/ESC. Guidelines for the Management of Patients with Atrial Fibrillation. www.americanheart.org/downloadable/heart/222_ja20017993p_1.pdf.

Levy S. Epidemiology and classification of atrial fibrillation. J Cardiovasc Electrophysiol 1998;9(8 Suppl):S78–S82. PMID 9727680.

Levy S. Classification system of atrial fibrillation. Curr Opin Cardiol 2000;15(1):54–57. PMID 10666661.

Prystowsky EN. Management of atrial fibrillation: therapeutic options and clinical decisions. Am J Cardiol 2000;85(10A):3D–11D.

ASTHMA RESOURCES

Jenkins C, Costello J, Hodge L. Systematic review of the prevalence of aspirin-induced asthma and its implications for clinical practice. BMJ 2004;328:434.

Leggett JJ, Johnson BT, Mills M, Gamble J, Heaney LG. Prevalence of gastroesophageal reflux in difficult asthma. Chest 2005;127(4):1227–1231.

Maddox L, Schwartz DA. The pathophysiology of asthma. Annu Rev Med 2002;53:477–498.

National Asthma Education and Prevention Program. Expert Panel Report: Guidelines for the Diagnosis and Management of Asthma. National Institute of Health, Bethesda, MD 1997;97–4051. http://www.nih.gov/guidelines/asthma/asthgdln.pdf.

National Heart, Lung and Blood Institute. Diseases and Conditions Index. http://www.nhlbi. nih.gov/health/dci/Diseases/Asthma/Asthma_Treatments.html

Rodrigo GJ, Rodrigo C, Hall JB. Acute asthma in adults: a review. Chest 2004; 125(3):1081–1102.

http://www.webmd.com/asthma/guide/lung-function-tests.

SMOKING CESSATION RESOURCES

CDC. How tobacco smoke causes disease: the biology and behavioral basis for smoking-attributable disease: a report of the Surgeon General. Atlanta, GA: US Department of Health and Human Services, CDC; 2010. Available at http://www.surgeongeneral.gov/library/tobaccosmoke/report/full_report.pdf.

CDC. Smoking and tobacco use: trends in current cigarette smoking among high school students and adults, United States, 1965–2010. Atlanta, GA: US Department of Health and Human Services, CDC; 2011. Available at http://www.cdc.gov/tobacco/data_statistics/tables/trends/cig_smoking/index.htm.

CDC. Smoking-attributable mortality, years of potential life lost, and productivity losses—United States, 2000–2004. MMWR 2008;57:1226–8.

Community Guide Task Force on Community Preventive Services. The guide to community preventive services: what works to promote health. Part 1: changing risk behaviors and addressing environmental challenges. Tobacco[Chapter 1]. New York, NY: Oxford University Press; 2005. Available at http://www.thecommunityguide.org/tobacco/tobacco.pdf.

Curry SJ, Sporer AK, Pugach O, Campbell RT, Emery S. Use of tobacco cessation treatments among young adult smokers: 2005 National Health Interview Survey. Am J Public Health 2007;97:1464–9.

Fiore MC, Jaen CR, Baker TB, et al. Treating tobacco use and dependence: 2008 update. Clinical practice guideline. Rockville, MD: US Department of Health and Human Services, Public Health Service; 2008. Available at http://www.surgeongeneral.gov/tobacco/treating_tobacco_use08.pdf.

http://www.fda.gov/downloads/advisorycommittees/committeesmeetingmaterials/tobaccoproductsscientificadvisorycommittee/ucm269697.pdf.

Million Hearts. millionhearts.hhs.gov.

National Institute on Drug Abuse. Research report series: tobacco addiction. Bethesda MD: National Institutes of Health, National Institute on Drug Abuse; 2009. Available at http://drugabuse.gov/researchreports/nicotine/addictive.html.

Shiffman S, Brockwell SE, Pillitteri JL, Gitchell JG. Use of smoking-cessation treatments in the United States. Am J Prev Med 2008;34:102–11.

The Joint Commission. http://www.jointcommission.org/tobacco_and_alcohol_measures.

COPD RESOURCES

Albert RK, Connett J, Bailey WC, et al. Azithromycin for prevention of exacerbations of COPD. N. Engl. J. Med. 2011;365(8):689–698 (2011).

Alía I, de la Cal MA, Esteban A, et al. Efficacy of corticosteroid therapy in patients with an acute exacerbation of chronic obstructive pulmonary disease receiving ventilatory support. Arch. Intern. Med. 2011;171(21):1939–1946 (2011).

Anandan C, Nurmatov U, van Schayck OC, Sheikh A. Is the prevalence of asthma declining? Systematic review of epidemiological studies. Allergy. 2010;65(2):152–167.

Barnes PJ. New therapies for asthma: is there any progress? Trends Pharmacol. Sci. 2010;31(7):335–343.

Bousquet J, Mantzouranis E, Cruz AA, et al. Uniform definition of asthma severity, control, and exacerbations: document presented for the World Health Organization Consultation on Severe Asthma. J. Allergy Clin. Immunol. 2010;126(5):926–938.

Camargo CA Jr, Gurner DM, Smithline HA, et al. A randomized placebo-controlled study of intravenous montelukast for the treatment of acute asthma. J. Allergy Clin. Immunol. 2010;125(2):374–380.

Casanova C, de Torres JP, Aguirre-Jaíme A, et al. The progression of chronic obstructive pulmonary disease is heterogeneous: the experience of the BODE cohort. Am. J. Respir. Crit. Care Med. 2011;184(9):1015–1021.

Chong J, Poole P, Leung B, Black PN. Phosphodiesterase 4 inhibitors for chronic obstructive pulmonary disease. Cochrane Database Syst. Rev. 2011;11(5):CD002309.

Corren J, Lemanske RF, Hanania NA, et al. Lebrikizumab treatment in adults with asthma. N. Engl. J. Med. 2011;365(12):1088–1098.

Criner GJ. Alternatives to lung transplantation: lung volume reduction for COPD. Clin. Chest Med. 2011;32(2);379–397.

Garcia-Aymerich J, Gómez FP, Benet M, et al.; on behalf of the PAC-COPD Study Group. Identification and prospective validation of clinically relevant chronic obstructive pulmonary disease (COPD) subtypes. Thorax. 2011;66(5):430–437.

Han MK, Agusti A, Calverley PM, et al. Chronic obstructive pulmonary disease phenotypes. The future of COPD. Am. J. Respir. Crit. Care Med. 2010;182(5);598–604.

National Institutes of Health. A–Z Index. Accessed from http://www.nhlbi.nih.gov/health/dci/Diseases/Copd/Copd_KeyPoints.html.

National Institutes of Health. What Is COPD? Accessed from http://www.nhlbi.nih.gov/health/dci/Copd/Copd_Treatments.html.

Nicolino Ambrosino N, Paggiaro P. The management of asthma and chronic obstructive pulmonary disease. Expert Rev Resp Med. 2012;6(1):117–127.

Oh CK, Geba GP, Molfino N. Investigational therapeutics targeting the IL-4/IL-13/STAT-6 pathway for the treatment of asthma. Eur. Respir. Rev. 2010;19(115):46–54.

Qaseem A, Wilt TJ, Weinberger SE, et al. Diagnosis and management of stable chronic obstructive pulmonary disease: a clinical practice guideline update from the American College of Physicians, American College of Chest Physicians, American Thoracic Society, and European Respiratory Society. Ann. Intern. Med. 2011;155(2):179–191.

Rabe KF, Wedzicha JA. Controversies in treatment of chronic obstructive pulmonary disease. Lancet. 2011;378(9795):1038–1047.

Ram FS, Rodriguez-Roisin R, Granados-Navarrete A, Garcia-Aymerich J, Barnes NC. Antibiotics for exacerbations of chronic obstructive pulmonary disease. Cochrane Database Syst. Rev. 2011;19(1):CD004403.

Soriano JB, Rodríguez-Roisin R. Chronic obstructive pulmonary disease overview: epidemiology, risk factors, and clinical presentation. Proc. Am. Thorac. Soc. 2011;8(4):363–367.

Rennard SI, et al. Reduction of exacerbations by the PDE4 inhibitor roflumilast - the importance of defining different subsets of patients with COPD. Respiratory Research 2011;12:18.

TUBERCULOSIS RESOURCES

American Thoracic Society/CDC. Infectious Diseases Society of America. Controlling tuberculosis in the United States. Am J Respir Crit Care Med 2005;172:1169–227.

American Thoracic Society/CDC. Targeted tuberculin testing and treatment of latent tuberculosis infection. Am J Respir Crit Care Med 2000;161:S221–S247. http://www.cdc.gov/nchstp/tb/.

CDC. Core curriculum on tuberculosis: what the clinician should know, 4th ed. Atlanta, GA: US Department of Health and Human Services, CDC. 2000. Available at http://www.cdc.gov/nchstp/tb/.

CDC. Update: Fatal and severe liver injuries associated with rifampin and pyrazinamide for latent tuberculosis infection, and revisions in American Thoracic Society/CDC recommendations—United States, 2001. MMWR 2001;50:733–735.

CDC. Centers for Disease Control and Prevention, Division of Tuberculosis Elimination. Core Curriculum on Tuberculosis: What the Clinician Should Know. 4th ed. (2000). Updated Aug 2003.

CDC. Morbidity and Mortality Weekly Report (MMWR)MMWR Weekly. December 9, 2011/60(48);1650–1653.

CDC. Severe isoniazid-associated liver injuries among persons being treated for latent tuberculosis infection—United States, 2004–2008. MMWR 2010;59:224–229.

CDC. Targeted tuberculin testing and treatment of latent tuberculosis infection. MMWR 2000;49(No. RR-6).

CDC. Update: adverse event data and revised American Thoracic Society/CDC recommendations against the use of rifampin and pyrazinamide for treatment of latent tuberculosis infection—United States, 2003. MMWR 2003;52:735–739.

CDC. Treatment of Tuberculosis American Thoracic Society, CDC, and Infectious Diseases Society of America. MMWR 2003;52(RR11);1–77.

CDC. CDC Issues Guidelines on Use of QuantiFERON TB Gold Test MMWR Morb Mortal Wkly Rep. 2005;54(RR-15):49–55.

Food and Drug Administration, Center for Devices and Radiological Health. QuantiFERON®-TB—P010033 [Letter]. Rockville, MD: Food and Drug Administration, 2002. http://www.fda.gov/cdrh/pdf/P010033b.pdf.

Geiter LJ, ed. Ending neglect: the elimination of tuberculosis in the United States. Institute of Medicine, Committee on Elimination of Tuberculosis in the United States. Washington, DC: National Academy Press; 2000. Available at http://www.nap.edu/catalog/9837.html.

Gostin LO. Controlling the resurgent tuberculosis epidemic: a 50 state survey of TB statutes and proposals for reform. JAMA 1993;269:255–261.

Horsburgh CR, Jr, Feldman S, Ridzon R. Practice guidelines for the treatment of tuberculosis. Clin Infect Dis. 2000;31:633–639.

Jasmer RM, Saukkonen JJ, Blumberg HM, Daley CL, Bernardo J, Vittinghoff E, King MD, Kawamura LM, Hopewell PC. Short-course rifampin and pyrazinamide compared with isoniazid for latent tuberculosis infection: a multucenter clinical trial. Short-Course Rifampin and Pyrazinamide for Tuberculosis Infection (SCRIPT) Study Investigators. Ann Intern Med 2002;137:640–647.

Mazurek GH, LoBue PA, Daley CL, et al. Comparison of a whole-blood interferon gamma assay with tuberculin skin testing for detecting latent *Mycobacterium tuberculosis* infection. JAMA 2001;286:1740–1747.

Martinson NA, Barnes GL, Moulton LH, et al. New regimens to prevent tuberculosis in adults with HIV infection. N Engl J Med 2011;365:11–20.

Saukkonen JJ, Cohn DL, Jasmer RM, et al. An official ATS statement: hepatotoxicity of antituberculosis therapy. Am J Respir Crit Care Med 2006;174:935–952.

Schechter M, Zajdenverg R, Falco G, et al. Weekly rifapentine/isoniazid or daily rifampin/pyrazinamide for latent tuberculosis in household contacts. Am J Respir Crit Care Med 2006;173:922–926.

Sterling TR, Villarino ME, Borisov AS, et al. Three months of once-weekly rifapentine and isoniazid for M. tuberculosis infection. N Engl J Med 2011;365:2155–2166.

Walley JD, Khan MR, Newell JN, Khan MH. Effectiveness of the direct observation component of DOTS for tuberculosis: a randomised controlled trial in Pakistan. Lancet 2001;357;664–669.

World Health Organization (WHO). Tuberculosis Fact sheet Number 104—Global and regional incidence. March 2006, Retrieved on October 6, 2006.

World Health Organization (WHO). What is DOTS? A guide to understanding the WHO-recommended TB control strategy known as DOTS. WHO/CDS/CPC/TB/99.270. Geneva, Switzerland: World Health Organization; 1999. http://www.who.int/gtb/dots.

HERBAL RESOURCES

ADA. Herbals May Interact With Anesthesia. 1698 JADA, Vol. 130, December 1999. Accessed from jada.ada.org/cgi/reprint/130/12/1700.pdf.

ADA Division of Communication. For the dental patient. How medications can affect your oral health. J Am Dent Assoc 2005;136;6:831. www.co-pulmonarymedicine.com/pt/re/copulmonary/fulltext.00063198-200705000-00006.htm;jsessionid=GL1D2Z0fZ.

Complementary & Alternative Medicine: Herbals, surgery, and anesthesia don't always mix. www.newsrx.com/newsletters/Pain-and-Central-Nervous-System-Week/2004-10-04.html.

ANTIRESORPTIVE AGENTS AND ARONJ RESOURCES

Aghaloo TL, Felsenfeld AL, Tetradis S. Osteonecrosis of the jaw in a patient on Denosumab. J Oral Maxillofac Surg 2010;68(5):959–963.

American Association of Oral and Maxillofacial Surgeons Position Paper on Bisphosphonate related Osteonecrosis of the Jaws, 2009 Update.

Barasch A, Cunha-Cruz J, Curro FA, et al. Risk factors for osteonecrosis of the jaws: a case-control study from the CONDOR dental PBRN. J Dent Res 2011;90(4):439–444.

Bashutski JD, Eber RM, Kinney JS, Benavides E, Maitra S, Braun TM, Giannobile WV, McCauley LK. Teriparatide and osseous regeneration in the oral cavity. N Engl J Med. 2010 Dec 16;363(25):2396-405.

Boonyapakorn T, Schirmer I, Reichart PA, Sturm I, Massenkeil G. Bisphosphonate-induced osteonecrosis of the jaws: prospective study of 80 patients with multiple myeloma and other malignancies. Oral Oncol 2008;44(9):857–869.

Cheng, ML, Gupta, V. Teriparatide—Indications beyond osteoporosis. Indian J Endocrinol Metab. 2012;16(3):343–348.

Chesnut CH III, Bell NH, Clark GS, et al. Hormone replacement therapy in post-menopausal women: urinary N-telopeptide of type I collagen monitors therapeutic effect and predicts response of bone mineral density. Am J Med. 1997 Jan;102(1):29–37.

Fleisher KE, Welch G, Kottal S, Craig RG, Saxena D, Glickman RS. Predicting risk for bisphosphonate-related osteonecrosis of the jaws: CTX versus radiographic markers. Oral Surg Oral Med Oral Pathol Oral Radiol Endod. 2010 Oct;110(4):509–516.

Harper RP, Fung E. Resolution of bisphosphonate-associated osteonecrosis of the mandible: possible application for intermittent low-dose parathyroid hormone [rhPTH(1–34)] (published correction appears in J Oral Maxillofac Surg 2007; 65[5]:1059. Dosage error in article text). J Oral Maxillofac Surg 2007;65(3):573–580.

Hellstein JW, Adler A, Roberts B, et al. Managing the care of patients receiving antiresorptive therapy for prevention and treatment of osteoporosis. Executive summary of recommendations from the American Dental Association Council on Scientific Affairs. JADA. 2011;142(11):1243–1251.

Lazarovici TS, Mesilaty-Gross S, Vered I, et al. Serologic bone markers for predicting development of osteonecrosis of the jaw in patients receiving bisphosphonates. J Oral Maxillofac Surg 2010;68(9):2241–2247.

Lee JJ, Cheng SJ, Jeng JH, et al. Successful treatment of advanced bisphosphonate-related osteonecrosis of the mandible with adjunctive teriparatide therapy. Head Neck 2011;33(9):1366–1371.

Liu L, Igarashi K, Haruyama N, Saeki S, Shinoda H, Mitani H. Effects of local administration of clodronate on orthodontic tooth movement and root resorption in rats. Eur J Orthod 2004;26(5):469–473.

Lo JC, O'Ryan FS, Gordon NP, et al. Predicting risk of osteonecrosis of the jaw with oral bisphosphonate exposure (PROBE) investigators. Prevalence of osteonecrosis of the jaw in patients with oral bisphosphonate exposure. J Oral Maxillofac Surg 2010;68(2):243–253.

Marx RE, Cillo JE Jr, Ulloa JJ. Oral bisphosphonate-induced osteonecrosis: risk factors, prediction of risk using serum CTX testing, prevention, and treatment. J Oral Maxillofac Surg. 2007 Dec;65(12):2397–2410.

Marx RE, Sawatari Y, Fortin M, Broumand V. Bisphosphonate-induced exposed bone (osteonecrosis/osteopetrosis) of the jaws: risk factors, recognition, prevention, and treatment. J Oral Maxillofac Surg. 2005 Nov;63(11):1567–1575.

Mavrokokki T, Cheng A, Stein B, Goss A. Nature and frequency of bisphosphonate-associated osteonecrosis of the jaws in Australia. J Oral Maxillofac Surg 2007; 65(3):415–423.

Montefusco V, Gay F, Spina F, et al. Antibiotic prophylaxis before dental procedures may reduce the incidence of osteonecrosis of the jaw in patients with multiple myeloma treated with bisphosphonates. Leuk Lymphoma 2008;49(11):2156–2162.

Narongroeknawin P, Danila MI, Humphreys LG Jr, Barasch A, Curtis JR. Bisphosphonate-associated osteonecrosis of the jaw, with healing after teriparatide: a review of the literature and a case report. Spec Care Dentist 2010;30(2):77–82.

Odvina CV, Zerwekh JE, Rao DS, Maalouf N, Gottschalk FA, Pak CY. Severely suppressed bone turnover: a potential complication of alendronate therapy. J Clin Endocrinol Metab 2005;90(3):1294–1301.

Phal, PM, Myall, RWT, Assael, LA, Weissman, JL. Imaging findings of bisphosphonate-associated osteonecrosis of the jaws. AJNR June 2007;28:1139–1145.

Rinchuse DJ, Rinchuse DJ, Sosovicka MF, Robison JM, Pendleton R. Orthodontic treatment of patients using bisphosphonates: a report of two cases. Am J Orthod Dentofacial Orthop 2007;131(3):321–326.

Ruggiero SL, Dodson TB, Assael LA, Landesberg R, Marx RE, Mehrotra B. American Association of Oral and Maxillofacial Surgeons position paper on bisphosphonate-related osteonecrosis of the jaws: 2009 update. J Oral Maxillofac Surg 2009;67(5 suppl):2–12.

Ruggiero SL, Mehrotra B, Rosenberg TJ, Engroff SL. Osteonecrosis of the jaws associated with the use of bisphosphonates: a review of 63 cases. J Oral Maxillofac Surg 2004;62(5):527–534.

Vescovi P, Nammour S. Bisphosphonate-related osteonecrosis of the jaw (BRONJ) therapy: a critical review (in English, Italian). Minerva Stomatol 2010;59:(4)181–203, 204–213.

Wang Z, Bhattacharyya, T. Trends in incidence of subtrochanteric fragility fractures and bisphosphonate use among the US elderly, 1996–2007. J Bone Miner Res. 2011 March;26(3):553–560.

Yarom N, Yahalom R, Shoshani Y, Hamed W, Regev E, Elad S. Osteonecrosis of the jaw induced by orally administered bisphosphonates: incidence, clinical features, predisposing factors and treatment outcome. Osteoporos Int 2007;18(10):1363–1370.

Zahrowski JJ. Optimizing orthodontic treatment in patients taking bisphosphonates for osteoporosis. Am J Orthod Dentofacial Orthop 2009;135(3):361–374.

ENDOCRINOLOGY RESOURCES

ADA. Women's oral health issues. Accessed from http://www.ada.org/prof/resources/topics/osteonecrosis.asp.

Arlt W, Allolio B. Adrenal insufficiency. Lancet 2003;361:1881–1893.

Drucker, DJ. The biology of incretin hormones. Cell Metab. 2006;3:153–165.

Howlett TA. An assessment of optimal hydrocortisone replacement therapy. Clin Endocrinol 1997;46:263–268.

Lenart, BA. Atypical fractures of the femoral diaphysis in postmenopausal women taking alendronate. N Engl J Med 2008;358:1304–1306.

Lovas K, Loge JH, Husebye ES. Subjective health status in Norwegian patients with Addison's disease. Clin Endocrinol 2002;56:581–588.

Monson JP. The assessment of glucocorticoid replacement therapy. Clin Endocrinol 1997;46:269–270.

Peacey SR, Guo CY, Robinson AM, et al. Glucocorticoid replacement therapy: are patients over treated and does it matter? Clin Endocrinol 1997;46:255–261.

Ten S, New M, Maclaren N. Clinical review 130: Addison's disease 2001. J Clin Endocrinol Metab 2001;86:2909–2922.

Society for Endocrinology. Accessed from http://www.endocrinology.org/education/ resource/summerschool/2004/ss04/ss04_arl.htm.

GLAUCOMA RESOURCES

Brooks AM, West RH, Gillies WE. The risks of precipitating acute angle-closure glaucoma with the clinical use of mydriatic agents. Med J Aust 1986;145:34–36.

Foster PJ, Oen FT, Machin D, et al. The prevalence of glaucoma in Chinese residents of Singapore: a cross-sectional population survey of the Tanjong Pagar district. Arch Ophthalmol 2000;118:1105–11.

Liew G. Fundoscopy: to dilate or not to dilate? BMJ 2006;332(7532):3.

Pandit RJ, Taylor R. Mydriasis and glaucoma: exploding the myth. A systematic review. Diabetic Med. 2000;17:693–699.

Patel KH, Javitt JC, Tielsch JM, et al. Incidence of acute angle-closure glaucoma after pharmacologic mydriasis. Am J Ophthalmology 1995;120: 709-17.

Wolfs RC, Grobbee DE, Hofman A, de Jong PT. Risk of acute angle-closure glaucoma after diagnostic mydriasis in nonselected subjects: the Rotterdam Study. Investigative Ophthalmology Visual Sci 1997;38: 2683–2687.

Wong TY, Saw SM, Tan DTH. The Singapore Malay eye study. Am J Ophthalmology 2005;139:S13.

SEIZURES RESOURCES

The Mayo Clinic. Grand mal seizure. www.mayoclinic.com/health/grand-mal-seizure/DS00222.

The Mayo Clinic. Petit mal seizure. www.mayoclinic.com/health/petit-mal-seizure/DS00216.

GASTROINTESTINAL DISEASES RESOURCES

Geller JL, Adams JS. Proton pump inhibitor therapy and hip fracture risk. JAMA 2007;297:1429.

MedlinePlus. Riboflavin deficiency (ariboflavinosis). National Institute of Health 2005.

National Cancer Institute. Colon cancer treatment. Accessed from http://www.cancer .gov/cancertopics/pdq/treatment/colon/patient.

National Digestive Diseases Information Clearinghouse. Colitus. Accessed from www.digestive.niddk.nih.gov/ddiseases/pubs/colitis/.

National Digestive Diseases Information Clearinghouse. Crohn's disease. Accessed from www.digestive.niddk.nih.gov/ddiseases/pubs/crohns/.

National Digestive Diseases Information Clearinghouse. GERD. http:// www. digestive.niddk.nih.gov/ddiseases/pubs/gerd/.

National Digestive Diseases Information Clearinghouse. Irritable bowel syndrome. Accessed from www.digestive.niddk.nih.gov/ddiseases/pubs/ibs/.

Mayo Clinic. Peptic ulcer. Accessed from www.mayoclinic.com/health/peptic-ulcer/DS00242.

Medline Plus. Celiac disease. Accessed from www.nlm.nih.gov/medlineplus/celiacdise ase.html.

Scully C. Apthous ulceration. NEJM 2006;355:165–172.

Scully C, Gorsky M, Lozada-Nur F. The diagnosis and management of recurrent aphthous stomatitis: a consensus approach. J Am Dent Assoc 2003;134:200–207.

Yang YX, Lewis JD, Epstein S, Metz DC. Long-term proton pump inhibitor therapy and risk of hip fracture. JAMA. 2006;296:2947–2953.

HEPATITIS AND CIRRHOSIS RESOURCES

AIDS Treatment Data Network. Liver Function Tests: A Simple Fact Sheet. Network www.atdn.org/simple/liverfun.html.

Arase Y, Ikeda K, Suzuki F, et al. Long-term outcome after interferon therapy in elderly patients with chronic hepatitis C. Intervirology. 2007;50(1):16–23.

Aronsohn A, Reau N. Long-term outcomes after treatment with interferon and ribavirin in HCV patients. J. Clin. Gastroenterol. 2009;43(7):661–671.

Asselah T, Estrabaud E, Bieche I, et al. Hepatitis C: viral and host factors associated with non-response to pegylated interferon plus ribavirin. Liver Int. 2010;30(9):1259–1269.

Awad T, Thorlund K, Hauser G, et al. Peginterferon alpha-2a is associated with higher sus—tained virological response than pegintereron alfa-2b in chronic hepatitis C. Hepatology. 2010;51(4):1176–1184.

Charlton M. Telaprevir, boceprevir, cytochrome P450 and immunosuppressive agents—a potentially lethal cocktail. Hepatology. 2011;54(1):3–5.

Cohen JA, Kaplan MM. The SGOT/SGPT ratio—an indicator of alcoholic liver disease. Dig Dis Sci 1979;24:835–838.

Department of Health and Human Services. Center for Disease Control and Prevention. National Immunization Program.

Diehl AM, Potter J, Boitnott J, Van Duyn MA, Herlong HF, Mezey E. Relationship between pyridoxal 5'-phosphate deficiency and aminotransferase levels in alcoholic hepatitis. Gastroenterol 1984;86:632–636.

Ghany MG, Strader DB, Thomas DL, Seeff LB. American Association for the Study of Liver Diseases. Diagnosis, management, and treatment of hepatitis C: an update. Hepatology 2009;49(4):1335–1374.

Giannini EG, Basso M, Savarino V, Picciotto A. Sustained virological response to pegylated interferon and ribavirin is maintained during long-term follow-up of chronic hepatitis C patients. Aliment. Pharmacol. Ther. 2010;31(4):502–508.

Goddard CJ, Warnes TW. Raised liver enzymes in asymptomatic patients: investigation and outcome. Dig Dis 1992;10:218–226.

Haber MM, West AB, Haber AD, Reuben A. Relationship of aminotranferases to liver histological status in chronic hepatitis C. Am J Gastroenterol 1995;90:1250.

Healey CJ, Chapman RW, Fleming KA. Liver histology in hepatitis C infection: a comparison between patients with persistently normal or abnormal transaminases. Gut 1995;37:274–278.

Jacobson IM, McHutchison JG, Dusheiko G, et al. Telaprevir for previously untreated chronic hepatitis C virus infection. N Engl J Med 2011;364(25):2405–2416.

Kamath PS. Clinical approach to the patient with abnormal liver function test results. Mayo Clin Proc 1996;71:1089–1094.

Keeffe EB, Sunderland MC, Gabourel JD. Serum gamma-glutamyl transpeptidase activity in patients receiving chronic phenytoin therapy. Dig Dis Sci 1986;31:1056–1061.

Kobayashi M, Suzuki F, Akuta N, et al. Development of hepatocellular carcinoma in elderly patients with chronic hepatitis C with or without elevated aspartate and alanine aminotransferase levels. Scand. J. Gastroenterol. 2009;44(8):975–983.

Kumada T, Toyoda H, Kiriyama S, et al. Incidence of hepatocellular carcinoma in hepatitis C carriers with normal alanine aminotransferase levels. J. Hepatol. 2009;50(4):729–735.

Lieberman D, Phillips D. "Isolated" elevation of alkaline phosphatase: significance in hospitalized patients. J Clin Gastroenterol 1990;12:415–419.

Lok AS, Everhart JE, Wright EC, et al. HALT-C Trial Group. Maintenance peginterferon therapy and other factors associated with hepatocellular carcinoma in patients with advanced hepatitis C. Gastroenterology. 2011;140(3):840–849.

Maylin S, Martinot-Peignoux M, Moucari R, et al. Eradication of hepatitis C virus in patients successfully treated for chronic hepatitis C. Gastroenterology 2008;135(3):821–829.

Mendis GP, Gibberd FB, Hunt HA. Plasma activities of hepatic enzymes in patients on anticonvulsant therapy. Seizure 1993;2:319–323.

MMWR. Hepatitis A vaccination coverage among children aged 24–35 months—United States, 2003. MMWR 2005;54(RR06);141–144.

MMWR. Prevention of Hepatitis A Through Active or Passive Immunization: Recommendations of the Advisory Committee on Immunization Practices (ACIP). MMWR 2006;55(No. RR-07).

Örmeci N, Erdem H. Basic Answers to complicated questions for the course of chronic hepatitis C treatment. Expert Rev Gastroenterol Hepatol. 2012;6(3):371–382.

Poordad F, McCone J Jr, Bacon BR, et al. Boceprevir for untreated chronic HCV genotype 1 infection. N Engl J Med. 2011;364(13):1195–1206.

Rothschild MA, Oratz M, Schreiber SS. Serum albumin. Hepatol 1988;8:385–401.

Scherzer TM, Reddy KR, Wrba F, et al. Hepatocellular carcinoma in long-term sustained virological responders following antiviral combination therapy for chronic hepatitis C. J. Viral Hepat. 2008;15(9):659–665.

Sherman KE, Flamm SL, Afdhal NH, et al. Response-guided telaprevir combination treatment for hepatitis C virus infection. N Engl J Med. 2011; 365(11):1014–1024.

Sherman KE. Alanine aminotransferase in clinical practice. Arch Intern Med 1991;151:260–265.

Sievert W, Dore GJ, McCaughan GW, et al. Virological response is associated with decline in hemoglobin concentration during pegylated interferon and ribavirin therapy in hepatitis C virus genotype 1. Hepatology. 2011;53(4):1109–1117.

Singal AK, Singh A, Jaganmohan S, et al. Antiviral therapy reduces risk of hepatocellular carcinoma in patients with hepatitis C virus-related cirrhosis. Clin. Gastroenterol. Hepatol. 2010;8(2):192–199.

Takata A, Kuromatsu R, Ando E, et al. HCC develops even in the early stage of chronic liver disease in elderly patients with HCV infection. Int. J. Mol. Med. 2010;26(2):249–256.

Theal RM, Scott K. Evaluating asymptomatic patients with abnormal liver function test results. Am Fam Physician 1996;53:2111–2119.

Westwood A. The analysis of bilirubin in serum. Ann Clin Biochem 1991;28:119–130.

Whitfield JB, Pounder RE, Neale G, Moss DW. Serum gamma-glutamyl transpeptidase activity in liver disease. Gut 1972;13:702–708.

Williams MJ, Lang-Lenton M. Trent HCV Study Group. Progression of initially mild hepatic fibrosis in patients with chronic hepatitis C infection. J. Viral Hepat. 2011;18(1):17–22.

OCCUPATIONAL POSTEXPOSURE PROPHYLAXIS (PEP) RESOURCES

HIV/AIDS Treatment Information Service: http://aidsinfo.nih.gov

Henderson DK, Dembry L, Fishman NO, et al. SHEA guideline for management of healthcare workers who are infected with hepatitis B virus, hepatitis C virus and/or human immunodeficiency virus. Infect Control Hosp Epidemiol. 2010;31:203–32.

Holmberg SD, Suryaprasad A, Ward JW. Updated CDC recommendations for the management of hepatitis B virus-infected health-care providers and students. MMWR. 2012;61(3):1–12.

PEPline: http://www.ucsf.edu/hivcntr/Hotlines/PEPline.

STD RESOURCES

CDC. CDC Guidelines for the Treatment of Sexually Transmitted Diseases: http://www.cdc.gov/nchstp/dstd.html.

CDC. Update to CDC's Sexually Transmitted Diseases Treatment Guidelines, 2006: Fluoroquinolones No Longer Recommended for Treatment of Gonococcal Infections. MMWR April 13, 2007.

CDC. Fact sheets. http://www.cdc.gov/std/healthcomm/fact_sheets.htm.

HIV RESOURCES

Aguirre JM, Echebarria MA, Ocina E, Ribacoba L, Montejo M. Reduction of HIV-associated oral lesions after highly active antiretroviral therapy. Oral Surg Oral Med Oral Pathol Oral Radiol Endod 1999;88:114–115.

AHRQ. Management of Dental Patients Who Are HIV Positive. Rockville, MD: Agency for Healthcare Research and Quality; 2001. AHRQ publication 01–E041.

Ball SC, Sepkowitz KA, Jacobs JL. Thalidomide for treatment of oral aphthous ulcers in patients with human immunodeficiency virus: case report and review. Am J Gastroenterol 1997;92:169–170.

Bartlett JG. Serologic tests for the diagnosis of HIV infection, in UpToDate.

Bell DM. Occupational risk of human immunodeficiency virus infection in healthcare workers: an overview. Am J Med 1997;102(5B):9–15. PMID 9845490.

Benson C, Kaplan J, Masur H. Treating opportunistic infections among HIV-infected adults and adolescents: recommendations from CDC, the National Institutes of Health, and the HIV Medicine Association/Infectious Diseases Society of America. Clin Infect Dis 2005;40:S131.

Burgess JA, Johnson BD, Sommers E. Pharmacological management of recurrent oral mucosal ulceration. Drugs 1990;39(1):54–65.

Cassolato, SF, Turnbull RS. Xerostomia: original articles: clinical aspects and treatment. Volume 20, No. 2. London: Blackwell Synergy-Geodontology.

Centers for Disease Control and Prevention. Interim guidance: preexposure prophylaxis for the prevention of HIV infection in men who have sex with men. MMWR Morb Mortal Wkly Rep. 2011;60(3):65–68.

Centers for Disease Control and Prevention (CDC). HIV/AIDS Surveillance Report. Atlanta: CDC; 2005.

Centers for Disease Control and Prevention: Guidelines for Preventing Opportunistic infections among HIV-infected persons—2002 Recommendations of the U.S. Public Health Service and the Infectious Disease Society of America. MMWR 2005;51RR-8:1–52.

Chen RY, Accortt NA, Westfall AO, et al. Distribution of health care expenditures for HIV-infected patients. Clin Infect Dis 2006;42L1003–10010.

Chou R, et al. Screening for HIV: A Review of the evidence for the U.S. Preventive Services Task Force. Annals of Internal Medicine 2005;143(1):55–73.

Cohen MS, Chen YQ, McCauley M, et al. HPTN 052 Study Team. Prevention of HIV-1 infection with early antiretroviral therapy. N Engl J Med. 2011;365(6):493–505.

Doyle T, Smith C, Vitiello P, et al. Plasma HIV-1 RNA detection below 50 copies/ml and risk of virologic rebound in patients receiving highly active antiretroviral therapy. Clin Infect Dis. 2012;54(5):724–732.

Farzadegan H, Vlahov D, Solomon L, et al. Detection of human immunodeficiency virus type 1 infection by polymerase chain reaction in a cohort of seronegative intravenous drug users. J Infect Dis 1993;168(2):327–331. PMID 8335969.

Grant RM, Lama JR, Anderson PL, et al. iPrEx Study Team. Preexposure chemoprophylaxis for HIV prevention in men who have sex with men. N Engl J Med. 2010; 363(27):2587–2599.

Grimes RM, Lynch DP. Frequently asked questions about the oral manifestations of HIV/AIDS. JAMA HIV/AIDS Information Center. Accessed April 2000. http://www.ama-assn.org/special/hiv/treatmnt/updates/oral.htm#q2.

Hansen AB, Gerstoft J, Kronborg G, et al. Incidence of low- and high-energy fractures in persons with and without HIV infection: a Danish population-based cohort study. AIDS. 2012;26(3):285–293.

Hare CB, Pappalardo BL, Busch MP, et al. Negative HIV antibody test results among individuals treated with antiretroviral therapy (ART) during acute/early infection. 2004. The XV International AIDS Conference: Abstract no. MoPeB3107.

HIVdent. Dental Treatment Considerations. Available at www.hivdent.org/DTC/dtctreatmen.htm.

Jacobsen JM, Greenspan JS, Spritzler J, et al. Thalidomide for the treatment of oral aphthous ulcers in patients with human immunodeficiency virus infection. National Institute of Allergy and Infectious Diseases AIDS Clinical Trials Group. N Engl J Med 1997;336:1487–1493.

Joint United Nations Programme on HIV/AIDS. 2006. Overview of the global AIDS epidemic 2006 report on the global AIDS epidemic.

Joint United Nations Programme on HIV/AIDS. AIDS epidemic update, 2005.

Levine AM, Karim R, Mack W, et al. Neutropenia in human immunodeficiency virus infection: data from the women's interagency HIV study. Arch Intern Med 2006;166:405–410.

Leynaert B, Downs AM, de Vincenzi I. Heterosexual transmission of human immunodeficiency virus: variability of infectivity throughout the course of infection. European

Study Group on Heterosexual Transmission of HIV. Am J Epidemiol 1998;148(1):88–96. PMID 9663408.

Marks G, Crepaz N, Senterfitt JW, Janssen RS. Meta-analysis of high risk sexual behavior in persons aware and unaware of their HIV status in the United States: implications for HIV prevention programs. J Acquir Immune Defic Syndr 2005;39:446.

McComsey GA, Kitch D, Daar ES, et al. Bone mineral density and fractures in antiretroviral-naive persons randomized to receive abacavir-lamivudine or tenofovir disoproxil fumarate-emtricitabine along with efavirenz or atazanavir-ritonavir: Aids Clinical Trials Group A5224s, a substudy of ACTG A5202. J Infect Dis. 2011;203(12):1791–1801.

McBride D. Management of aphthous ulcers. Am Fam Physician 2000;62:149–154,160.

Palella FJ, Jr, Delaney KM, Moorman AC, et al. Declining morbidity and mortality among patients with advanced human immunodeficiency virus infection. HIV Outpatient Study Investigators. N Engl J Med 1998;338(13):853–860. PMID 9516219.

Reeves JD, Doms RW. Human Immunodeficiency Virus Type 2. J Gen Virol 2002;83 (Pt 6):1253–1265. PMID 12029140.

Ridzon R, Gallagher K, Ciesielski C, et al. Simultaneous transmission of human immunodeficiency virus and hepatitis C virus from a needle-stick injury. N Engl J Med 1997;336:919–922.

Seattle and King County Public Health Department. Update on the HIV Antibody Test Window Period.

Smith DK, Grohskopf LA, Black RJ, et al. Antiretroviral Postexposure Prophylaxis After Sexual, Injection-Drug Use, or Other Nonoccupational Exposure to HIV in the United States. MMWR 2005;54(RR02):1–20.

Sullivan PS, Lansky A, Drake A. HITS-2000 Investigators. Failure to return for HIV test results among persons at high risk for HIV infection: results from a multistate interview project. J Acquir Immune Defic Syndr 2004;15;35:511–518.

Tappuni AR, Flemming GJ. The effect of antiretroviral therapy on the prevalence of oral manifestations in HIV-infected patients: a UK study. Oral Surg Oral Med Oral Pathol Oral Radiol Endod 2001;92:623–628.

Thompson MA, Aberg JA, Cahn P, et al. International AIDS Society–USA. Antiretroviral treatment of adult HIV infection: 2010 recommendations of the International AIDS Society–USA panel. JAMA. 2010;304(3):321–333.

Thompson MA, Aberg JA, MD; Hoy JF, et al. Antiretroviral Treatment of Adult HIV Infection: 2012 Recommendations of the International Antiviral Society–USA Panel. JAMA. 2012;308(4):387–402. doi:10.1001/jama.2012.7961.

Thompson MA, Mugavero MJ, Amico KR, et al. Guidelines for improving entry into and retention in care and antiretroviral adherence for persons with HIV: evidence-based recommendations from an International Association of Physicians in AIDS Care panel. Ann Intern Med. 2012;156(11):817–833.

US FDA. FDA approves first over-the-counter home-use rapid HIV test. Accessed from http://www.fda.gov/NewsEvents/Newsroom/PressAnnouncements/ucm310542.htm?source=govdelivery.

LYME DISEASE RESOURCES

Aguero-Rosenfeld ME, Wang G, Schwartz I, Wormser GP. Diagnosis of Lyme borreliosis. Clin Microbiol Rev. 2005;18:484–509.

Auwaerter PG, Aucott J, Dumler JS. Lyme borreliosis (Lyme disease): molecular and cellular pathobiology and prospects for prevention, diagnosis and treatment. Expert Rev Mol Med. 2004;6(2):1–22.

CDC. Lyme disease. http://www.cdc.gov/Lyme/.

Correspondence. The presenting manifestations of Lyme disease and the outcomes of treatment. N Engl J Med 2003;348:2472–2474.

Infectious Diseases Society of America. Practice guidelines for the treatment of Lyme disease. Clin Infect Dis. 2006;43:1089–1134.

Marques, A. Chronic Lyme disease: a review. Infect Dis Clin North Am 2008;22: 341–60.

Nadelman RB, Nowakowski J, Fish D, et al. Prophylaxis with single-dose doxycycline for the prevention of Lyme disease after an Ixodes scapularis tick bite. N Engl J Med 2001;345:79–84.

Steere AC, Coburn J, Glickstein L. The emergence of Lyme disease. J Clin Invest. 2004; 113(8): 1093–1101.

Wormser, GP. Clinical practice: early Lyme disease. N Engl J Med 2006;354:2794–801.

Treatment of Lyme disease. The Medical Letter, Inc. Volume 47 (Issue 1209) May 23, 2005. (Article reproduced with special permission of The Medical Letter.)

Walsh CA, Mayer EW, Baxi LV. Treatment of Lyme disease. (Abstract) Lyme disease in pregnancy: case report and review of the literature. Obstet Gynecol Surv. 2007 Jan;62(1):41–50.

Wormser GP, et al. Clinical Infectious Diseases 2006;43:1089–1134.

MRSA RESOURCES

Altieri KT, et al. Effectiveness of two disinfectant solutions and microwave irradiation in disinfecting complete dentures contaminated with methicillin-resistant Staphylococcus aureus. JADA 2012;143:270–277.

American Dental Association. Methicillin resistant Staphylococcus aureus. Available at http://www.ada.org/3080.aspx?currentTab=1#top.

Boyce JM, Pittet D. Healthcare Infection Control Practices Advisory Committee; HICPAC/SHEA/APIC/IDSA Hand Hygiene Task Force. Guideline for hand hygiene in health-care settings: recommendations of the Healthcare Infection Control Practices Advisory Committee and the HICPAC/SHEA/APIC/IDSA Hand Hygiene Task Force—Society for Healthcare Epidemiology of America/Association for Professionals in Infection Control/Infectious Diseases Society of America. MMWR Recomm Rep 2002;51(RR-16):1–45.[Medline].

Buonavoglia A, Latronico F, Greco MF. Methicillin-resistant staphylococci carriage in the oral cavity: a study conducted in Bari (Italy). Oral Dis. 2010;16:465–468.

CDC. MRSA. Accessed from http://www.cdc.gov/mrsa/.

CDC. Personal protective equipment (PPE) in healthcare settings. www.cdc.gov/ncidod/dhqp/ppe.html.

Gorwitz R, Kruszon-Moran D, McAllister SK, et al. Changes in the prevalence of nasal colonization with Staphylococcus aureus in the United States, 2001-2004. J Infect Dis. 2008;197:1226–1234.

Infection Control in Practice. OSAP Checkup: 2003 CDC Guidelines. 2004;3:1-9. Available at http://www.osap.org/resource/resmgr/Publications/OSAP_CheckUp_2003_CDC_Guidel.pdf.

Jarvis WR, Schlosser J, Chinn RY, et al. National prevalence of methicillin-resistant Staphylococcus aureus in inpatients at US health facilities in 2006. Am J Infect Control. 2007;35:631–637.

Kallen AJ, Mu Y, Bulens S, et al. Healthcare associated invasive MRSA infections, 2005-2008. JAMA. 2010;304:641–648.

Klevens RM, Gorwitz RJ, Collins AS. Methicillin-resistant Staphylococcus aureus: a primer for dentists. J Am Dent Assoc. 2008;139:1328–1337.

Kohn WG, Collins AS, Cleveland JL, et al. Guidelines for infection control in dental health-care settings—2003. MMWR Recomm Rep 2003;52(RR-17):1–61.

Kurita H, Kurashina K, Honda T. Nosocomial transmission of methicillin-resistant Staphylococcus aureus via the surfaces of the dental operatory. Br Dent J. 2006; 201:297–300.

Liu C, et al. Clinical practice guidelines by the Infectious Diseases Society of America for the treatment of methicillin resistant Staphylococcus aureus infections in adults and children. Clin Infect Dis. 2011;52(3):e18–e55.

Rautemaa R, Nordberg A, Wuolijoki-Saaristo K, Meurman JH. Bacterial aerosols in dental practice—a potential hospital infection problem. J Hosp Infect. 2006;64: 76–81.

Rybak MJ, Lomaestro BM, Rotschafer JC, et al. Vancomycin therapeutic guidelines: a summary of consensus recommendations from the Infectious Diseases Society of America, the American Society of Health-System Pharmacists, and the Society of Infectious Diseases Pharmacists. Clin Infect Dis 2009;49:325–7.

Schmitz GR, Bruner D, Pitotti R, et al. Randomized controlled trial of trimethoprim-sulfamethoxazole for uncomplicated skin abscesses in patients at risk for community-associated methicillin-resistant Staphylococcus aureus infection. Ann Emerg Med 2010;56:283–287.

Siegel JD, Rhinehart E, Jackson M, Chiarello L; Healthcare Infection Control Practices Advisory Committee. Guideline for isolation precautions: preventing transmission of infectious agents in healthcare settings 2007. www.cdc.gov/ncidod/dhqp/pdf/guidelines/Isolation2007.pdf.

ORAL LESIONS RESOURCES

Ball SC, Sepkowitz KA, Jacobs JL. Thalidomide for treatment of oral aphthous ulcers in patients with human immunodeficiency virus: case report and review. Am J Gastroenterol 1997;92:169–170.

Burgess JA, Johnson BD, Sommers E. Pharmacological management of recurrent oral mucosal ulceration. Drugs 1990;39(1):54–65.

Grimes RM, Lynch DP. Frequently asked questions about the oral manifestations of HIV/AIDS. JAMA HIV/AIDS Information Center. Accessed April 2000. http://www.ama-assn.org/special/hiv/treatmnt/updates/oral.htm#q2.

Jacobsen JM, Greenspan JS, Spritzler J, Ketter N, Fahey JL, Jackson JB, et al. Thalidomide for the treatment of oral aphthous ulcers in patients with human immunodeficiency virus infection. National Institute of Allergy and Infectious Diseases AIDS Clinical Trials Group. N Engl J Med 1997;336:1487–1493.

McBride D. Management of Aphthous Ulcers. Am Fam Physician 2000;62:149–154,160.

Verpilleux MP, Bastuji-Garin S, Revuz J. Comparative analysis of severe aphthosis and Behçet's disease: 104 cases. Dermatol 1999;198:247–251.

PREGNANCY, LACTATION, AND CONTRACEPTION RESOURCES

Academy of General Dentistry. Pregnancy and Gingivitis. http://www7.agd.org/consumer/topics/pregnancy/pregnancy_gingivitis.asp.

American Academy of Periodontology. Baby Steps to a Healthy Pregnancy and On-Time Delivery. http://www.perio.org/consumer/pregnancy.htm.

American Academy of Periodontology. Periodontal (Gum) Disease. http://www.ada.org/public/resources/glossary.asp#d.

American Dental Association FAQs: Pregnancy. http://www.ada.org/public/topics/pregnancy_faq.asp.

American Dental Association: Treating Periodontal Disease: Scaling and Root Planing. http://www.ada.org/prof/resources/pubs/jada/patient/patient_23.pdf.

American Pregnancy Association: Pregnancy and Dental Work. http://www.americanpregnancy.org/pregnancyhealth/dentalwork.html.

Baccaglini L. A meta-analysis of randomized controlled trials shows no evidence that periodontal treatment during pregnancy prevents adverse pregnancy outcomes. J Am Dent Assoc. 2011;142(10):1192–1193.

Burroughs KE, Chambliss ML. Antibiotics and Oral Contraceptive Failure. Arch Fam Med. 2000;9:81–82.

Cleveland Clinic. Dental Care During Pregnancy. http://www.clevelandclinic.org/health/health-info/docs/3200/3235.asp.

Dickinson BD, Altman RD, Nielsen NH, Sterling ML. Drug interactions between oral contraceptives and antibiotics. Obstet Gynecol. 2001;98(5 Pt 1):853–860.

Dogterom P, van den Heuvel MW, Thomsen T. Absence of pharmacokinetic interactions of the combined contraceptive vaginal ring NuvaRing with oral amoxicillin or doxycycline in two randomised trials. Clin Pharmacokinet. 2005;44(4):429–438.

Fazio A. Oral contraceptive drug interactions: important considerations. South Med J. 1991;84:997–1002.

Gaffield ML, Gilbert BJ, Malvitz DM, Romaguera R. Oral health during pregnancy: an analysis of information collected by the pregnancy risk assessment monitoring system. JADA 2001;132(7):1009–1016.

Helms SE, Bredle DL, Zajic J, et al. Oral contraceptive failure rates and oral antibiotics. J Am Acad Dermatol. 1997 May;36(5 Pt 1):705–710.

JADA, Feb 2001: An update on radiographic practices: Information and recommendations. http://www.ada.org/prof/resources/pubs/jada/reports/report_radiography.pdf.

JAMA. Dental Radiography Study Bolsters ADA Recommendations. http://www.ada.org/prof/resources/pubs/adanews/adanewsarticle.asp?articleid=853.

Novak MJ, et. al. Periodontal bacterial profiles in pregnant women: response to treatment and associations with birth outcomes in the obstetrics and periodontal therapy (OPT) study. J Periodontol. 2008 Oct;79(10):1870-9.

Michalowicz BS, et al. Serum inflammatory mediators in pregnancy: changes after periodontal treatment and asso-ciation with pregnancy outcomes. J Periodontol. 2009 Nov;80(11):1731-41.

Michalowicz BS, et al. Change in periodontitis during pregnancy and the risk of preterm birth and low birthweight. J Clin Periodontol. 2009 Apr;36(4):308-14.

Michalowicz BS, DiAngelis AJ, Novak MJ, et al. Examining the safety of dental treatment in pregnant women. J Am Dent Assoc. 2008;139(6):685–695.

Michalowicz BS, Hodges JS, DiAngelis AJ, et al. OPT Study. Treatment of periodontal disease and the risk of preterm birth. N Engl J Med. 2006;355(18):1885–1894.

Murphy AA, Zacur HA, Charache P, Burkman RT. The effect of tetracycline on levels of oral contraceptives. Am J Obstet Gynecol. 1991 Jan;164(1 Pt 1):28–33.

Polyzos NP, Polyzos IP, Zavos A, et al. Obstetric outcomes after treatment of periodontal disease during pregnancy: systematic review and meta-analysis. BMJ. 2010 Dec 29;341:c7017.

Taylor J, Pemberton MN. Antibiotics and oral contraceptives: new considerations for dental practice. British Dental Journal. 2012;212:481–483.

Toh S, Mitchell AA, Anderka M, et al. Antibiotics and oral contraceptive failure—a case-crossover study. Contraception. 2011 May;83(5):418–425.

MALIGNANT HYPERTHERMIA RESOURCES

Denborough MA, Ebeling P, King JO, Zapf PW. Myopathy and malignant hyperpyrexia. Lancet 1970;I:1138–1140.

Larach MG, for the North American Malignant Hyperthermia Group. Standardization of the caffeine halothane muscle contracture test. Anesth Analg 1989;69:511–515.

Malignant Hyperthermia Association of United States. www.mhaus.org/.

Nelson TE, Flewellen EH. The malignant hyperthermia syndrome. New Eng J Med 1983;309:416–418. www.hkpp.org/physicians/mh_hyper.html.

Nelson TE, Flewellen EH. Malignant hyperthermia: A pharmacogenetic disease of Ca^{++} regulating proteins. Curr Mol Med 2002;2:347–369.

PAGET'S DISEASE RESOURCES

Delmas PD, Meunier PJ. The management of Paget's disease of bone. N Engl J Med 1997;336:558.

Mayo Clinic. Paget's Disease of the Bone. Mayoclinic.com www.mayoclinic.com/health/pagets-disease-of-bone/DS00485.

MedlinePlus. Paget's disease of Bone. www.nlm.nih.gov/medlineplus/pagetsdiseaseof bone.html.

METHOTREXATE RESOURCES

Albrecht K, Müller-Ladner U. Side effects and management of side effects of methotrexate in rheumatoid arthritis. Clin. Exp. Rheumatol. 2010;28(Suppl. 61),S95–S101.

Boers M. The COBRA trial 20 years later. Clin. Exp. Rheumatol. 2011;29(5 Suppl. 68):S46–S51.

Braun J. Optimal administration and dosage of methotrexate. Clin. Exp. Rheumatol. 2010;28(Suppl. 61):S46–S51.

Breedveld FC, Weisman MH, Kavanaugh AF et al. A multicenter, randomized, double-blind clinical trial of combination therapy with adalimumab plus methotrexate versus methotrexate alone or adalimumab alone in patients with early, aggressive rheumatoid arthritis who had not had previous methotrexate treatment. Arthritis Rheum. 54,26–37 (2006).

Brinker RR, Ranganathan P. Methotrexate pharmacogenetics in rheumatoid arthritis. Clin. Exp. Rheumatol. 2010;28(Suppl. 61):S33–S39.

Coury FF, Weinblatt ME. Clinical trials to establish methotrexate as a therapy for rheumatoid arthritis. Clin. Exp. Rheumatol. 2010;28(Suppl 61):S9–S12.

Cronstein B. How does methotrexate suppress inflammation? Clin. Exp. Rheumatol. 2010;28(Suppl. 61):S21–S23.

Fiehn C. Methotrexate transport mechanisms: the basis for targeted drug delivery and ß-folate-receptor-specific treatment. Clin. Exp. Rheumatol. 2010;28(Suppl. 61):S40–S45.

Gossec L, Smolen JS, Gaujoux-Viala C, et al. European League Against Rheumatism recommendations for the management of psoriatic arthritis with pharmacological therapies. Ann. Rheum. Dis. 2011;71(1):4–12

Hochberg MC, Johnston SS, John AK. The incidence and prevalence of extraarticular and systemic manifestations in a cohort of newly-diagnosed patients with rheumatoid arthritis between 1999 and 2006. Curr. Med. Res. Opin. 2008;24:469–480.

Kaltsonoudis E, Papagoras C, A Drosos AA. Current and Future Role of Methotrexate in the Therapeutic Armamentarium for Rheumatoid Arthritis. Int J Clin Rheumatol. 2012;7(2):179–189.

Keystone E, Heijde D, Mason D Jr, et al. Certolizumab pegol plus methotrexate is significantly more effective than placebo plus methotrexate in active rheumatoid arthritis: findings of a fifty-two-week, Phase III, multicenter, randomized, double-blind, placebo-controlled, parallel-group study. Arthritis Rheum. 2008;58:3319–3329.

Krüger K. [Combination therapy using methotrexate with DMARDs or biologics-current status]. Z. Rheumatol. 2011;70:114–122

Morgan SL, Baggott JE. Folate supplementation during methotrexate therapy for rheumatoid arthritis. Clin. Exp. Rheumatol. 2010;28(Suppl. 61):S102–S109

Mühl H, Pfeilschifter J. [Pharmacogenetics and pharmacogenomics of methotrexate. Current status and novel aspects]. Z. Rheumatol. 2011;70:101–107.

Rath T, Rubbert A. Drug combinations with methotrexate to treat rheumatoid arthritis. Clin. Exp. Rheumatol. 2010;28(Suppl. 61):S52–S57.

Rau R. Efficacy of methotrexate in comparison to biologics in rheumatoid arthritis. Clin. Exp. Rheumatol. 2010;28(Suppl. 61):S58–S64.

Reiss AB, Carsons SE, Anwar K, et al. Atheroprotective effects of methotrexate on reverse cholesterol transport proteins and foam cell transformation in human THP-1 monocyte/macrophages. Arthritis Rheum. 2008;58:3675–3683.

Visser K, Katchamart W, Loza E, et al. Multinational evidence-based recommendations for the use of methotrexate in rheumatic disorders with a focus on rheumatoid arthritis: integrating systematic literature research and expert opinion of a broad international panel of rheumatologists in the 3E Initiative. Ann. Rheum. Dis. 2009;68:1086–1093.

Yazici Y. Long-term safety of methotrexate in the treatment of rheumatoid arthritis. Clin. Exp. Rheumatol. 2010;28(Suppl. 61):S65–S67.

GOUT RESOURCES

Medicinenet.com. Gout (gouty arthritis) and hyperuricemia. Accessed from medicinenet.com/gout/article.htm.

MedlinePlus. Gout and pseudogout. Accessed from www.nlm.nih.gov/medlineplus/goutandpseudogout.html.

POLYMYOSITIS AND DERMATOMYOSITIS RESOURCES

Amato AA, Barohn RJ. Idiopathic inflammatory myopathies. Neurol Clin 1997;(3):615–648.

Briani C, Doria A, Dalakas MC. Update on idiopathic inflammatory myopathies. Autoimmunity 2006;39(3):161–170.

Christopher-Stine L, Plotz PH. Myositis: an update on pathogenesis. Curr Opin Rheumatol 2004;16(6):700–706.

Dalakas MC, Hohlfeld R. Polymyositis and dermatomyositis. Lancet 2003; 362(9388):971–982.

Dalakas MC, Sivakumar K. The immunopathologic and inflammatory differences between dermatomyositis, polymyositis and sporadic inclusion body myositis. Curr Opin Neurol 1996;9(3):235–239.

Oddis CV. Idiopathic inflammatory myopathies: a treatment update. Curr Rheumatol Rep 2003;5(6):431–436.

Olsen NJ, Park JH. Inflammatory myopathies: issues in diagnosis and management. Arthritis Care Res 1997;Jun;10(3):200–207.

Salomonsson S, Lundberg IE. Cytokines in idiopathic inflammatory myopathies. Autoimmunity 2006;39(3):177–190.

Schnabel A, Hellmich B, Gross WL. Interstitial lung disease in polymyositis and dermatomyositis. Curr Rheumatol Rep 2005;7(2):99–105.

PARKINSON'S DISEASE RESOURCES

Nutt JG, Wooten GF. Supplement to: Diagnosis and initial management of Parkinson's disease. N Engl J Med 2005;353:1021–1027. content.nejm.org/cgi/content/full/353/10/1021/DC1

National Institute of Neurological Disorders and Stroke. Parkinson's disease Research web overview. Accessed from http://www.ninds.nih.gov/research/parkinsonsweb/.

MYASTHENIA GRAVIS RESOURCES

Juel VC. Myasthenia gravis: management of myasthenic crisis and perioperative care. Semin Neurol. 2004;24(1):75–81.

Keesey JC. Clinical evaluation and management of myasthenia gravis. Muscle Nerve 2004;29(4):484–505.

Mehta S. Neuromuscular disease causing acute respiratory failure. Respir Care 2006;51(9):1016–1021; discussion 1021–1023.

National Institute of Neurological Disorders and Stroke. Myasthenia Gravis Fact Sheet. www.ninds.nih.gov/disorders/myasthenia_gravis/detail_myasthenia_gravis.htm.

Palace J, Vincent A, Beeson D. Myasthenia gravis: diagnostic and management dilemmas. Curr Opin Neurol 2001;14(5):583–589.

Pascuzzi RM. The edrophonium test. Semin Neurol 2003;23(1):83–88.

Saperstein DS, Barohn RJ. Management of myasthenia gravis. Semin Neurol 2004;24(1):41–48.

Vincent A, Palace J, Hilton-Jones D. Myasthenia gravis. Lancet 2001;357(9274):2122–2128.

MedlinePlus. Myasthenia gravis. www.nlm.nih.gov/medlineplus/myastheniagravis .html.

MULTIPLE SCLEROSIS RESOURCES

Chemaly D, Lefrançois A, Pérusse R. Oral and maxillofacial manifestations of multiple sclerosis. J Can Dent Assoc 2000;66:600–611.

Commins DJ, Chen JM. Multiple sclerosis: a consideration in acute cranial nerve palsies. Amer J Otol 1997;18:590–595.

Confavreux C, Hutchinson M, Hours MM, et al. Rate of pregnancy-related relapse in multiple sclerosis. Pregnancy in Multiple Sclerosis Group. N Engl J Med 1998;339(5):285–291.

Dumas M, Pérusse R. Trigeminal sensory neuropathy: a study of 35 cases. Oral Surg Oral Med Oral Pathol Oral Radiol Endod 1999;87:577–582.

Durelli L, Verdun E, Barbero P, et al. Every-other-day interferon beta-1b versus once-weekly interferon beta-1a for multiple sclerosis: results of a 2-year prospective randomised multicentre study (INCOMIN). Lancet 2002; 359(9316):1453–1460.

Fukazawa T, Moriwaka F, Hamada K, et al. Facial palsy in multiple sclerosis. J Neurol 1997;244:631–633.

Goodin DS, Frohman EM, Garmany GP, et al. Disease modifying therapies in multiple sclerosis: report of the Therapeutics and Technology Assessment Subcommittee of the American Academy of Neurology and the MS Council for Clinical Practice Guidelines. Neurol 2002;58(2):169–178.

Johnson KP, Brooks BR, Cohen JA, et al. Copolymer 1 reduces relapse rate and improves disability in relapsing-remitting multiple sclerosis: results of a phase III multicenter, double-blind placebo-controlled trial. The Copolymer Multiple Sclerosis Study Group. Neurol 1995;45(7):1268–1276.

Lublin FD, Whitaker JN, Eidelman BH, et al. Management of patients receiving interferon beta-1b for multiple sclerosis: report of a consensus conference. Neurol 1996;46(1):12–18.

McDonald WI, Compston A, Edan G, et al. Recommended diagnostic criteria for multiple sclerosis: guidelines from the International Panel on the diagnosis of multiple sclerosis. Ann Neurol 2001;50(1):121–127.

McGrother CW, Dugmore C, Phillips MJ, et al. Multiple sclerosis, dental caries and fillings: a case-control study. Br Dent J 1999;187:261–264.

Meaney JF, Watt JW, Eldridge PR, et al. Association between trigeminal neuralgia and multiple sclerosis: role of magnetic resonance imaging. J Neurol Neurosurg Psychiatry 1995;59:253–259.

National Institute of Neurological Disorders and Stroke. NINDS multiple sclerosis information page. www.ninds.nih.gov/disorders/multiple_sclerosis/multiple_sclerosis .htm.

Noseworthy JH, Lucchinetti C, Rodriguez M, Weinshenker BG. Multiple sclerosis. N Engl J Med 2000; 343(13):938–952.

Penarrocha Diago P, Bagan Sebastian JV, Alfaro Giner AA, Escrig Orenga VE. Mental nerve neuropathy in systemic cancer. Report of three cases. Oral Surg Oral Med Oral Pathol 1990;69:48–51.

PRISMS Study Group: Randomised double-blind placebo-controlled study of interferon beta-1a in relapsing/remitting multiple sclerosis. PRISMS (Prevention of Relapses and Disability by Interferon beta-1a Subcutaneously in Multiple Sclerosis) Study Group. Lancet 1998;352(9139):1498–1504.

Sellebjerg F, Frederiksen JL, Nielsen PM, Olesen J. Double-blind, randomized, placebo-controlled study of oral, high-dose methylprednisolone in attacks of MS. Neurol 1998;51(2):529–534.

Thompson AJ, Polman CH, Miller DH, et al. Primary progressive multiple sclerosis. Brain 1997;120(Pt 6):1085–1096.

Vastag B. Not so fast: research on infectious links to MS questioned. JAMA 2001; 285(3):279–281.

Weiner HL, Hohol MJ, Khoury SJ, et al. Therapy for multiple sclerosis. Neurol Clin 1995;13(1):173–196.

Weinshenker BG. The natural history of multiple sclerosis. Neurol Clin 1995;13(1):119–146.

SJÖGREN'S SYNDROME RESOURCES

American Dental Association. NIDCR announces new Sjögren's syndrome classification criteria. ADA News. May 7, 2012;**43**:8. http://www.ada.org/news/7050.aspx Accessed June 1, 2012.

Antoniazzi RP, Miranda LA, Zanatta FB, et al. Periodontal conditions of individuals with Sjögren's syndrome. J Periodontol. Mar 2009;80(3):429–435.

Fox RI. Sjögren's syndrome. Lancet. Jul 23-29 2005;366(9482):321–331.

Gálvez J, Sáiz E, López P, et al. Diagnostic evaluation and classification criteria in Sjögren's Syndrome. Joint Bone Spine. Sep 29 2008.

Giuca MR, Bonfigli D, Bartoli F, Pasini M. Sjögren's syndrome: correlation between histopathologic result and clinical and serologic parameters. Minerva Stomatol. Apr 2010;59(4):149-54, 154–157.

Gøransson LG, Herigstad A, Tjensvoll AB, et al. Peripheral neuropathy in primary Sjögren's syndrome: a population-based study. Arch Neurol. Nov 2006;63(11):1612–1615.

Haldorsen K, Moen K, Jacobsen H, et al. Exocrine function in primary Sjögren syndrome: natural course and prognostic factors. Ann Rheum Dis. Jul 2008;67(7):949–954.

Hammar O, Ohlsson B, Wollmer P, Mandl T. Impaired gastric emptying in primary Sjögren's syndrome. J Rheumatol. Nov 2010;37(11):2313–2318.

Helmick CG, Felson DT, Lawrence RC, et al. Estimates of the prevalence of arthritis and other rheumatic conditions in the United States. Part I. Arthritis Rheum. Jan 2008;58(1):15–25.

Katayama I, Kotobuki Y, Kiyohara E, Murota H. Annular erythema associated with Sjögren's syndrome: review of the literature on the management and clinical analysis of skin lesions. Mod Rheumatol. Apr 2010;20(2):123–129.

Langegger C, Wenger M, Duftner C, et al. Use of the European preliminary criteria, the Breiman-classification tree and the American-European criteria for diagnosis of primary Sjögren's Syndrome in daily practice: a retrospective analysis. Rheumatol Int. Jun 2007;27(8):699–702.

Lemp MA. Advances in understanding and managing dry eye disease. Am J Ophthalmol. Sep 2008;146(3):350–356.

Meijer JM, Meiners PM, Vissink A, et al. Effectiveness of rituximab treatment in primary Sjögren's syndrome: a randomized, double-blind, placebo-controlled trial. Arthritis Rheum. Apr 2010;62(4):960–8.

Ng KP, Isenberg DA. Sjögren's syndrome: diagnosis and therapeutic challenges in the elderly. Drugs Aging. 2008;25(1):19–33.

Parambil JG, Myers JL, Lindell RM, et al. Interstitial lung disease in primary Sjögren's syndrome. Chest. Nov 2006;130(5):1489–1495.

Parkin B, Chew JB, White VA, et al. Lymphocytic infiltration and enlargement of the lacrimal glands: a new subtype of primary Sjögren's syndrome? Ophthalmology 2005;112(11):2040–2047.

Pflugfelder SC. Antiinflammatory therapy for dry eye. Am J Ophthalmol. 2004; 137(2):337–342.

Ramachandiran N. Apparently persistent weakness after recurrent hypokalemic paralysis: a tale of two disorders. South Med J. Sep 2008;101(9):940–942.

Ren H, Wang WM, Chen XN, et al. Renal involvement and followup of 130 patients with primary Sjögren's syndrome. J Rheumatol. Feb 2008;35(2):278–284.

Shiboski SC, Shiboski CH, Criswell L, et al. American College of Rheumatology Classification Criteria for Sjögren's Syndrome: a data-driven, expert consensus approach in the Sjögren's International Collaborative Clinical Alliance Cohort. Arthritis Care Res. 2012;64:475–487.

Thanou-Stavraki A, James JA. Primary Sjogren's syndrome: current and prospective therapies. Semin Arthritis Rheum. Apr 2008;37(5):273–92.

Theander E, Vasaitis L, Baecklund E, et al. Lymphoid organisation in labial salivary gland biopsies is a possible predictor for the development of malignant lymphoma in primary Sjögren's syndrome. Ann Rheum Dis. Aug 2011;70(8):1363–1368.

Versura P, Frigato M, Cellini M, et al. Diagnostic performance of tear function tests in Sjögren's syndrome patients. Eye. Feb 2007;21(2):229–237.

Vitali C, Bombardieri S, Jonsson R, et al. Classification criteria for Sjögren's syndrome: a revised version of the European criteria proposed by the American-European Consensus Group. Ann Rheum Dis. 2002;61:554–558.

HEAD AND NECK CANCERS RESOURCES

American Cancer Society. Cancer Facts and Figures 2006. Atlanta, GA: American Cancer Society; 2007.

Armitage JO. Treatment of non-Hodgkin's lymphoma. N Engl J Med 1993;328(14):1023–1030.

Bastion Y, Sebban C, Berger F, et al. Incidence, predictive factors, and outcome of lymphoma transformation in follicular lymphoma patients. J Clin Oncol 1997;15(4):1587–1594.

Browman GP, Wong G, Hodson I, et al. Influence of cigarette smoking on the efficacy of radiation therapy in head and neck cancer. N Engl J Med 1993;328(3):159–163.

Cabanillas F, Velasquez WS, Hagemeister FB, et al. Clinical, biologic, and histologic features of late relapses in diffuse large cell lymphoma. Blood 1992;79(4):1024–1028.

Close LG, Brown PM, Vuitch MF, et al. Microvascular invasion and survival in cancer of the oral cavity and oropharynx. Arch Otolaryngol Head Neck Surg 1989;115(11):1304–1309.

Consensus conference. Magnetic resonance imaging. JAMA 1988;259(14):2132–2138.

Day GL, Blot WJ. Second primary tumors in patients with oral cancer. Cancer 1992;70(1):14–19.

Jones KR, Lodge-Rigal RD, Reddick RL, et al. Prognostic factors in the recurrence of stage I and II squamous cell cancer of the oral cavity. Arch Otolaryngol Head Neck Surg 1992;118(5):483–485.

Langendijk JA, de Jong MA, Leemans ChR, et al. Postoperative radiotherapy in squamous cell carcinoma of the oral cavity: the importance of the overall treatment time. Int J Radiat Oncol Biol Phys 2003;57(3):693–700.

Lip and oral cavity. In: American Joint Committee on Cancer: The AJCC Cancer Staging Manual and Handbook. 6th ed. New York: Springer; 2002; pp 23–32.

National Cancer Institute. Non-hodgkin lymphoma. Accessed from www.cancer .gov/cancertopics/types/non-hodgkin.

Po Wing Yuen A, Lam KY, Lam LK, et al. Prognostic factors of clinically stage I and II oral tongue carcinoma—A comparative study of stage, thickness, shape, growth pattern, invasive front malignancy grading, Martinez-Gimeno score, and pathologic features. Head Neck 2002;24(6):513–520.

Pui CH, Evans WE. Treatment of acute lymphoblastic leukemia. N Engl J Med 2006; 354(2):166–178

Van der Tol IG, de Visscher JG, Jovanovic A, et al. Risk of second primary cancer following treatment of squamous cell carcinoma of the lower lip. Oral Oncol 1999;35(6):571–574.

Yuen AR, Kamel OW, Halpern J, et al. Long-term survival after histologic transformation of low-grade follicular lymphoma. J Clin Oncol 1995;13(7):1726–1733.

MULTIPLE MYELOMA RESOURCES

Alexanian R, Dimopoulos MA, Delasalle K, Barlogie B. Primary dexamethasone treatment of multiple myeloma. Blood 1992;80(4):887–890.

Alyea EP, Anderson KC. Allogeneic bone marrow transplantation in the treatment of multiple myeloma. PPO Updates 2000;14:1–10.

Attal M, Harousseau JL, Stoppa AM, et al. A prospective, randomized trial of autologous bone marrow transplantation and chemotherapy in multiple myeloma. Intergroupe Francais du Myelome. N Engl J Med 1996;335(2):91–97.

Barlogie B, Shaughnessy J, Munshi N, Epstein J. Plasma cell myeloma. In: Beutler E, Lichtman M, Coller B, Kipps T, Seligsohn U, eds. Williams Hematology (6th ed.). New York: McGraw-Hill; 2001:1279–1304.

Billadeau D, Ahmann G, Greipp P, Van Ness B. The bone marrow of multiple myeloma patients contains B cell populations at different stages of differentiation that are clonally related to the malignant plasma cell. J Exp Med 1993;178:1023–1031.

Bloomfield DJ. Should bisphosphonates be part of the standard therapy of patients with multiple myeloma or bone metastases from other cancers? An evidence-based review. J Clin Oncol 1998;16(3):1218–1225.

Cooper MR, Dear K, McIntyre OR, et al. A randomized clinical trial comparing melphalan/prednisone with or without interferon alfa-2b in newly diagnosed patients with multiple myeloma: a Cancer and Leukemia Group B study. J Clin Oncol 1993;11(1):155–160.

Dimopoulos MA, Moulopoulos A, Smith T, et al. Risk of disease progression in asymptomatic multiple myeloma. Am J Med 1993;94(1):57–61.

Gerull S, Goerner M, Benner A, et al. Long-term outcome of nonmyeloablative allogeneic transplantation in patients with high-risk multiple myeloma. Bone Marrow Transplant 2005;36(11):963–969.

Kuehl WM, Bergsagel PL. Multiple myeloma: evolving genetic events and host interactions. Nat Rev Cancer 2002;2:175–187.

Kumar A, Loughran T, Alsina M, et al. Management of multiple myeloma: a systematic review and critical appraisal of published studies. Lancet Oncol 2003;4(5):293–304.

Kyle RA, Greipp PA. Plasma cell dyscrasias: current status. Crit Rev Oncol Hematol 1988;8(2):93–152.

Kyle RA, Rajkumar SV. Multiple Myeloma. N Engld J Med 2004;351:1860–1873.

Kyle RA, Therneau TM, Rajkumar SV, et al. A long-term study of prognosis in monoclonal gammopathy of undetermined significance. N Engl J Med 2002;346:564–569.

Lokhorst HM, Sonneveld P, Cornelissen JJ, et al. Induction therapy with vincristine, adriamycin, dexamethasone (VAD) and intermediate-dose melphalan (IDM) followed by autologous or allogeneic stem cell transplantation in newly diagnosed multiple myeloma. Bone Marrow Transplant 1999;23(4):317–322.

Ludwig H, Fritz E, Kotzmann H, et al. Erythropoietin treatment of anemia associated with multiple myeloma. N Engl J Med 1990;14;322(24):1693–1699.

Ludwig H, Kumpan W, Sinzinger H. Radiography and bone scintigraphy in multiple myeloma: a comparative analysis. Br J Radiol Mar;1982;55(651):173–181.

Moreau P, Hullin C, Garban F, et al. Tandem autologous stem cell transplantation in high-risk de novo multiple myeloma: final results of the prospective and randomized IFM 99–04 protocol. Blood 2006; 107(1):397–403.

Nordic Myeloma Study Group. Interferon-alpha 2b added to melphalanprednisone for initial and maintenance therapy in multiple myeloma. A randomized, controlled trial. The Nordic Myeloma Study Group. Ann Intern Med 1996;124(2):212–222.

Ross ME, Zhou X, Song G, et al. Classification of pediatric acute lymphoblastic leukemia by gene expression profiling. Blood 2003;102:2951–2959.

Samson D, Gaminara E, Newland A, et al. Infusion of vincristine and doxorubicin with oral dexamethasone as first-line therapy for multiple myeloma. Lancet 1989;2(8668):882–885.

Schreiman JS, McLeod RA, Kyle RA, Beabout JW. Multiple myeloma: evaluation by CT. Radiology 1985;154(2):483–486.

Singhal S, Mehta J, Desikan R, et al. Antitumor activity of thalidomide in refractory multiple myeloma. N Engl J Med 1999;341(21):1565–1571.

Van de Berg BC, Lecouvet FE, Michaux L, et al. Stage I multiple myeloma: value of MR imaging of the bone marrow in the determination of prognosis. Radiol Oct 1996;201(1):243–246.

Yeoh EJ, Ross ME, Shurtleff SA, et al. Classification, subtype discovery, and prediction of outcome in pediatric acute lymphoblastic leukemia by gene expression profiling. Cancer Cell 2002;1:133–143.

PSYCHIATRIC CONDITIONS RESOURCES

American Psychiatric Association Work Group on Eating Disorders. Practice guideline for the treatment of patients with eating disorders (revision). Amer J Psychiatry 2000;157(1 Suppl):1–39.

Andreasen NC, Arndt S, Alliger R, et al. Symptoms of schizophrenia. Methods, meanings, and mechanisms. Arch Gen Psychiatry 1995;52(5):341–351.

Atri A, Shaughnessy LW, Locascio JJ, Growdon JH. Long-term course and effectiveness of combination therapy in Alzheimer disease. Alzheimer Dis Assoc Disord. 2008;22(3):209–221.

Becker AE, Grinspoon SK, Klibanski A, Herzog DB. Eating disorders. N Engl J Med 1999;340(14):1092–1098.

Benazzi F. Bipolar II disorder: epidemiology, diagnosis, and management. CNS Drugs. 2007;21(9):727–740.

Black SE, Doody R, Li H, et al. Donepezil preserves cognition and global function in patients with severe Alzheimer disease. Neurology. 2007;69(5):459–469.

Bowden CL. Anticonvulsants in bipolar disorders: current research and practice and future directions. Bipolar Disord. 2009;11(suppl 2):20–33.

Bruce B, Agras WS. Binge eating in females: a population-based investigation. Intl J Eating Disorders 1992;12:365–373.

Bullock R, Dengiz R. Cognitive performance in patients with Alzheimer's disease receiving cholinesterase inhibitors for up to 5 years. Int J Clin Pract. 2005;59:817–822.

Clifford R. Jack Jr, et al. Introduction to the recommendations from the National Institute on Aging—Alzheimer's Association workgroups on diagnostic guidelines for Alzheimer's disease. Alzheimer's & Dementia: The Journal of the Alzheimer's Association 2011;7(3):257–262.

Complete guide to bipolar disorder symptoms, diagnosis, and treatment. Understanding mania. 2012. http://www.bipolarhome.org/understanding-mania/.

Courtney C, Farrell D, Gray R, et al. AD2000 collaborative group. Long-term donepezil treatment in 565 patients with Alzheimer's disease (AD2000): randomised double-blind trial. Lancet. 2004;363(9427):2105–2115.

Cummings JL, Frank JC, Cherry D, Kohatsu ND, Kemp B, Hewett L, et al. Guidelines for managing Alzheimer's disease: part I. Assessment. Am Fam Physician 2002;65:2263–2272.

Cummings JL, Frank JC, Cherry D, Kohatsu ND, Kemp B, Hewett L, et al. Guidelines for managing Alzheimer's disease: part II. Treatment. Am Fam Physician 2002;2525–2534.

Davidson JR. Trauma: the impact of post-traumatic stress disorder. J Psychopharmacol 2000;14(2Suppl1):S5–S12.

De Deyn PP, Katz IR, Brodaty H, et al. Management of agitation, aggression, and psychosis associated with dementia: a pooled analysis including three randomized, placebo-controlled double-blind trials in nursing home residents treated with risperidone. Amer J Alzheimer's Dis & Other Dementias 2006;21;2:101–108. DOI: 10.1177/153331750602100209

Delagarza VW. Pharmacologic treatment of Alzheimer's disease: an update. Am Fam Physician 2003;68:1365–1372.

Doody RS, Geldmacher DS, Gordon B, et al. Open-label, multicenter, phase 3 extension study of the safety and efficacy of donepezil in patients with Alzheimer disease. Arch Neurol. 2001;58:427–433.

Doody RS, Stevens JC, Beck C, et al. Practice parameter: management of dementia (an evidence-based review). Report of the Quality Standards Subcommittee of the American Academy of Neurology. Neurology. 2001;56(9):1154–1166.

Folstein MF, Folstein SE, McHugh PR. "Mini-mental state": a practical method for grading the cognitive state of patients for the clinician. J Psychiatr Res. 1975;12:189–198.

Frances A, Mack AH, Ross R, First, MB. 2000. The DSM-IV Classification and Psychopharmacology.

Frank E. Interpersonal and social rhythm therapy: a means of improving depression and preventing relapse in bipolar disorder. J Clin Psychol. 2007;63(5):463–473.

Jagust W, Reed B, Mungas D, et al. What does fluorodeoxyglucose PET imaging add to a clinical diagnosis of dementia? Neurology. 2007;69(9):871–877.

Kane JM. Schizophrenia. N Engl J Med 1996;334(1):34–41.

Kelly MJ, ed. End of life: a nurses' guide to compassionate care. Ambler, PA: Lippincott, Williams and Wilkins; 2007.

Keltner NL, Folks DG. Psychotropic drugs. 4th ed. St. Louis, MO: Elsevier Mosby; 2005.

Kornhuber J, Weller M, Schoppmeyer K, et al. Amantadine and memantine are NMDA receptor antagonists with neuroprotective properties. J Neural Transm Suppl. 1994;43:91–104.

Lagomasino I, Daly R, Stoudemire A. Medical assessment of patients presenting with psychiatric symptoms in the emergency setting. Psychiatr Clin North Am 1999;22(4):819–850, viii–ix.

Lehne RA. Pharmacology for nursing care. 6th ed. St. Louis, MO: Elsevier Saunders; 2007.

McKhann GM, et al. The diagnosis of dementia due to Alzheimer's disease: Recommendations from the National Institute on Aging – Alzheimer's Association workgroups on diagnostic guidelines for Alzheimer's disease. Alzheimer's & Dementia: The Journal of the Alzheimer's Association 2011;7(3):263–269.

MedlinePlus. Dementia. www.nlm.nih.gov/medlineplus/dementia.html.

Mintzer J, Greenspan A, Caers I, et al. Risperidone in the treatment of psychosis of Alzheimer disease: results from a prospective clinical trial. Amer J Geriatr Psychiatry 2006;14(3):280–291.

National Institute of Mental Health. Symptoms of bipolar disorder may go undiagnosed in some adults with major depression. http://www.nimh.nih.gov/science-news/2010/symptoms-of-bipolar-disorder-may-go-undiagnosed-in-some-adults-with-major-depression.shtml.

Novartis. Tegretol (carbamazepine) Prescribing information. East Hanover, NJ: Novartis Pharmaceuticals; 2011. http://www.pharma.us.novartis.com/product/pi/pdf/tegretol.pdf.

Noven Therapeutics. Lithobid (lithium carbonate) prescribing information. Miami, FL: Noven Therapeutics; 2011. http://lithobid.net/pdfs/LithobidPI.pdf.

Patterson CE, Todd SA, Passmore AP. Effect of apolipoprotein E and butyrylcholinesterase genotypes on cognitive response to cholinesterase inhibitor treatment at different stages of Alzheimer's disease. The Pharmacogenomics J. 2011;11:444–450.

Physician's Desk Reference 2010. 64th ed. Montvale, NJ: Physician's Desk Reference; 2009.

Reisberg B, Doody R, Stöffler A, et al. Memantine in moderate-to-severe Alzheimer's disease. N Engl J Med. 2003;348(14):1333–1341.

Saddock BJ, Saddock VA. Kaplan and Sadock's concise textbook of clinical psychiatry. 3rd ed. Philadelphia, PA: Wolters Kluwer/Lippincott Williams and Wilkins; 2008.

Shaldubina A, Agam G, Belmaker RH. The mechanism of lithium action: state of the art, ten years later. Prog Neuropsychopharmacol Biol Psychiatry. 2001;25(4):855–866.

Small GW, Rabins PV, Barry PP, et al. Diagnosis and treatment of Alzheimer disease and related disorders. Consensus statement of the American Association for Geriatric Psychiatry, the Alzheimer's Association, and the American Geriatrics Society. JAMA 1997;278:1363–1371.

Spitzer RL, Yanovski S, Wadden T, et al. Binge eating disorder: its further validation in a multisite study. Intl J Eating Disorders 1993;13(2):137–153.

Spratto G, Woods AL. 2011 Delmar nurse's drug handbook. Clifton Park, NY: Delmar Cengage Learning; 2011.

Strober M, Freeman R, Lampert C, et al. Controlled family study of anorexia nervosa and bulimia nervosa: evidence of shared liability and transmission of partial syndromes. Amer J Psychiatry 2000;157(3):393–401.

Stovall J. Bipolar disorder in adults: pharmacotherapy for acute mania, mixed episodes, and hypomania. UpToDate. 2012. http://www.uptodate.com/contents/bipolar-disorder-in-adults-pharmacotherapy-for-acute-mania-mixed-episodes-and-hypomania.

Sullivan PF. Mortality in anorexia nervosa. Amer J Psychiatry 1995;152(7):1073–1074.

Tariot PN, Farlow MR, Grossberg GT, et al. Memantine treatment in patients with moderate to severe Alzheimer disease already receiving donepezil: a randomized controlled trial. JAMA. 2004;291(3):317–324.

Varcarolis EM, Halter MJ. Foundations of psychiatric mental health nursing: a clinical approach. 6th ed. St. Louis, MO: Saunders/Elsevier; 2010.

Watkins PB, Zimmerman HJ, Knapp MJ, et al. Hepatotoxic effects of tacrine administration in patients with Alzheimer's disease. JAMA. 1994;271(13):992–998.

Whitehouse PJ, Price DL, Struble RG, et al. Alzheimer's disease and senile dementia: loss of neurons in the basal forebrain. Science. 1982;215(4537):1237–1239.

ORGAN TRANSPLANT

Aker S, Ivens K, Guo Z, et al. Cardiovascular complications after renal transplantation. Transplant Proc 1998; 30(5):2039–2042.

al-Asfari R, Fahdi L, Hadidy S, et al. Medical complications of renal transplantation. Transplant Proc 1999; 31(8):3218.

al-Aasfari R, Hadidy S, Yagan S. Infectious complications of kidney transplantation. Transplant Proc 1999; 31(8):3204.

Hricik DE, Whalen CC, Lautman J, et al. Withdrawal of steroids after renal transplantation—clinical predictors of outcome. Transplantation 1992;53(1):41–45.

Jordan ML, Shapiro R, Vivas CA, et al. The use of tacrolimus in renal transplantation. World J Urol 1996;14(4):239–242.

Kozaki K, Takeuchi H, Hirano T, et al. Withdrawal or reduction of steroids based on pharmacodynamics assessed by antilymphocyte action after renal transplantation. Transplant Proc 1996;28(3):1300–1301.

Kramer BK, Krager B, Mack M, et al. Steroid withdrawal or steroid avoidance in renal transplant recipients: focus on tacrolimus-based immunosuppressive regimens. Transplant Proc 2005;37(4):1789–1791.

Levitsky J, Cohen SM. The liver transplant recipient: what you need to know for long-term care. J Fam Pract 2006;55(2):136–144.

Mark W, Berger N, Lechleitner M, et al. Impact of steroid withdrawal on metabolic parameters in a series of 112 enteric/systemic-drained pancreatic transplants. Transplant Proc 2005;37(4):1821–1825.

McCaughan GW, Koorey DJ. Liver transplantation. Aust N Z J Med 1997;27(4):371–378.

Middleton PF, Duffield M, Lynch SV. Living donor liver transplantation—adult donor outcomes: a systematic review. Liver Transpl 2006;12(1):24–30.

Morris, PJ. Transplantation—A medical miracle of the 20th century. N Engl J Med 2004;351:2678–2680. PMID 15616201.

Muñoz SJ. Long-term management of the liver transplant recipient. Med Clin North Am 1996;80(5):1103–1120.

Oberholzer J, John E, Lumpaopong A, et al. Early discontinuation of steroids is safe and effective in pediatric kidney transplant recipients. Pediatr Transplant 2005;9(4):456–463.

Ojo AO, Meier-Kriesche HU, Hanson JA, et al. Mycophenolate mofetil reduces late renal allograft loss independent of acute rejection. Transplantation 2000;69(11):2405–2409.

Organ Procurement and Transplantation Network. Waiting list candidates: Liver. Transplants: Liver. Organ Procurement and Transplantation Network. http://optn.transplant.hrsa.gov/latestData/step2.asp.

Perry I, Neuberger J. Immunosuppression: towards a logical approach in liver transplantation. Clin Exp Immunol 2005;139(1):2–10.

Ponticelli C, Tarantino A, Montagnino G, Vegeto A. Use of steroids in renal transplantation. Transplant Proc 1999;31(6):2210–2211.

Puig i Mari JM. Induction treatment with mycophenolate mofetil, cyclosporine, and low-dose steroids with subsequent early withdrawal in renal transplant patients: results of the Spanish Group. Spanish Group of the Cell Cept Study. Transplant Proc 1999;31(6):2256–2258.

Shapiro R, Jordan ML, Scantlebury VP, et al. Tacrolimus in renal transplantation. Transplant Proc 1996;28(4):2117–2118.

Tintinalli, JE. Liver transplantation. In: Emergency medicine: a comprehensive study guide. 5th ed. 2004:587–588.

Transplantation Proceedings. Tacrolimus in renal transplantation: a comparison of induction vs noninduction therapy (triple therapy): three-month results. Transplant Proc 1999;31(1–2):330–331.

US Mycophenolate Mofetil Study Group. Mycophenolate mofetil for the prevention of acute rejection of primary cadaveric kidney transplants: status of the MYC 1866 study at 1 year. Transplant Proc 1997;29(1–2):348–349.

Varon NF, Alangaden GJ. Emerging trends in infections among renal transplant recipients. Expert Rev Anti Infect Ther 2004;2(1):95–109.

Index

Dentist's Guide to Medical Conditions, Medications, and Complications, Second Edition. Kanchan M. Ganda.
© 2013 John Wiley & Sons, Inc. Published 2013 by John Wiley & Sons, Inc.